BRAIN TUMORS - CURRENT AND EMERGING THERAPEUTIC STRATEGIES

Edited by **Ana Lucia Abujamra**

Brain Tumors - Current and Emerging Therapeutic Strategies
Edited by Ana Lucia Abujamra

Published by InTech
Janeza Trdine 9, 51000 Rijeka, Croatia

Publishing Process Manager Iva Simcic

Technical Editor Teodora Smiljanic

Cover Designer InTech Design Team

Additional hard copies can be obtained from orders@intechopen.com

Brain Tumors - Current and Emerging Therapeutic Strategies,
Edited by Ana Lucia Abujamra
p. cm.
ISBN 978-953-307-588-4

For EU product safety concerns:
IN TECH d.o.o., Prolaz Marije Krucifikse Kozulić 3, 51000 Rijeka, Croatia,
info@intechopen.com or visit our website at intechopen.com.

Meet the editor

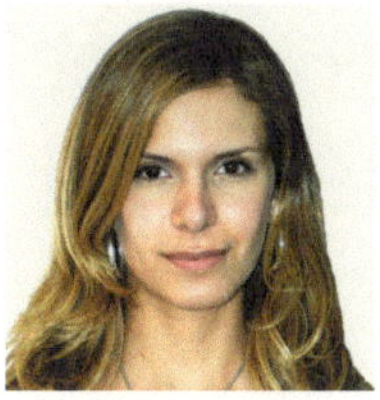

Ana Lucia Abujamra received her training at Boston University School of Medicine, where she was awarded her doctorate degree. Later she worked at Beth Israel Deaconess Medical Center and at Boston Medical Center, Boston, Massachusetts, USA. She currently lives in Porto Alegre, Brazil, working as translational research coordinator at the Children's Cancer Institute and principal investigator of the Cancer Research Laboratory, University Hospital, Federal University of Rio Grande do Sul. She holds a teaching position at the Department of Medical Sciences, Federal University of Rio Grande do Sul, and is partner and co-founder of Ziel Biosciences, a biotech start-up focusing on individualized therapy for cancer patients.

Contents

Preface

Tumors of the central nervous system are extensively complex, not only because of their location, but because of the intricate cellular and molecular mechanisms involved in their pathogenesis. Special emphasis must be given to diagnose these tumors correctly, and to treat them as efficiently, albeit as conservatively as possible, in order to preserve the surrounding healthy tissue. Understanding the molecular mechanisms that give rise to this disease, and how this knowledge can be applied to diagnosis and treatment, has been a research focus for many years.

With this in mind, the book is divided into three sections: The first section addresses the tumor models currently available to study brain tumors, new diagnostic methods and the molecular mechanisms that are frequently involved in the pathogenesis of brain tumors. Established and novel therapeutic strategies are described in section two, with a special focus of gene therapy and immunotherapy in section three.

The main focus of this book is the gliomas, given their incidence and dismal prognosis, but other brain tumors, including medulloblastoma and brain metastases, are also discussed. Written by experts in brain tumor research and in managing brain tumors, this book provides the most up-to-date information regarding tumor models, clinical diagnostic methods and therapeutic strategies.

The chapters here presented aim in contributing to the understanding of brain tumor pathogenesis, tumor behavior within the cellular niche, and of the new therapeutic methods for managing brain tumors. All topics possess translational potential in the hopes that the health care professional in the field can benefit not only by increasing knowledge, but increasing clinical applicability as well.

Sincerely,

Dr. Ana Lucia Abujamra
Hospital de Clínicas de Porto Alegre
Oncologia Pediátrica- Terceiro Leste
R. Ramiro Barcelos, 2350
Bairro Rio Branco
Porto Alegre, Rio Grande do Sul 90035-903
Brasil

Part 1

Tumor Models, Molecular Mechanisms and Diagnostics

1

Xenograft Model of Human Brain Tumor

Chen Hua[1,2], Dong Jun[1] and Huang Qiang[1]
[1]*Department of Neurosurgery, 2nd Affiliated Hospital of Suzhou University*
[2]*Department of Neurosurgery, Nanjing First Hospital, Nanjing Medical University*
China

1. Introduction

In the life sciences, scientists are paying more and more attention to the human brain, the essential center of the body. The gliomas in human brains are especially unique challenges for doctors due to the difficulties of identifying early cancer lesions and little effective treatments. Gliomas account for about half of the central nervous system tumors. Due to its invasive growth and other malignant behaviors, gliomas are difficult to be radically cured; moreover, most of gliomas are difficult to be early detected, even they are discovered, it is difficult to cure them because of their resistance to radiation or chemotherapy. Therefore, developing animal models of human gliomas is essential for us to explore the mechanisms of occurrence and development of brain tumor and promote clinical research. From past to future, the far-sighted men attached and will continue to attach importance to the development of animal models of human gliomas. Judging from the research and development process, human beings have, after a hundred years' efforts, moved from the development and application of animal models of spontaneous and induced brain tumor to the generation of the experimental platform of various animal models of human brain tumors. Now we are trying to improve the simulation of the animal models to the human diseases. For the human glioma, the early model was the solid tumors formed by directly inoculating in vitro passaged cell lines to animals; then, human glioma tissue were successfully inoculated into animals. In recent years, with the progress of tumor molecular biology, transgenic or gene knockout procedures are used to generate genetic engineering mouse brain tumor model, which meet the requirement of finding the molecular etiology of human brain tumors through specific molecular genetics. After the successful cloning of glioma stem cells, the establishment of animal models retaining the characteristics of glioma stem cells is on the agenda. In short, although we face difficulty building up animal models of brain tumor, we have tried to imitate the models to diseases from the system-cell level to the system-cells -molecular level.

2. The types of tumor model

2.1 Allogeneic graft model of mouse brain tumor

Although allogeneic grafting of animals' spontaneous tumors succeeded before, this method had been abandoned because of its poor simulation such as the low incidence, the early stage occult and short survival period of tumor-bearing animals. It has been replaced by the development of induced animal brain tumor model. The most commonly used cancer-inducing methods are by chemical carcinogen or by viruses. Back to 1939, Seligman et al reported that implantation the pill made of the polycyclic aromatic hydrocarbons methylcholanthrene in mice brain induced glioma and sarcoma. From the middle of last century, the systemic administration of pro-nerve alkylating agent was proved to induce nervous system tumors. Since then, the polycyclic aromatic hydrocarbons-induced method has been gradually replaced by nitrosourea derivatives-induced methods, especially by the methods using nitrosourea and ethyl nitrosourea which have higher rates of inducing central nervous system tumors. Nitrosourea can induce tumor effectively in adult mice. It can induce astrocytoma, oligodendrocytes, ependymal tumor or the most commonly glioma, which is the mixture of all the previous tumor cell types. The intravenous injection of ethyl nitrosourea to the 20 days pregnant rats induced the central nervous system tumors in all the offsprings. The widely used P494, C6, 9L and G422 animal glioma models are all produced by the similar methods. The sensitivity to carcinogen of rat central nervous system is formed 10 days before birth, and reaches the peak at birth (50 times sensitize than the adult). One month after birth, the sensitivity drops to the adult level.

In addition to the chemical carcinogen, oncogenic virus is also used to induce gliomas. The virus can induce two types of brain tumors: RNA viruses, such as Rous sarcoma virus or DNA viruses, such as adenovirus. Concentrated Rous sarcoma virus (0.01ml) have been injected into the brains of newborn dogs, which all had gliomas after a period of latency. (Bigner et al, 1970) It was also reported that direct injection of AD12 virus into the brain of mouse that had been born for 24 hours induced brain tumors after an incubation period of several months, most of which are medulloblastoma. Usually for the newborn rats, tumor is formed 9-100 days after birth, the longest one takes about a year to mature after viral transfection. Tumor cells were implanted by intracerebral inoculation of 4×10^7 chick embryo fibroblasts infected with the Schmidt-Ruppin strain of Rous sarcoma virus (RSV). With a 15 to 67 day latency, brain tumors were induced in 11 (73.3%) of 15 RSV-inoculated monkeys. (Tabuchi et al, 1985) Scientist also found that inoculating the viruses isolated from brain tissue of progressive multifocal leukoencephalopathy (PML) patients into hamsters' or monkeys' brains could induce cerebellum medulloblastoma, hypothalamic gliomas, pinealomas, intraventricular ependymoma and many other types of brain tumors in various locations. Brain tumors caused by viruses can only be produced into models with stable biological characteristics by cloning, such as the RT2 glioma model induced by the chicken tumor virus.

These chemical carcinogens and oncogenic viruses are prevalent in the human environment, which which imitates the natural occurrence of spontaneous human gliomas. The induced tumors in animals will be continuously passed through generations and the biological characteristics of tumors are relatively stable, which play active roles in understanding the tumor development and in preventing tumors. However, animal models of brain tumors induced by oncogenic have different cycles and different pathological types. Compared to human brain tumors, the induced brain tumors in animals were different in genetics, cell biology and histology. Researchers hope to develop the xenograft model of human brain tumor to improve the simulation.

2.2 Xenograft model of human brain tumor

2.2.1 Animal strains

Typically, it is impossible for the human tumors to grow in the animal due to strong immune rejection. So the tumor is usually inoculated in the anterior chamber or parts of the hamster cheek pouch where immune cells can not reach. But these tumors have very unstable biological characteristics such as spontaneous regression, so the above method is only used for tumorigenicity testing. We have injected immunosuppressive agents dexamethasone in newborn rats to successfully inoculate the human glioma cell line SHG44 into the brain of Westar rats, which is the first experiment to use human glioma cells for in situ animal tumorigenicity experiments. Later, due to the appearance and wide usage of immune-deficient animals, the injection methods of immunosuppressive agents have been abandoned.

Internationally, there are more than 30 kinds of pure T cell deficient nude mice with clear genetic background available, as well as T cells and B cells combined deficient mice -- (Lasat), SCID (severe combined immunodeficiency), NOD-SCID, CBA / I mice, and Beige mice with T cells and NK cells double deficiencies. The nude mice currently used in China -- Balb / C, Swiss, and NC strains -- were imported from abroad in the early 80s of last century. The NC strain mice introduced from Japan in 1981 are non-inbred nude mice with high reproductive rate; they are resistant to pathogens and easy to manage. They are still used for establishing human glioma models NHG-1.

The recent established green fluorescent protein (GFP) transgenic mice C57BL/6J-GFP are very popular because it is easy to trace the green fluorescence in the host tissue or cells of tumor xenograft models. However, tumor xenografts could not be established because of their normal immune function. To apply them in human cancer model transplantation, Yang and colleagues (Yang et al, 2004) successful hybridized them with nude mice to produce immunocompromised nude mice expressing GFP which are suitable for human cancer transplantation. We have also successfully cultured the NC nude mice expressing GFP (Figure 1), and these mice have been used in human glioma xenograft experiment.

2.2.2 Method of transplantation

Commonly, tumor cell lines cultured in vitro, tumor tissue or the cell suspension digested from tumor tissue are used for eatablish xenograft model. Usually, the implantation sites can be subcutaneous space, foot, abdomen, renal capsule, intracranial brain parenchyma, ventricles or spinal subarachnoid space, depending on the experimental need. In the early stage, we established the NHG-1 solid tumor subcutaneously in nude mice model using the human brain malignant astrocytic tumor cell lines implantation, the NHE-2 nude mice xenograft model using human ependymoblastoma tissue implantation and the mouse - human chimeric immune mice model of human glioma using human peripheral blood mononuclear cells SCID transfusion. By subcutaneous xenograft, it is not only convenient to observe the tumor volume by visual or dynamic measurement, but also easy to evaluate the effects of anticancer drugs. However, the tumor formed in this way is not in the brain and the blood-brain barrier, the macro- and micro- environment of tumor cells are quite different from those in clinical diseases. Therefore, the orthotopic transplantation model of human brain glioma in nude mice is a better model for imitating the clinical diseases.

The animal model of glioma orthotopic transplantation used in previous researches usually applied cell suspension cranial injection or tissue inoculation with craniotomy (Antunes L et al, 2000, Bradley NJ et al, 1978, DeArmond SJ et al, 1994, Horten BC et al, 1981, Rana MW et al, 1977, Taillandier L et al, 2003). The former method can be used to generate the tumor model, but the procedure is too complicated. There are lots of issues, for example: (1) the tumor cells for inoculation are usually cultured in vitro for several generations, which are damaged during the trypsin digestion. It is difficult to get enough living cells; (2) the injection volume and speed are restricted by automatic pump because of the small compensatory volume. It will take a long time to make the model; (3) the inoculation cells are out of the incubator for too long to keep all alive because the operation takes too much time. Although the same amount of cells was used in different batches of xenograft, it is hard to get about the same number of alive cells in every experiment, which have impact on the tumor-inducing rate and latency. Although the later method can avoid the above problems, there are still lots of concerns such as large craniotomy injury to mice, complicated operation and other issues. We used needle for transplanting tumor tissue in either subcutaneous or intracerebral space, as shown in Figure 2. In such way, the trauma was relatively small. Compared with the cell suspension, tissue transplantation inoculated suitable environment (stroma) at the same time. It is better in maintaining the original parental tumor structure, tumor biology or molecular phenotype.

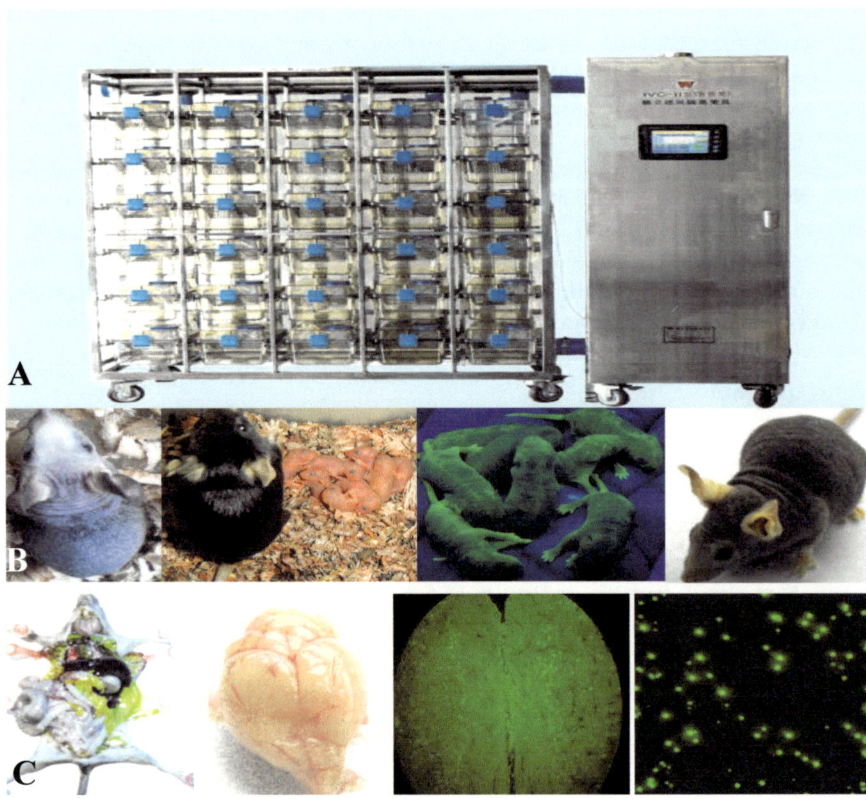

Fig. 1. The proliferation and fluorescent protein expression in nude mice transfected GFP: A row, IVC system, an independent air supply cage for mice, produced in Suzhou, consists of 4 parts: the air supply system, exhaust system, cage, mouse box. Fan is imported from German; high efficiency filter is produced by Aetna, a chinese-Japanese jointed venture; differential pressure gauge is imported from the United States. The cage is made of imported stainless steel tubes 304. The rat box is made of polysulfone transparent material. B row, from left to right are NC male mice used for breeding, neonatal of GFP/C57 female mice, bred GFP/C57/NC nude mice and adult mice. C row, from left to right are GFP/C57/NC nude mice under anatomy, eye view of mice brains, the cerebral hemispheres and bone marrow biopsy under fluorescence microscopy.

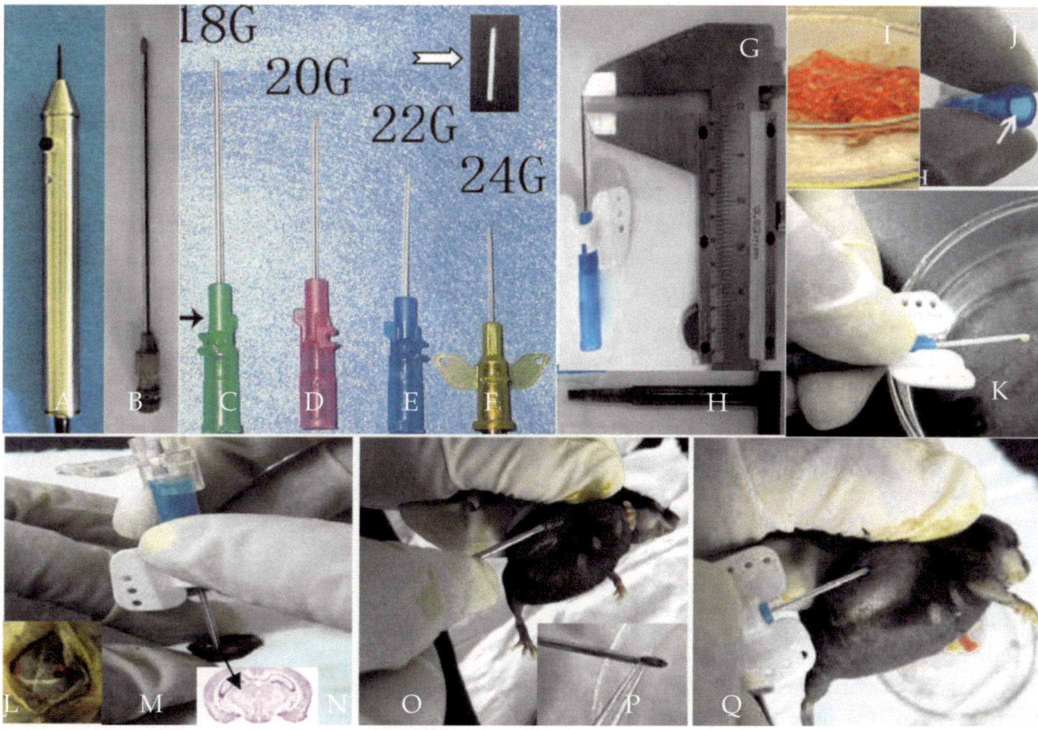

Fig. 2. The diagram of intracerebral and subcutaneous tumor xenograft transplantation: A-K: the surgical instruments, including micro-cranial drill (A), a metal trocar for subcutaneous inoculation (B), plastic trocars (C, D) and plastic trocars for intracerebral inoculation (E, F). For intracerebral inoculation, an external pin 2mm or 3mm shorter than the inner sleeve of the jacket tube (F, white arrow) must be used to control the depth of the puncture (if necessary, use the caliper G for measurement). Use the forceps to move the tumor tissue (I) on the top of the trocar (J, arrow), then use propeller (H) to push the tumor tissue into the casing, any extra tissue will overflow automatically from the needle end, and then place the core needle, push ahead to the second stent level (2-3mm length of tumor tissue is still left in the casing, at this piont, K). In intracranial inoculation, the anesthetized animals should have scalp incision, and drilled at 2.5mm right to the sagittal suture, 1.0mm to the cranial coronal suture (L), the needle to be vertically inserted into the brain (2mm or 3mm) and the inner core is pushed slowly until the tumor tissue be removed from the casing into the caudate nucleus (M, N arrow). If the tissue need to be inoculated subcutaneously in the puncture site (usually in the right armpit), use ordinary needle to puncture a hole, and then put the metal casing filled with tumor tissue (P) in the puncture holes, push the core of the casing to move the tumor tissue into the subcutaneous (O), slowly remove the needle. Plastic trocar also can be used for inoculation (Q).

There are essential indicators for evaluating the inoculation quality: transplantation success rate and the stability of parent tumor characteristics. According to the author's experience, the success rate of brain tumor xenografts is determined by the following factors. (1) For the subcutaneous inoculation, the nearer the location is to the head, the easier it is to generate the model. (2) Compared with using human tumor tissue, it is easy to generate the model by using the established tumor cell lines. The *in vitro* cultured tumor cell lines have stable biological characteristics and proliferate very fast, which make it ideal for establishing xenograft model. The tumor tissue inoculation keeps the original tumor characteristics in simulating the blood supply, interstitial structure and growth characteristics. (3) It is more successful to use tumor tissue inoculation than using trypsin digested tumor cells inoculation. The latter method can provide the exact amount of inoculation cells. (4) The more cells inoculated, the shorter the incubation period would be (no less than 1×10^7 cells in the initial inoculation). But Singh's group (Singh et al, 2003, 2004) has reported that it was the number of tumorigenic stem cells, rather than the number of total cells, that has decisive effect. The study also showed that 10^2 tumorigenic stem cells are sufficient for tumor generation, while 10^5 non-tumorigenic stem cells would not. (5) Compared with inoculating in subcutaneous space and in the abdominal cavity, it is easier to generate the model by inoculating in the peri-renal adipose capsule with relatively low immunity or in intracerebral space.

To determine the stability of transplantation tumor biologic characteristics, the models must be evaluated by the following indicators: (1) maintain the genetic characteristics: the chromosome of transplanted tissue is same as the primary inoculated human tumor tissues; (2) maintain the morphological features: the morphology, mitotic status, tumor stroma and vascular structures of transplanted tissue are identical to the primary inoculated human tumor tissues under the light and electron microscopy; (3) maintain the tumor markers: the specific qualitative biochemical indicators or quantitative biochemical indicators of transplanted tumor tissues are consistent with those of the primary inoculated human tumor tissues; (4) maintain the stability of the biological characteristics of tumor-bearing animals: after several generations, when the transplant success rate reaches 100%, there are less difference in spontaneous regression, tumor size and the survival rate between tumor-bearing animals; (5) maintain the proliferation kinetics of tumor cells: the mitotic index, phase, cell cycle and doubling time are almost the same. According to the above criteria, we have successfully established a primary malignant glioma and lung cancer brain metastases orthotopic transplantation nude mice models.

With the progress in the cancer stem cell research, it seems the quality control of animal models should be focused on the probability of replicating the parent tumor stemness characteristics. As is mentioned above (Singh et al, 2003, 2004), Singh's group found that there are inconsistent cellular renewal and proliferation rate in human brain tumors. They have isolated CD133+ tumor stem cell, the only subtype that can cause intracranial tumors, and proved that CD133+ cells are the tumorgenic cells in human brain. These findings make the generation of stem cell-induced brain tumor animal model possible. XioNan Li's group had generated the real animal models using human brain stem cells (Shu et al, 2008). 17 cases of pediatric glioma specimens were grounded into single cells or 3-5 cells suspension, and were injected into the NOD-SCID mice brain or cerebellum using the needle. He built 10 animal models for human glioma xenograft. Evaluated by HE staining and the critical markers, especially CD133 immunohistochemistry, the transplanted tumor retained the parental tumor characteristics, like invasion, histological type and BTSCs and stem cell pool expressing CD133 +. In the tumor neovascular, the human specific CD31 and CD34 were negative, while the human /mouse shared vWF was positive. The results indicated that the tumor neovascular was provided by the host. It is controversial, because previous report indicated that BTSCs provide the neovascular. BTSCs originated angiogenesis have been found *in vitro* and *in vivo*. Our results were different from those of Li' team, because we used tissue inoculation while Li et al. used single-cell or 3-5 cells cluster inoculation; these two methods may provide different micro-environment for BTSCs. We think that tissue transplantation will better maintain the characteristics of origin tumor.

2.3 Genetic engineering model of mouse brain tumor

In 1984, Brinster et al fused the promoter (MK) with polyomavirus SV40 gene. After enzyme digestion, he microinjected the DNA fragments into male pronucleus of fertilized eggs to built transgenic mice. The transgenic mice developed a variety of tumors, such as choroid plexus papilloma, thymoma and tumors in endocrine system. In 1988, Reynold et al. used H-2kb/ SV40 infusion to generate the transgenic mice, which provided results similar to Bringster's. Later, Vogel et al fused HTIV-LTR with tat gene, the injected transgenic mice can spontaneously develop neurofibroma. In 1990s, the transgenic glioma model was finally generated. Studies showed that there were lots of similarities between the making of glioma model and other tumor models. Some important DNA elements, such as the promoters and enhancers, modulated the transfected gene; the foreign genes fused with promoter and enhancer promoted a strong expression of target genes. The promoter or enhancer can be located in the upper stream or down stream of the genome, or it can be inserted in the non-transcribed DNA fragments (introns). There are constructed transgenic mice with astrocytoma, medulloblastoma, oligodendroglioma and multiforme glioblastoma.

2.3.1 Genetic engineering mouse of astrocytoma

Bachoo et al (Bachoo et al, 2002, Xiao et al, 2002) developed the mouse glioma model using retroviral carrying the active EGFR to infect astrocytes. They confirmed that injection of Ink4a/Arf-/- astrocytes expressing EGFR formed spheres into the animal's brain induced the formation of the high invasive astrocytoma. To simulate the RB mutations, Terry Van Dyke et al generated mouse astrocytoma model by introducing SV40T antigen (T121) which bind with RB and RB family members, P107 and P130 under the control of glial fibrillary acidic protein (GFAP) promoter. In 1995, Andrew Danks et al reported GFAP/SV40 TAg transgenic low-grade astrocytoma model. GFAP is the primary marker to identify the origin of the tumor, while SV40 TAg binds to P53 and inhibits its activity. After these two proteins were combined, the former regulated SV40 TAg and promoted its development of astrocytic tumors, while the latter suppressed the activity of wild-type p53 and promoted tumor development. As was shown in morphology and immunohistochemistry, astrocytes mainly were located in the subependymal zone in GFAP/SV40 TAg transgenic mice. Consistent with the characteristics of astrocytomas, some were located in the brain parenchyma or around neurons and blood vessel with GFAP expression. Chinese researcher Li HD reported that transfection myc andSV40TAg would promote cerebellum neuroblastoma and pancreatic cancer development.

2.3.2 Genetic engineering mouse of oligodendroglioma

Myelin basic protein (MBP) is an over-expressed protein during the formation of nerve myelin, which located in oligodendrocytes in the central nervous system or in Schwann cells in the peripheral nerves system. Oncogene neu was highly expressed in the majority of gliomas. In 1992, Hayes recombined Neu gene isolated from PSV2neu NT plasmid with MBP isolated from Cosmid (cos138) clones, and implanted it into C57BL / 6 × DBA / 2 F2 fertilized eggs. Of the 93 fertilized eggs injected with the recombined DNA, 14 of them had offspring. Four of the neonatal had brain tumors, which appeared in the underside of the brain, the thalamus and the posterior fossa and compressed the brain stem. Under the light microscope, the brain tumors of three mice had the characteristic morphology of glioblastoma multiforme, and had extensive leptomeningeal invasion. Under the electron microscope, there were some characteristics of undifferentiated cells. To identify the origin of tumor cells, they used NF, GFAP, MBP and Leu 7 immunohistochemical staining. The results showed that there were GFAP, MBP and Leu 7 positive staining in relatively well-differentiated tumor cells, while in low differentiated tumor cells, less GFAP, MBP, and LEU 7 positive staining were found. None of the cells had NF positive staining. For the morphological analysis, Hayes's experiment did not successfully induce typical oligodendrocyte tumor, although the expression of MBP and Leu 7 indicated the presence of oligodendrocytes. The hybridization analysis was further used to clarify its origin, the results showed that a large number of neu gene presented in tumor cells, but not in normal brain cells. In addition, the results also showed that RNA level of myelin specific proteins MBP, PLP, MAG and CNP were 5-10 times higher in tumor cells than in the control group, which suggested that the myelin-forming cells was enriched in the tumor. There was no myelination protein Po found in peripheral nerve, indicating that tumor cells were derived from oligodendrocytes, but not from Schwann cells. Moreover, there was no NF detected in brain tumor cells, indicating that there was no neuron present in the tumors. Analyzed by the solid tumor markers, Hayes had established the transgenic mice of oligodendrocyte cell tumors.

2.3.3 Genetic engineering mouse of glioblastoma

Injection of the combination of activated Ras and AKT into an Ntv-a transgenic mice induced glioblastoma tumor (Holland et al, 2000). When the DNA mixture was injected into Ntv-a mice with inactivate NK4a-ARF, the formation of the glioblastoma was accelerated. Ras and Akt work on the downstream signaling pathways of several growth factor receptors. In most of the glioblastoma multiforme tumors (GBMs), Ras and Akt are activated simultaneously. It has been proved that the abnormal expression of Ras can inhibit p53/RB pathway which induced the transformation of astrocytes into anaplastic astrocytoma cells that finally obtained GBMs characteristics after transfection AKT in the cells. These results confirmed the combined action of Ras and AKT in malignant glioma. Another GBMs model is generated in Nf1 and p53 double-silent mouse mated by the p53 knockout mice and the heterozygous of Nf1 and Cis (Reilly et al, 2000). Transplantation cells from such mice into other mice induced glioma or GBMs, which was caused by a depletion of a tumor suppressor gene instead of overexpression oncogene. Despite the molecular differences in previous GBMs models, they have something in common. Nf1 (nerve fiber) suppresses Ras activity, Nf1 knockout would lead to RAS activation. Nf1 alone is not sufficient to induce tumor formation, Nf1 combined with p53 deletion or lack of cell cycle regulation will induce tumor formation.

2.3.4 Genetic engineering mouse of medulloblastoma

Generation of Ptch heterozygous mice is essential for the development of medulloblastoma transgenic mouse model. It is well known that Ptch receptor suppress proliferation through SHH / GLI signaling pathway. Inactivated Ptch receptor increases the risk for medulloblastoma, about 14% to 19% of the Ptch +/- mice develop medulloblastoma within 12 months, indicating that retained Ptch locus still function. When these mice were mated with the p53 deficient mice, the tumor incidence of their offspring increase to 95%, all

affected mice die within 12 weeks (Zurawel et al, 2000, Wetmore, 2001), suggesting that P53 plays an important role in this model.
The systemic experiment on the retroviral model and RCAS/tv-a indicated that SHH pathway was related to the formation of medulloblastoma. Under the guidance of ultrasound, utero injection of retroviral SHH directly into the cerebellum could induce medulloblastoma (Weiner et al, 2002). Fults et al over-expressed SHH in newborn mouse cerebellum using RCAS / tv-a system, which induced the formation of medulloblastoma. c-Myc over-expression enhanced the induction. SHH's activities require the participation of Ptch. Inactivation of p53 and RB genes in neural progenitor cells in cerebellar granule cell layer developed brain tumor, indicating that RB family proteins may work on the tumorgenesis. P53 and RB conditional knockout mouse can produce a medulloblastoma, while single inactivated p53 or RB genes has no such effect. Some studies have shown (Tong et al, 2001) that adenosine diphosphate ribose polymerase (ADRP) is an early DNA damage response molecule. The mouse lack of ADP-ribose polymerase mate with the p53 gene deficient mice to generate ADRP and p53 double deletion mouse. Half of the mice have medulloblastoma located in the cerebellum.

3. Pathological features of transplantation tumor

When human cancer tissue or cells are transplanted into animals, the micro-ecological environment has undergone tremendous changes. The cell morphology, molecular biology, host survival period, clinical symptoms of tumor are difficult to keep consistent with those of original tumors in many ways. Tumors developed with single cell suspension or ectopic transplantation have the interstitial and vascular components provided by the host (mouse), which is significantly different from clinical disease. For example, in human glioma subcutaneous xenografts model, the tumor weight up to 5-6 grams is not life-threatening to the 25 grams weighted nude mice. For the intracranial tumor, even when the inoculated tumors cover the entire cerebral hemisphere, or grow into the contralateral hemisphere, the cranial tumor-bearing mice are still alive (Figure 3). Therefore, to study the pathology of transplant tumor, we have to link them with clinical as closely as possible. There is no much references available, so we shared a few research data with all the readers here.

3.1 Homogeneity

Xenografts inoculated in nude mice can induce the transplant tumor having pathological features similar to the clinical specimens. Usually, the subcutaneous xenografts in nude mice are different from the original tumor. Brain glioblastoma multiforme tumor (GBM) transplanted subcutaneously in nude mice does not have the typical GBM features, but more like "fibrosarcoma". When the xenograft is inoculated in the brain, some invasive characteristics and molecular markers are consistent with the parental tumor. Our data proved that the parental tumor is non-invasive and overexpression of CEA, with acidic mucus secretion, the brain tumor metastases from lung cancer in nude mice can mimic these characteristics. While the highly invasive GBM with high expression of EGFR inoculated into nude mice brain showed highly invasive and EGFR over-expression characteristics. For morphology analysis, it is rarely identical. The morphology of implanted tumor has different characteristics depending on different locations, such as cerebral cortex, white matter, gray matter, ventricles and cerebellum.

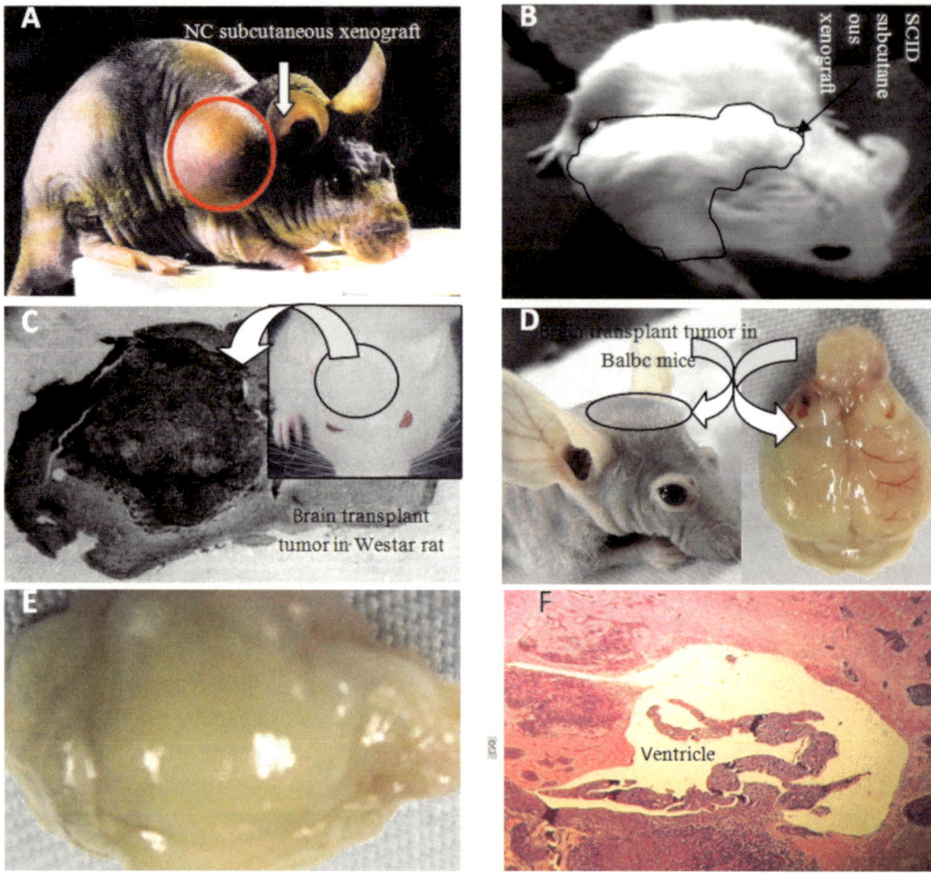

Fig. 3. NC glioma in nude mice, SCID mice transplanted subcutaneously, dexamethasone immunosuppressed Wistar rats and brain transplantation model in Balbc nude mice: the cells in subcutaneous space and in brain grow into large tumors due to unlimited proliferation. Intracranial skull uplifting can be observed in some mice (C, D black circle). Observed with cranial dissecting microscope or bear eye, the transplanted tumors almost covered the entire hemisphere (C arrow), or reached the olfactory lobe and the contralateral frontal lobe (D arrow). If spread to the choroid plexus, the tumor will cause hydrocephalus, both hemispheres are highly swollen (E) and ventricular expansion (F) will be noticed.

3.2 Mimesis

In the tissue repair process involving neural stem cells, the amplified daughter cells must have the same type of repair tissue to rebuild the function of cells, a phenomenon known as mimesis of neural stem cells, which had already been confirmed. We only focus on what the xenograft grows like and the tissue types of the parental tumor. When the glioma stem cells were implanted, we only checked whether the xenograft had neurons and glial cells features, rather than clarifying the subtype of the tissue. Our experiments have shown that stem cells derived from GBM grew diffusely, when it is located in the choroid plexus, it developed into choroid plexus carcinoma (Jun et al, 2010); when it settled in the ventricle wall, it developed into the ependymal neuroblastoma; when it settled in the brain surface and spinal table, it developed into uniform small round cells (do not know the subtype). In short, stem cells derived from GBM implantation has no typical GBM characteristics, the type of transplant tumor highly depends on the location. We believe that glioma stem cells, like neural stem cells, have mimesis growing characteristics.

3.3 Remodeling

The tissue remodeling during the development is very common. In tumor development and progression, it is not conclusive whether there is remodeling between tumor and the host tissue cells, such as interstitial and vascular. Tumor vessel remodeling was first discovered in the malignant retina melanoma and the xenograft (Maniotis et al, 1999, Zhang et al, 2006). The vessels composed of tumor cells are called vessel memisis; while the vessels composed of tumor cells and endothelial cells are called mosaic blood vessels. We have made detailed observation on tumor vessel in malignant glioma (Yue et al, 2005). In human glioma transplanting into nude mice, the glioma stem cells migrated and proliferated around the host blood vessels. Besides relying on the host for the blood supplies, the tumor had spontaneous vascular memisis and mosaic blood vessels to provide nutrition for rapidly proliferating tumor. Moreover, some vascular wall cells had both host protein and tumor protein expression, indicating that in the process of tumor angiogenesis, the tumor stem cells as well as tumor-derived endothelial cells were directly involved.

There are several types of cancer stem cells and host cells remodeling. Besides the vascular remodeling, it is possible that the individual suspension glioma stem cells could remodel with host cells. There are following possibilities: (1) individual tumor cell relies on the host stromal cells for nutrition supply, therefore remodeling with the host vessel; (2) individual tumor cells fuse with host cells or other tumor cells to form multinucleated giant cells or aneuploid cells, which use the fusion cells to rebuild tumor blood vessels; (3) in very few cases, individual tumor cells, in particular disseminated tumor cells, transdifferentiate into vascular endothelial cells and build stem cell niche (Niche), which expand to form a distal distribution of tumor cells block. With the tumor progression, the host tissue gradually disappears among tumor mass.

3.4 Tumor imaging

The earlier imaging study about the animals bearing human brain tumor used single photon emission computed tomography (PET). Using tumor monoclonal antibody labeled with iodine radionuclides, the biological imaging of subcutaneous tumor had been collected by the γ camera and SPECT (single photon emission computer-aided tomography) machine in tumor-bearing mice, which may guide the diagnosis (Haubner et al, 2001, Herschman et al, 2003 Massoud & Gambhir, 2003,). ^{18}F Radionuclide labeled glucose associated with tumor cell metabolism is also been used to trace tumor proliferation activity. Since most of the tumor-bearing animals are rats or mice, inoculated brain tumors are difficult to distinguish, both methods only work for the subcutaneous tumors. With the improvement in scientific technology, foreign researchers have used animal-specific high magnetic field MR (3-17.6T) on rats or mice for conducting imaging studies of intracranial tumors (Beck et al, 2002, Lewis et al, 2002, Pirko et al, 2005). Chinese researchers are still using ordinary field MR (1.5T) for imaging studies of rat intracranial tumors. Recently, we used rats and mice specific small coil 1.5T MR machine for imaging studies of orthotopic glioma in nude mice. We got some satisfactory results, which can be used for monitoring tumor and adjacent structures and

calculating tumor volume. But it will take a long imaging time and can not mimic the patient pictures.
Tumor vessel imaging is part of the tumor imaging. Percutaneous transcatheter and intravascular injection of contrast agents, and digital subtraction angiography (DSA) are used to get tumor microvascular data. However, the transplanted tumors mostly use small rodent animals, on which the DSA technology can not be applied. The vascular endothelial cell marker, such as CD34 + was used to calculate the vascular density and evaluate the number of tumor blood vessels, and the therapeutic effect of anti-tumor angiogenesis drugs. However, this method can not be used to evaluate the transporting function of these vessels. The cancer stem cell self-generated blood vessels (vasculogenesis) different from the host vascular endothelial cells formed blood vessels (angiogenesis). We established the activated carbon granular heart chamber perfusion method, which confirmed that various types of tumor vessels are involved in tumor-bearing animal systemic circulation (Figure 4) (Dong et al, 2010). The detailed procedures are as following: (1) producing activated carbon suspension: activated carbon particles were ground into powder and added to the PBS to make the suspension. Then the mixture was filtered through 40-micron net (U.S. BD Company). After rested for 1 min, the carbon particle was sucked by a flat cut, polished needle; (2) infusing activated carbon suspension: the tumor-bearing mice were anesthetized by 10% chloral hydrate. The syringe was pierced through the left ventricle of mice, while a small hole was cut in the right atrial appendage of the heart to facilitate the replacement of circulating blood. After 2-3 ml of carbon suspension was infused, the tumor tissue was removed, fixed in 4% paraformaldehyde and embedded in paraffin; (3) analyzing the perfusion results: active carbon particle suspension in left ventricular cavity went into host circulation and the tumor blood circulation. The active carbon particle distribution was related to the blood density. There were small carbon particles in host large vessels and new bleeding necrotic area, and integrated condensate active carbon particles in the medium-sized blood vessels, aggregated carbon particles in the tumor microvascular. It is worthy to mention that the active carbon particles would leak out of the lumen because the carbon particle is less than 40 microns in diameter, smaller than the red blood cells. It is interesting that the carbon particles were present in the marker of highly malignant tumor "false daisy group" and "tumor necrosis". For the former one, few carbon particles were observed in the central lumen, while in the latter structure, large piece of carbon particles were scattered in the gap of sparse distributed tumor cells. Since there is no red blood cells or other tangible materials found, suggesting that this change existed after tumor necrosis. The present carbon particles indicated that there was nutrition supply, suggesting that necrotic tumors tissue might have a micro-environment promoting "self-healing" process.
Imaging of fluorescent protein tracer is a newly developed technology. We had inoculated human glioma stem cells SU3 transfected with red fluorescent protein (RFP) into BAlbc nude mice brains to trace its location (Fig. 5). Hoffman (Hoffman, 2002) had inoculated U87 glioma cells transfected with RFP into the brains of nude mice expressing green fluorescent protein (GFP). Farin et al (Farin et al, 2006) had injected C6 glioma cells labeled with eGFP and DsRed-2 into the forebrains of neonatal rats, and used fluorescence imaging to observe dynamic tumor growth *in vivo*. Although clarity of the imaging, precision of the display of tumor size, location and depth are still not satisfying, this method will be widely used with the development of technology. In this platform, the outstanding finding was that glioma cells invaded brain tissue along the cavity of blood vessels. Tumor cell intruded into the endothelial cells and the pseudo foot of astrocytes, not the vascular cavity. In addition, glioma cells jumped forward sometimes slowly and sometimes rapidly, with the maximum

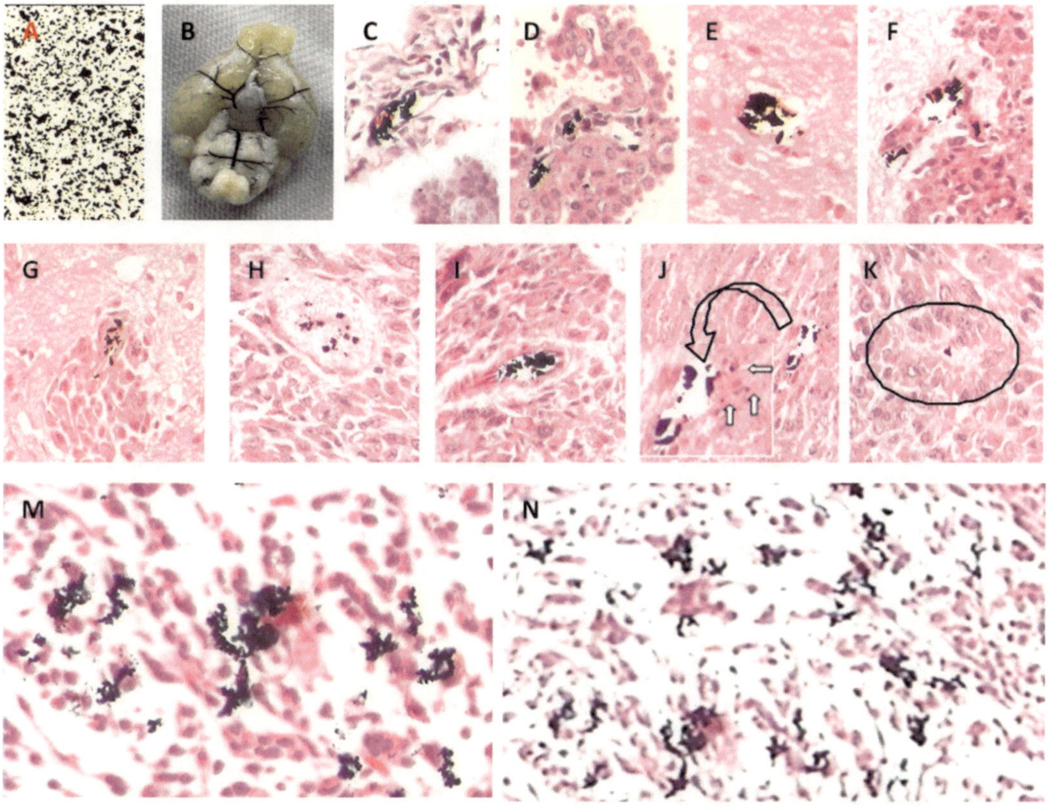

Fig. 4. Carbon particles ventricular perfusion in tumor-bearing mice, to trace blood flow of new Integrated tumor vessels. When carbon particles are perfused in tumor-bearing mice hearts, the blood flow of new tumor vessels is showed as following: A: suspension of carbon particles by light microscopy; B: the ventral surface profile of brain tumor, showing the basilar artery and Willis ring filled with carbon particles; C-K: the HE sections, showing that the carbon particles go into the following vascular tissue: subarachnoid space (C); choroid plexus (D); normal brain tissue (E); tumor margin (F); tumor foci (G); massive tumor tissue, including some endothelial-dependent blood vessels (H, host blood vessels) and some blood vessels formed by tumor cells (I, vascular mimesis); carbon particles leaking from tumor-origin blood vessels (J, arrow in magnified square); carbon particles in the central vessel of false daisy (K, circle); besides, carbon particles existing outside of vessels in the tumor necrosis, in acute necrotizing period, carbon particles and floating red blood cells coexist (M); after the acute period, carbon particles exist in absorbed lesions (N), indicating that there are blood supply even in the repair period of tumor necrosis.

speed over 100um per second; the migrated cells would go through proliferation and division. Cells divided at or near the vascular bifurcation. This was the first time the comprehensive kinetic data about glioma cell infiltration in vivo was recorded, which indicated that the proliferation and migration of glioma cells related closely with host vascular system. Considering from the reconstruction of tumor tissue, host's own tissues and cells also play an important role and provide nutrition for the growth of tumor. Yang (Yang et al, 2004) and we had inoculated human glioma stem cells non-transfected and transfected with RFP into nude mice brains. The former model (Jun et al, 2010) had proved that cancer stem cells involved in tumor blood vessel formation and fusion with host cells; In the latter model, host cells were proliferating actively around the tumor, and active host cells cultured in vitro have immortalized features (Figure 6).

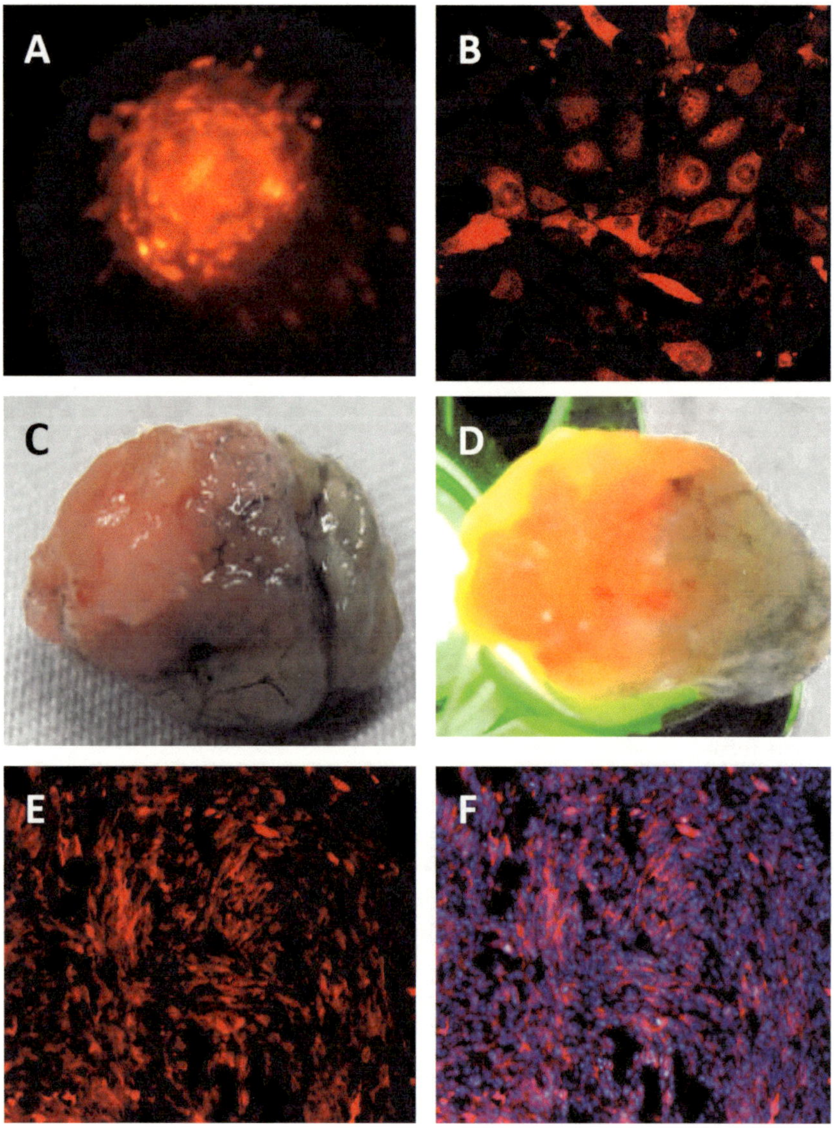

Fig. 5. Tracing human glioma stem cells SU3 and orthotopic transplantation tumor in Balbc nude mice with red fluorescent protein (RFP)mice: A and B: the SU3 with RFP transfection cultured with growth factors or serum under optical phase contrast microscope; C and D: the brain tumor observed in natural light and excitation light, red swollen tumor in th front of the brain; E and F: the tumor tissue sections under confocal microscope, the red tumor cells (E) and the nuclear staining (F) crowdedly arranged, suggesting a high degree of malignancy.

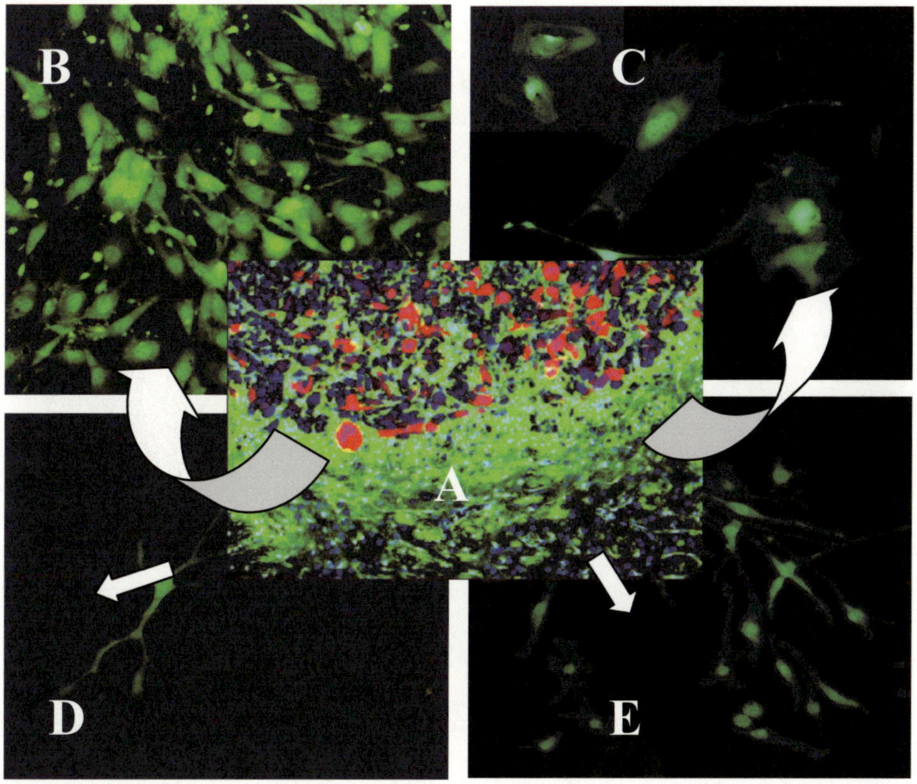

Fig. 6. The image of RFP / GFP brain tumor biopsy under fluorescence scanning confocal microscopy. RFP/GFP brain tumor biopsy under fluorescence scanning confocal microscope (A), human glioma stem cells (SU3) transfectded with RFP is red, host (NC/C57BL/6J-GFP nude mice transfected with GFP) tissues and cells is green, the nucleus is blue. There are host tissues in tumor interstitial and around the active zone, where the high proliferative host cells crowed together. The morphology are diverse among the cell suspension cultured from the tissue taken from the active zone under the the fluorescent microscope. Some of them are pleomorphic tumor cells, with several features: star shape, highly proliferative, rapidly covering the culture bottom, monoclonal passaged (B); others are macrophages with putiplnucleus (C); neurons (D) and fiberblast (E).

The establishment of fluorescent protein transfected tumor cells and transgenic mouse tumor model has made a significant contribution to the medical research. There are lots of application followed by pitfalls: (1) although fluorescent protein is less toxic to cells, it has cytotoxic effects to liver, heart and nervous stem cells (Huang et al, 2000]; (2) tumor cells expressing fluorescent protein may be engulfed by phagocytic cells invaded into the tumor area, it is impossible to distinguish them using current technology, which may lead to a false judgment of the experimental results; (3) limited by the current technology, the method can not fully meet the needs of interpreting fluorescent tracer image. However, we have every reason to believe that with the introduction of new imaging technologies, fluorescent tractor will make greater contribution to cancer research. For example, neural stem cells and cancer stem cells transfected with different colors of fluorescent protein are likely to help distinguish the origin of tumor cells; in the tumor micro-ecology research, the improved technology will help to dissect the components of cancer stem cell niche; in tumor evolution, it is known that anaplastic cell is the basis for malignant tumor, tumor cells and host cells transfected with different colors will help to elucidate whether cell fusion could contribute to the malignant progression. Finally, during the reconstruction process of transplant tumor, the donor and receptor with different fluorescent proteins are expected to be used to record their roles non-invasively.

4. Acknowledgments

This chapter is supported by National Basic Research Program of China (973 program, 2010CB529403), National Natural Science Foundation of China (No. 30872654, 81071766), Natural Science Foundation of Jiangsu Province (NO. BK2008173, 2010227) and the Foundation of Suzhou YJ S0950.

5. References

Antunes L, Angioi-Duprez KS, Bracard SR, et al. Analysis of tissue chimerism in nude mouse brain and abdominal xenograft models of human glioblastoma multiforme: what does it tell us about the models and about glioblastoma biology and therapy? J Histochem Cytochem 2000; 48:847-58.

Bachoo RM, Maher EA, Ligon KL, et al. Epidermal growth factor receptor and Ink4a/Arf:convergent mechanisms governing terminal differentiation and transformation along the neural stem cell to astrocyte axis. Cancer Cell, 2002, 1: 269–277.

Beck B, Plant DH, Grant SC, et al. Progress in high field MRI at the University of Florida. MAGMA, 2002, 13:152-157.

Bigner DD, Kvedar JP, Vick NA, et al. An improved method of preparing Schmidt-Ruppin Rous sarcoma virus for brain tumor induction in mammals. Neurology. 1970 ,20:413.

Bradley NJ, Bloom JG, Dawies AJS, et al. Growth of human gliomas in immune-deficient mice: a possible model for pre-clinical therapy studies. Br J Cancer, 1978, 38:263-272.

DeArmond SJ, Stowring L, Amar A, et al. Development of a non-selecting, non-perturbing method to study human brain tumor cell invasion in murine brain. J Neurooncol, 1994, 20:27-34.

Farin A, Suzuki SO, Weiker M, et al. Transplanted glioma cells migrate and proliferate on host brain vasculature：a dynamic analysis. Glia, 2006, 53:799-808 ·

Haubner R, Wester HJ, Weber WA, et al. Non-invasive imaging of alpha(v)beta3 integrin expression using 18F-labeled RGD-containing glycopeptide and positron emission tomography. Cancer Res, 2001, 61:1781–1785.

Herschman HR. Micro-PET imaging and small animal models of disease. Curr Opin Immunol, 2003, 15: 378–384.

Hoffman RM. Green fluorescent protein imaging of tumor cells in mice. Lab Anim. 2002, 31: 34–41.

Holland EC, Celestino J, Dai C, et al. Combined activation of Ras and Akt inneural progenitors induces glioblastoma formation in m ice . Nat Genet, 2000, 25: 55- 57.

Horten BC, Basler GA, Shapiro WR,et al. Xenograft of human malignant glial tumors into brains of nude mice. J Neuropathol Exp Neurol 1981, 40:493-511.

Huang WY, Aramburu J, Douglas PS, et al. Transgenic expression of green fluorescence protein can cause dilated cardimyophthy. Nat Med 2000, 6:482-483 ·

Jun Dong, QuanBin Zhang, Qiang Huang, et al. Glioma stem cells invoived in tumor tissue remordeling in a xenograft model. J Neurosurg. 2010, 113:249-60

Lewis JS, Achilefu S, Garbow JR, et al. Small animal imaging current technology andperspectives for oncological imaging. Eur. J. Cancer, 2002, 38:2173–2188.

Maniotis AJ , Folbcrg R , Hess A , et a1 · Vascular channel formation by human melanoma cells in vivo and in vitro, vasculogenic mimicry. Am J Patho1, 1999, 155:739-752.

Massoud TF, Gambhir SS. Molecular imaging in living subjects: seeing fundamental biological processes in a new light. Genes Dev, 2003,17: 545–580.

Pirko I, Fricke ST, Johnson AJ, et al. Magnetic resonance imaging, microscopy, and spectroscopy of the central nervous system in experimental animals. NeuroRx , 2005, 2: 250-264.

Rana MW, Pinkerton H, Thornton H,et al. Heterotransplantation of human glioblastoma multiforme and meningioma to nude mice. Proc Soc Exp Biol Med, 1977, 155:85-88.

Reilly KM, Loisel DA, Bronson RT, et al. Nf1, Trp53 mutant mice develop glioblastoma with evidence of strain-specific effects. Nat Genet, 2000, 26 : 109- 113.

Shu Q, Wong KK, Su JM, et al. Direct Orthotopic Transplantation of Fresh Surgical Specimen Preserves CD133+Tumor Cells in Clinically Relevant Mouse Models of Medulloblastoma and Glioma. Stem Cells, 2008, 26: 1414-1424.

Singh SK, Hawkins C, Clare ID, et al. Identification of human brain tumor initiating cell.Nature. 2004, 432:396-401.

Singh SK, Ian DC, Mizuhiko T, et al. Identification of a cancer stem cell in human brain tumors. Cancer Res , 2003; 63:5821- 5828.

Tabuchi K, Nishimoto A, Matsumoto K, et al. Establishment of a brain-tumor model in adult monkeys. J Neurosurg. 1985, 63:912-6.

Taillandier L, Antunes L, Angioi-Duprez KS. Models for neuro-oncological preclinical studies:solid orthotopic and heterotopic grafts of human gliomas into nude mice. J Neurosci Methods. 2003, 125:147-157.

Tong WM, Cortes U, Wang ZQ. Poly (ADP-ribose)polymerase: A guardian angel protecting the genome and suppressing tumorigenesis, Bioch im Biophys Acta, 2001, 20 : 8167-8174.

Weiner HL, Bakst R, HurlbertM S, etal. Induction of medulloblastomas in mice by sonic hedgehog independent of Glil. Cancer Res, 2002, 62 :6385- 6389.

Wetmore C, Eberhart DE, Curran T. Loss of p53 but not ARF accelerates medulloblastoma in mice heterozygous for patched. Cancer Res, 2001, 61 : 513- 516.

Xiao A., Wu H, Pandolfi PP, et al. Astrocyte inactivation of the pRb pathway predisposes micetomalignant astrocytoma developmentthat is accelerated by PTEN mutation. Cancer Cell, 2002, 1:157–168.

Yang M, Reynoso J, Jiang P, et al. Transgenic nude mouse with ubiquitous green fluorescent protein expression as a host for human tumors. Cancer Res, 2004, 64:8651-8656.

Yue WY, Chen ZP. Does Vasculogenic Mimicry Exist in Astrocytoma? J Histochem Cytochem. 2005, 53:997-1002

Zhang S, Guo H, Zhang D ,et al. Microcirculation patterns in different stages of melanoma. Oncol Rep, 2006, 15:15-20

Zurawel RH, Allen C, Wechsler-Reya R, ,et al. Evidence that haploinsufficiency of Ptch leads to medulloblastoma in mice. Genes Chromosomes Cancer. 2000, 8:77–81.

2

Experimental Brain Tumors: Current Concepts

Jesús Vaquero and Mercedes Zurita
Neuroscience Research Unit, Hospital Puerta de Hierro-Majadahonda, Madrid Spain

1. Introduction

The possibility of having experimental models of brain tumors allows for testing therapies applicable to human brain tumors. They can be induced by viruses, chemicals or radiation. Radiation-induced brain tumors have seldom been used, but diverse virus groups have been used to induce brain tumors. Among DNA viruses, both adenoviruses and papovaviruses have been shown to induce brain tumors in animals. The RNA viruses causing experimental brain tumors have consistently belonged to the retrovirus group, and have been generally limited to the murine sarcoma virus, the avian sarcoma virus, and the murine sarcoma virus. In these models, brain tumors are induced in rodents after intracerebral inoculation, with a variable latency, and the induced tumors are generally classified as gliomas, sarcomas, ependymomas or choroid plexus tumors.

On the other hand, the heterotransplantation of human brain tumors into immunodeprived animals gained great interest after the development of the nude mouse model, a thymus-deficient animal that provided the possibility for the xenografting of human brain tumors. It is known that human meningiomas and glioblastomas can grow after subcutaneous transplantation into the nude mouse, maintaining its original morphology. Nevertheless, at present, diverse chemical agents provide the best models of experimental neurocarcinogenesis.

2. Viral neurocarcinogenesis

The role of viruses in human oncology is a question that has interested for many years to researchers and clinicians (Bigner and Pegram, 1976). However, despite the intense research that has been developed over the last decades in this field, we still can not establish a clear etiological association between the presence of certain viruses and tumor development in humans, with some exceptions, such as the case of Epstein-Barr virus associated to Burkitt's lymphoma, although there has never been any conclusive proof that this virus causes the tumor.

From an experimental point of view, one of the models used to trigger the development of neural tumors in experimental animals is inoculation by different routes of virus with oncogenic capacity (Bullard and Bigner, 1980). The potential value of virus-induced gliomas has been questioned, however the information obtained from these experimental models has enabled significant progress in the treatment of human cancers. This experimental model of virus-induced neurocarcinogenesis offers the advantage that some of the viruses used will induce the development of tumors in a short period of time, the tumors are specifically located at the Central Nervous System (CNS) or Peripheral Nervous System (PNS), so that we can not rule out the possible viral etiology of certain types of brain tumors in humans. However, at present, numerous studies failed to establish any etiological association between viruses and humans brain tumors (Minn et al, 2002).

We now know different animal viruses that can act as transforming agents in normal cells, since they are capable of causing malignant transformation of a cell through its ability to integrate genetic information. It is well known that, for example, intracerebral inoculation of retroviruses can induce brain tumors in a wide variety of animals. Viral carcinogenesis allows us to induce experimental tumors with a short latency period and with a more specific location that offers radiation carcinogenesis, location depends on the route of administration, animal age and the amount of virus inoculated. However, it is obvious that experimental models of viral neurocarcinogenesis have the inconvenience and risks involved in the handling of virus particles.

Numerous studies have shown that RNA viruses (retroviruses) are able to induce the development of tumors in the CNS of experimental animals. Within this group, we highlight the avian sarcoma virus, murine sarcoma virus and simian sarcoma virus, being the most widely used in experimental neuro-oncology. Avian sarcoma virus (ASV) has been one of the most used in the literature to induce experimental brain tumors. The tumors are usually induced in chickens by intracerebral inoculation, and intracerebral tumors originated showed characteristics of sarcomas. There have been studies of ASV inoculation in the brains of monkeys because of their similarity to man, and tumors induced were fibrosarcomas. Interestingly, no author has reported the existence of glial tumors, but it has shown the ability of this virus to infect and replicate in glial cells when they grow in tissue culture.

Murine sarcoma virus (MSV) with its three strains: Moloney MSV, Kirsten and Harvey, can cause leukemia and sarcomas when inoculated subcutaneously in rodents and also is capable of inducing brain tumors in rats when inoculated intracerebrally. Neoplasms that may result show usually the aspect of glioblastomas, gemistocytic astrocytomas, oligodendrogliomas and hemangioblastomas, depending on the age of the animal and the dose of virus inoculated.

The simian sarcoma virus (SSV), after intracerebral inoculation in marmosets (Sanguinus nigricolli) induces the development of tumors that are morphologically similar to human glioblastoma multiforme, being able to demonstrate the presence of virus particles within tumor cells.

Among the known DNA virus, adenovirus and papovavirus have proved very effective in inducing brain tumors after intracerebral inoculation in animals, preferably in neonatal age.

Intracerebral inoculation of polyoma virus induces a high incidence of intracranial sarcomas in experimental animals, increasing their impact in terms of age of the animal (Rabson and Kirschstein, 1960). However, when inoculated cells transformed in vitro with the same virus, tumors of astrocytic aspect can be seen.

The SV-40 virus shows no oncogenic effect in monkeys, a species from which it was originally obtained, but it is one of the more capable oncogenic virus in rodents. Intracerebral inoculation in hamsters induces the development of ventricular tumors that were classified as ependymoma, choroid plexus papillomas and meningeal sarcomas. The induction of brain tumors by this type of virus depends very heavily on the dose. The role of SV-40 virus in human tumor development, not only brain tumors but also bone tumors and mesothelioma, has been subject of discussion for decades, but now there is conclusive evidence. Furthermore, human adenoviruses can cause meningeal tumors when inoculated intracerebrally into experimental animals, with tumor development after latent periods of 35 to 40 days.

While most existing data in the literature refer to the oncogenic virus ASV virus and SV-40, other viruses whose first guest is the man also play an important role in viral neurocarcinogenesis, such as Ad12 virus, BKV and JCV, three DNA viruses that have been widely used in experimental studies designed to establish a possible relationship between virus inoculation and the development of brain tumors. The human adenovirus Ad12 is able to induce brain tumors in rats after intracerebral inoculation, with a greater susceptibility of neonatal animals, where the range of incidence may vary between 8 and 100%. Furthermore, induced tumors develop after periods of latency between 31 and 235 days. The human papovavirus BK is capable of inducing brain tumors with different histological features, when inoculated into experimental animals. This virus is specifically used to induce choroid plexus papillomas and ependymomas after being inoculated intracerebrally.

The JC virus (JCV), when inoculated subcutaneously or intraperitoneally into young hamsters, induces the development of a variety of tumors, especially mesenchymal neoplasms, and may even induce the development of peripheral neuroblastomas. Moreover, intracerebral inoculation can induce the development of malignant astrocytomas. In human neuro-oncology, this virus has been associated with the development of medulloblastomas and more recently, with recurrence of glioblastomas.

On the other hand, it is important to note that in recent years, a new focus on the use of viruses has emerged in experimental neuro-oncology, and currently the use of viruses, or parts of them, are used as therapeutic vectors. Although some success has been reached using oncolytic viruses in experimental treatments for malignant gliomas in humans, the fact is that so far the results with these new techniques do not appear to meet the initial expectations (Zemp et al, 2010).

3. Chemical neurocarcinogenesis

The discovery of chemical carcinogens has stimulated neuro-oncology research because, after systemic application, these compounds induce a high incidence of tumors in the CNS and PNS, such as demonstrated Druckrey et al. in 1965, with the N-methyl-N-nitrosourea (MNU). Subsequently, we have found a greater number of chemical compounds, with equal effectiveness. Some of these compounds only occasionally induce tumors in the CNS of adult animals, but they represent, however, powerful neuro-oncogenic agents when administered transplacentally or during the early stages of postnatal life. Compounds, such as N-propyl-N-nitrosourea, N-butyl-N-nitrosourea, N-dimethyl-N-nitrosourea, and N-Trimethyl-N-nitrosourea, have been used. However, at present, N-ethyl-N-nitrosourea (ENU) is considered the best chemical agent to induce experimental brain tumors, because it is capable of inducing a high incidence of tumors, with known latency and morphology.

3.1 Mechanism of tumor induction in chemical neurocarcinogenesis

Most carcinogenic compounds actually represent precarcinogens which are converted in the host. The final product of this transformation is an electrophilic group that is capable of reacting with various cell constituents. It is clear that neuro-oncogenic compounds exhibit biological effects as alkylating metabolites which are formed during processing in vivo. The molecular basis of malignant transformation is not fully clarified, and at present, the cell being the target for the initiation of carcinogenesis has not identified. Most investigations are based on the interaction of carcinogens with nucleic acids and proteins.

Recent studies suggest the possibility that the induction of neural tumors by nitrosourea compounds may be related to a deficiency in DNA repair mechanisms in the Nervous System. When applied 14C-ENU in neonatal rats, the loss of O6-ethylguanina in liver DNA is very rapid. However, it persists for several days in the cerebral DNA (Goth and Ralewsky, 1974). In the non-target organs for carcinogenic action, the O6-alkylation excision is repaired during replication, or alteration remains in the sequence of DNA bases.

It is assumed that the inability of the neuro-oncogenic agents to induce neuronal tumors may be because neurons represent a cell population that has no capacity to divide. The permanent genetic alterations are the result of a mutation (transition) and this requires DNA replication. On the other hand, no direct evidence exists to affirm that the alkylation of nucleic acids is the cause that triggers the initiation of malignant tumors development.

3.2 Factors affecting the induction of experimental brain tumors in chemical neurocarcinogenesis

In chemical neurocarcinogenesis, the incidence, distribution, histology of tumors, and survival time of animals are influenced by the species and age of animals, in addition to dose and mode of application of the carcinogen.

3.2.1 Species

The susceptibility of different species to the carcinogenic activity of nitrosoureas has been investigated by several authors. Thus, Druckrey et al. (1970) observed that strains of rats such as Sprague-Dawley and Fischer, Long-Evans and Wistar, were susceptible to the carcinogenic action, producing a high number of tumors in the CNS. However, the response was not uniform, for example, male Sprague-Dawley rats treated with MNU only developed brain tumors, while male Fischer rats showed a high incidence of PNS tumors (Swenberg et al. 1972).

3.2.2 Age of animals

There is evidence that the response to neuro-oncogenic agents in fetuses and newborn rats differs significantly from the response in adult animals. The main characteristics of the perinatal induction of tumors in the nervous system by chemical agents can be summarized in the following points:

1. In adult animals, repeated doses of the carcinogen is needed to obtain a high incidence of neurogenic tumors. In the perinatal carcinogenesis, however, a single dose is sufficient to induce tumors in the nervous system, approximately in 90-100% of the experimental animals. On the other hand, some compounds such as 1,2-dimethylhydrazine, only induce tumors in fetuses and newborn rats, but never produce neurogenic tumors in adults.
2. Transplacental induction of neurogenic tumors in rats is possible only after day 11 of gestation. This is not due to lack of penetration of the carcinogen in fetal tissue, because embryotoxic and teratogenic effects occur after treatment, during the early stages of development. Nervous system susceptibility to chemical carcinogens increases sharply after day 11 of gestation and peaks during late intrauterine development period (Druckrey et al. 1969). After the first month of postnatal development, the response to neuro-oncogenic agents is broadly similar to that obtained in adult animals.

3. In adult animals, the tumors are located mainly in the brain (Denlinger et al, 1973). However, after perinatal application, tumors typically occur at the level of the spinal cord and the PNS. Trigeminal nerve tumors occur more frequently when the carcinogen is administered at the end of gestation, whereas in this case, the number of brain tumors is less than when the carcinogen is administered on day 15 of intrauterine development (Kahle, 1970).
4. The prenatal administration of these compounds increases the neurospecific carcinogenic effect. After transplacental administration tumors are located almost exclusively in the CNS. Postnatal application also produces a significant number of extraneural tumors (Schreiber et al, 1972).

3.2.3 Dosage and application

The incidence and latency period of experimental tumors is highly influenced by the dose of carcinogen. The number of tumors transplacentally induced by ENU can vary between 100% and 63% when the carcinogen dose is reduced from 80 mg / kg to 5 mg / kg. Moreover, the latency period is increased from 180 days to 500 days, when the dose of ENU administered in neonatal rats is reduced in the same way. The mode of application of the carcinogen plays a key role in the location and type of tumor that will be induced. Thus, local application of nitrosoureas can induce the formation of local tumors, but when these compounds are administered by intravenous injection, they can produce tumors that are spread throughout the body.

3.2.4 Hormonal and immunological factors

The possible influence of hormones on chemical carcinogenesis was first indicated by Ivankovic (1969) and Alexandrov (1973). They found that pregnant mice, when injected one or more doses of MNU, developed a high incidence of tumors of the uterus, vagina and breast cancer, however, when similar doses were administered in non-pregnant rats the results were different. Schreiber et al. (1972) found an increase in the number of extraneural tumors induced by MNU in rats to which previously had undergone ovariectomy. However, neither the execution of ovariectomy, or the application of testosterone or other oral contraceptives, have altered the oncogenic results (Schreiber et al. 1972; Thomas et al. 1972).

Regarding the role of immunological factors in the development of nervous system tumors, there is very little data. Delinger et al. (1973) studied the effect of the suppression of cell-mediated immunity in carcinogenesis with MNU in Fischer rats. They used a treatment with anti-lymphocyte serum and observed no change in the incidence of neurogenic tumors.

3.3 Morphology and biology of nitrosourea-induced brain tumors

There are a number of compounds able to induce tumors in the nervous system. However, all studies have been directed toward understanding the morphology of tumors induced by repeated doses of MNU in adult animals, or just for perinatal injection of ENU (Schiffer et al. 1970; Koestner et al. 1971; Lantos, 1972; Swenberg et al. 1972, Jones et al. 1973).

3.3.1 Tumor location

Regardless of the type of carcinogen used, preferably tumors develop in a number of specific regions of the nervous system. For example, in the brain, they are located mainly in the periventricular region, in the subcortical white matter of the cerebral hemispheres, and hippocampus. The periventricular tumors usually develop around the lateral ventricles, including the caudate nucleus and corpus callosum. Tumors rarely appear localized in the cerebellum. In the spinal cord, are normally at cervical and lumbar segments. These tumors are also developed on the cranial nerves, of which the trigeminal nerve is the most frequent location (Mennel and Zulch, 1971; Ivankovic, 1972, Schreiber et al. 1972).

3.3.2 Morphology

Tumors induced by chemical carcinogenesis in the nervous system are tumors with similar morphology to that presented gliomas and malignant schwannomas in humans.

After numerous histological studies on a large number of tumors induced in rats by nitrosoureas (Wechsler et al. 1969, Druckrey et al. 1970), unequivocal neuronal tumors were not found. After studies by light and electron microscopy of neurogenic tumors induced by ENU, Koestner et al. (1971) and Swenberg et al. (1972) established a classification for them that correlated with human tumors, but using different terminology. Thus, these authors classified the experimental brain tumors induced by ENU as: 1) Mixed gliomas (oligodendro-astrocytomas). 2) Anaplastic gliomas, tumors that show great cellular pleomorphism with high mitotic activity and regressive changes. 3) Glioependymomas, tumors with ependymoma features that contained pleomorphic glial cells. 4) Gliosarcomas, containing neoplastic glial cells and mesodermal cells. In 1973, Jones et al. provide another classification showing distinct groups (in order of frequency of occurrence) of ENU-induced tumors: 1) Gliomas of periventricular subependymal plate, they are divided in turn into ependymomas and ependymoma-oligoastrocytomas. 2) Astrocytic and oligodendrocytic tumors. 3) Neural tumors of the spinal cord and intracranial nerve ganglia. 4) Neuronal-like tumors and 5) Meningeal tumors.

Gliomas of periventricular subependymal plate are the first tumors are the first tumors that develop, they are identical to the anaplastic glioependymomas, and almost equivalent to the periventricular pleomorphic gliomas originating from the undifferentiated cells of the subependymal plate described by Lantos (1972). The presence of true ependymomas between the ENU-induced tumors is controversial, and generally they have been considered as such, either by their intraventricular location, or due to their histological features, reminiscent of ependymomatous tumors of humans. Unequivocal ependymomas were not seen in series of mice exposed transplacentally to ENU, but according to accepted classifications, approximately 20% of the ENU-induced brain tumors could be diagnosed as ependymomas, anaplastic ependymomas, or mixed glial tumors with ependymoma areas (Mandybur and Alvira, 1982). In many classifications, ependymomatous tumors were termed as "anaplastic glioependymomas" due to the presence of ependymoma-like cells, but these tumor cells coexist with other glial-like cells, pleomorphic cells and generally with rounded cells being very similar to those of human oligodendrogliomas. In any case, the histopathological diagnosis of the ENU-induced ependymomas is based on the existence of tumor cells arranged in rosettes around blood vessels. Ultrastructurally, there are two cell types: a small undifferentiated cell, and a larger type, more differentiated. Transitional forms between these two cell types can be seen. Undifferentiated cells are small, with a relatively large nucleus and little cytoplasm. The more differentiated tumor cells have a pleomorphic nucleus in an eccentric position, surrounded by abundant cytoplasm. Overall neoplastic ependymal cells do not possess cilia or blepharoplasts, and are not equipped with junctional complexes. Studies by Mandybur and Alvira (1982) supported that the named

"ENU-induced ependymomas" are not true ependymal tumors and that differ from the human ependymomas, because none of the ultrastructural features of normal or tumoral ependymal cells were present. Therefore these authors suggested that these tumors may actually be regarded as undifferentiated tumors, with some features of ependymomas.

On the other hand, the histology of tumors induced by ENU and MNU are similar. There are however some differences that were highlighted by Swenberg et al. (1972). These authors found that ENU-induced gliomas are better differentiated than the MNU-induced tumors, and that ENU produces a greater number of anaplastic schwannoma-like tumors. In animals treated with MNU, gliosarcoma can be found in 10% of cases, however, this type of tumor is completely absent in the treatments with ENU, a carcinogen that produced almost exclusively oligodendroglioma-like tumors and malignant schwannoma-like tumors, as was pointed out by Schiffer et al. (1970). This criterion has been confirmed in numerous studies later and most of the reviews about the morphology of the ENU-induced brain tumors reflected the observation that most tumors can be considered as malignant oligodendroglioma-like tumor or malignant schwannoma-like tumors (Vaquero et al, 1994).

The oligodendroglioma-like tumors are characteristically located at the subcortical white matter of the cerebral hemispheres, showing macroscopic appearance of well-defined tumors, often with hemorrhagic characteristics and foci of necrosis. Sometimes these tumors develop large cystic cavities.

In light microscopy studies, the oligodendroglioma-like tumors show a fairly uniform cell population. They are composed of small cells, which show a dark and small nucleus, and a clear cytoplasm. Regressive changes are absent and there are small hemorrhagic foci. Outlying areas of these tumors have a cellular isomorphism, which is not appreciated in the central areas, where the existing cell population shows more pleomorphism, containing giant cells, occasionally multinucleated. Ultrastructural studies reveal the presence of neoplastic cells with an elongated or oval dark nucleus, and a small, clear cytoplasm, poor in organelles. However, some neoplastic cells show a dark nucleus and a dense cytoplasm. These findings suggest that these tumors are primitive undifferentiasted tumors with some oligodendroglial features, and their undifferentiated character is supported by immunohistochemical studies. On immunohistochemistry, there is a concordance between our results and those of other authors regarding the expression of the protein S-100, PGA and vimentin (Conley, 1979, Mauro et al. 1983; Mennel and et al. 1990; Raju, 1990; Reifenberg et al. 1989) but importantly we have obtained strong synaptophysin positivity in most of these tumors. Considering that in human pathology, this marker is useful for the recognition of primitive neuroectodermal tumors such as medulloblastoma (Molenaar et al, 1991) and also for the neuronal characterization of brain tumors, it is logical to suppose that the majority of ENU-induced brain tumors can be regarded as undifferentiated neuroectodermal tumors with possible neuronal differentiation, regardless of their morphological appearance. Furthermore, in our studies, most of the ENU-induced oligodendroglioma-like tumors show immunopositivity to the neuroblastic marker NB-84. This finding agrees with some of the previous classifications of these neoplasms, such as that of Jones et al. (1973), who first identified the ENU-induced tumors as neuroblastomas.

The schwannoma-like tumors generally developed at the skull base, on the zone of the Gasser ganglion. They can be also located in the spinal root, with usually solid and sometimes cystic consistency. In our studies, these malignancies began to show neurological symptoms after a latent period ranging between 3 and 7 months after carcinogen administration. After 8 months of postnatal life, the development of these tumors is more infrequent, and after this time, intracerebral neoplasms, mainly of oligodendroglioma-like type, started to become symptomatic.

The microscopical study of these tumors with hematoxylin-eosin technique suggests that they can be classified "malignant schwannomas". They generally show a cell population highly isomorphous, consisting of small cells with dark and more or less rounded nucleus, usually in a central position, with the typical appearance of undifferentiated cells. Furthermore, a great number of mitotic figures can be seen. Moreover, in these tumors there is a large blood supply, with hyperplasia of the vessels and the formation of large cystic spaces. Sometimes is possible to find areas of necrosis. Despite the large cellular isomorphism that characterizes these tumors, is possible see compact areas showing cells with fusiform aspect, arranged in palisade, or sometimes areas with looser reticular aspect. When the tumors are located in the region of trigeminal ganglion, is frequent the presence of large neuron-like cells interspersed with the small undifferentiated cells, which supposedly correspond to trigeminal ganglion neurons that are trapped between tumor cells, but the possibility of actually correspond to a gangliocytic differentiation of the tumor can not be ruled out.

In the ultrastructural study of these tumors, at least two cell types can be found. On the one hand, there was a cell type with dark nucleus, whose chromatin is condensed to form a ring around the nuclear membrane and cytoplasmic features suggesting a neoplastic Schwann-cell. The other cell type shows a small, dark and round nucleus usually with a central position and chromatin that was condensed at the nuclear periphery. These cells showed a dense cytoplasm, with abundant rough endoplasmic reticulum, free ribosomes and polyribosomes, microtubules, primary lysosomes and a large quantity of mitochondria with dense matrix. Some of these cells show cytoplasmic granular vesicles, suggesting neuronal differentiation.

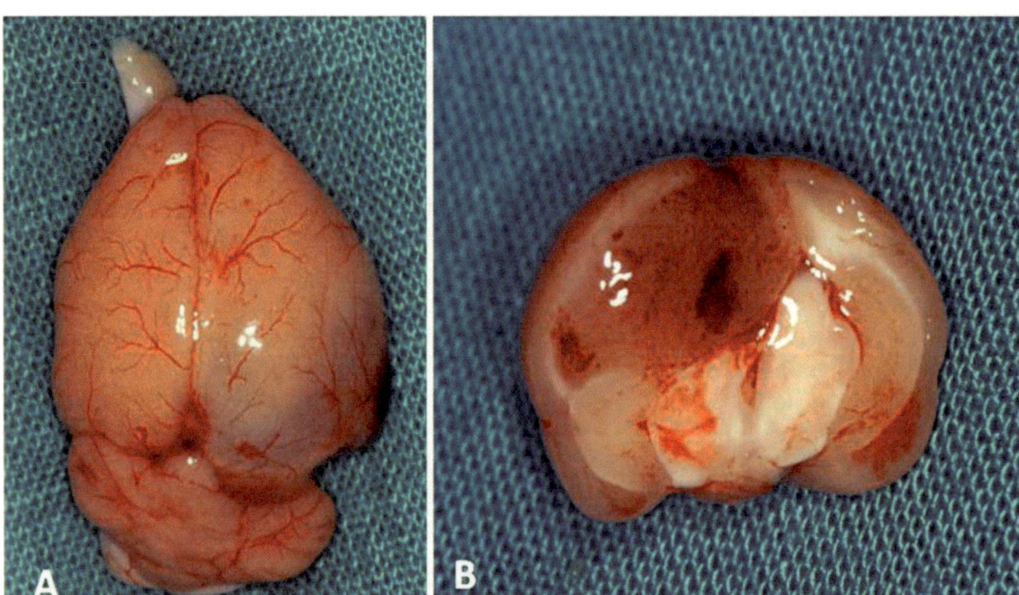

Fig. 1. Macroscopic appearance of an ENU-induced intraparenchymatous brain tumor

Finally, interspersed with these two cell types, it is possible to observe the existence of small cells, with scant cytoplasm and much more irregular nuclear configuration, which were interpreted as undifferentiated tumor cells.
The immunohistochemical study of these tumors shows a clear positivity for S-100 protein and synaptophysin. Furthermore, neuroblastic specific markers, such as NB-84 are positive in all cases. Vimentin is strongly positive in only some cases, and finally, the detection of GFAP is negative in all cases.

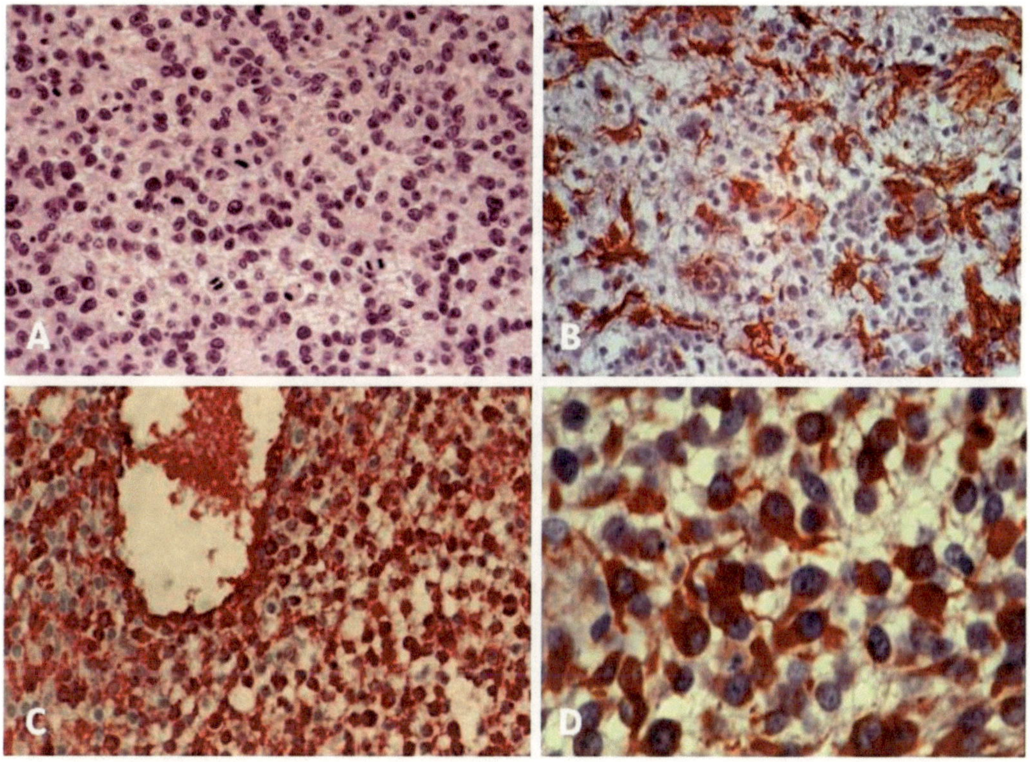

Fig. 2. Microscopic aspects of ENU-induced brain tumors. A: Tumor with oligodendroglial aspect showing abundant mitoses. B: Expression of GFAP in astrocytes trapped in the tumor. C: Expression of synaptophysin in an ENU-induced brain tumor with oligodendroglial appearance. D: Tumor cells showing positivity to the neuroblastic marker NB-84.

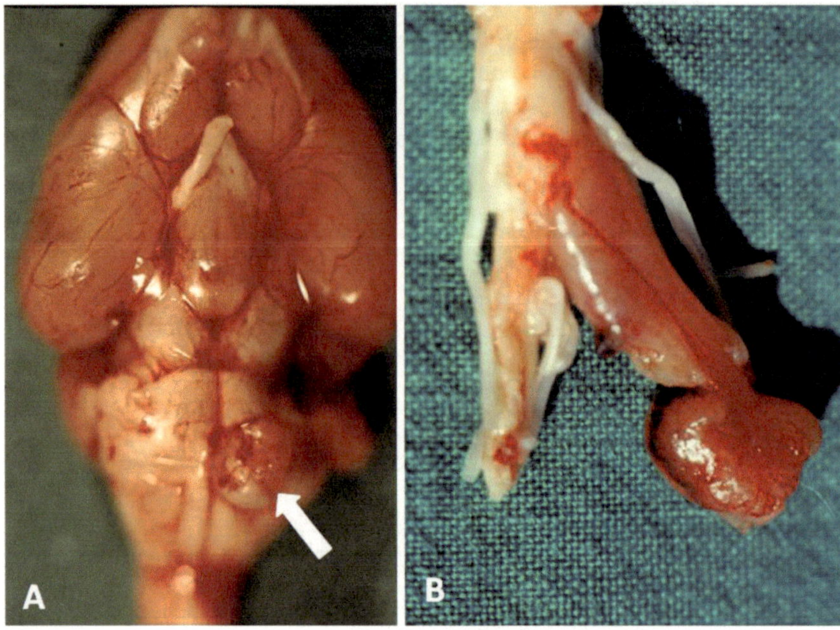

Fig. 3. Macroscopic appearance of ENU-induced tumors at level of trigeminal ganglion (A) and lumbar roots (B).

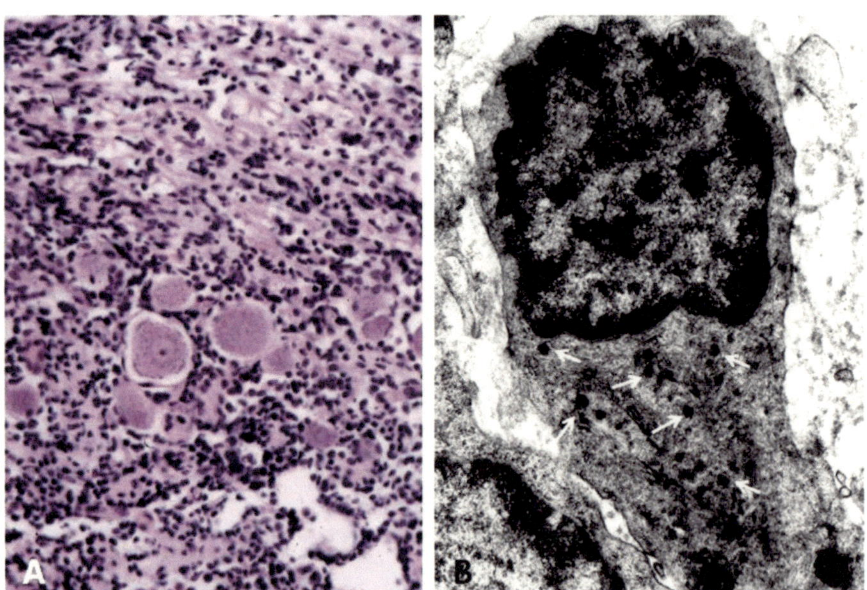

Fig. 4. A: Microscopic appearance of an ENU-induced tumor at level of trigeminal ganglion. Mature neurons can be seen, generally interpreted as trapped neurons from trigeminal ganglion. B: Ultrastructural aspect of tumor cells show undifferentiated aspect with dense granules (arrows), suggesting the neuroblastic nature of the tumor cells.

3.3.3 Development

The first sequence of the development of brain tumors induced by transplacental administration of ENU in rats was studied by Lantos and Cox in 1976. There is a latency period that it is the time between birth and the first neurological manifestations. This period has generally been estimated between 5 or 6 months. When animals are killed during this period of time, tumor lesions can be observed with different levels of development.

The different stages of development of tumors induced by administration of ENU transplacentally in rats were also studied by Shiffer in 1991. This author adopted the terms proposed by Koestner et al (1971), and reported various lesions which differed in size and that called as "early neoplastic proliferations" (less than 300 microns), microtumors (between 300 - 500 microns) and "tumors" (greater than 500 microns in diameter). The first "early neoplastic proliferations" appear about two months after birth. These lesions represent early stages of tumor development, and are generally located in the white matter at the level of the lateral ventricles, and the angle of the ventricle, between the caudate nucleus and corpus callosum, or in the subcortical white matter. The tumors that develop from these microtumors retain their morphology, including proliferation centers, but occasionally may have an increased cellular pleomorphism. At four-five months, they show a polymorphic aspect. In many proliferative centers, the cells develop a cytoplasm showing a clear appearance of astrocytes, which subsequently can be gemistocytic. In these neoplasms a central zone showing avascular necrosis, and a peripheral vascular zone can be observed. In most vessels, hyperplasia at level of endothelial cells (Nishio et al. 1983), and an increase in the number of capillaries can be seen.

3.3.4 Possibility of diagnostic "in vivo"

In our studies, we have obtained clear evidence that ENU-induced brain tumors in Wistar rats can be detected in vivo using conventional Magnetic Resonance Image (MRI). With this technique, the experimental brain tumors are characteristically hypointense on T1-phase, and hyperintense on T2-phase. They show intense and homogeneous enhancement after paramagnetic contrast administration (gadolinium). It is obvious that using this experimental model, MRI can identify effectiveness of different experimental therapeutic protocols with potential application to human neuro-oncology.

3.3.5 Transplantation

Transplantation and culture *in vitro* of chemically induced brain tumors have provided important information about their biological characteristics. In addition, transplantation on syngeneic newborn animals can get a great number of brain tumor-bearing animals in a short period of time. On the other hand, tumor lines derived from chemically induced brain tumors are often used, especially for studies of drug response, such as the glioma C-6 of rats, the 9L gliosarcoma, the T9 tumor, the RG2 and F98 gliomas, or the RN-2 glioma.

The C-6 tumor is a glioma induced by methyl nitrosourea in Wistar-Furth rats by Benda et al, in 1968. Usually it shows S-100-positivity. However, this line has the disadvantage of its frequent sarcomatous degeneration, so it is rarely used as a transplantable tumor model, although it has been used occasionally with success in the nude mouse.

The murine 9L gliosarcoma possibly developed natively in an animal crossing Wistar rats and CD Fischer, through the administration of methyl-nitrosourea.

The T9 tumor was induced in F344 rats by methyl-nitrosourea and do not have enough information about its stability in successive passes or transplants.

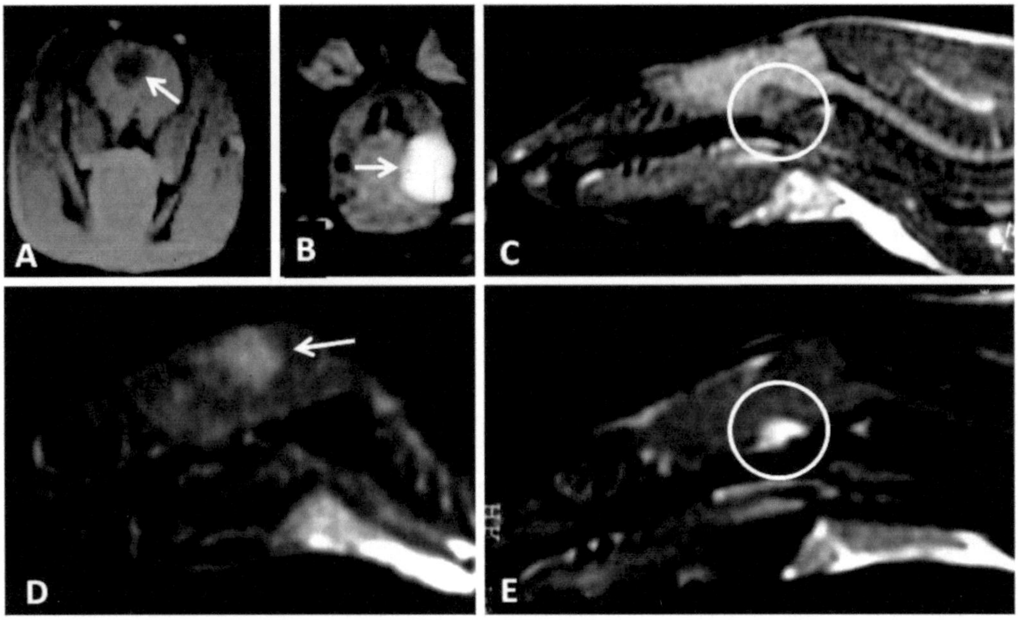

Fig. 5. Magnetic Resonance Images showing ENU-induced brain tumors. A, B and D were intraparenchymatous oligodendroglial-like tumors. C and D were extraparenchymatous tumors with features of malignant schwannomas.

The RG2 and F98 gliomas were both chemically induced by administering ENU to pregnant rats, the progeny of which developed brain tumors that subsequently were propagated *in vitro* and cloned. They have an invasive pattern of growth and uniform lethality, which make them particularly attractive models to test new therapies.

The murine glioma RN-2 derived from the induction by ethyl-nitrosourea in F344 rats. It transplanted well and has a stable glial population, many expressing antigenic markers.

These and other models are commonly used in experimental neuro-oncology, but it is essential to know the limitations of each of the experimental brain tumor models, and depending upon the nature of the study to be conducted, it is important that the appropiate model be selected (Barth and Kaur, 2009). In any case, the achievement of stable tumor cell lines, capable of growing in immunocompetent animals, is of great importance to study the efficacy of new antitumor drugs or biological agents capable of modifying the biological response in presence of a brain tumor.

3.4 Biological similarities of enu-induced brain tumors with human tumors

Although the ENU-model of neurocarcinogenesis offers the possibility to study many aspects of the biology of brain tumors, the fact is that there are many differences when establishing morphological similarities between the ENU-induced brain tumors and the different types of brain tumors in man. In human neuropathology it is accepted that certain tumors of neuronal nature, such as the so-called "central neurocytoma" may present an appearance of oligodendroglioma, but immunohistochemical and ultrastructural studies provide the correct classification (Hassoun et al. 1982). It is very similar to what happens in the case of ENU-induced oligodendroglioma-like tumors, and similar considerations can be applied to the ENU-induced malignant schwannomas. In our opinion, the immunostain and ultrastructural pattern of these experimental tumors suggests that, regardless of their histologic appearance with conventional hematoxylin-eosin staining, ENU-induced tumors can be regarded as undifferentiated neuroectodermal tumors with a tendency to neuronal differentiation.

On the other hand, we consider interesting the discussion about the etiological relationships between human brain tumors and experimental ENU-induced tumors. Although there are no reliable data on the etiological factors that determine the beginning of a human brain tumor, and the possibility of a multifactorial mechanism is considered, is interesting the finding that prenatal exposure to a carcinogen can lead to tumor development several months after birth. Moreover, considering the lifetime of rodents, the age that experimental brain tumors become manifest (mean age of the life of the rat) corresponds to the higher frequency of brain tumor development in humans (adult age). If some types of human brain tumor may be caused by exposure to certain carcinogens in the prenatal period, is an open question (Huncharek, 2010).

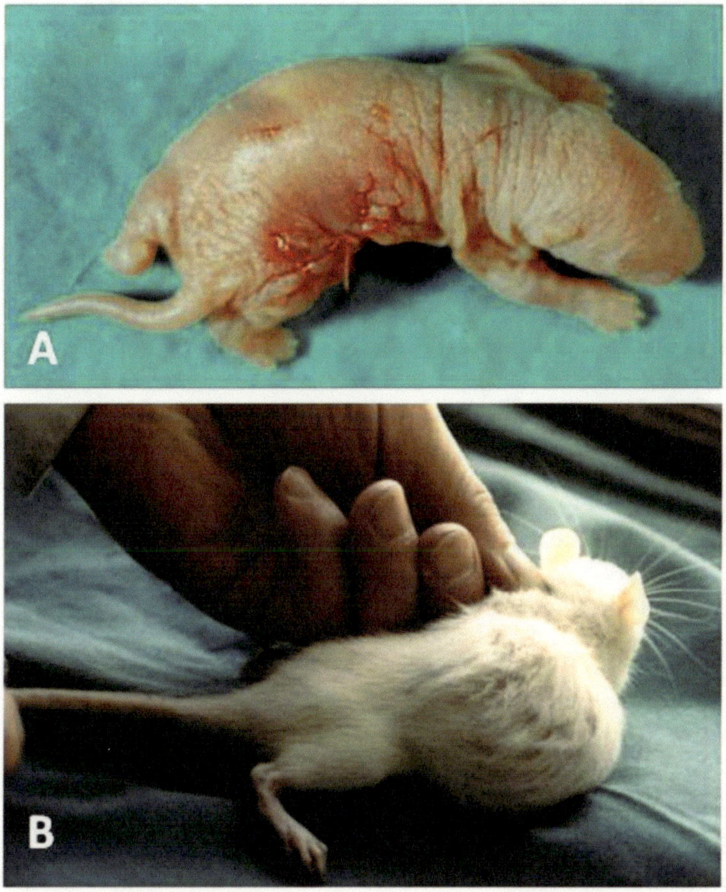

Fig. 6. A: Subcutaneous transplantation of an ENU-induced brain tumor in immunocompetent newborn rat. B: Tumor growth one month later.

4. References

Alexandrov, V. A. (1973). In: *Transplacental Carcinogenesis*. Tomatis L. and Mohr, eds.). IARC Sci. 4:112-126, Lyon, 1973.

Barth, R.F., Kaur, B. (2009). Rat brain tumor models in experimental neuro-oncology: the C6, 9L, T9, RG2, F98, BT4C, RT-2 and CNS-1 gliomas. *J. Neurooncol.* 94: 299-312.

Bigner, D.D., Pegram, C.N. (1976). Virus-induced experimental brain tumors and putative associations of viruses with human brain tumors: a review. *Adv. Neurol.*, 15: 57-83.

Bullard, D.E.B., Bigner, D.D. (1980). Animal models and virus induction of tumours. In: *Brain Tumours. Scientific Basis, Clinical Investigation and Current Therapy*. Thomas D.G.T., and Graham, D.I. (Eds). Butterworth and Co., pp: 51-84.

Conley, F. K. (1979). The immunocytochemical localization of GFA protein in experimental murine CNS tumors. *Acta Neuropathol.*, 45, 9-16.

Delinger, R. H., Koestner, A., Swenberg, J. A. (1973). An experimental model for selective production of neoplasms of the peripheral nervous system. *Acta Neuropathol.*, 23, 219-228.

Druckrey, H., Preussmann, R., Ivankovic, S. (1969). N-nitroso compounds in organotropic and transplacental carcinogenesis. *Ann. N. Y. Acad. Sci.* 163,676-696.

Druckrey, H., Schagen, B., Ivankovic, S. (1970). The induction of neurogenic malignancies by single dosage of ENU to newborn and young BD IX rats. *Z. Krebsforsch.* 74, 141-161.

Goth, R., Rajewsky, M. F. (1974). Persistence of 06-ethylguanine in rat-brain DNA: Correlation with nervous system-specific carcinogenesis by ethylnitrosourea. *Proc. Natl. Acad. Sci. USA* 71, 639-643.

Hassoun, J., Gambarelli, D., Grisoli, F., Pellet, W., Salamon, G., Pelissier, J. F., Toga, M. (1982). Central neurocytoma. An electron microscopic study of two cases. *Acta Neuropathol.* 56, 151-156.

Huncharek, M. (2010). Maternal intake of N-nitroso compounds from cured meat and the risk of pediatric brain tumors: a review. *J. Environ. Pathol. Toxicol. Oncol.* 29: 245-253.

Ivankovic, S. (1969). Induction of genital cancer in pregnant rats. *Arzneim Forsch* 19, 1040-1041.

Ivankovic, S. (1972). Induction of malignances in rats following the transplacental action of N-isopropyl-alfa-2-(methylamydrazine)-p-toluamide. *Arzneim Forsch,* 22, 905-907.

Jones, E. L, Searle, C. E, Smith, W. T. (1973). Tumours of the nervous system induced in rats by the neonatal administration of N-ethyl-N-nitrosourea. *J. Pathol.* 109, 123-139.

Kahle, W. (1970). Embryogenetic aspects of diaplacental induction of gliomata. *Proc. VI Int Congr Neuropath Paris*: Masson et Cie, 556-557.

Koestner, A., Swenberg, J. A., Wechsler, W. (1971). Transplacental production with ethylnitrosourea of neoplasms of the nervous system in Spraguer-Dawley rats. *Am. J. Pathol.* 63, 37-56.

Lantos, P. L. (1972). The fine structure of periventricular pleomorphic gliomas induced transplacentally by N-ethyl-N-nitrosoureas in BD-IX rats. With a note on their origin. *J. Neurol. Sci.* 17, 443-460.

Lantos, P. L, Cox D.J. (1976). The origin of experimental brain tumours: a sequential study. *Experientia*, 32, 1457-1468.

Mandybur, T. I., Alvira, M. M. (1982). Ultrastructural findings in so-called ependymal rat tumors induced by transplacental administration of ethylnitrosourea (ENU). *Acta Neuropathol.* 57, 51-58.

Mauro, A., Giordana, M.T., Migheli, A., Schiffer, D. (1983). Glial fibrillary acidic protein (GFAP) in rat brain tumors transplacentally induced by ethylnitrosourea (ENU). *J. Neurol. Sci.* 61, 349-355.

Mennel, H. D., Dreyhaupt, T. (1990). Immunohistochemical investigations in experimentally induced tumors of the nervous system. *Exp. Pathol.,* 40, 45-53.

Mennel, H.D, Zülch, K.J. (1971). The morphology of malignant tumors of the pripheral nerves. *Zentralbl. Neurochir.* 32, 11-24.

Minn, Y., Wrensch, M., Bondy, M.L. (2002). Epidemiology of primary brain tumors. In: *Brain Cancer.* Prados M, Atlas of Clinical Oncology, Steele, G.D., Phillips, T., L., Chabner, B.A. (Eds). American Cancer Society, BC Decker Inc., Hamilton, London. pp: 1-15.

Molenaar, W. M., Baker, D. L., Pleasure, D. (1990). The neuroendrocrine and neural profiles of neuroblastomas, ganglioneuroblastomas and ganglioneuromas. *Am. J. Pathol.,* 136, 375-382.

Nishio, S., Ohta, M., Abe, M., Kitamura, K. (1983). Microvascular abnormalities in Ethylnitrosourea (ENU)-induced rat brain tumors: Structural basis for altered blood-brain barrier function. *Acta Neuropathol.* 59, 1-10.

Rabson, A.S., Kirschstein, R.L. (1960). Intracranial sarcomas produced by polyoma virus in Syrian hamsters. *Arch. Pathol.* 69: 663-671.

Raju, N.R. (1990). Immunohistochemical characterization of the rat central and peripheral nerve tumors induced by ethylnitrosourea. *Toxicol. Pathol.* 18, 18-23.

Reifenberger, G., Bilzer, T., Seitz, R.J., Wechsler, W. (1989). Expression of vimentin and glial fibrillary acidic protein in ethylnitrosourea-induced rat glioma and glioma cell lines. *Acta Neuropathol.,* 78, 270-282.

Schiffer, D. (1991). Patterns of tumor growth. In: *Neurobiology of brain tumors.* Salcman M. ED. Concepts in Neurosurgery, Vol 4, Willians and Wilkins, Baltimore. pp: 85-210.

Schiffer, D., Fabiani, A., Grossi-Paoletti, Paoletti, P. (1970). Experimental brain tumours induced in rats by nitrosourea derivatives. Part 1. Morphological aspects of methylnitrosourea tumours. *J. Neurol Sci.* 11, 559-572.

Schreiber, D., Warzok, R., Scholtze, P., Schneider, J., Lageman, A., Batka, H. (1972). The spectrum of extraneural tumors of the rat after administration of MNU. *Zentralbl. Allg. Pathol.,* 115, 48-61.

Swenberg, J. A., Koestner, A., Wechsler, W., Denlinger, R. H. (1972). Quantitative aspects of transplacental tumor induction with ethylnitrosourea in rats. *Cancer Res.* 32, 2656-2660.

Thomas, C., Rogg, H., Bücheler, J. (1972). The cancer-inducing effect of MNU after administration of hormonal contraceptives. Beitr Pathol. *Anat. Allgem Pathol.* 146, 332-338.

Vaquero, J., Oya, S., Coca, S., Zurita, M. (1994). Experimental induction of primitive neuroectodermal tumours in rats: A re-appraisement of the ENU-model of neurocarcinogenesis. *Acta Neurochir. (Wien)* 131, 294-301, 1994.

Wechsler, W., Kleihues, P., Matsumoto, D., Zülch, K. J., Ivankovic, S., Preussmann, R., Druckrey, H. (1969). Pathology of experimental neurogenic tumors chemically induced during prenatal and postnatal life. *Ann. N.Y. Acad. Sci.,* 159, 360-408.

Zemp, F.J., Corredor, J.C., Lun, X., Muruve, D.A., Forsyth, P.A. (2010). Oncolytic viruses as experimental treatments for malignant gliomas: using a scourge to treat a devil. *Cytokine Growth Factor Rev.* 21: 103-117.

3

Molecular Diagnostics of Brain Tumours by Measuring the 5-Methylcytosine Level in Their DNA

Anna-Maria Barciszewska[1], Stanisław Nowak[1], Iwona Gawrońska[2] and Mirosława Barciszewska[2]
[1]*Department of Neurosurgery and Neurotraumatology Karol Marcinkowski University ,School of Medical Sciences, Poznan*
[2]*Institute of Bioorganic Chemistry of the Polish Academy of Sciences, Poznan Poland*

1. Introduction

Brain tumours form a group of neoplasms with distinct histological characteristics and different malignancies [Maher 2001]. Various molecular alterations occurring in brain tumors may have diagnostic and predictive values as they are connected with histologically determined tumour types and malignancy grades [Martinez et al. 2009; Martinez and Esteller 2010; Sciume et al. 2010]. Methylation of DNA cytosine residue at the carbon 5 position (m^5C) is a common epigenetic marker in many eukaryotes and is often found in the sequence context of CpG. It is assumed that ca 5% of all cytosine residues, i.e. 1% of the nucleic bases, in mammalian genomes are methylated. Although DNA methylation has been viewed as a stable epigenetic mark, studies in the past decade have revealed that this modification is not as static [Wu and Zhang 2010]. In fact, loss of DNA methylation (DNA hypomethylation), has been observed in the specific context and can occur through active, passive or random modification mechanisms. Although the genome in each cell within the body is identical, cell- and tissue-specific profiles of gene transcription, posttranscriptional modification, modifications and translation are specifically regulated by epigenetic mechanisms that include DNA methylation, histone modification and noncoding RNAs [Robertson 2005]. In the central nervous system epigenetic mechanisms serve as main regulators of homeostasis and plasticity development, which are sensitive to local and global environmental, vascular and systemic factors [Martinez and Esteller 2010].

It is generally accepted that cancer initiation and progression are linked to the disruption of red-ox balance of the cell [Grek and Tew 2010]. Current evidences support an idea that cancer cells are generated by enhanced reactive oxygen species (ROS) generation, their accumulation, and down regulation of antioxidant enzymes [Essick and Sam 2010]. The oxidative damage to the cell caused by ROS plays a critical role in the etiology and progression of different neoplasms in humans [Johnstone and Baylin 2010; Jomova and Valko 2011].

Oxygen radicals cause damage to DNA and chromosomes, induce epigenetic alterations, interact with oncogenes or tumour suppressor genes, and finally change the immunological mechanisms [Robertson 2005; Pelizzola and Ecker 2010].

5-methylcytosine (m^5C), along with other DNA constituents and the cell components, are targets for ROS, of which the most reactive species is the hydroxyl radical (•OH). Hydroxyl radical causes a wide range of DNA lesions including base modifications, deletions and strands breakage. Radical oxidation of m^5C leads to its modification including demethylation and deamination (Fig. 1). It results in decreasing the global (genomic) m^5C content in cellular DNA (hypomethylation). Therefore DNA methylation (m^5C status) is a sensitive marker of the neoplasm formation effected by the oxidative damage reactions and very characteristic for cancer cells [Robertson 2005].

Measurements of m^5C in DNA can be done either by analysing the pattern of methylated target sequences along individual DNA molecules or as an average methylation level at a single genomic locus across many DNA molecules [Rao and Balachandran 2002].

One should remember that 5% of m^5C deaminates to thymine under moderately acidic conditions and 2-5% is converted to thymine during the standard overnight incubation with sodium bisulfite [Wu and Zhang 2010].

One can also measure the global DNA methylation changes [Li et al. 2009; Pelizzola and Ecker 2010]. To investigate whether hypomethylation has a causal role in tumour formation, we have analyzed the level of m^5C in DNA of human brain tumour tissues using two-dimensional thin layer chromatography (TLC) analysis of [^{32}P] postlabelled DNA components. We have found a correlation of m^5C global content in DNA of tumour tissues with their malignancy. We have shown that as m^5C amount decreases, the tumour grade of malignancy increases. The elaborated method has a practical application potential in the clinical diagnostics and also as the DNA quality test.

2. Materials and methods

Patients

Patients with brain tumours have been operated at the Department of Neurosurgery and Neurotraumatology of Poznań University of Medical Sciences. Brain tumour samples from 577 patients were collected between 2007 and 2010 and stored at -80°C. Histopatological analysis was done in the Neuropathology Laboratory and tumours classified according to the 2007 WHO rules [Louis et al. 2007]. Informed consent for samples and data analysis was obtained from each patient.

Isolation of DNA from brain tumor tissue

DNA was isolated from tumour tissue according to the method described earlier [Miller et al. 1988] or with a commercial kit (A&A Biotechnology, Poland).

DNA hydrolysis, labeling and analysis

Dried DNA (1 μg) was digested with 0.02 U of micrococcal nuclease (MN) and 0.001 U spleen phosphodiesterase II (SPD) to mononucleotides (Np) in 50 mM succinate buffer pH 6 containing 10 mM $CaCl_2$ in 3.5 μl total volume for 5 h at 37°C. Mononucleotides (0.17 μg) were labelled with 0.1 μCi [γ-^{32}P] ATP (6000 Ci $mmol^{-1}$, USB) and T4 polynucleotide kinase (1.5 U) in 3 μl of 10 mM bicine-NaOH pH 9.7 buffer containing 10 mM $MgCl_2$, 10 mM dithiothreitol and 1 mM spermidine for 30 min at 37°C.

To remove inorganic phosphate (PPi) 3 μl (10 U ml^{-1}) of apyrase (Sigma) in the same 10 mM bicine-NaOH buffer pH 9.7 was added and incubation was continued for 30 min. Finally the 3′ phosphate was cleaved off with 0.2 μg RNase P1 in 500 mM ammonium acetate buffer pH 4.5 [Barciszewska 2007].

Separation of [γ-^{32}P]m^5C from other nucleotides was performed with thin layer chromatography (TLC) on cellulose plates (Merck) using isobutyric acid:NH_4OH:H_2O (66:1:17 vol/vol) in the first dimension and 0.1 M sodium phosphate pH 6.8 - ammonium sulfate - n-propanol (100 ml/ 60 g/ 2 ml) in the second dimension. The chromatogram was analyzed with Phosphoimager using Image Quant Software. The amount of m^5C was calculated as of the spot intensities ratio of [$m^5C/(m^5C+C+T)$] ×100 and expressed as R coefficient. The analysis was repeated 3 times for each probe and results were evaluated.

3. Results and discussion

Low level of some reactive oxygen species (ROS) as superoxide, hydroxyl radical or hydrogen peroxide can enhance cellular survival and stimulate proliferation. However, when that is a concominant with chronic ROS production, redox homeostasis can become imbalanced and normal cells may undergo transformation [Rao and Balachandran 2002]. In the last years many data have been collected that link cell stress to various diseases including cancer, cardiovascular disease, diabetes and neurodegenerative disorders. Current evidence support the hypothesis that cancer cells are characterized by enhanced ROS generation, increased ROS accumulation and the degradation of antioxidant enzymes. There are many explanations how cellular stress induces a disease. It is known that the cell stress causes genetic and epigenetic changes and results in an altered cellular "memory" that drives diseases pathology [Robertson 2005]. The main risk for cancer is a chronic exposure and increasing DNA damage. There is a wealth of data which supports the idea that cancerous cells have aberrant patterns of epigenetic modifications. The best studied epigenetic modification is DNA methylation, which consists of the methyl group at carbon 5 of the cytosine. Methylation of cytosine residues in DNA provides a mechanism for a gene control expression.

DNA methylation in promotor region as well as coding sequences inhibits binding of regulatory protein and causes gene silencing [Frigola et al. 2005]. It has been estimated that up to 5% of cytosines are methylated in normal tissues and that this DNA methylation is necessary for controlling gene expression of tissue-specific housekeeping or imprinted genes and for maintaining genomic stability through silencing transposable elements of the genome. Genomic DNA can undergo changes not only in the sequence level but also by the addition or removal of chemical groups. Aberrant DNA methylation, appeared as either hyper-, or hypomethylation, is associated with changes in the phenotype of various diseases including brain tumours [Frigola et al. 2005].

The brain and other points of the nervous system are particularly vulnerable to the free radical damage for a number of reasons. The membrane lipids in brain contain high level of polyunsaturated fatty acid side chains, which are prone to free radical damage. Brain also takes up large quantities of oxygen contributing to the formation of reactive oxygen species. At the same time brain contains low level of antioxidant enzymes such as catalase, superoxide dismutase and glutathione peroxidase. Presence of iron, copper and manganese in the brain contribute significantly to the production of a highly reactive and very short living ROS via Fenton reaction [Kehrer 2000; Essick and Sam 2010]. Free radicals, and •OH in particular, cause damaging of DNA, proteins and lipids. They include for example 8-hydroxy-2-deoxyguanosine, 4-hydroxy-2-nonenal and others [Fraga et al. 2002; Tudek et al. 2010].

Gliomas are the most common primary tumours affecting the human central nervous system (CNS). They are classified in accordance with their histopatological features and clinical presentation. The most abundance gliomas are astrocytomas, oligodendrogliomas and oligoastrocytomas [Louis et al. 2007]. Astrocytomas occur with an incidence of 80-85% of all gliomas and glioblastoma multiforme (GBM) represent the most frequent malignant primary brain tumours. Various genes with frequent tumour related promoter hypermethylation have been identified in glioma [Martinez and Esteller 2010]. Gene regulation in tumours by promoter methylation has been established [Robertson 2005]. It has a prognostic and predictive potential in cancers. Therefore one can expect DNA methylation analysis to become an important diagnostic tool for many types of cancer.

Oxidative stress from aberrant accumulation of ROS over time can damage of proteins, lipids and nucleic acids and forms the molecular basis of free-radical background of cancer. It is well established that the oxidative stress is linked directly to cancer [Essick and Sam 2010; Grek and Tew 2010; Johnstone and Baylin 2010]. Although ROS modification to DNA has been broadly discussed in the past, its activity towards 5-methylcytosine, a main epigenetic marker, causing DNA demethylation has been overlooked for a long time [Berdasco and Esteller 2010].

Although DNA methylation has been recognized as a stable epigenetic mark, recently many data on loss of DNA methylation (DNA demethylation) has been collected. It can be that DNA demethylation is an active, enzymatic or chemical process of the methyl group removal through breaking a carbon-carbon bond. Genome-wide and gene-specific demethylation events are observed [Trewick et al. 2002; Martinez et al. 2009; Martinez and Esteller 2010]. The first occurs at specific times during early development, whereas the latter occurs in somatic cells responding to specific signals.

Many enzymes and various mechanisms have been proposed to carry out active DNA demethylation [Wu and Zhang 2010]. They include base m^5C excision repair, deamination of m^5C to T, nucleotide excision repair, oxidative demethylation and radical S-adenosylmethionine-based demethylation [Wu and Zhang 2010; Klug et al. 2010].

In addition to that, it is also possible for DNA to be demethylated randomly with very active hydroxyl radical [Kehrer 2000]. It is known that DNA molecule is subjected to a broad range of free radicals and oxidative injuries *in vivo* [Ulrey et al. 2005]. The oxidation reaction of with $-CH_3$ group of m^5C hydroxyl radical causes spontaneous demethylation or deamination leading to C or T, respectively (Fig. 1).

The demethylation of m^5C proceeds through 5-hydroxymethylcytosine intermediate [Guo et al. 2011]. The mechanism of this reaction is similar to that of radical SAM [Wu and Zhang 2010]. Imbalance of red-ox state in tumor cells affects the genomic methylation patterns what can be used to distinguish cancerous from normal brain cells, and to find correlations with their pathological features [Bart et al. 2005].

There are evidences which support the existence of DNA demethylation in vertebrate cells, although the mechanism of that process is not clear [Wu and Zhang 2010].

A low amount of m^5C in human DNA and a limited availability of brain tumour tissues, prompted us to look for a new and suitable method of m^5C determination with diagnostic potential. We have applied a nucleic acid postlabelling approach with $[\gamma\text{-}^{32}P]$-ATP and T4 polynucleotide kinase (T4 PNK) to analyze DNA components with the thin layer two dimensional chromatography (TLC) and particularly for a quantitative assessment of the modified nucleotides (Fig. 2).

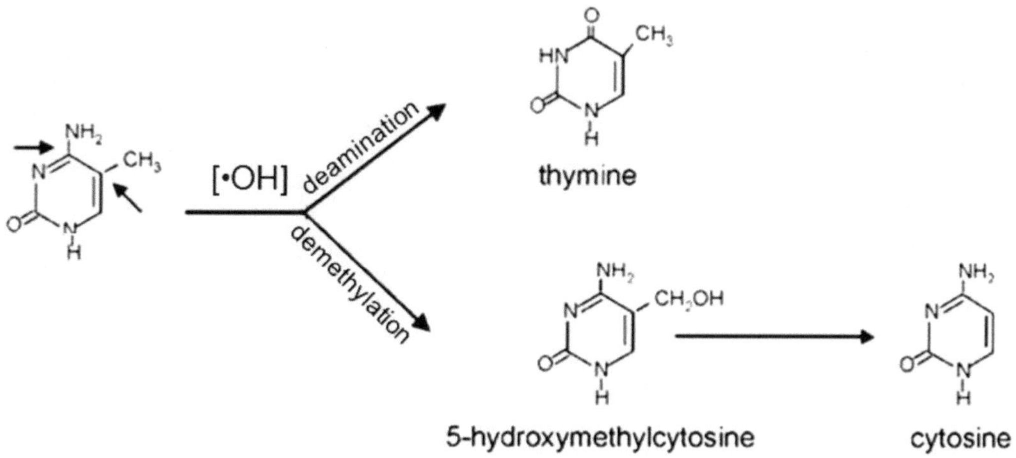

Fig. 1. Formation of thymine and cytosine in the reaction of m5C in DNA with hydroxyl radical.

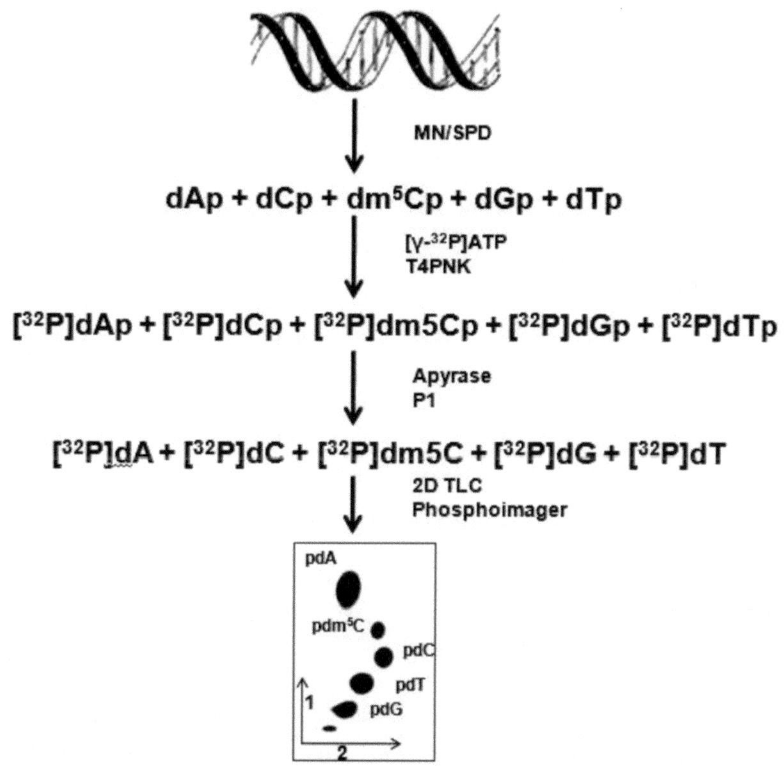

Fig. 2. Flow chart of m5C analysis in DNA hydrolyzed to 3'mononucleotides (Np). They are furthermore labelled with [γ-32P] ATP, dephosphorylated of 3' phosphate and separated with TLC in two dimensions (1 and 2).

It seems that deamination and demethylation of m^5C effected with hydroxyl radical oxidation, leads to thymine (T) and cytosine (C) formation, respectively (Fig. 1). These bases obtained from m^5C are naturally occurring in DNA and therefore we included them in the equation: $R= [m^5C/ (m^5C+C+T)] \times 100$, for m^5C assessment. In this way R represents the amount of m^5C in relation to all pyrimidines (basic bases) present in DNA. We assume R as global methylation coefficient.
Before we began the analysis of m^5C in human brain tumours DNA, we have checked the effect of tissue samples handling on the assignment of m^5C. Tumour tissues were resected and handled in three different conditions. For the same tissue sample, one part was freshly frozen (FF), immediately put on dry ice, the other was formalin-fixed, paraffin embedded (FFPE) and the third one was stored for 3 hrs at room temperature on the bench. For DNA isolation, the tissue from FFPE was recovered as described previously [Sanchez-Navarro et al. 2010]. DNA isolated from all differently treated tissue samples showed changes in global amount of m^5C (Fig. 3).

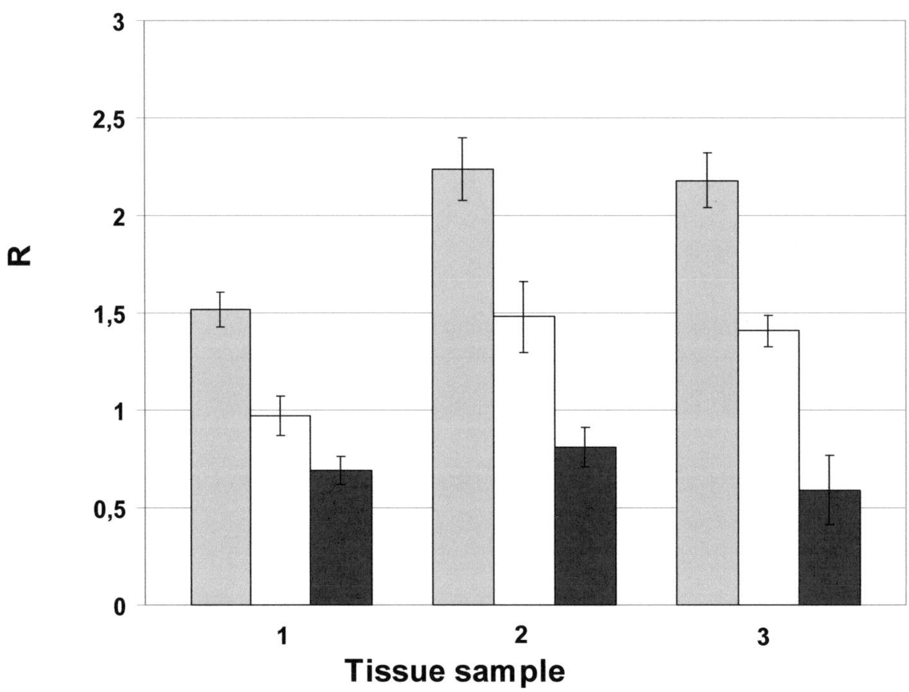

Fig. 3. The level of cytosine methylation (m^5C) in DNA isolated from resected meningioma tissues and stored at -80°C (grey), formaldehyde fixed, paraffin embedded (FFPE) (white) and exposed at room temperature for 3 hrs (black).

It is known that the development of molecular tests for clinical use has been limited by the lack of good available clinical samples for validation of candidate biomarkers. FF samples are difficult to collect and store for large scale studies, but FFPE samples on the other hand are stable at room temperature and easily to store. However the last approach has some disadvantages. Recently, it has been shown that RNA isolated from FFPE is a poor material for gene expression analysis due to its deep degradation [Farragher et al. 2006; Sanchez-Navarro et al. 2010].

Formalin fixation and paraffin embedding is the most commonly used method worldwide for tissue storage. This method preserves the tissue integrity but causes extensive damage to nucleic acids within the tissue. There is a huge resource of FFPE tissues specimens held in histopathology departments around the world. The samples provide an invaluable resource for studying the molecular basis of disease, making it possible to perform large retrospective studies correlation molecular features with therapeutic response and clinical out come [Farragher et al. 2008]. We have clearly showed that DNA in FFPE samples is degraded (Fig. 3) and observed significant demethylation in cellular DNA is due to oxidative damage [Tudek et al. 2010]. The highest DNA methylation level we observed for DNA isolated from fresh frozen tissues. The majority of studies to date have used high quality RNA from FF samples, however those studies have been restricted due to the small number of samples [Farragher et al. 2008]. Significantly lower amount of m^5C was observed for FFPE tissues and severe hypomethylation for DNA from the cells stored at room temperature. One can conclude that m^5C demethylation is effected by cellular oxidative damage which is reduced by deep freezing of a tissue sample immediately after tumor resection. A cellular damage occurring during embedding in paraffin, which includes heating up step in liquid paraffin, significantly stimulates demethylation has been observed earlier [Barciszewska et al. 2006; Blow 2007]. One can conclude that the decrease of DNA m^5C is a consequence of severe DNA oxidation including m^5C with •OH.

The goal of our studies was to understand the biology of malignant gliomas on the level that leads to the development of new diagnostic method.

We have analyzed the global level m^5C in DNA samples from 577 individuals with brain tumours aged 11 - 80. Histopatological analysis of brain tumours was done according to WHO 2007 rules [Louis at al. 2007]. There were 285 males (49.5%) and 292 (50.5%) females.

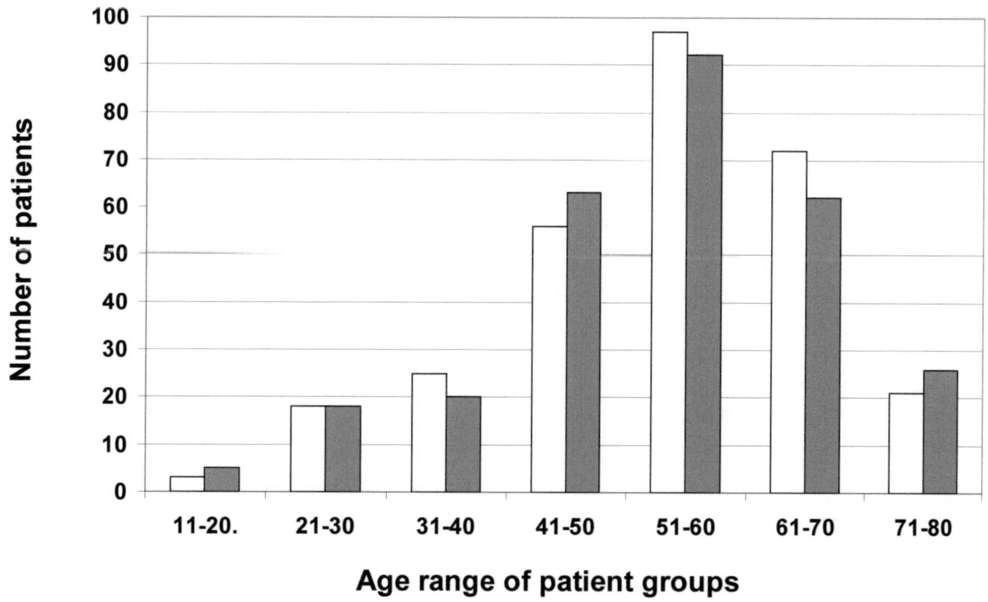

Fig. 4. Number of patients in the different age groups. Men – black bars, women – white bars.

The biggest group included patients of 41-70 years old. The highest ratio of patients at the time of diagnosis showed a group aged 51-60 years. The median age of patients at the time of diagnosis was 53.4±13.2 years (Fig. 4).
To correlate human brain tumours malignancy established with pathomorphological analysis with global DNA methylation, we have analyzed the genomic m5C content in DNA from human brain tissues of different gliomas. (Fig. 5, Table 1).

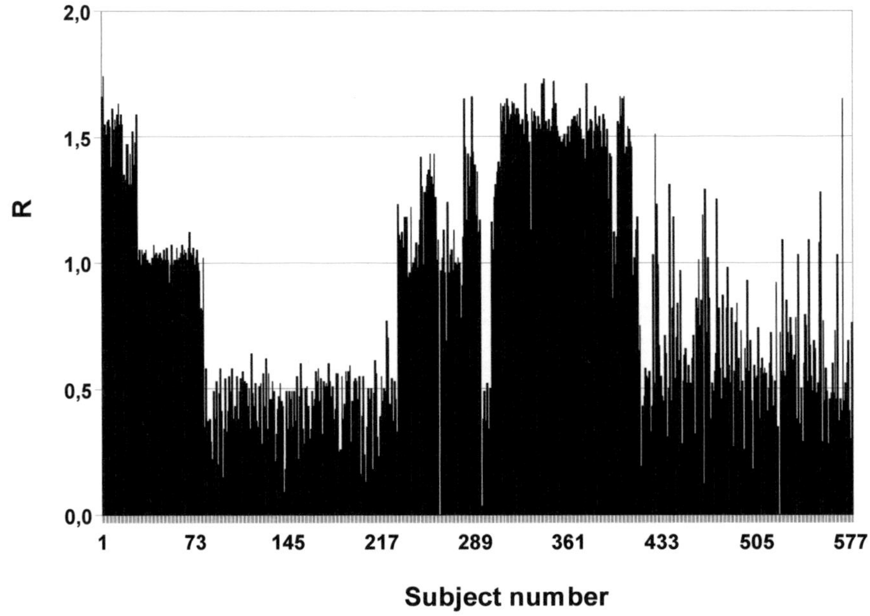

Fig. 5. 5-methylcytosine contents in DNA from patients with brain tumors.

Human tumours often display genome-wide DNA hypomethylation, which promotes cancer through the effect on chromosomal stability [Gaudet et al. 2003; Eden 2003; Yamada et al. 2005; Nishiyama et al. 2005].
One can see that m5C content in different human brain tumours varies very much (Fig. 5, Table 1). It is known that hydroxylation of m5C promotes active DNA demethylation in the adult brain [Guo et al. 2011]. Analysis patients' groups with high grade glioma shows that m5C content (R) decrease as malignancy increases (Fig. 6). The most abundant are gliomas astrocytomas, oligodendrogliomas or tumours with morphological features of both astrocytes and oligodendrocytas called oligoastrocytomas (Table 1). The histological classification is followed by grading (from I to IV) which expresses the tumour malignancy with IV being the most malignant. Astrocytic tumours are subsequently graded with I (pilocytic astrocytoma), II e.g. diffuse astrocytoma, III (anaplastic astrocytoma) and IV (glioblastoma multiforme). Oligodendrogliomas and astrocytomas are graded furthermore as with grade II or III (anaplastic). The highest DNA demethylation is observed for glioblastoma multiforme (Fig. 6).
These results are in agreement with previous observations done for a smaller group of patients [Zukiel 2004]. Importantly these data are supported by others, showed that primary glioblastoma and established glioma cell lines show significant reduction of m5C content

compared with normal brain tissue [Cadieux et al. 2006]. Furthermore one can see that grade III shows R in the range 1 - 1.2, but for WHO IV R coefficient is below 0.5 (Fig. 6). This is the lowest level of DNA methylation observed ever, not only for high grade gliomas. Because the correlation of m5C content (R) and WHO grade is linear (Fig. 6), therefore R can be used as a probe of tumorgenesis. One can clearly see that the global DNA methylation analysis easily differentiate low and high grade tumours as well as metastatic (Fig. 7). Different relations occur for meningeomas (Fig. 8, Table 2).

No.	Brain tumor histological type	Malignancy WHO grade	No. of cases	R
	Astrocytic tumours			
1	Pilocytic astrocytoma	I	4	1.62
2	Diffuse astrocytoma	II	24	1.49
3	Anaplastic astrocytoma	III	52	1.02
4	Glioblastoma	IV	139	0.44
5	- Giant cell glioblastoma	IV	5	0.46
6	- Gliosarcoma	IV	1	0.46
7	Gliomatosis cerebri	IV	1	0.33
	Oligodendroglial tumours			
8	Oligodendroglioma	II	11	1.10
9	Anaplastic oligodendroglioma	III	6	1.02
	Oligoastrocytic tumours			
10	Oligoastrocytoma	II	13	1.30
11	Oligoastrocytoma	III	8	0.98
12	Anaplastic oligoastrocytoma	III	10	1.04
	Ependymal tumours			
13	Subependymoma	I	3	0.93
14	Ependymoma	II	4	1.43
15	Anaplastic ependymoma	III	1	1.30
	Neuronal and mixed neuronal-glial tumours	I	2	1.54
16	Dysembryoplastic neuroepithelial tumour	II	2	1.42
17	Ganglioglioma	III	1	1.19
18	Anaplastic ganglioglioma	II	3	1.22
19	Central neurocytoma			
	Tumours of the pineal region	IV	1	0.38
20	Pineoblastoma			
	Embryonal tumours	IV	6	0.45
21	Medulloblastoma			

Table 1. The list of human brain tumours of neuroepithelial origin (total number 297) identified in patients. For each of them malignancy and m5C content [R] were established.

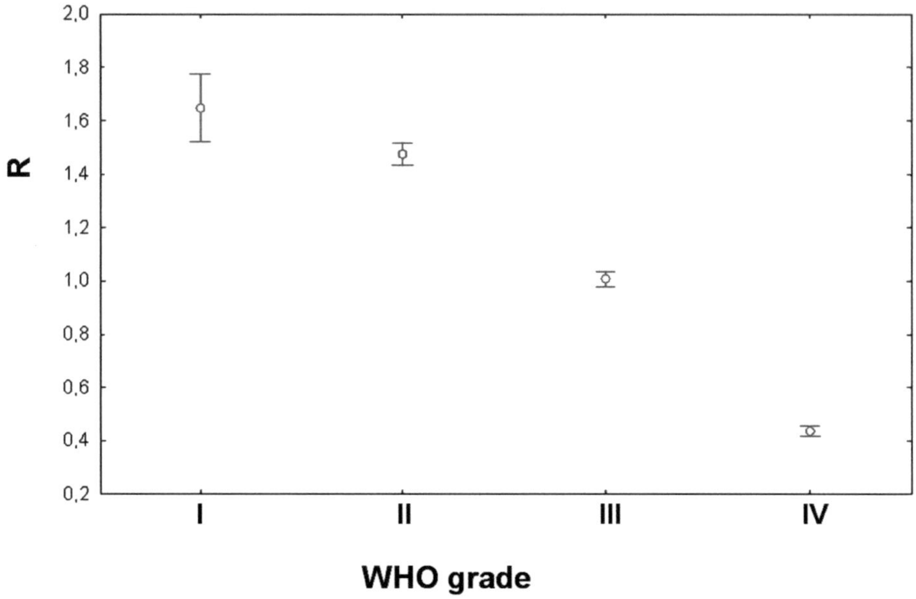

Fig. 6. The mean values (p< 0.0002-0.0003) of global DNA (m^5C) methylation expressed as R for different human gliomas with different malignancy grades (I-IV). See Table 1.

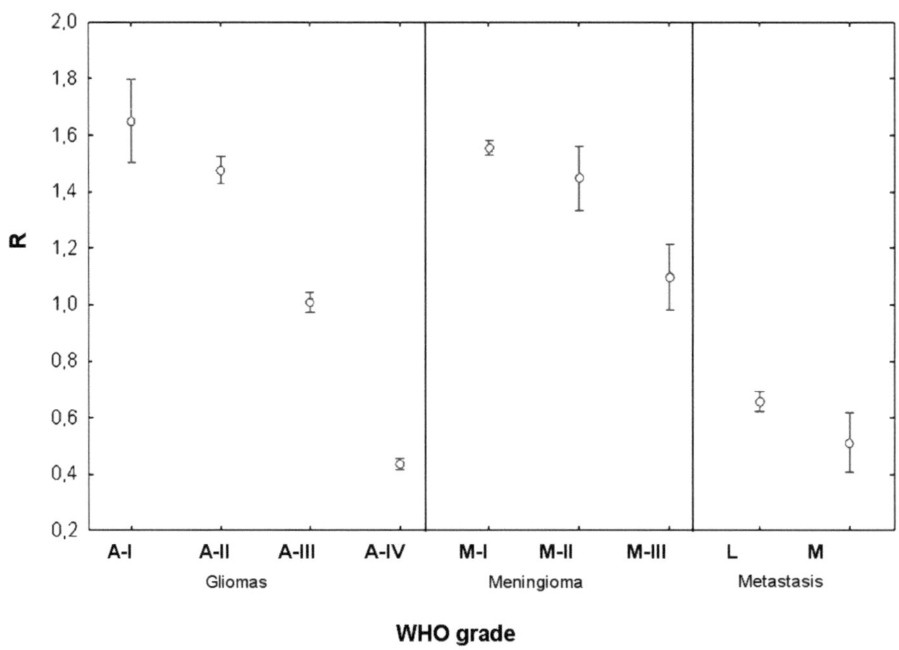

Fig. 7. The mean values (p<0,0002 – 0.0003) of m^5C in DNA for gliomas (A-I – AIV), meningeomas (M-I – M-III) and metastasis (L-from lung, M-from melanoma skin cancer).

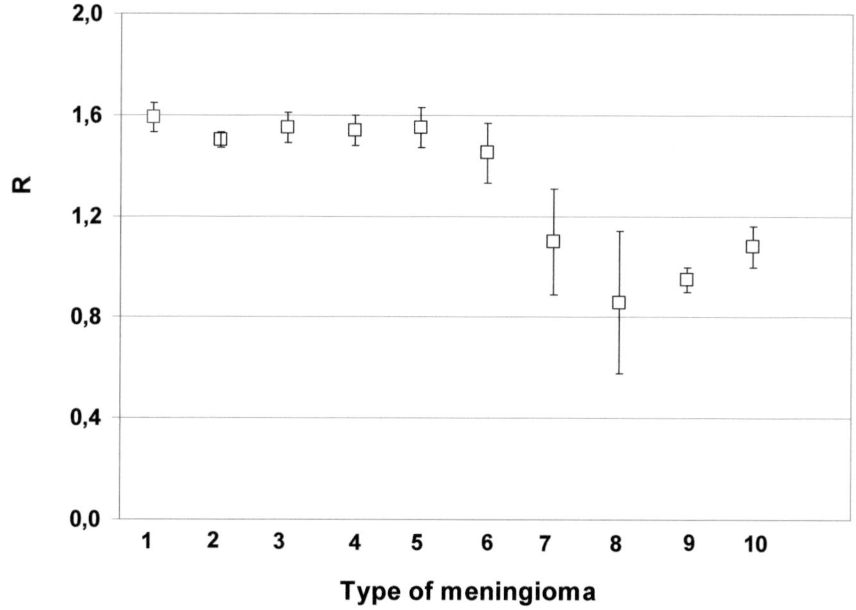

Fig. 8. The mean value of DNA methylation (m^5C) for different meningiomas. 1 – meningotheliale meningioma I; 2 – angiomatosum meningioma I; 3 – fibrosum meningioma I; 4 – psammomatous meningioma I; 5 – transitional meningioma II; 6 – atypical meningioma II; 7 –anaplastic meningioma III; 8 – haemangioblastoma I; 9 – haemangioma I; 10 – haemangiopericytoma III.

No.	Brain tumor histological type	Malignancy WHO grade	No. of cases	R
	Tumours of meningothelial cells			
1	Meningothelial meningioma	I	48	1.59
2	Fibrous meningioma	I	22	1.55
3	Transitional (mixed)meningioma	I	15	1.55
4	Psammomatous meningioma	I	4	1.54
5	Angiomatous meningioma	I	13	1.50
6	Atypical meningioma	II	5	1.45
7	Anaplastic (malignant) meningioma	III	5	1.10
	Mesenchymal tumours			
8	Haemangioma	I	1	0.95
9	Haemangiopericytoma	III	2	1.08
	Other neoplasms related to the meninges	I	3	0.86
10	Haemangioblastoma			

Table 2. The list of meningioma and their malignancies identified in patients as well as the amount of m5C determined.

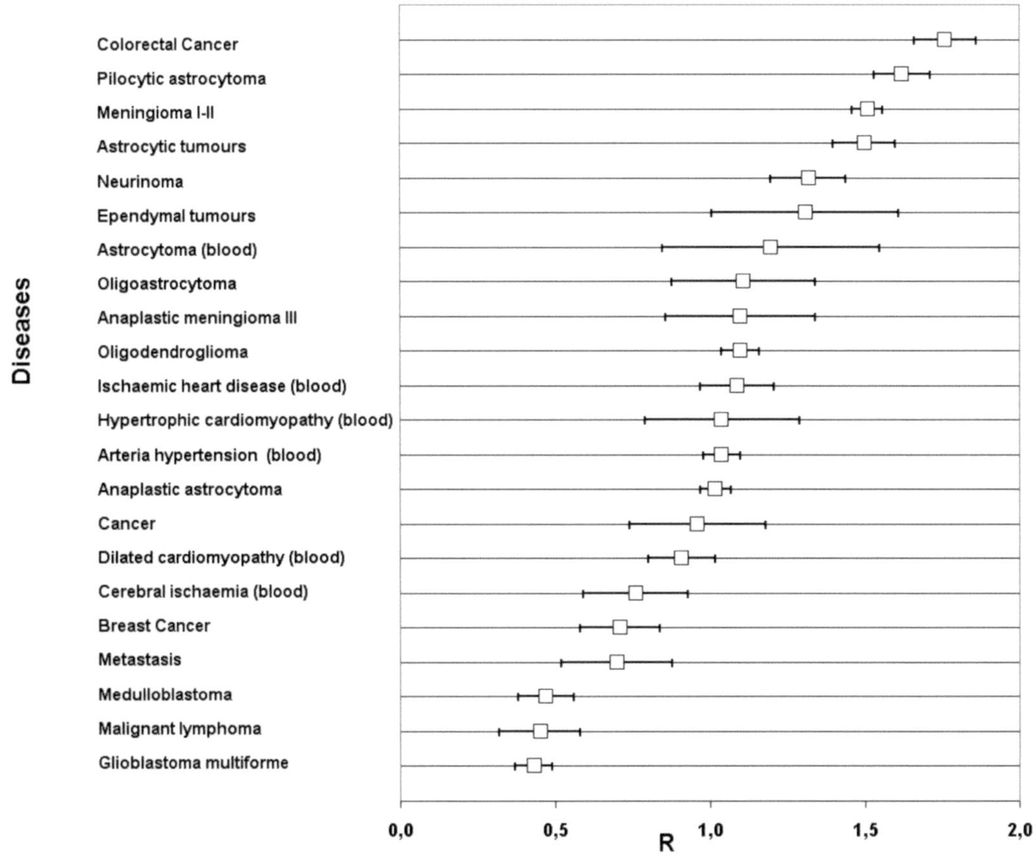

Fig. 9. R values for DNA isolated from tissues of different diseases.

The DNA methylation in meningiomas is on very similar level. The R value is between 0.86 and 1.59. It means that red-ox processes in these tumour cells are not so intensive.

If so, one can ask whether genomic methylation level can be a good diagnostic marker for the early tumour detection in the clinical practice [Hatada et al. 2006]. We have found that the extent of DNA demethylation process is different and specific for various diseases (Fig. 9). The lowest level of DNA methylation is observed for very aggressive tumours like glioblastoma and anaplastic astrocytoma. On the other hand methylation of DNA in colorectal cancer or pilocytic astrocytoma is higher. One can also see different m^5C content in DNA from blood of patients with other diseases. It means that the global methylation analysis can be used as diagnostic tool [Widschwendter and Jones 2002; Lavon et al. 2010]

This method of nucleic acid compounds analysis can be also used as a quality control test of DNA. Currently for DNA isolation from different tissues, various isolation kits are used. Usually such material is good for cloning and enzymatic analysis However for molecular characteristic DNA should be RNA free. A contamination with RNA can be easily established with our method.

Mechanisms of regulation of DNA methylation are an important question, which has elicited much attention over the past decade. Recently many ideas have been proposed for mechanism of DNA demethylation. In addition to that, we have proposed a genomic one effected with hydroxyl radical oxidative damage. It turned out that the global methylation level of DNA provides information on grade cancer and progress of a disease.

4. Acknowledgements

This work was supported with the research grant from Ministry of Science and Informatization (MNII) Nr N N401 066338 (to M.B.) and N N403 219637 (to S.N.)

5. References

Barciszewska A-M, Murawa D, Gawronska I, Murawa P, Barciszewska MZ (2007) Analysis of 5-methylcytosine in DNA of breast and colon cancer tissues. IUBMB Life 59:1-6

Barciszewska A-M, Nowak S, Żukiel R i in (2006) Wpływ przechowywania tkanki nowotworowej na zawartość 5-metylocytozyny w DNA guzów mózgu. Neuroskop 8:160-162 (Poland)

Bart A, van Passel MW, van Amsterdam K, van der Ende A (2005) Direct detection of methylation in genomic DNA. Nucleic Acids Res 33:e124

Berdasco M, Esteller M (2010) Aberrant epigenetic landscape in cancer: how cellular identity goes awry. Dev Cell 19:698-711

Blow N (2007) Tissue issues. Nature 448: 959-962

Cadieux B, Ching TT, VadenBerg SR et al (2006) Genome-wide hypomethylation in human glioblastomas associated with specific copy number alteration, methylenetetrahydrofolate reductase allele status, and increased proliferation. Cancer Res 66:8469-8476

Eden A, Gaudet F, Waghmare A, Jaenisch R (2003) Chromosomal instability and tumors promoted by DNA hypomethylation. Science 300:455

Essick EE, Sam F (2010) Oxidative stress and autophagy in cardiac disease, neurological disorders, aging and cancer. Oxid Med Cell Longev 3:168-177

Farragher SM, Tanney A, Kennedy RD, Harkin DP (2008) RNA expression analysis from formalin fixed paraffin embedded tissues. Histochem Cell Biol 130:435-445

Fraga MF, Uriol E, Borja Diego L, Berdasco M, Esteller M, Cañal MJ, Rodríguez R (2002) High-performance capillary electrophoretic method for the quantification of 5-methyl 2'-deoxycytidine in genomic DNA: application to plant, animal and human cancer tissues. Electrophoresis 23:1677-1681

Frigola J, Sole X, Paz MF, Moreno V, Esteller M, Capella G, Peinado MA (2005) Differential DNA hypermethylation and hypomethylation signatures in colorectal cancer. Human Molecular Genetics 14:319-326

Gaudet F, Hodgson JG, Eden A, Jackson-Grusby L, Dausman J, Gray JW, Leonhardt H, Jaenisch R (2003) Induction of tumors in mice by genomic hypomethylation. Science 300:489-492

Grek CL, Tew KD (2010) Redox metabolism and malignancy. Curr Opin Pharmacol 10:362-368

Guo JU, Su Y, Zhong Ch, Guo-li Ming G, Song H (2011) Hydroxylation of 5-methylcytosine by TET1 promotes active DNA demethylation in the adult brain. Cell 145:1-12

Hatada I, Fukasawa M, Kimura M, Morita S, Yamada K, Yoshikawa T, Yamanaka S, Endo C, Sakurada A, Sato M, Kondo T, Horii A, Ushijima T, Sasaki H (2006) Genome-wide profiling of promoter methylation in human. Oncogene 25:3059-3064

Johnstone SE, Baylin SB (2010) Stress and the epigenetic landscape: a link to the pathobiology of human diseases? Nat Rev Genet 11:806-812

Jomova K, Valko M (2011) Advances in metal-induced oxidative stress and human disease. Toxicology 283:65-87

Kehrer JP (2000) The Haber-Weiss reaction and mechanisms of toxicity. Toxicology 149:43-50

Klug M, Heinz S, Gebhard C, Schwarzfischer L, Krause SW, Andreesen R, Rehli M (2010) Active DNA demethylation in human postmitotic cells correlates with activating histone modifications, but not transcription levels. Genome Biol 11:R63

Lavon I, Refael M, Zelikovitch B, Shalom E, Siegal T (2010) Serum DNA can define tumor-specific genetic and epigenetic markers in gliomas of various grades. Neuro Oncol 12:173-180

Li M, Hu S, Shen Z, He X, Tao S, Dong L, Zhu Y (2009) High-performance capillary electrophoretic method for the quantification of global DNA methylation: Application to methotrexate-resistant cells. Anal Biochem 387:71-75

Louis DN, Ohgaki H, Wiestler OD, Cavenee WK, Burger PC, Jouvet A, Scheithauer BW, Kleihues P (2007) The 2007 WHO classification of tumours of the central nervous system. Acta Neuropathol 114:97-109

Maher EA, Furnari FB, Bachoo RM, Rowitch DH, Louis DN, Cavenee WK, DePinho RA (2001) Malignant glioma: genetics and biology of a grave matter. Genes Dev 15:1311-1333

Martinez R, Esteller M (2010) The DNA methylome of glioblastoma multiforme. Neurobiol Dis 39:40-46

Martinez R, Martin-Subero JI, Rohde V, Kirsch M, Alaminos M, Fernandez AF, Ropero S, Schackert G, Esteller M (2009) A microarray-based DNA methylation study of glioblastoma multiforme. Epigenetics 4:255-264

Miller SA, Dykes DD, Polesky HF (1988) A simple salting out procedure for extracting DNA from human nucleated cells. Nucleic Acids Res. 16:1215

Nishiyama R, Qi L, Tsumagari K, Weissbecker K, Dubeau L, Champagne M, Sikka S, Nagai H, Ehrlich M (2005) A DNA repeat, NBL2, is hypermethylated in some cancers but hypomethylated in others. Cancer Biol Ther 4:440-448

Pelizzola M, Ecker JR (2010) The DNA methylome. FEBS Lett. 2010 Nov 5. [Epub ahead of print

Rao AV, Balachandran B (2002) Role of oxidative stress and antioxidants in neurodegenerative diseases. Nutr Neurosci 5:291-309

Reale A, Matteis GD, Galleazzi G, Zampieri M, Caiafa P (2005) Modulation of DNMT1 activity by ADP-ribose polymers. Oncogene 24:13-19

Robertson KD (2005) DNA methylation and human disease. Nat Rev Genet 6:597-610

Sánchez-Navarro I, Gámez-Pozo A, González-Barón M, Pinto-Marín A, Hardisson D, López R, Madero R, Cejas P, Mendiola M, Espinosa E, Vara JA (2010) Comparison of gene expression profiling by reverse transcription quantitative PCR between fresh frozen and formalin-fixed, paraffin-embedded breast cancer tissues. Biotechniques 48:389-397

Sciumè G, Santoni A, Bernardini G (2010) Chemokines and glioma: invasion and more. J Neuroimmunol 224:8-12

Soh Y, Shin MH, Lee JS, Jang JH, Kim OH, Kang H, Surh YJ (2003) Oxidative DNA damage and glioma cell death induced by tetrahydropapaveroline. Mutat Res 544:129-142

Trewick SC, Henshaw TF, Hausinger RP, Lindahl T, Sedgwick B (2002) Oxidative demethylation by Escherichia coli AlkB directly reverts DNA base damage. Nature 419:174-178

Tudek B, Winczura A, Janik J, Siomek A, Foksinski M, Oliński R (2010) Involvement of oxidatively damaged DNA and repair in cancer development and aging. Am J Transl Res 2:254-284

Ulrey CL, Liu L, Andrews LG, Tollefsbol TO (2005) The impact of metabolism on DNA methylation. Hum Mol Genet 14:R139-147

Widschwendter M, Jones PA (2002) DNA methylation and breast carcinogenesis. Oncogene 21:5462-5482

Widschwendter M, Jones PA (2002) The potential prognostic, predictive, and therapeutic values of DNA methylation in cancer. Clin Cancer Res 8:17-21

Wu SC, Zhang Y (2010) Active DNA demethylation: many roads lead to Rome. Nat Rev Mol Cell Biol 11:607-620

Yamada Y, Jackson-Grusby L, Linhart H, Meissner A, Eden A, Lin H, Jaenisch R (2005) Opposing effects of DNA hypomethylation on intestinal and liver carcinogenesis. Proc Natl Acad Sci USA 102:13580-13585

Zukiel R, Nowak S, Barciszewska A-M, Gawrońska I, Keith G, Barciszewska MZ (2004) A simple epigenetic method for the diagnosis and classification of brain tumors. Mol Can Res 2:196-202

4

The Bevacizumab "Pseudoresponse" in Glioma: Disappointment or Opportunity?

Piia Thomas, Daniel Spielman and Lawrence Recht
Departments of Neurology, Radiology and Electrical Engineering
Stanford University School of Medicine, Stanford CA
USA

1. Introduction

Cancer biology has focused for years on better characterizing what makes cancer distinctive relative to normal tissue so as to better define targets for treatment. This has resulted in our current cancer paradigm in which cancers arise through an essentially cell autonomous series of variable cellular genetic and epigenetic events that drives the malignant process [1, 2]. The corollary of this model is that cancer is a highly complex process with no two individual cancers being identical leading in turn to the current trend towards "personalizing" therapy. We propose that there is a much simpler way to view cancer, one in which it is viewed from a tissue rather than a cellular perspective. From this vantage point, properties are "distributed" among cell populations, creating a highly integrated cell population and that treatment is better aimed at perturbing the system as a whole rather than a particular gene or receptor target. This physiological approach thus focuses on two universal attributes of malignancy that have not yet been linked experimentally: (i) the need for growing tumors to establish an adequate blood supply, i.e., neoangiogenesis [3, 4]; and (ii) the unique metabolism of tumor tissue in which an inordinate amount of energy is derived through glycolysis (GLY) rather than oxidative phosphorylation (OXPHOS) even in the presence of adequate oxygen (aerobic glycolysis) [5, 6]. Although much research has focused on these two topics, the impact they have upon each other has not been addressed to any extent in living organisms, despite there being substantial information on the relationship between flow and metabolism in normal tissues. Admittedly, one major reason for this lack of study has been technical, i.e., although flow can be assessed, there has not until recently been a way to assess tumor metabolism in intact animals in real time.

The recent introduction of the anti-VEGF monoclonal antibody bevacizumab into the field of brain tumor therapeutics has resulted in an unprecedented rapid improvement in MRI abnormalities and mass effect which led to its fast track approval by the FDA in 2009 based on Phase II studies [7, 8]. While dramatic, this response is transient and associated with late failures that are largely resistant to salvage therapies (Figure 1). This phenomenon has been recently labeled a "pseudoresponse" [9, 10] and has generated a second wave of studies that have been much less optimistic about the prospects of this therapy [11].

In this review, we will develop the argument that when viewed from the tissue perspective, the pseudoresponse reflects the effect of blood flow changes that result in a depletion of nutrients, especially glucose and lactate, that results in increased tissue OXPHOS to maintain energy needs. This results in a "starvation" state within the cancer tissue that temporarily opens a therapeutic window that closes as the tumor tissue adapts to this crisis. We term this the "Warburg-Folkman" effect and postulate that its magnitude will be proportional to the real time lactate/bicarbonate level observed within tumor tissue after anti-angiogenic therapy that can now be visualized in the intact organism with the recent refinement in $^{13}C_1$-pyruvate MRS technologies.

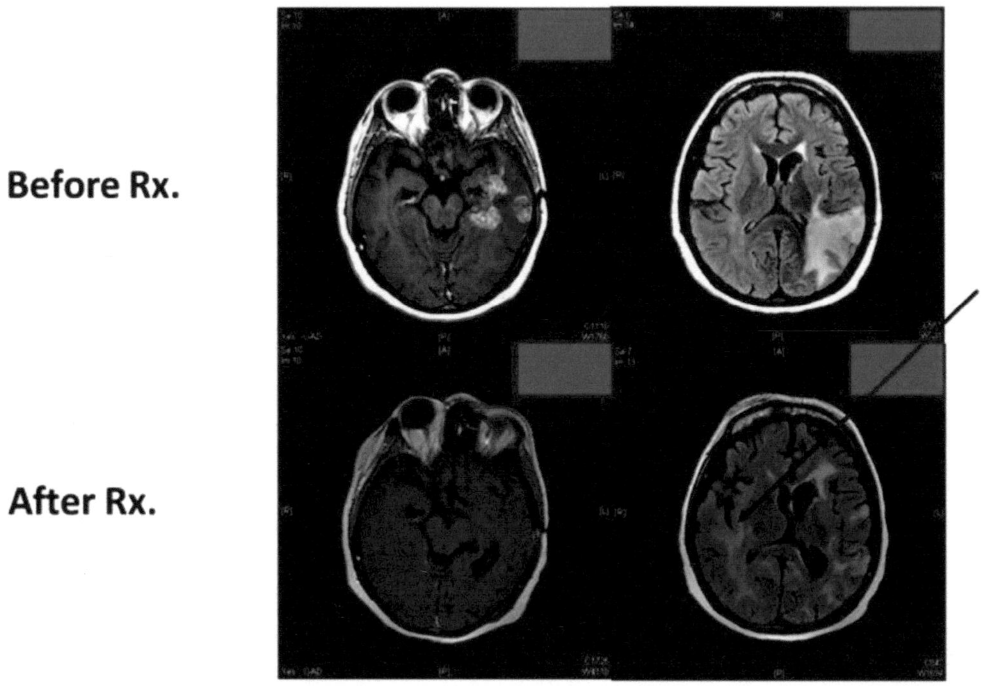

Fig. 1. Demonstration of response to bevacizumab in recurrent glioblastoma. Top two panels reflect an axial T1 enhanced and axial FLAIR image from a 43 year old woman with recurrent GBM before first infusion of BEV while the bottom two panels represent imaging performed after third infusion. Note the marked improvement in enhancement and amount of mass effect after treatment. However, there is now an increased area of T2 FLAIR abnormality distant from original site of relapse (Arrow). This represents new infiltrative tumor.

2. Neoangiogenesis in GBM

Four decades ago, Folkman proposed that all solid tumors are dependent on the formation of new blood vessels (angiogenesis) based on the observation that experimental solid tumors otherwise entered a dormant state or died once their size reached 2-3 mm [4]. In this and subsequent papers (for a review of this work, consult [12-14]), he noted a strong interaction and counterdependency between endothelium and tumor cells that suggested the presence of a diffusible messenger released from tumor cells was transitioning endothelial cells from a resting state to one capable of forming new capillaries.

Though his hypothesis was initially met with a high level of skepticism, subsequent studies confirmed the relationship between neoangiogenesis and cancer progression as well as characterizing several cytokines that were important in mediating these effects. Numerous pro- and anti-angiogenic mediators are now known that respond to adverse conditions such as hypoxia so that the balance is tipped in favor of angiogenesis (i.e., the "angiogenic switch"). Although a number of these factors have been identified including bFGF and members of the EGF receptor family [15, 16], the most prominent factor mediating angiogenesis is the family of vascular endothelial growth factor (VEGF) molecules. The VEGF family consists of the VEGF ligands VEGF-A, VEGF-B, VEGF-C, VEGF-D, platelet derived growth factor (PDGF) and placental growth factor. These ligands bind to the VEGF receptor (VEGFR) tyrosine kinases VEGFR-1 and VEGFR-2. The most important of these ligands is VEGF-A which by primarily binding to VEGFR-2 regulates endothelial cell survival, proliferation, vascular permeability and migration. In hypoxic conditions, VEGF-A is primarily induced via hypoxic inducible factor (HIF-1α), which in the presence of a hypoxic environment is dissociated from the Von Hippel Lindau protein allowing it to bind to promoter regions of several pro-angiogenic factors including VEGF [17].

Among cancers, glioblastoma (GBM) is among the most highly vascularized, the extent of which correlates closely with tumor proliferation and aggressiveness [18]. Vascularization occurs via three mechanisms: arteriogenesis (utilizing collaterals from a pre-existing blood supply to augment metabolic demands), vasculogenesis (formation of new vessels via the migration and differentiation of progenitor cells into endothelial cells) and angiogenesis (the production of new blood vessels from pre-existing ones). When the angiogenic cascade is triggered in GBMs, a wide range of cells can become tumor endothelial cells, including circulating progenitor cells that are mobilized from the bone marrow and other tissues as well as other hematopoietic cells and even glioma cells themselves [19-23].

While it is not clear how much tumor vascularization is due to co-option of other vessels relative to the creation of new ones, it is widely accepted that angiogenesis is a key factor in tumor proliferation. Neoangiogeneic vessels are tortuous, leaky, and dilated with aberrant interconnections and abnormal basement membranes resulting in inefficient and heterogeneous blood flow as well as increased blood volume within the tumor [24]. The endothelial cells lining these vessels are abnormal with loosely attached or absent pericytes and basement membranes are often absent or abnormally thickened.

3. Anti-VEGF therapy and the pseudoresponse

The discovery that cancer angiogenesis is dependent on cytokines released by tumor cells spurred interest in developing agents that could interrupt these cytokine loops so as to impact tumor growth via inhibiting vessel formation. After VEGF's identification as perhaps the most important mediator of this process (including one of the seminal papers describing its high concentration in GBM [25]), a number of strategies were designed to block VEGF's contribution to this process. This led to the development of bevacizumab, the first anti-angiogenic agent to be approved and be widely used.

Bevacizumab is a recombinant humanized monoclonal antibody that selectively binds with high affinity to VEGF ligand preventing its interaction with the VEGF-1 and VEGF-2 receptor on the surface of endothelial cells, thus preventing VEGF induced endothelial cell migration, proliferation and vascular permeability [26]. Bevacizumab (and other anti-VEGF therapies) exerts its effects via multiple mechanisms that block the development of new aberrant vessels and induce regression of existing aberrant vasculature, thus resulting in tumor growth arrest. This so-called "normalization" of mature vasculature at least theoretically also results in improved susceptibility to treatment via improved delivery of chemotherapeutic agents and via radiosensitization from improved oxygen delivery [24].

Bevacizumab was approved in 2004 for first line use in people with metastatic colon cancer but despite the observation that GBMs were associated with the highest VEGF levels among cancers, its use was delayed in brain tumor patients because of the fear of increasing hemorrhagic risk. The dramatic, immediate effect of bevacizumab on MRI enhancement and clinical status noted when it was finally utilized [27, 28] generated an unprecedented initial enthusiasm that led to a fast-track FDA approval for recurrent glioma based on two pivotal Phase II studies [7, 8].

Unfortunately, and perhaps not unexpectedly, despite the impressive radiologic responses with corresponding clinical benefit seen early after BEV treatment, these results were not sustained over long intervals, resulting in only a modest overall survival benefit. What was especially disappointing was the observation of an increased glioma invasiveness that often resulted in the development of a gliomatosis picture [29]. This disappointing outcome has tempered enthusiasm concerning the overall role of BEV in GBM therapies and led to intensive research aimed at understanding why this failure occurs. Among the mechanisms invoked for this observation is an up regulation of alternative pro-angiogenic factors such as the pro-angiogenic fibroblast growth factor [30], increased protection of tumor vasculature by increasing pericyte coverage, recruitment of pro-angiogenic inflammatory cells and a cooption of normal vessels by the invading tumor cells [31]. At the root of most of the explanation for why anti-VEGF therapy is ultimately ineffective is that, by diminishing flow, intratumoral hypoxia is increased, inducing tumor cells to become more aggressive and invasive [32-34].

While the clinical observation of a worsening MRI occurring as a result of treatment effect rather than tumor progression has been well characterized (i.e., pseudoprogression [35]), the introduction of anti-angiogenic therapies such as BEV produced a diametrically opposite effect of rapid resolution of MRI abnormalities that, despite its magnitude, is as much of a function of blocking VEGF's effect on permeability as it is on a cytotoxic response. This phenomenon has therefore been labeled a "pseudoresponse" [9], in part to reflect the impression that it is similar to what is occasionally seen when steroids are administered to brain tumor patients and is supported by several observations including its association with increased invasive nonenhancing tumor seen on T2/FLAIR imaging representing dispersion of the tumor in an infiltrating pattern [10] and the demonstration of a rapid radiologic response, rebound enhancement on discontinuation and rapid re-response on recontinuation with anti-VEGF therapy [33, 36, 37].

Within the framework of neoangiogenesis, the pseudoresponse is felt to be a manifestation of an initial "normalization" of perfusion that increases hypoxia, both increasing apoptosis initially as well as upregulating the HIF1 axis. It is through this latter activation that cancer cells initiate cellular programs that increase invasiveness and ultimately lead to a more resistant tumor [38]. Such observations have cast a pall over the early excitement generated by the introduction of BEV and have led many workers to question its ultimate value in GBM treatment [11, 32].

While it is certainly valid and reasonable to assess the effects of anti-VEGF therapies in terms of hypoxia, it should be noted that a growing tumor is already adapted to a very low oxygen tension. It is therefore unclear why any change in oxygen delivery should have such a profound impact. We believe that this concept is misleading and unproven and offer a fundamentally more logical explanation that relates to the cancer's peculiar metabolism, which we next address.

4. Cancer's peculiar metabolism

The drive to acquire cell mass and proliferate requires an adequate energy supply and building blocks, underscoring the need for ample amounts of energy in the form of ATP. There are two general ways in which this can be accomplished. Oxidative phosphorylation (OXPHOS), which takes place in the mitochondria, is an oxygen-dependent process in which pyruvate (which can be derived from a number of sources, especially glucose) is converted to acetyl-CoA which is then oxidized to CO_2 and H_2O producing NADH. NADH is further oxidized via the electron transport chain using oxygen as the final electron acceptor, ultimately generating a net of 36 ATP/glucose molecule. Alternatively, cells may use glycolysis (GLY), in which glucose is converted to pyruvate, generating 2 ATP/glucose molecule, completely bypassing the mitochondria. In normal cells, the balance between these two pathways is highly oxygen dependent; in the presence of adequate amounts of oxygen, cells utilize the more efficient OXPHOS while when oxygen is inadequate, the cell transitions to the less efficient GLY (Pasteur Effect) [39].
Under optimal conditions, cells derive ninety percent of their energy from OXPHOS and ten percent from GLY. Over 80 years ago, Otto Warburg observed that tumor cells generate an inordinate amount of ATP via GLY, even in the presence of adequate oxygen levels (aerobic glycolysis) [5, 6, 40]. This preferential shift to the glycolytic pathway is not absolute, instead representing a shift from a baseline glycolytic rate of 10% seen in normal cells to over fifty percent[41] (Figure 2). In association with this shift towards GLY, tumors rely almost exclusively on glucose relative to other substrates (such as fatty acids) for energy needs.
Although it remains unexplained why tumors overutilize GLY, its universal presence that persists even under normal oxygenation and its close correlation with tumor aggressiveness suggests a survival and growth benefit that exceeds the apparent inefficiency of the glycolytic pathway [39]. Despite its persistence under normal oxygen levels, several studies still point to an important role of hypoxia in this process, perhaps because the byproducts of GLY lead to acidification of the micro-environment. An acidic environment is toxic to adjacent normal cells, assists in destruction of extracellular matrix and triggers angiogenesis, suggesting that the glycolytic shift is necessary for evolution into invasive cancer [39, 42]. Moreover, as tumor cells proliferate they physically increase their distance from their vascular supply creating additional areas of low oxygen tension that results in activation of HIF1, which in turn upregulates genes that code for proteins important in cancer development and proliferation including glucose metabolism, apoptosis resistance, invasion, angiogenesis and metastasis [43].
As tumors become vascularized, the glycolytic phenotype persists despite improved oxygenation. Although the reasons for this remain unclear, one potential explanation relates to the fact that while aerobic glycolysis is much less efficient than oxidative respiration, its kinetics are such that in the presence of excess substrate, it may result in more ATP production as a function of time than can be obtained with OXPHOS [43, 44]. Vasquez *et al.* studied a model of ATP flux demonstrating that glucose uptake capacity and solvent

capacity of the cytoplasm are important factors. They proposed that at lower levels of glucose uptake OXPHOS is most efficient but once a threshold has been reached, a gradual decrease in OXPHOS relative to GLY results in more efficient ATP production [44]. Alternatively, the reasons underlying the persistent dependence on GLY may be related to the fact that rapidly dividing cells become dependent on this pathway for production of nutrients such as amino acids, nucleotides and lipids needed for development of new cells at a sufficient rate for a rapidly dividing tumor [45].

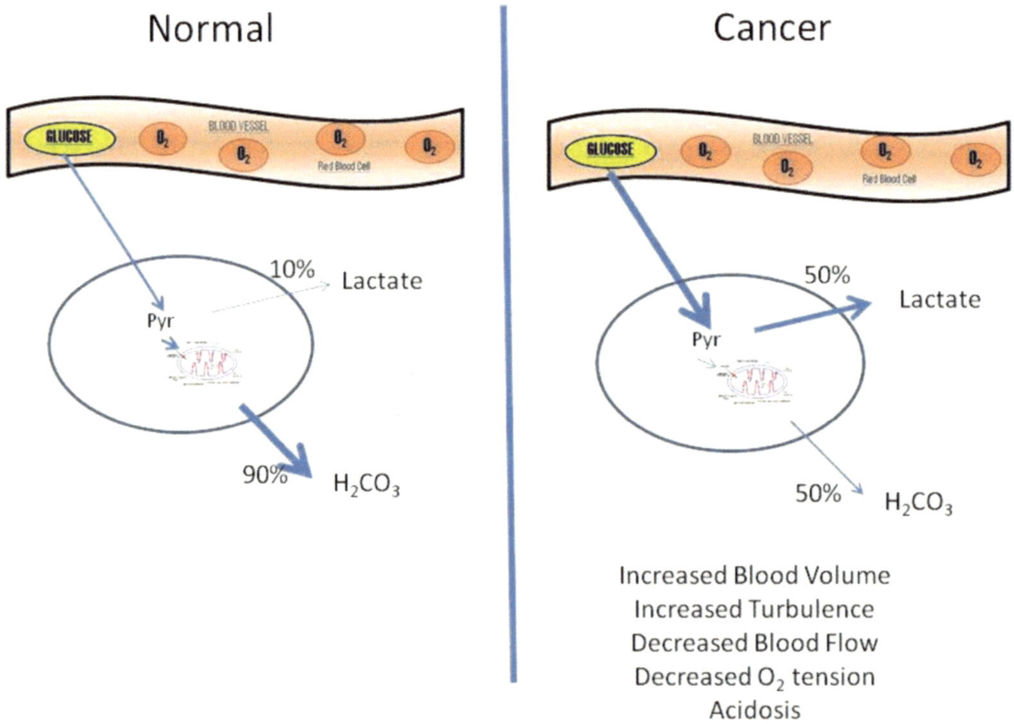

Fig. 2. Simplified graphic that demonstrates some key features of Warburg effect. Under normal conditions, approximately 90% of glucose and other energy substrates are efficiently metabolized via the mitochondria. Only 10% of glucose is metabolized via glycolysis to lactate. In solid cancers, however, there is a shift towards increased glycolysis and now over 50% of ATP is generated through glycolysis. In association with this, the tumor environment is characterized by increased blood volume, stasis and low O2 tension and pH. For more detailed recent descriptions of tumor metabolism, the reader is referred to [39, 42, 46, 60].

Although Warburg proposed that the glycolytic shift related to defective mitochondria, this has proven to be an oversimplification in that this organelle definitely functions in cancer cells, albeit not always at a normal level[46]. In fact, since GLY is a characteristic of normal rapidly proliferating tissues, this shift can occur even in the presence of normally functioning mitochondria [45]. Instead, it is more likely that this shift results from a number of cytokines and oncogenic mutations that combine to effect increased GLY. For instance, HIF1 increases GLY and down regulates mitochondrial function by activating genes involved in glucose uptake such as GLUT1 as well as enzymes responsible for the glycolytic breakdown of glucose such as phosphofructokinase, aldolase and pyruvate dehydrogenase [41]. Mutations that either inactivate p53 or activate NF-kβ can also result in a shift towards producing energy via GLY as do environmental triggers such as acidosis and increased extracellular lactate [47].

5. Linking blood flow with metabolism to explain the BEV pseudoresponse

In the modern era, cancer is viewed as essentially a cell autonomous phenomenon. In this context, the Warburg effect has therefore been addressed primarily through attempting to ascertain what genetic mutations underlie the shift towards GLY. This has also led many to question its universality for all cancers since it is well documented that at least some cancer cells definitely harness energy via OXPHOS.

In our view, however, the Warburg effect is a tissue not a cell phenomenon, meant to connote the net activity of GLY vs. OXPHOS in the tissue, not the cell. This is in keeping with Warburg's original descriptions of the process in which he utilized animal preparations to demonstrate the effect [6]. In fact, within the tumor itself, it would be advantageous from the point of view of distributing energy substrates if certain cells used GLY to increase extracellular lactate concentrations that can then be used by other cells for OXPHOS (similar to the astrocyte/neuron relationship [48]; interestingly, a similar distribution of function has been proposed for breast cancers [49]). In steady state, therefore, within cancers including those of the brain, this environment is associated with increased blood volume, increased lactate and decreased blood flow, which results in a substrate "excess", which as is predicted by models that examine energy utilization within tissues, favors GLY [44].

Such a steady state requires an adequate amount of blood flow to deliver adequate amounts of glucose to support the process, as well as a high amount of stasis to keep lactate available. It follows therefore that in addition to supporting adequate blood vessel formation to support the growing tumor, VEGF should also be crucial to supporting the cancer's metabolism. We propose therefore that it is this linkage between VEGF, blood vessel maintenance and tumor metabolism that explains the profound initial effects of BEV on GBM and suggest it be named the **Warburg-Folkman effect** to honor the two scientists whose concepts provide its foundation. We propose that the paring of the tumor vasculature (or "normalization") after BEV results in a period of acute tumor "starvation" resulting from lowered glucose (delivery of which is decreased due to vascular constriction lowering flow) and lactate (removal of which is increased due to decreased stasis) levels (Figure 3). This creates a situation wherein cells within the cancer must resort to the more efficient OXPHOS in the presence of decreased substrate. This forced utilization of mitochondria results in the exposure of cells to pro-apoptotic factors such as cytochrome C and apoptosis inducing factor and increases reactive oxygen species, increasing susceptibility of these cells to apoptosis [4550].

In effect, therefore, we believe the observed clinical pseudoresponse represents an acute crisis for the cancer tissue, which responds over time by adaptations that favor "dispersion", a term we prefer to invasion since we believe this represents a compensatory process in which tumor cells migrate to areas where the supply of energetic substrates is more favorable rather than an evolution to a more aggressive tumor. Such a model would suggest that while the effect may be transient, the acute removal of VEGF creates a period in which tumors should be extremely vulnerable to further metabolic perturbations, perhaps to the point where they can be induced to "collapse".

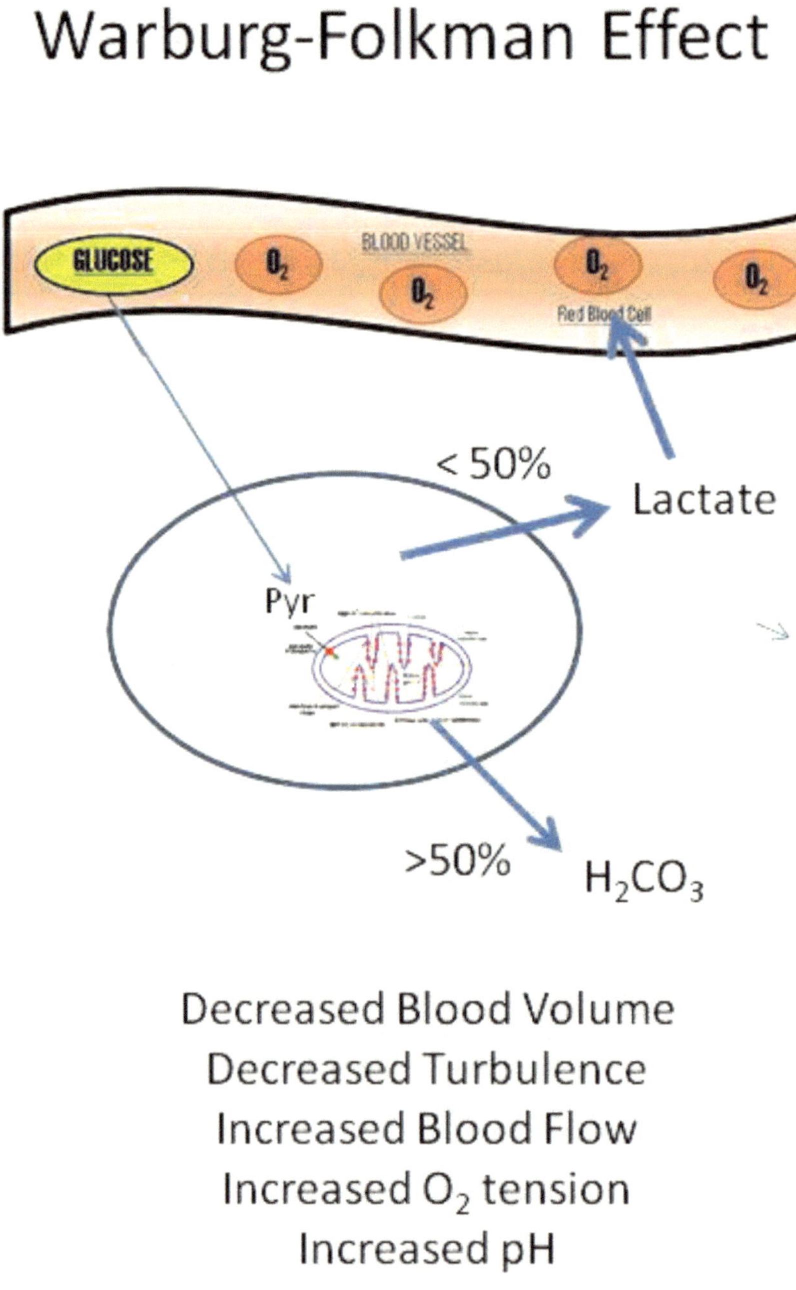

Fig. 3. Proposed early effect of VEGF blockage on the tumor environment: the Warburg-Folkman effect. The effect of removing VEGF is to cause a vessel "paring" that has been proposed to "normalize" flow. We propose that this has the effect of acutely depleting energy substrates—both glucose and lactate—through decreased delivery and increased removal, respectively. This results in increase mitochondrial utilization that results in increased OXPHOS as well as increased ROS production.

6. Measuring OXPHOS and GLY in intact organisms; MRS of hyperpolarized $^{13}C_1$-pyruvate

Since our proposal predicts a change in tumor metabolism at the tissue level with the introduction of anti-VEGF therapy, its proof depends on a tool in which the relative amounts of GLY and OXPHOS can be ascertained in the living organism. Until recently, therefore, this question could not easily be addressed. On first glance, one could consider using FDG PET scanning, the importance of which in cancer diagnostics is derived from Warburg's observations and is dependent upon the upregulation of glucose uptake mechanisms in neoplasms compared to normal surrounding tissue. FdG is an analogue of glucose and areas of increased FDG uptake indicate increased tissue metabolic activity and the amount of uptake correlates with tumor aggressiveness [51]. However, while FDG PET scanning also indirectly reflects the Warburg effect (because cancers must up regulate glucose transporters to maintain their metabolism), it does not provide a real time picture of the cancer's metabolism and does not measure either OXPHOS or GLY. A similar problem exists with conventional MRI techniques; thus, one can measure total lactate using proton MRS, but this only reflects the total pool, not the throughput.

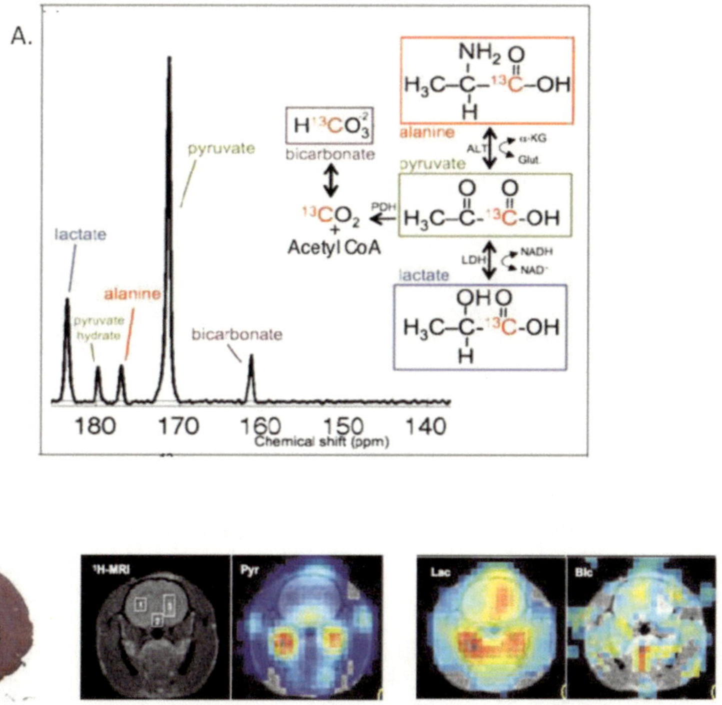

Fig. 4. (A) Single acquisition in vivo ^{13}C spectrum from a rat heart following the injection of hyperpolarized $^{13}C_1$-Pyr. ^{13}C-Pyr and its products ^{13}C-Lac, ^{13}C-Ala, and ^{13}C-BiC are easily visualized. A small fraction of the ^{13}C-Pyr is in equilibrium with metabolically inactive ^{13}C-Pyr-hydrate. (B) (left) H&E stained cross-section of rat brain with implanted glioma. (right) Dynamic ^{13}C metabolic imaging results: TR = 3 s, 2.7x2.7x5 mm^3 nominal voxels. ROIs selected for further analysis are shown on the proton images. Elevated lactate is clearly visualized within the tumor.

A novel technology has being developed that can address these important questions, however. *In vivo* hyperpolarized ^{13}C MRS achieves dramatically enhanced signal to noise ratios, thus enabling the real-time investigation of metabolism with more than 10,000-fold signal increase over conventional ^{13}C methods [52]. It provides unprecedented opportunities for real-time imaging of in vivo metabolic pathways critical to the identification and evaluation of cancer [53-57]. In terms of studying the Warburg-Folkman effect, it enables the quantitative assessment of the fate of labeled pyruvate, a key nodal point in the metabolic pathway in which glucose is either converted to lactate (which reflects GLY) or acetyl CoA (which then enters the Krebs cycle, resulting in bicarbonate production, which reflects OXPHOS) (Figure 4). With this technology, the amount of lactate and bicarbonate produced during a 60-90 second period after a labeled injection of pyruvate can be measured, thus permitting generation of a lactate/HCO_3^- ratio (the Glycolytic Index). Two published studies have already demonstrated increased lactate production in brain cancers this way [58, 59], and this technology is already being tested in the clinic.

This technology therefore offers the prospect of being able to obtain a metabolic "snapshot" at multiple times during the course of cancer and offers an ideal way to assess the BEV's impact on glioma metabolism. Our prediction is that the Glycolytic Index produced after a pyruvate probe will be significantly decreased during a finite time interval after exposure to BEV. We would also predict that as treatment fails, this ratio will once again increase towards lactate production and believe that the extent to which the ratio trends towards "normal" (i.e., that seen in normal tissue) would correlate with outcome (i.e., it will be a reliable gauge of treatment response).

Ultimately, one could envision such an approach leading to a therapeutic strategy based on physiology rather than genetics. Thus, while it is well known that cancer tissues have a high rate of GLY, it remains unclear whether lowering the amount of GLY relative to OXPHOS would correlate with decreased aggressiveness or whether if the relative amounts were lowered to "normal", growth would "stall". We believe this ratio (which can be mathematically expressed as $\text{Cancer aggressiveness} = k * \dfrac{1}{bicarbonate / lactate}$) will be a *highly sensitive and rapid readout* from which one can repeatedly assess both aggressiveness and treatment effect. In effect therefore, the opportunity is to use this ratio in a way that other physicians may use blood pressure to gauge cardiovascular health.

7. References

[1] Nowell PC. The clonal evolution of tumor cell populations. Science. 1976;194:23-28
[2] Hahn WC, Weinberg RA. Modelling the molecular circuitry of cancer. Nature Reviews/Cancer. 2002;2:331-341
[3] Folkman J. What is the evidence that tumors are angiogenesis dependent? J Natl Cancer Inst. 1990;82:4-6
[4] Folkman J. Tumor angiogenesis: therapeutic implications. New Engl J Med. 1971;285:1182-1186
[5] Warburg O. The metabolism of tumours. London: Arnold Constable, 1930

[6] Warburg O, Wind F, Negelein E. The metabolism of tumors in the body. J General Physiol. 1927;8:519-530

[7] Vredenburgh JJ, Desjardins A, Herndon JE et al. Phase II trial of bevacizumab and irinotecan in recurrent malignant glioma. Clinical Canc Res. 2007;13:1253-1259

[8] Vredenburgh JJ, Desjardins A, Herndon JE et al. Bevacizumab plus irinotecan in recurrent glioblastoma multiforme. J Clinical Oncology. 2007;25:4722-4729

[9] Reardon DA, Galanis E, DeGroot J et al. Clinical trial endpoints for high-grade glioma: the evolving landscape. Neuro-Oncology. 2011

[10] Wen PY, Macdonald D, Reardon DA et al. Updated response assessment criteria for high-grade gliomas: Response assessment in Neuro-Oncology Working Group. J Clinical Oncology. 2010;28:1963-1972

[11] Verhoeff J, van Tellingen O, Claes A et al. Concerns about anti-angiogenic treatment in patients with glioblastoma multiforme. BMC Cancer. 2009;9:444

[12] Folkman J. Angiogenesis: an organizing principle for drug discovery? Nature Reviews Drug Discovery. 2007;6:273-286

[13] Folkman J. Angiogenesis. Annu Rev Med. 2006;57:1-18

[14] Folkman J, Kalluri R. Cancer without disease. Nature. 2004;427:787

[15] Folkman J, Klagsbrun M. Angiogenic factors. Science. 1987;235:442-447

[16] Kerbel RS. Tumor angiogenesis: past, present and the near future. Carcinogenesis. 2000;21:505-515

[17] Rahman R, Smith S, Rahman C, Grundy R. Antiangiogenic therapy and mechanisms of tumor resistance in malignant glioma. J Oncology. 2010

[18] Argyriou AA, Giannopoulou E, Kalofonos HP. Angiogenesis and anti-angiogenic molecularly targeted therapies in malignant gliomas. Oncology 2009;77:1-11

[19] Wang R, Chadalavada K, Wilshire J et al. Glioblastoma stem-like cells give rise to tumour endothelium. Nature. 2010;468:829-833

[20] Soda Y, Marumoto T, Friedmann-Morvinski D et al. Transdifferentiation of glioblastoma cells into vascular endothelial cells. Proc Natl Acad Sci U S A. 2011;108:4274-4280

[21] Ricci-Vitiani L, Pallini R, Biffoni M et al. Tumour vascularization via endothelial differentiation of glioblastoma stem-like cells. Nature. 2010;468:824-828

[22] Semenza GL. Vasculogenesis, angiogenesis, and arteriogenesis: mechanisms of blood vessel formation and remodeling. J Cell Biochem. 2007;102:840-847

[23] Kioi M, Vogel H, Schultz G et al. Inhibition of vasculogenesis, but not angiogenesis, prevents the recurrence of glioblastoma after irradiation in mice. J Clinical Investigation. 2010;120:694-705

[24] Jain RK. Normalization of tumor vasculature: An emerging concept in antiangiogenic therapy. Science. 2005;307:58-62

[25] Plate KH, Breier G, Weich HA, Risau W. Vascular endothelial growth factor is a potential tumour angiogenesis factor in human gliomas in vivo. Nature. 1992;359:845-847

[26] Eicholz A, Sairoz M, Gaya AM. Anti-angiogenesis therapies: their potential in cancer management. Onco Targets and Ther. 2010;3:69-82

[27] Pope WB, Lai A, Nghiemphu P et al. MRI in patients with high-grade gliomas treated with bevacizumab and chemotherapy. Neurology. 2006;66:1258-1260

[28] Stark-Vance V. Bevacizumab and CPT-11 in the treatment of relapsed malignant glioma. Neuro-Oncology. 2005;7:369, Abstract 342

[29] Norden AD, Young GS, Setayesh K et al. Bevacizumab for recurrent malignant gliomas. Efficacy, toxicity, and patterns of recurrence. Neurology. 2008;70:779-787

[30] Crawford Y, Ferrara N. Tumor and stromal pathways mediating refractoriness/resistance to anti-angiogenic therapies. Trends in Pharmacological Sciences. 2009;30:624-630

[31] Bergers G, Hanahan D. Modes of resistance to anti-angiogenic therapy. Nat Rev Cancer. 2008;8:592-603

[32] Paez-Ribes M, Allen E, Hudock J et al. Antiangiogenic therapy elicits malignant progression of tumors to increased local invasion and distant metastasis. Cancer Cell. 2009;15:220-231

[33] Keunen O, Johansson M, Oudin A et al. Anti-VEGF treatment reduces blood supply and increases tumor cell invasion in glioblastoma. Proc Natl Acad Sci USA. 2011

[34] Lucio-Eterovic AK, Piao Y, de Groot JF. Mediators of glioblastoma resistance and invasion during antivascular endothelial growth factor therapy. Clinical Cancer Res. 2009;15:4589-4599

[35] Brandsma D, Stalpers L, Taal W et al. Clinical features, mechanisms, and management of pseudoprogression in malignant gliomas. Lancet Oncol. 2008;9:453-461

[36] Batchelor PE, Sorensen AG, di Tomaso E et al. AZD2171, a pan-VEGF receptor tyrosine kinase inhibitor, normalizes tumor vasculature and alleviates edema in glioblastoma patients. Cancer Cell. 2007;11:83-95

[37] Kamoun WS, Ley CD, Farrar CT et al. Edema control by cediranib, a vascular endothelial growth factor receptor-targeted kinase inhibitor, prolongs survival despite persistent brain tumor growth in mice. J Clinical Oncology. 2009;27:2542-2552

[38] Kim W-Y, Lee H-Y. Brain angiogenesis in developmental and pathological processes: mechanism and therapeutic intervention in brain tumors. FEBS J. 2009;276:4653-4664

[39] Gatenby RA, Gillies RJ. Why do cancers have high aerobic glycolysis. Nature Reviews Cancer. 2004;4:891-899

[40] Warburg O. On the origin of cancer cells. Science. 1956;123:309-314

[41] Denko NC. Hypoxia, HIF1 and glucose metabolism in the solid tumour. Nat Rev Cancer. 2008;8:705-713

[42] Cairns R, Harris IS, Mak TW. Regulation of cancer cell metabolism. Nature Reviews Cancer. 2011;11:85-95

[43] Lopez-Lazaro M. The Warburg effect: Why and how do cancer cells activate glycolysis in the presence of oxygen? Anti-Cancer Agents in Med Chem. 2008;8:305-312

[44] Vazquez A, Liu J, Zhou Y, Oltvai ZN. Catabolic efficiency of aerobic glycolysis: The Warburg effect revisited. BMC Systems Biology. 2010;4:58

[45] Vander Heiden MG, Cantley LC, Thompson CB. Understanding the Warburg effect: The metabolic requirements of cell proliferation. Science. 2009;324:1029-1034

[46] Solaini G, Sgarbi G, Baracca A. Oxidative phosphorylation in cancer cells. Biochimica et Biophys Acta. 2010

[47] Ak P, Levine AJ. p53 and NF-kB: different strategies for responding to stress leads to a functional antagonism. FASEB J. 2010

[48] Turner DA, Adamson DC. Neuronal-astrocyte metabolic interactions: Understanding the transition into abnormal astrocytoma metabolism. J Neuropathol Exp Neurology. 2011;70:167-176

[49] Pavlides S, Whitaker-Menezes D, Castello-Cros R et al. The reverse Warburg effect. Aerobic glycolysis in cancer associated fibroblasts and the tumor stroma. Cell Cycle. 2009;8:3984-4001

[50] Michelakis ED, Webster L, Mackey JR. Dichloroacetate (DCA) as a potential metabolic-targeting therapy for cancer. Br J Cancer. 2008;99:989-994

[51] Kunkel M, Reighert TE, Benz P et al. Overexpression of Glut-1 and increased glucose metabolism in tumors are associated with a poor prognosis in patients with oral squamous cell carcinoma. Cancer. 2003;97:1015-1024

[52] Ardenkjaer-Larsen JH, Fridlund B, Gram A et al. Increase in signal-to-noise ratio of > 10,000 times in liquid-state NMR. Proc Natl Acad Sci U S A. 2003;100:10158-10163

[53] Chen AP, Albers MJ, Cunningham CH et al. Hyperpolarized C-13 spectroscopic imaging of the TRAMP mouse at 3T-initial experience. Magn Reson Med. 2007;58:1099-1106

[54] Day SE, Kettunen MI, Gallagher FA et al. Detecting tumor response to treatment using hyperpolarized 13C magnetic resonance imaging and spectroscopy. Nat Medicine. 2007;13:1382-1387

[55] Gallagher FA, Kettunen MI, Hu DE et al. Production of hyperpolarized [1,4-13C2]malate from [1,4-13C2]fumarate is a marker of cell necrosis and treatment response in tumors. Proc Natl Acad Sci U S A. 2009;106:19801-19806

[56] Golman K, Ardenkjaer-Larsen JH, Petersson JS et al. Molecular imaging with endogenous substances. Proc Natl Acad Sci U S A. 2003;100:10435-10439

[57] Golman K, Zandt RI, Lerche MH et al. Metabolic imaging by hyperpolarized 13C magnetic resonance imaging for in vivo tumor diagnosis. Cancer Research. 2006;66:10855-10860

[58] Park I, Larsen PE, Zierhut ML et al. Hyperpolarized 13C magnetic resonance imaging: application to brain tumors. Neuro Oncology. 2010;12:133-144

[59] Day SE, Kettunen MI, Cherukuri MK et al. Detecting response of rat C6 glioma tumors to radiotherapy using hyperpolarized [1-(13)C] magnetic resonance spectroscopic imaging. Magn Reson Med. 2010

[60] Dang CV, Hamaker M, Sun P et al. Therapeutic targeting of cancer cell metabolism. J Mol Med. 2011

5

The Molecular Mechanism for Differentiation Therapy of Malignant Glioma

Wenbo Zhu and Guangmei Yan
Zhongshan School of Medicine, Sun Yat-sen University
People's Republic of China

1. Introduction

Gliomas are the most common malignant cancer affecting the CNS, accounting for 60% of primary brain tumors (DeAngelis, 2001; Yiu&He, 2006). The majority of gliomas in adults are highly malignant with a poor prognosis, in particular with high-grade tumors such as glioblastoma multiforme. Current therapy with surgery, radiation, and chemotherapy rarely, if ever, cures the disease and infrequently prolongs life for 1 year (Curran et al., 1993; Bao et al., 2006). Additional considerations focus on developing novel modalities to increase anti-glioma effects and decrease side-effects.

Differentiation therapy, using agents that modify cancer cell differentiation, has shown promise in the spectrum of agents used against tumors (Leszczyniecka et al., 2001). Wang and Chen demonstrated the clinical application for differentiation therapy by introducing all-trans-retinoic acid to clinical use for the treatment of acute promyelocytic leukemia (APL) (Huang et al., 1988; Wang&Chen, 2000). Notably, the inorganic toxicant arsenic trioxide (As2O3), a well known environmental carcinogen, has been also proven to be an effective drug in the treatment of APL patients by triggering apoptosis and differentiation of APL cells in a dose-dependent manner (Shen et al., 1997; Kinjo et al., 2000). Such excellent effects, however, were not reproduced in other hematological and, particularly, solid tumors. Differentiation agents for malignant gliomas remain a real challenge.

In this chapter, we base on our research and mainly discuss proteins or molecules capable of inducing differentiation via targeting cAMP/cAMP-dependent protein kinase A (PKA) signal pathway and crucial factors such as glycogen synthase kinase-3β (GSK-3β) and hypoxia-inducible factor-1α (HIF-1α) determining the efficiency of these drugs. Although agents for differentiation therapy have wide application prospect, their real therapeutic potentiality remains to be further realized.

2. The molecular mechanism for differentiation therapy of malignant glioma

2.1 cAMP/PKA signaling activators induce malignant glioma cell differentiation

cAMP/PKA signaling has been reported to play important roles in multiple physiological processes, including growth, differentiation, gene regulation, and apoptosis (Walsh&Van Patten, 1994). Disruption of the PKA catalytic subunit causes destabilization of the diploid cell cycle, and the cells start meiosis under conditions repressive for wild-type meiosis (Maeda et al., 1994). Ample evidences indicate that cAMP-elevating stimuli such as N-substituted cAMP analogues and cAMP-increasing reagents can induce cell differentiation in gliomas (Takanaga et al., 2004; Van Kolen&Slegers, 2004).

2.1.1 Biotoxin-cholera toxin

Cholera toxin is the major virulent factor of *Vibrio cholerae* and is the most recognizable enterotoxin causing diarrhea, the disease second only to cardiovascular disease as causes of death (Goodman&Segreti, 1999). Cholera toxin catalyzes ADP-ribosylation of Gs protein and results in accumulation of cellular cAMP (Moss&Vaughan, 1979; Guerrant et al., 1994). Guerrant *et al.* reports that active whole cholera toxin, but not inactive choleragenoid, produces elevation of cAMP and parallel morphological changes in CHO cells (Guerrant et al., 1974). Ganglioside GM1 reaction with the B subunit of cholera toxin is reported to induce neuron-like differentiation of PC12 and neuroblastoma cells (Masco et al., 1991; Kimura et al., 2001). All of the findings mentioned above reveal the potential of cholera toxin, a kind of biotoxin, in the differentiation induction of tumor cells.

In Li's study (Li et al., 2007), rat malignant glioma cell line C6 cells in conjunction with primary cultured human glioma cells, which are much more clinically relevant, are used to characterize the effect of cholera toxin on the key malignant phenotypes of malignant glioma cells to see whether it induces differentiation in them. Cholera toxin triggers cell transformation indicative of the cells' differentiation into a more mature astrocytic state (Figure 1a and 1c). This differentiation potential is further confirmed by an increased

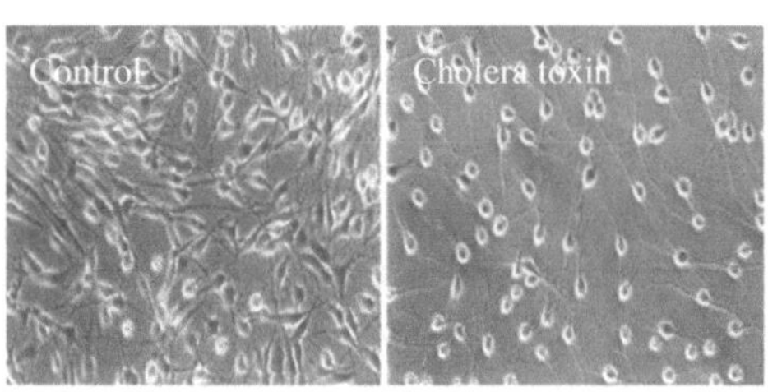

(a) Morphological transformation induced by cholera toxin in rat glioma cell line C6 cells. (Original magnification: ×200.)

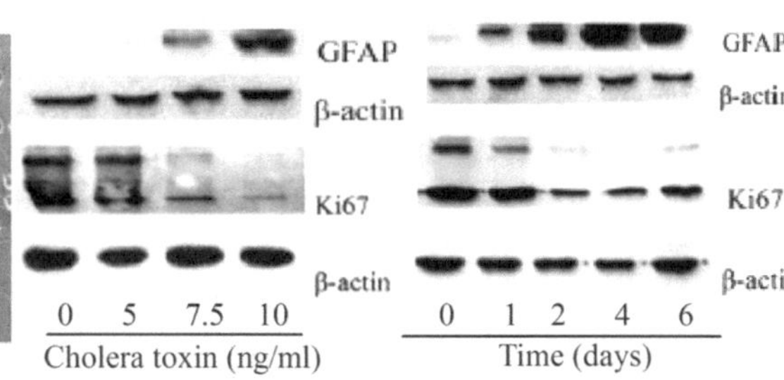

(b) Concentration- and time-dependent effect of cholera toxin on GFAP and Ki-67 expression in C6 cells.

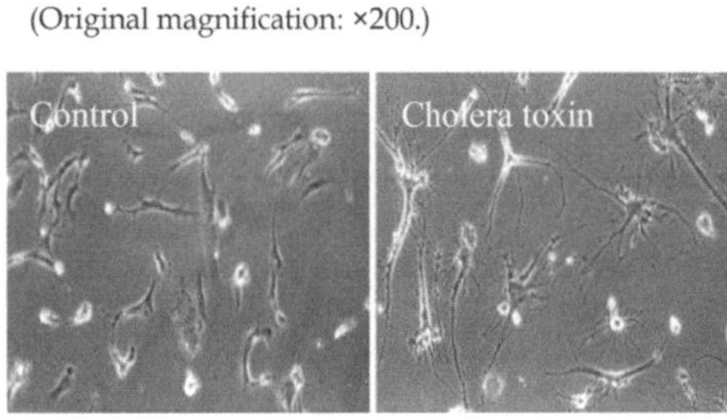

(c) Morphological transformation induced by cholera toxin in primary cultured human glioma cells. (Original magnification: ×200.)

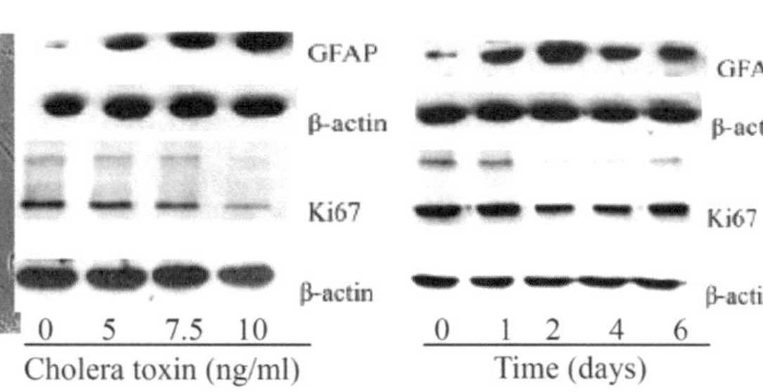

(d) Concentration- and time-dependent effect of cholera toxin on GFAP and Ki-67 expression in primary cultured human glioma cells.

Fig. 1. Morphological transformation, GFAP and Ki-67 expression induced by cholera toxin in rat glioma cell line C6 cells and primary cultured human glioma cells.

expression of GFAP, a 50-kDa type III intermediate filament protein considered to be a reliable differentiation marker of normal astrocytes (Roymans et al., 2001), and a lowered amount of Ki-67 protein (Figure 1b and 1d). The Ki-67 antigen presents during all active phases of the cell cycle but is absent from resting cells exclusively in the nuclei of cycling cells; the defined period of nuclear expression makes it a reliable marker of malignant proliferating cells (Schluter et al., 1993; Shachaf et al., 2004). In further experiments (Shu et al., 2011), the cholera toxin-induced GFAP expression is proved to be mediated by an oncogenic pathway interleukin-6/janus kinase 2/signal transducer and activator of transcription 3 (IL-6/JAK2/STAT3) cascade, implies that a survival-promoting signal may also play a differentiation-supporting role in malignant gliomas (Figure 2). However, the B subunit of cholera toxin (choleragenoid) at a dose of 10 ng/ml and even 10 μg/ml does not cause any alterations on cell morphology, GFAP expression and proliferation in C6 glioma cells (Figure 3). A mechanism that cholera toxin specifically activates ganglioside GM1 and induces differentiation in C6 glioma cells is therefore eradicated.

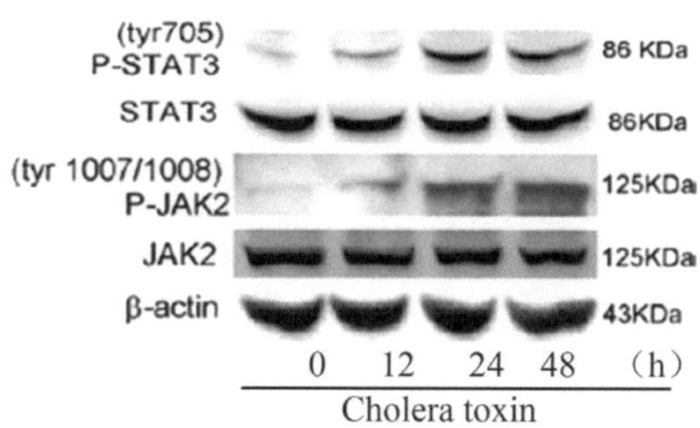

(a) Time-dependent effects of cholera toxin on phosphorylation of STAT3 (tyr705) and JAK2 (tyr1007/1008).

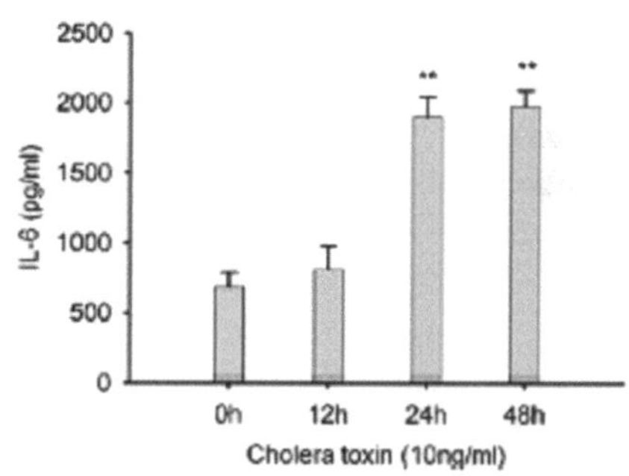

(b) Time-dependent effects of cholera toxin on IL-6 protein expression.

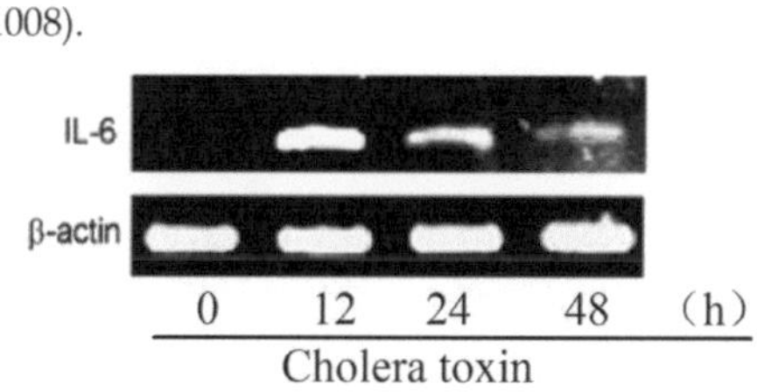

(c) Time-dependent effects of cholera toxin on IL-6 mRNA level.

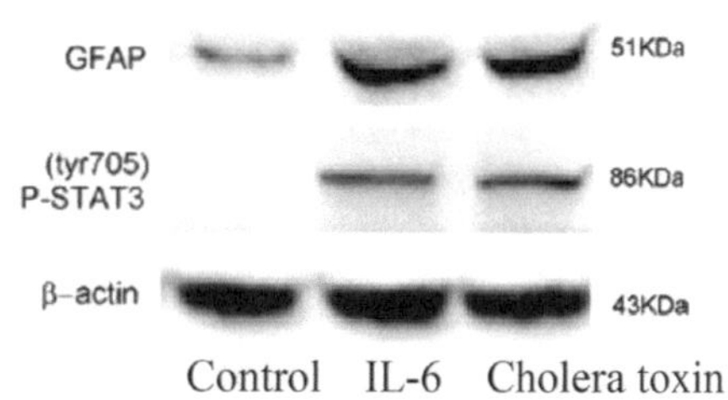

(d) IL-6 induces GFAP expression.

Fig. 2. Activation of IL-6/JAK2/STAT3 contributes to GFAP induction during the cholera toxin-induced differentiation in C6 glioma cells.

The regulation of cell proliferation and terminal differentiation is a critical aspect of normal development and homeostasis, but is frequently disturbed during tumorigenesis. Cell proliferation and differentiation are specifically controlled in the G1 phase and the G1/S phase transition in the cell cycle (Nurse, 2000). In differentiation triggered by cholera toxin, cellular proliferation inhibition is observed but not significant cell death and accumulation of cells in the G0/G1 phase of the cell cycle at multiple points within the machinery governing the G1/S transition is concurrent (Figure 4a-c and Table 1). The expression of G1 control proteins cyclin D1 and Cdk2 is down-regulated and associated with profound increased $p21^{Cip1}$ and $p27^{Kip1}$ protein levels (Figure 4d). Cyclin D1 is a critical regulator involved in cell-cycle progression through the G1 phase into the S phase, thereby contributing to cell proliferation. Cyclin D1 expression is significantly correlated with the degree of malignancy, invasion and prognosis of patients in a variety of human carcinomas, including glioma (Arato-Ohshima&Sawa, 1999; Lamb et al., 2003). The Cdk inhibitors $p21^{Cip1}$ and $p27^{Kip1}$ play an important role in mediating growth arrest and are thought to function as brakes of the cell cycle (Sherr&Roberts, 1999). The downregulation of cyclin D1 and overexpression of $p21^{Cip1}$ and $p27^{Kip1}$ might therefore be a pivotal candidate for the perturbed cell-cycle progression and differentiation induced by cholera toxin.

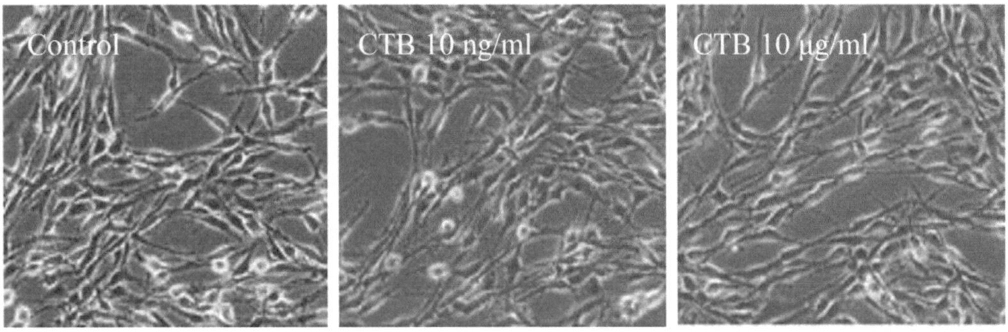

(a) Morphological transformation induced by the B subunit of cholera toxin (CTB) in C6 cells. (Original magnification: ×200.)

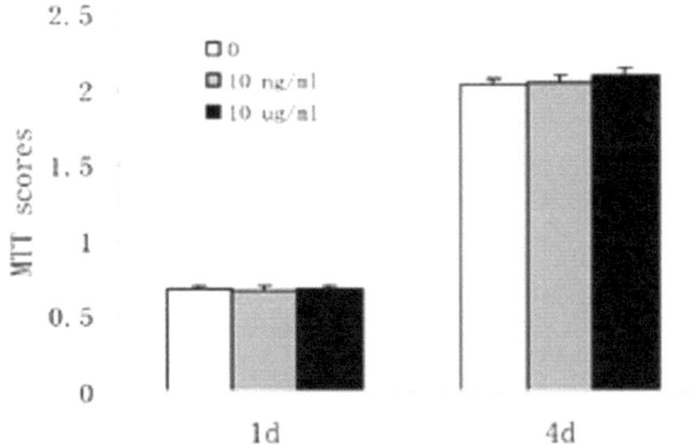

(b) Effect of the B subunit of cholera toxin (CTB) on cell viability in C6 cells.

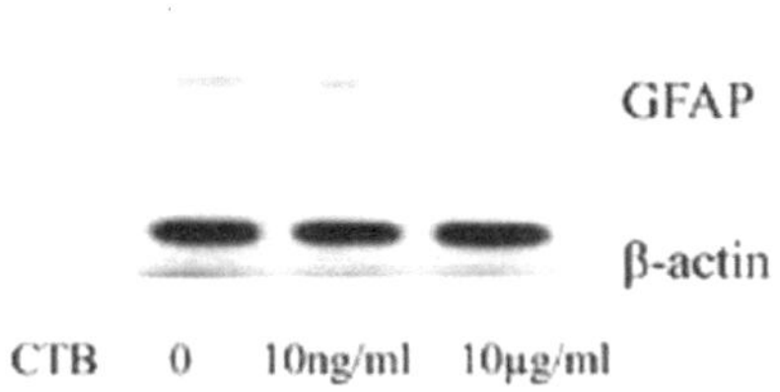

(c) Effect of the B subunit of cholera toxin (CTB) on GFAP protein expression in C6 cells.

Fig. 3. The B subunit of cholera toxin does not cause any alterations on cell morphology, GFAP expression, and proliferation in C6 glioma cells.

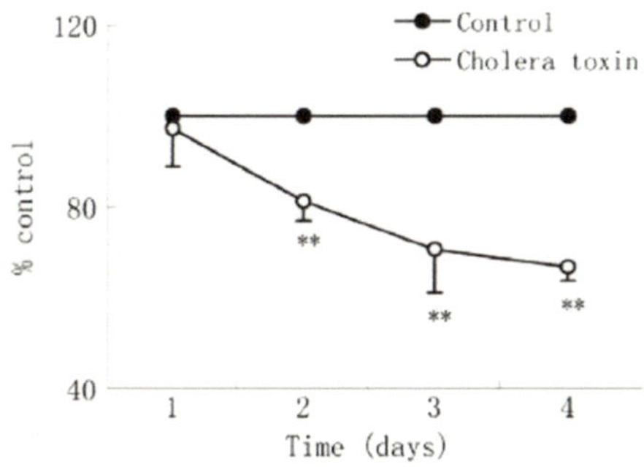

(a) Time-dependent effect of cholera toxin on cell viability in C6 cells.

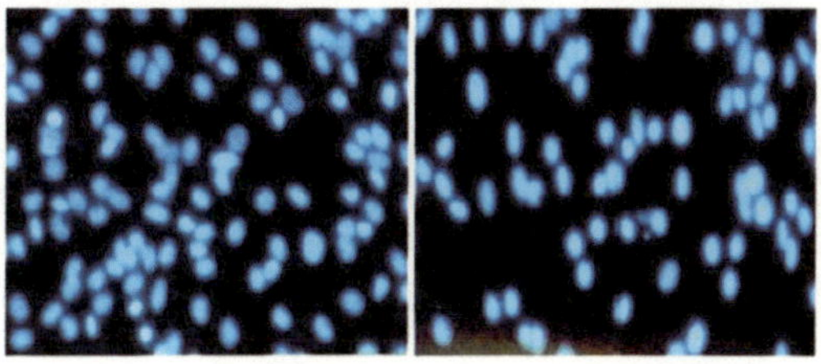

(b) Effect of cholera toxin on cell apoptosis in C6 cells (Hoechst 33258 staining).

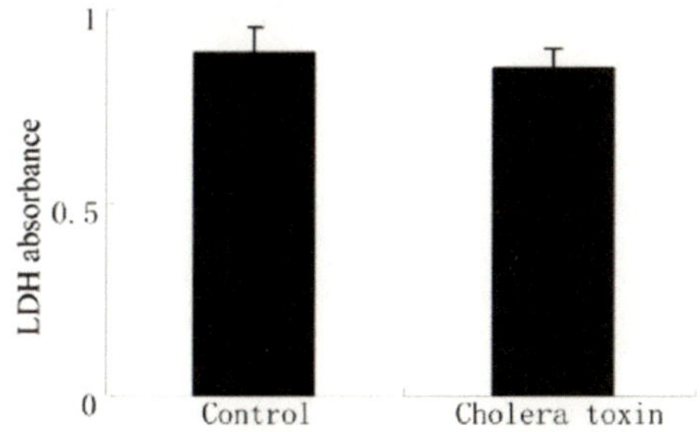

(c) Effect of cholera toxin on LDH release in C6 cells.

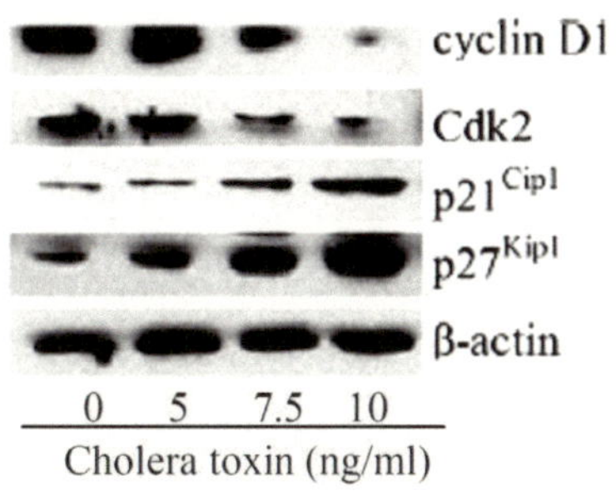

(d) Effect of cholera toxin on cell-cycle regulatory molecules in C6 cells.

Fig. 4. Cholera toxin inhibits cell proliferation and alters the protein expressions of cell-cycle regulatory molecules in C6 glioma cells.

	C6 glioma cells		Human primary glioma cells	
Groups	G0/G1	S	G0/G1	S
Control	63.6±7.4	27.7±5.9	51.5±11.8	36.0±8.2
Cholera toxin	88.2±6.8*	7.9±3.9**	81.3±3.1**	7.7±2.9**

Results are expressed as means ±SD (n=3) for control and cholera toxin groups. *, $p<0.05$; **, $p<0.01$ compared with control, respectively.

Table 1. Cholera toxin causes a G0/G1-phase cell cycle arrest in C6 and human primary glioma cells.

One of the potential downstream signaling targets of PKA is the CREB protein, an inducible transcription factor. Phosphorylation of Ser-133 is a critical event in CREB activation, leading to an increase of transcriptional activation by the recruitment of additional coactivators. The phosphorylation of CREB by PKA-mediated cAMP-dependent signaling cascade responds to a variety of external signals and appears to play crucial roles in differentiation and neurite outgrowth in multiple cell lines (Masson et al., 1993; Impey et al., 2004; Sato et al., 2006). Cells from transgenic mice expressing a dominant-negative form of CREB show a profound proliferative defect and G1 cell-cycle arrest in response to a number of different activation signals (Barton et al., 1996). It remains to be explored, however, whether PKA/CREB signaling participates in the differentiation of malignant glioma cells. In cholera toxin-treated glioma cells, a cholera toxin-induced cAMP increase is able to trigger the activation of downstream effectors, as evidenced by PKA activation and CREB transcription factor phosphorylation (Figure 5a). In addition, the essential role of PKA

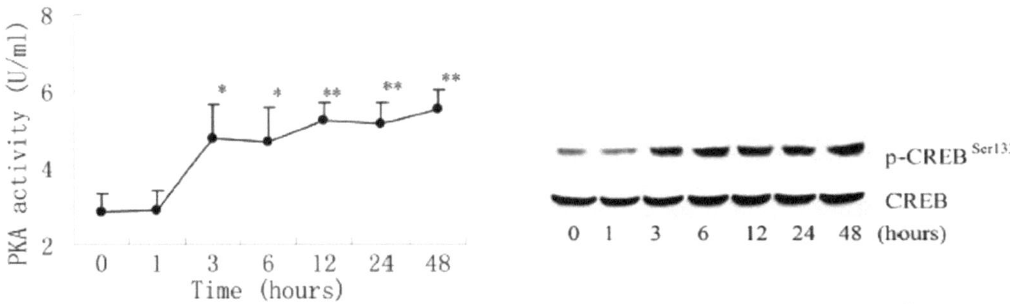

(a) Cholera toxin-induced cAMP increase is able to trigger the activation of downstream effectors, as evidenced by PKA activation and CREB transcription factor phosphorylation.

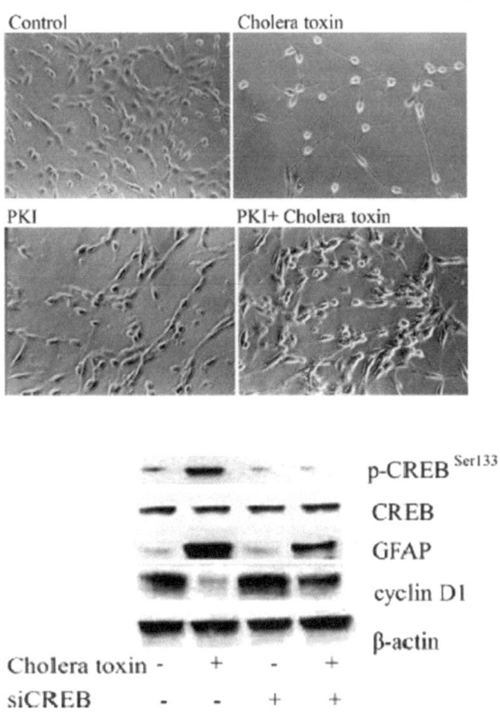

(b) PKA activity mediates for cholera toxin-induced differentiation in C6 cells.

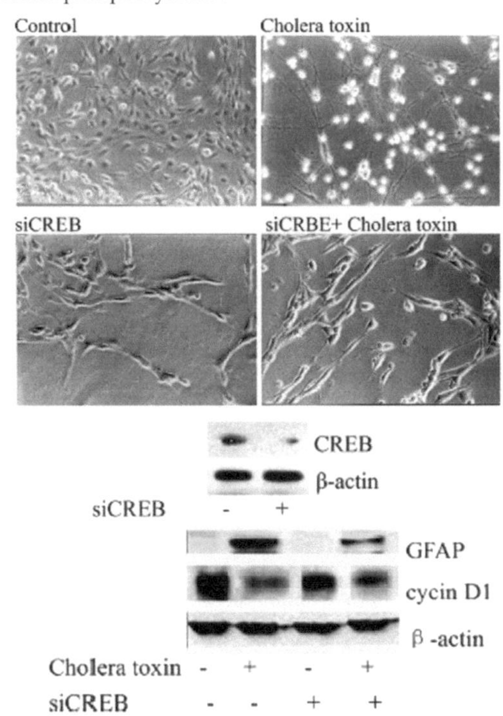

(c) Up-regulation of CREB is required for cholera toxin-induced differentiation in C6 cells.

Fig. 5. Cholera toxin-induced differentiation is inhibited by PKI or depletion of CREB.

activation in the cholera toxin-induced differentiation process is supported by experiments showing that differentiation is impaired if PKA activity is inhibited by PKI added before the differentiating agent cholera toxin or depletion of CREB by siRNA (Figure 5b and 5c). These data indicate that differentiation triggered by cholera toxin is effected through the PKA/CREB pathway and suggest the requisite role of PKA and transcription factor CREB for cholera toxin-induced differentiation.

In conclusion, cholera toxin might be an astrocytic differentiation-inducing agent in rat C6 and primary cultured human glioma cells of intensified therapeutic interest in the treatment of glioma. This effect may be caused by G1 arrest in the cell cycle ascribed to the restrain of cyclin D1 and Cdk2 activities by augmented expression of $p21^{Cip1}$ and $p27^{Kip1}$ proteins. Of the various possibilities for cholera toxin-induced differentiation, elevated PKA/CREB signaling pathway represents a plausible candidate. Significantly, cholera toxin, the traditional bacterial toxin, may be a novel agent with substantial differentiation potential in the therapy of malignant glioma. Future studies, however, should extend these findings to in vivo tumor models.

2.1.2 Forskolin and other PKA activators

Forskolin, a diterpene extracted from the roots of the plant Coleus forskohlii, directly activates adenylate cyclase (AC) and catalyzes synthesis of cAMP from ATP to activate PKA. Accumulating evidences have reported that forskolin induces the differentiation of human monoblast U937 cells, neurocytoma cells and neuroblastoma x rat glioma cell line NG108-15 cells via elevating cAMP (Ammer&Schulz, 1997; Brodsky et al., 1998; Kim et al., 2004) , suggesting forskolin to be a potential candidate of differentiation inducing agents for glioma. In accordance with previous reports, forskolin represses cell growth via cell cycle arrest in the G0/G1 phase and induces cell differentiation characteristic with elongated processes and restoration of GFAP expression when administrated to malignant glioma C6 cells (Figure 6a and 6b) (Lu et al., 2009; He et al., 2011). In mechanisms, forskolin promotes C6 cell differentiation via regulating the transcription and proteolysis of cyclin D1, and maintenance of low cyclin D1 expression is required for its effects on differentiation as demonstrated by gain and loss of function studies (Figure 6c and 6d). All the information supports the notion that forskolin can be developed into a candidate for the future in differentiation therapy of glioma, and cyclin D1 is a promising target for pro-differentiation strategy.

All data mentioned above also indicates that other cAMP/PKA signaling activators should have the same potential to induce cell differentiation and proliferation inhibition. Data in Figure 7 show that db-cAMP mimics forskolin's differentiation effects of cholera toxin on cell morphology, GFAP expression, cell proliferation, and cell-cycle distributions in C6 glioma cells.

2.2 GSK-3β controls differentiation of malignant glioma cells

GSK-3 is an evolutionary conserved, ubiquitous serine/threonine kinase that is highly enriched in the brain and consists of 2 distinct isoforms, α and β, in mammals (Woodgett, 1991). One of the most notable qualities of GSK-3 is the vast number of signaling pathways that converge on this enzyme and subsequently an even greater number of biological targets (Cohen&Frame, 2001; Jope&Johnson, 2004). Numerous studies have indicated that GSK-3 is involved in key functions of the brain and is associated with dysfunction in multiple neurological diseases (Grimes&Jope, 2001). More recent studies indicate a role for GSK-3 in the control of neoplastic transformation and tumor development, suggesting that GSK-3 is a potential therapeutic target in human cancers. However, most attention has focused on the β-isoform of GSK-3 and the exact role of GSK-3β in malignancies remains highly controversial due to the conflicting results from different tumor models. Although some studies found that GSK-3β is a part of a tumor suppressor complex that phosphorylates the oncoprotein β-catenin and that GSK-3β inactivation could possibly lead to tumor promotion (Hinoi et al., 2000; Rask et al., 2003), other studies have shown that inhibition of GSK-3β suppresses cancer cell proliferation and induces apoptosis by abrogating nuclear factor NF-κB mediated gene transcription (Ougolkov et al., 2005; Ougolkov et al., 2007). In addition, the vast majority of research on GSK-3β has been focused on the aspects of proliferation and apoptosis, and little is known about its possible role involved in the process of cancer cell differentiation.

In differentiation-sensitive C6 and U87-MG malignant glioma cells, intensive GSK-3β is highly expressed and activated during the cholera toxin-induced differentiation, whereas the GSK-3α activity remains stable. In differentiation-resistant U251 and T98G glioma cells, GSK-3β is lowly expressed (Figure 8a). Inhibition of GSK-3β activity or knockdown of its expression by small interfering RNA (siRNA) suppresses this differentiation (Figure 8b), whereas constitutively active S9A-GSK-3β initiates robust differentiation in differentiation-resistant U251 glioma cells (Figure 8c). These results indicate that GSK-3β overexpression and activation possibly is a contributory event in the process of cellular differentiation in malignant gliomas. In addition, ubiquitin/proteasome-dependent degradation is identified the major pathway responsible for cyclin D1 reduction and sequential differentiation. By further experiments, GSK-3β is confirmed to regulate differentiation by triggering cyclin D1 translocation and degradation (Figure 9).

To extend these findings to clinical malignant gliomas, a series of 10 primary cell cultures grown from 7 Grade III and 3 Grade IV malignant astrocytoma explants are further prepared. Exposure to the differentiation agent cholera toxin also results in differentiated characteristics with a stellar shape with filamentous processes and increased GFAP expression in all the primary cultures examined (Figure 10a). Furthermore, the phosphorylated form of GSK-3β shows the same alteration panel as in the rat C6 cell line and GSK-3β inhibitors LiCl and SB216732 could block the increased GFAP and decreased PCNA levels induced by differentiation agent cholera toxin (Figure 10b). These results confirm the findings in C6 cells and, moreover, suggest a general correlation of GSK-3β activity with differentiation in malignant glioma cells.

To further confirm the possibility that GSK-3β expression is associated with sensitivity to differentiation therapy, GSK-3β expression in human glioma tissue samples (WHO Grade III and IV) is examined by immunohistochemical staining. Tissues are scored on the basis of the percentage of GSK-3β-positive tumor cells. As shown in Figure 10c, overexpression of GSK-3β is observed frequently in the cytoplasm of tumor cells (representative immunostaining image from Grade IV malignant glioma tissues), whereas weak expression only is observed in the cytoplasm of cells from normal brain. p-GSK-3β^{Y216} that represents the active kinase form of GSK-3β is also detected to assess the activation state of the protein. Figure 10c shows a higher expression of p-GSK-3β^{Y216} in malignant gliomas compared with normal brain tissues (representative image from Grade IV malignant glioma tissues). The immunohistochemical results of GSK-3β expression and its Y216 phosphorylation in patients are summarized in Figure 10d. Together, it is likely that overexpression of active GSK-3β is a pathological characteristic of clinical malignant gliomas, which are sensitive to the induced-differentiation.

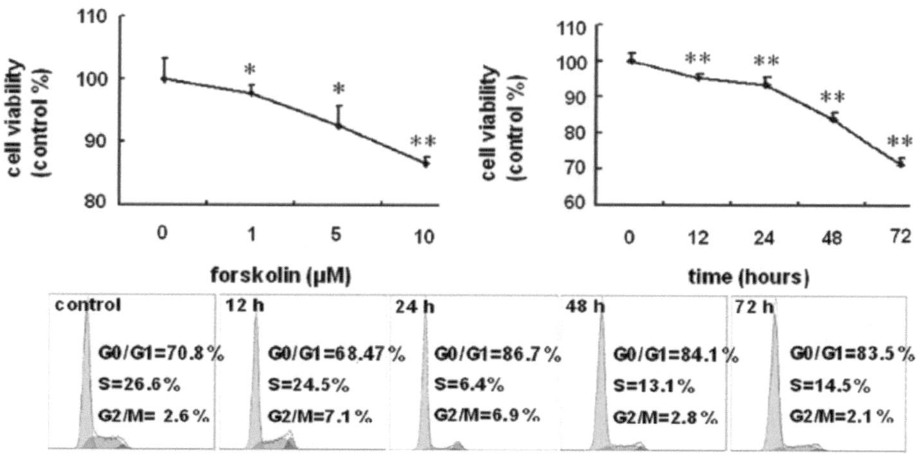

(a) Forskolin inhibits cell proliferation and induces G0/G1-phase cell cycle arrest in C6 cells.

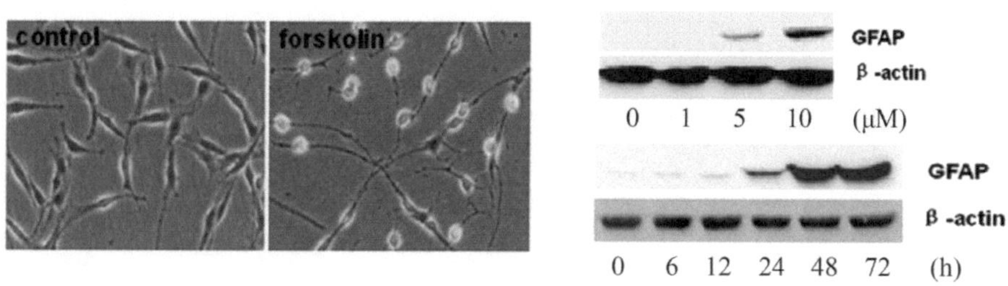

(b) Forskolin induces morphological transformation into astrocytic state and upregulation of GFAP protein expression in C6 cells.

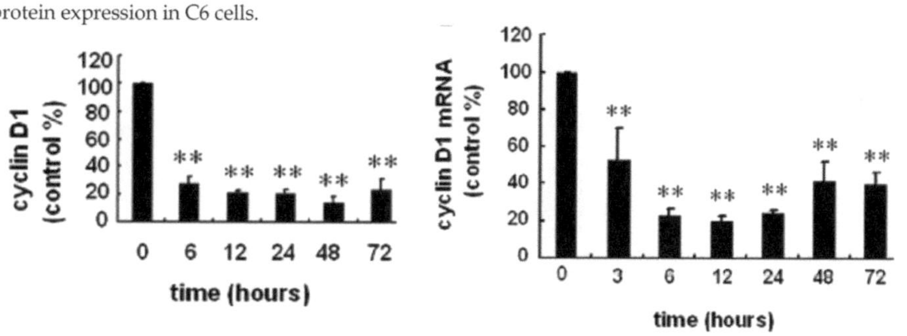

(c) Forskolin decreases the protein and mRNA levels of cyclin D1 in C6 cells.

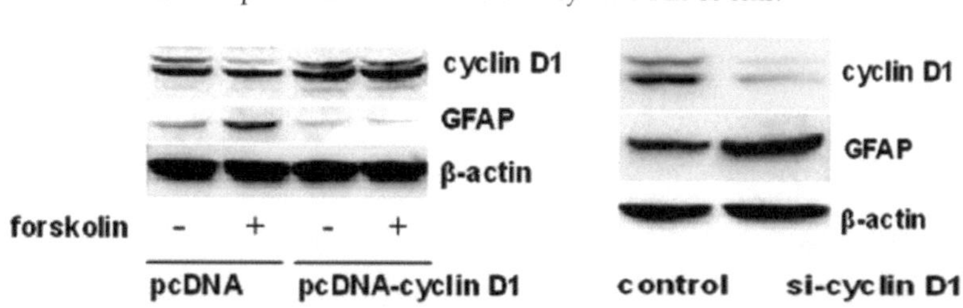

(d) Cyclin D1 down-regulation is requisite for forskolin-induced differentiation in C6 glioma cells.

Fig. 6. Forskolin induces differetiation via downregulation of cyclin D1.

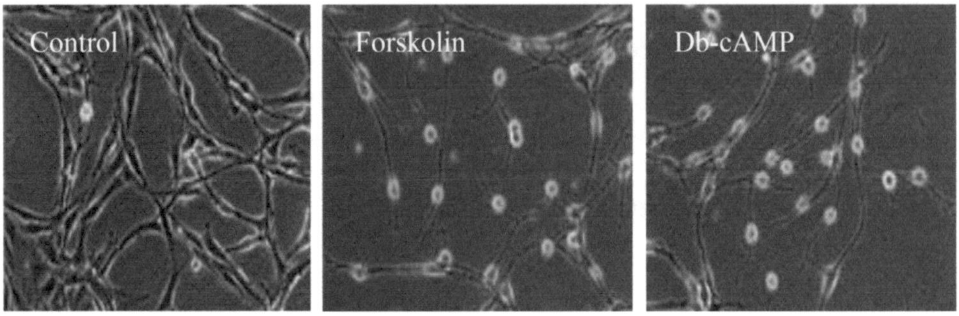

(a) Morphological transformation induced by forskolin and db-cAMP in C6 cells. (Original magnification: ×200.)

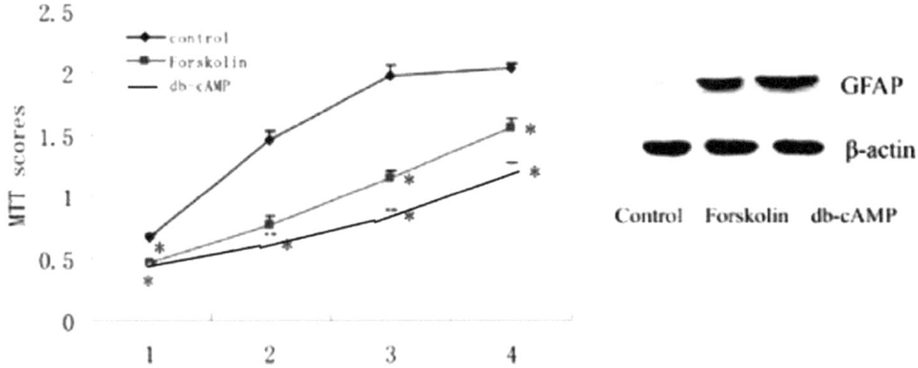

(b) Forskolin and db-cAMP induce cell proliferation inhibition and upregulation of GFAP protein expression in C6 cells.

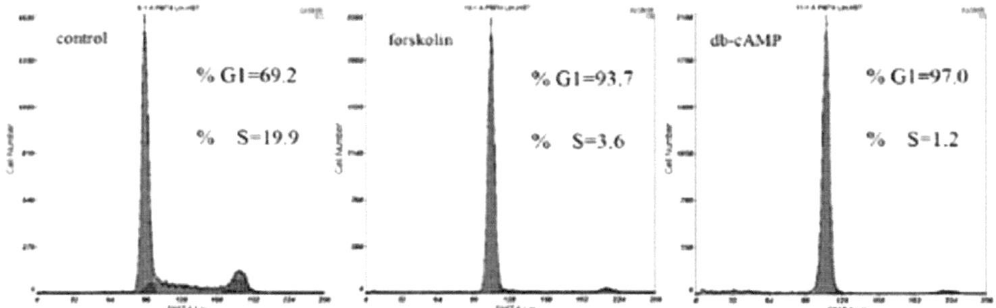

(c) Forskolin and db-cAMP induce G0/G1-phase cell cycle arrest in C6 cells.

Fig. 7. Forskolin and db-cAMP induce cell proliferation inhibition and cell differentation in C6 glioma cells.

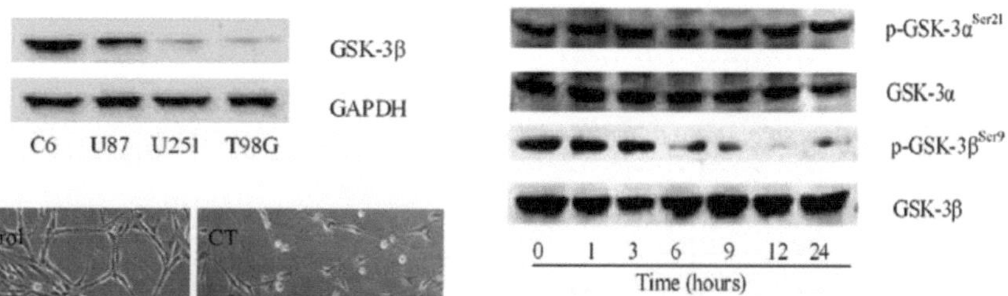

(a) GSK-3 is highly expressed in C6 and U87 cells and activated by cholera toxin.

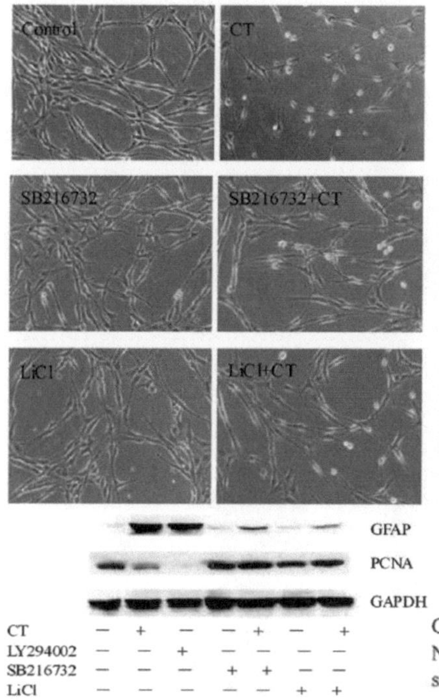

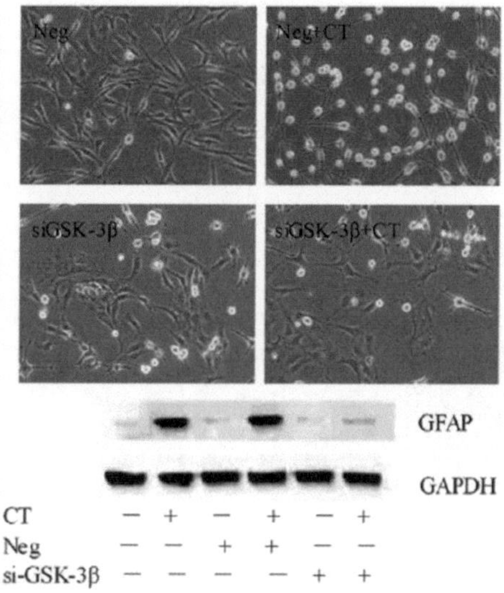

(b) Inhibition of GSK-3β activity or knockdown of its expression by small interfering RNA (siRNA) suppresses cholera toxin (CT)-induced differentiation.

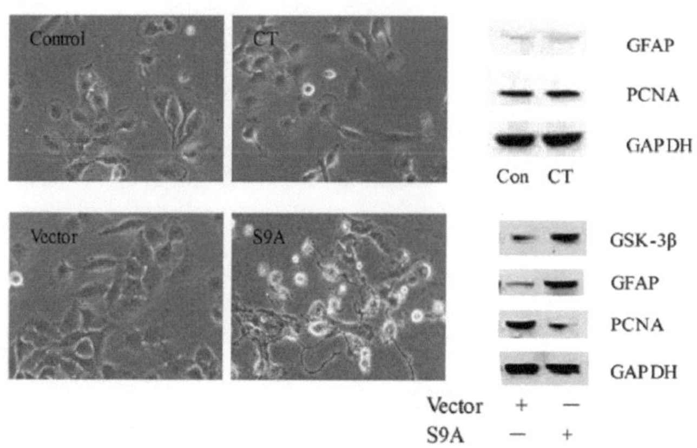

(c) Constitutively active S9A-GSK-3β initiates robust differentiation in differentiation-resistant U251 glioma cells.

Fig. 8. GSK-3β may be a determinant of cellular differetiation in malignant tumor as a pathological characteristic of differentiation-sensitive glioma cells.

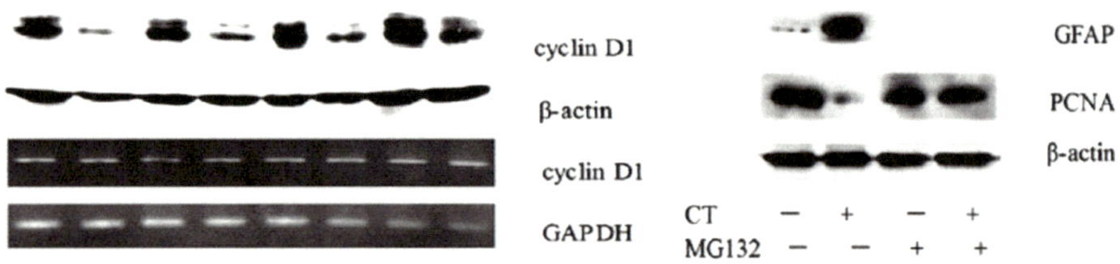

(a) Cholera toxin downregulates the protein level of cyclin D1 but not mRNA level and upregulation of GFAP and downregulation of PCNA induced by cholera toxin are attenuated by proteasome inhibitor MG132.

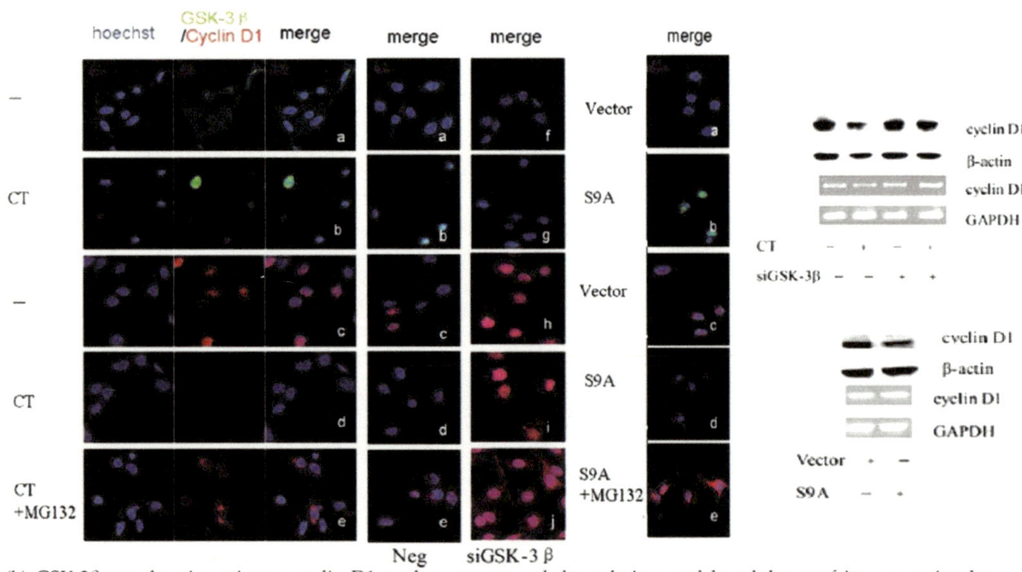

(b) GSK-3β translocation triggers cyclin D1 nuclear export and degradation, and knockdown of its expression by small interfering RNA (siRNA) suppresses this effect while constitutively active S9A-GSK-3β initiates this effect in differentiation-resistant U251 glioma cells.

Fig. 9. GSK-3β regulates differentiation by triggering cyclin D1 translocation and degradation.

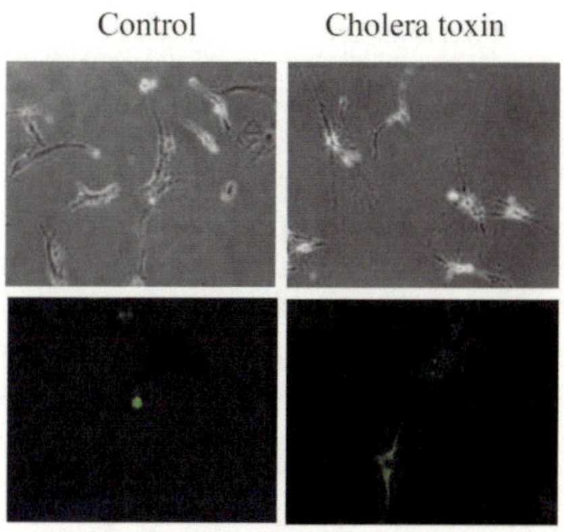

(a) Morphology and GFAP immunofluorescence in human primary cultured malignant glioma cells treated by cholera toxin.

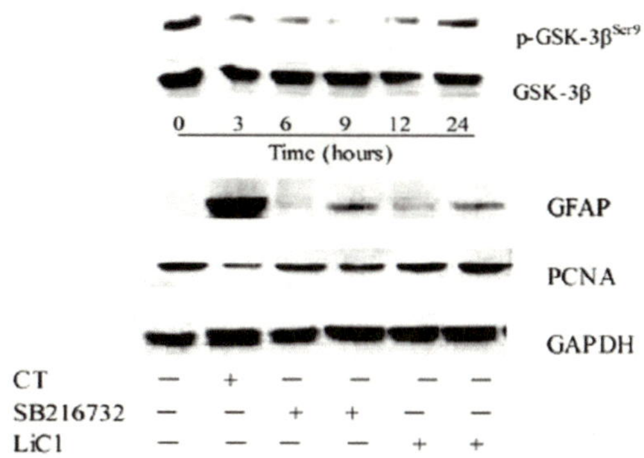

(b) Immunoblot of p-GSK-3β^{ser9} and GSK-3β levels in cholera toxin (CT)-treated human primary cultured malignant glioma cells and GSK-3β inhibitors LiCl and SB216732 block the increased GFAP and decreased PCNA levels induced by cholera toxin.

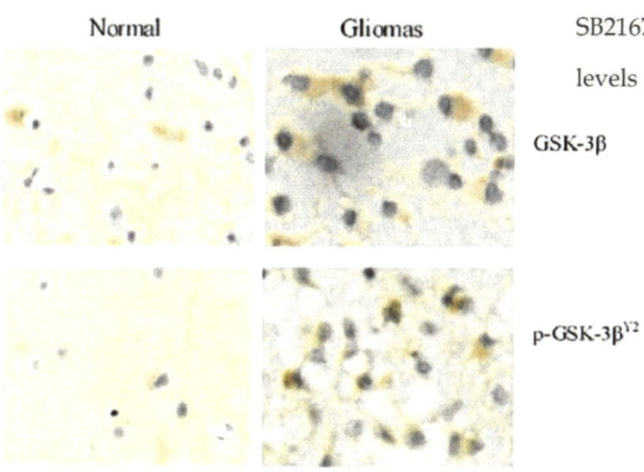

(c) GSK-3β and p-GSK-3β^{Y216} immunocytochemistry of stained sections from representative tissues of primary gliomas and normal brains.

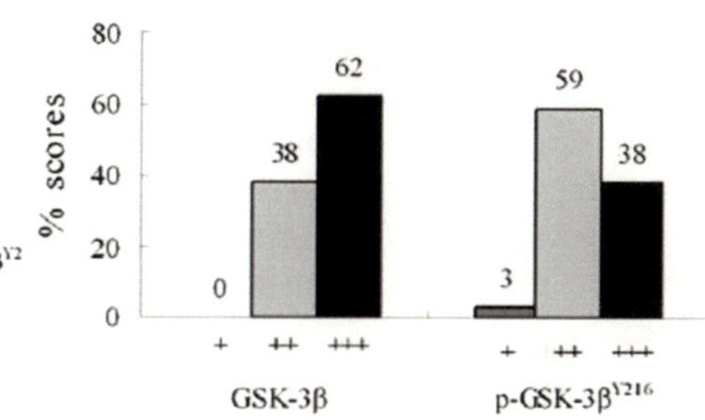

(d) Percentage of patients with malignant gliomas in their GSK-3β and p-GSK-3β^{Y216} immunostaining scored + (positive staining for <10%), ++ (positive staining for 10–60%), or +++ (positive staining for >60%)

Fig. 10. Expression and phosphorylation of GSK-3β in primary human malignant gliomas.

In summary, GSK-3β initiates resistant glioma cells susceptible to differentiation and loss of GSK-3β activity interrupts cyclin D1 proteolysis necessary for the astrocytic differentiation of malignant glioma cells. These data provide strong evidence that GSK-3β acts as a tumor suppressor to induce cellular differentiation, and thus suppresses tumor development. As a pathological characteristic of differentiation-sensitive glioma cells, GSK-3β may be a novel therapeutic target and a determinant of cellular differentiation in malignant tumors. The data also show that GSK-3α and GSK-3β have distinct biological roles, as the former is not involved in the differentiation-inducing mechanism of cholera toxin in malignant gliomas.

2.3 HIF-1α blocks differentiation of malignant gliomas

Solid tumors frequently develop in regions with hypoxia because of an imbalance in oxygen supply and consumption. Recent reports indicate that hypoxic microenvironments contribute to cancer progression by activating adaptive transcriptional programs that promote cell survival, motility and tumor angiogenesis (Harris, 2002; Pouyssegur et al., 2006). Histopathological analyses frequently reveal the spatial overlap of hypoxia and dedifferentiation within solid tumors, suggesting the role of hypoxia in tumor cell differentiation (Jogi et al., 2002; Helczynska et al., 2003). However, it is unclear whether hypoxia plays a causal role in this relationship.

Cells within hypoxic regions adapt to this environment by altering their gene-expression program, and thus their phenotype (Leszczyniecka et al., 2001). One of the transcription factors primarily responsible for this change is the HIF-1 (Semenza, 2003). HIF-1 is a heterodimer that consists of a constitutively expressed β subunit (HIF-1β or ARNT) and a catalytic a subunit (HIF-1α) (Harris, 2002; Semenza, 2003). At normoxia, HIF-1α is hydroxylated at specific proline residues by oxygen-dependent prolyl hydroxylases, leading to an interaction with the von Hippel-Lindau tumor suppressor protein (pVHL) /E3 ligase complex and subsequent ubiquitin mediated destruction (Maxwell et al., 1999; Ivan et al., 2001; Jaakkola et al., 2001). Under hypoxic conditions, HIF-1α escapes from hydroxylation and translocates to the nucleus, where it forms a complex with HIF-1β and the cAMP-responsive element binding protein (CREB)-binding protein (CBP) / p300 co-activator, binds to hypoxia-response elements and transcriptionally modulates target genes (Semenza, 2002). HIF-1 has been shown to play critical roles in tumor angiogenesis, glucose metabolism, invasion / metastasis, and response to radiation and chemotherapy (Moeller et al., 2005; Fulda&Debatin, 2007; Lin et al., 2008; Rankin&Giaccia, 2008; Yang et al., 2008). However, little is known about its possible role in the process of cellular differentiation in solid tumors.

Gliomas are the most common and malignant primary brain tumors in humans and are among the most hypoxic tumors known (DeAngelis, 2001; Rong et al., 2006). Glioblastoma multiforme, the highest-grade glioma, is characterized by large necrotic areas within the tumor mass, which correlates with enhanced resistance to therapy, increased invasiveness and a poor prognosis for the patient (Rong et al., 2006). In addition, malignant glioma cells could be induced to undergo differentiation towards their normal counterparts and thus serve as a faithful model to study molecular mechanisms underlying differentiation defects in solid tumors (Takanaga et al., 2004; Li et al., 2007).

In the present study, cobalt chloride and deferoxamine (DFO) are used to mimic an intratumoral mild hypoxia condition, and the data shows that differentiation induced by forskolin in rat C6 and primary cultured human malignant glioma cells is reversibly inhibited (Figure 11). Deletion of the endogenous HIF-1α gene restores the differentiation capacities, even in the presence of cobalt chloride (Figure 12a). In contrast, stabilization of HIF-1 with small interfering RNA (siRNA) against VHL, which leads to proteosomal degradation of HIF-1α, shows differentiation blockage similar to that induced by cobalt chloride (Figure 12b). Furthermore, inhibition of HIF-1α binding to its transcriptional co-activator CBP/ p300 by chetomin abolishes the differentiation-inhibitory effect of HIF-1 and attenuates tumor growth in combination with forskolin (Figure 13).

Analyses of human glioma tissues have suggested a strong correlation between the expression of HIF-1α and malignancy (World Health Organization grade). Expression of HIF-1α protein is found in all 95 samples (representative immunostaining images are shown in Figure 14a), and no obvious staining is observed in the five normal brain samples (a representative image is

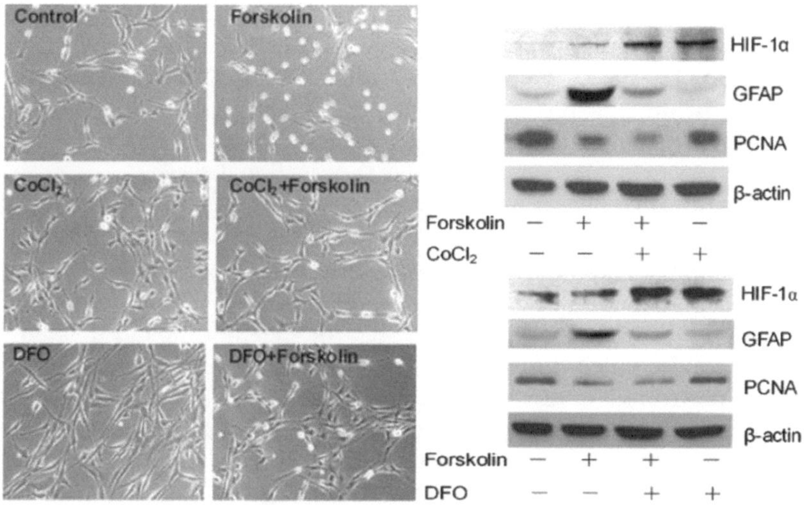

(a) Morphological transformation of C6 cells pretreated with 100 μM $CoCl_2$ or 100 μM DFO for 2 h and then treated with 10 μM forskolin for a further 24 h. (Original magnification: ×200.)

(b) HIF-1α, GFAP and PCNA expression of C6 cells pretreated with 100 μM $CoCl_2$ or 100 μM DFO for 2 h and then treated with 10 μM forskolin for a further 24 h.

Fig. 11. Cobalt chloride ($CoCl_2$) and DFO inhibit differentiation induced by forskolin in C6 glioma cells.

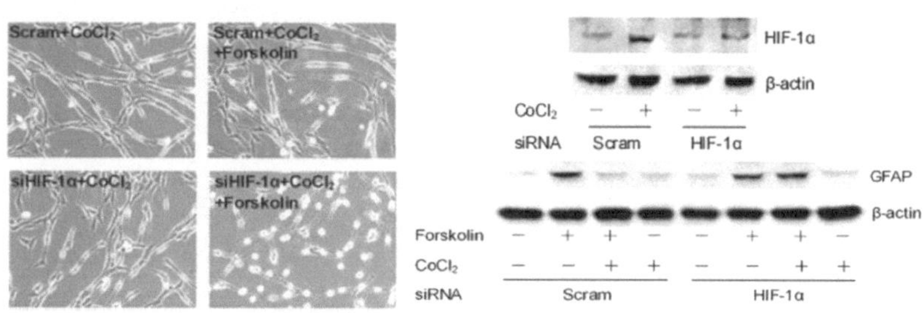

(a) Cobalt chloride ($CoCl_2$) fails to induce HIF-1α accumulation in C6 cells transfected with siHIF-1α.

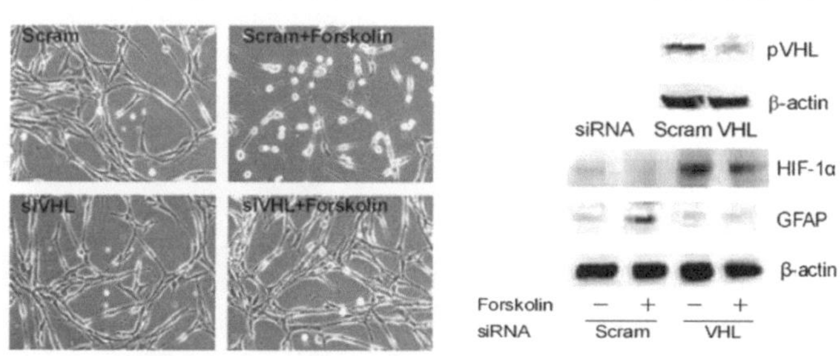

(b) VHL knockdown blocks differentiation of C6 cells.

Fig. 12. HIF-1α is required for the differentiation-inhibitory effect of cobalt chloride ($CoCl_2$) in C6 cells.

shown in Figure 14a). Statistical evaluation reveals that the amount of HIF-1α is significantly increased in parallel with increasing glioma grade (Figure 14a). The percentage of HIF-1α-positive cells in Grade I is 19.4%, while one in Grade II, III and IV is 32.5%, 46.1% and 70.5% respectively. Thus, HIF-1α is demonstrated to be broadly accumulated in glioma cells and its overexpression is correlated with glioma malignance grading, in other words, higher levels of expression of HIF-1α suggest a greater degree of differentiation defects.
Then, to test the generality of the inhibitory effects of HIF-1α, primary cultured human glioma cells are exposured to the differentiation agent forskolin. The result shows that forskolin also results in differentiated characteristics, of a stellar shape with filamentous processes and increased GFAP expression in the primary glioma cells (Figure 14b). However, co-incubation with cobalt chloride blocks the morphological alterations and increased the amount of GFAP induced by forskolin (Figure 14b). Quantitative analysis indicates that the percentage of GFAP-expressing cells is significantly up-regulated upon treatment with forskolin. Moreover, the up-regulation is reversed by cobalt chloride (Figure 14b). These results confirm the findings in C6 cells and, moreover, suggest a general correlation of HIF-1α activity with differentiation in malignant glioma cells.Taken together, HIF-1α negatively regulates the differentiation of malignant gliomas and provides new insights into the differentiation therapy by targeting the HIF-1α pathway in solid tumors.

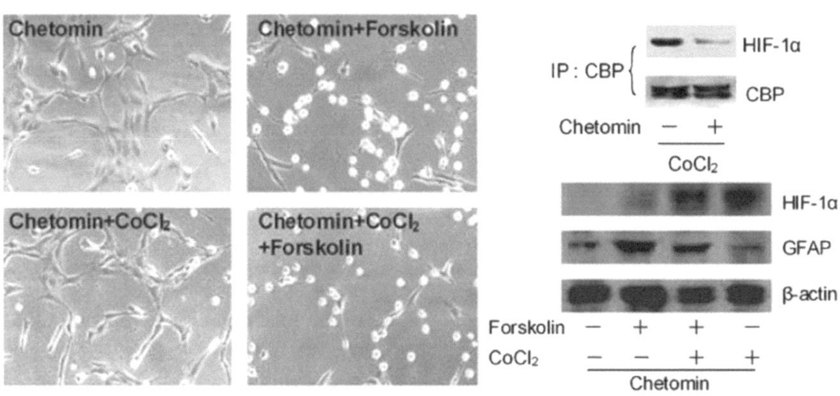

(a) Targeting HIF-1 by chetomin abolishes the differentiation-inhibitory effect of cobalt chloride ($CoCl_2$) in vitro.

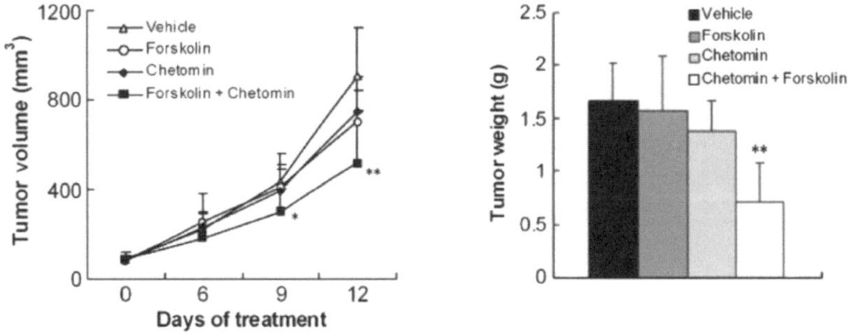

(b) Targeting HIF-1 by chetomin cooperates with forskolin to attenuate glioma growth in vivo.

Fig. 13. Chetomin abrogates the differentiation-inhibitory effect of cobalt chloride in vitro and combination of chetomin and forskolin attenuates tumor growth in vivo.

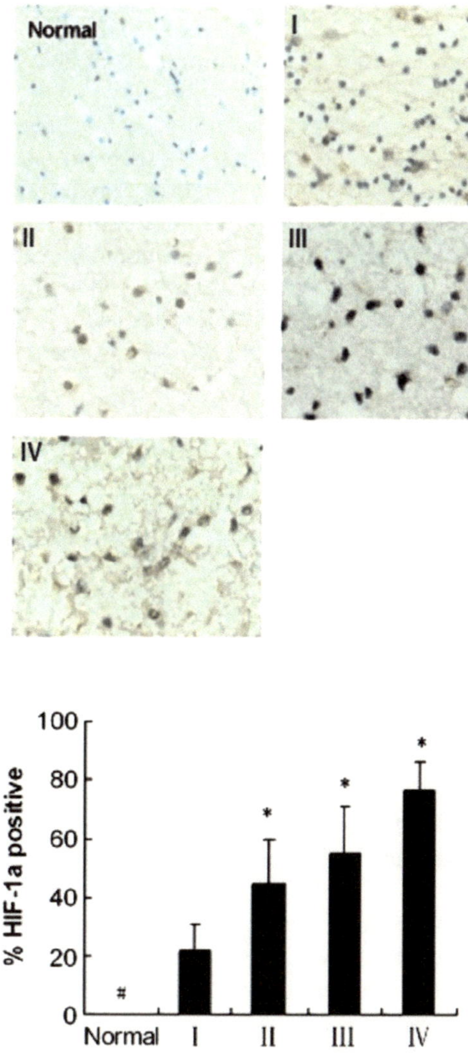

(a) HIF-1a expression increases with tumor grade.

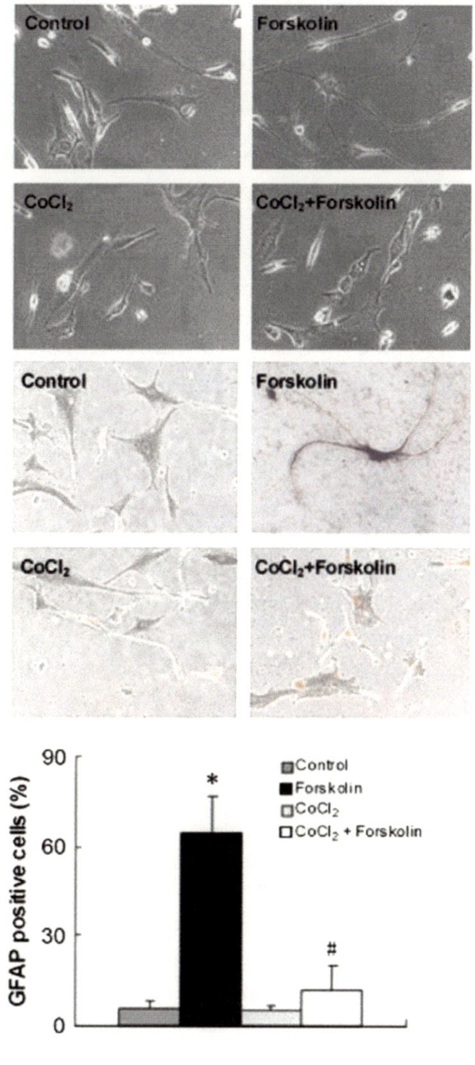

(b) HIF-1a blocks differentiation in primary human malignant glioma cells.

Fig. 14. HIF-1α activity is generally correlated with differentiation in malignant gliomas.

3. Conclusion

Deviation from the tissue/lineage-specific differentiation program is one of the fundamental aspects of tumorigenesis (Scott, 1997). The aberrantly differentiated cells show abnormal growth characteristics and distinct invasive and metastatic properties (Sell, 2004). Treating malignant tumors through the induction of cell differentiation has been an attractive concept, but clinical development of differentiation-inducing agents, especially for solid tumors, has been limited to date (Leszczyniecka et al., 2001). Several cell lines established from solid tumors are also reported to be differentiated by respective differentiation-inducers in vitro (Chintharlapalli et al., 2004; El-Metwally et al., 2005; Li et al., 2007; Choi et al., 2009). However, this differentiation has not been verified in in vivo animal models or clinically, and there exists little convincing explanation for this finding.

Based on information mentioned above, cAMP/PKA signaling activators such as cholera toxin and foskolin is capable of inducing the differentiation of glioma cells highly expressing GSK-3β, and overexpression of active GSK-3β can restore differentiation capacity of resistant glioma cells. In addition, HIF-1α is confirmed as a negative regulator of the differentiation in malignant gliomas, and targeting the HIF-1α pathway can potentiate the inhibitory effect of differentiation inducer in solid tumors. We have reasons to believe that all information above not only provide reasonable explanation in molecular mechanisms for the previous difficulty of differentiation therapy, but also will promote the development of differentiation therapy of glioma even solid tumor in future.

4. Acknowledgment

We thank Dr. Wei Yin, Yan Li, Huimin Lu, Songmin He, Minfeng Shu, Yijun Huang, Lijun Chen, Jun Hu, Dong Xu, Jun Xie and all other members of this laboratory for their excellent assistances to this work.

The project was supported by National Natural Science Foundation of China (No. 30830111).

5. References

Ammer, H. & Schulz, R. (1997). Regulation of stimulatory adenylyl cyclase signaling during forskolin-induced differentiation of mouse neuroblastoma x rat glioma (NG108-15) cells, Neurosci Lett 230(3): 143-146.

Arato-Ohshima, T. & Sawa, H. (1999). Over-expression of cyclin D1 induces glioma invasion by increasing matrix metalloproteinase activity and cell motility, Int J Cancer 83(3): 387-392.

Bao, S., Wu, Q. & McLendon, R. (2006). Glioma stem cells promote radioresistance by preferential activation of the DNA damage response, Nature 444(7120): 756-760.

Barton, K., Muthusamy, N. & Chanyangam, M. (1996). Defective thymocyte proliferation and IL-2 production in transgenic mice expressing a dominant-negative form of CREB, Nature 379(6560): 81-85.

Brodsky, A., Davio, C. & Shayo, C. (1998). Forskolin induces U937 cell line differentiation as a result of a sustained cAMP elevation, Eur J Pharmacol 350(1): 121-127.

Chintharlapalli, S., Smith, R. & Samudio, I. (2004). 1,1 - Bis(3'-indolyl) - 1 - (p-substitutedphenyl) methanes induce peroxisome proliferator-activated receptor gamma-mediated growth inhibition, transactivation, and differentiation markers in colon cancer cells, Cancer Res 64(17): 5994-6001.

Choi, E., Oh, H. & Wee, H. (2009). Eupatilin exhibits a novel anti-tumor activity through the induction of cell cycle arrest and differentiation of gastric carcinoma AGS cells, Differentiation 77(4): 412-423.

Cohen, P. & Frame, S. (2001). The renaissance of GSK3, Nat Rev Mol Cell Biol 2(10): 769-776.

Curran, W., Scott, C. & Horton, J. (1993). Recursive partitioning analysis of prognostic factors in three Radiation Therapy Oncology Group malignant glioma trials, J Natl Cancer Inst 85(9): 704-710.

DeAngelis, L. (2001). Brain tumors, N Engl J Med 344(2): 114-123.

El-Metwally, T., Hussein, M. & Pour, P. (2005). High concentrations of retinoids induce differentiation and late apoptosis in pancreatic cancer cells in vitro, Cancer Biol Ther 4(5): 602-611.

Fulda, S. & Debatin, K. (2007). HIF-1-regulated glucose metabolism: a key to apoptosis resistance?, Cell Cycle 6(7): 790-792.

Goodman, L. & Segreti, J. (1999). Infectious diarrhea, Dis Mon 45(7): 268-299.

Grimes, C. & Jope, R. (2001). The multifaceted roles of glycogen synthase kinase 3beta in cellular signaling, Prog Neurobiol 65(4): 391-426.

Guerrant, R., Brunton, L. & Schnaitman, T. (1974). Cyclic adenosine monophosphate and alteration of Chinese hamster ovary cell morphology: a rapid, sensitive in vitro assay for the enterotoxins of Vibrio cholerae and Escherichia coli, Infect Immun 10(2): 320-327.

Guerrant, R., Fang, G. & Thielman, N. (1994). Role of platelet activating factor in the intestinal epithelial secretory and Chinese hamster ovary cell cytoskeletal responses to cholera toxin, Proc Natl Acad Sci U S A 91(20): 9655-9658.

Harris, A. (2002). Hypoxia--a key regulatory factor in tumour growth, Nat Rev Cancer 2(1): 38-47.

He, S., Zhu, W. & Zhou, Y. (2011). Transcriptional and post-transcriptional downregulation of cyclin D1 contributes to C6 glioma cell differentiation induced by Forskolin, J Cell Biochem 112(5)：in press.

Helczynska, K., Kronblad, A. & Jogi, A. (2003). Hypoxia promotes a dedifferentiated phenotype in ductal breast carcinoma in situ, Cancer Res 63(7): 1441-1444.

Hinoi, T., Yamamoto, H. & Kishida, M. (2000). Complex formation of adenomatous polyposis coli gene product and axin facilitates glycogen synthase kinase-3 beta-dependent phosphorylation of beta-catenin and down-regulates beta-catenin, J Biol Chem 275(44): 34399-34406.

Huang, M., Ye, Y. & Chen, S. (1988). Use of all-trans retinoic acid in the treatment of acute promyelocytic leukemia, Blood 72(2): 567-572.

Impey, S., McCorkle, S. & Cha-Molstad, H. (2004). Defining the CREB regulon: a genome-wide analysis of transcription factor regulatory regions, Cell 119(7): 1041-1054.

Ivan, M., Kondo, K. & Yang, H. (2001). HIFalpha targeted for VHL-mediated destruction by proline hydroxylation: implications for O2 sensing, Science 292(5516): 464-468.

Jaakkola, P., Mole, D. & Tian, Y. (2001). Targeting of HIF-alpha to the von Hippel-Lindau ubiquitylation complex by O2-regulated prolyl hydroxylation, Science 292(5516): 468-472.

Jogi, A., Ora, I. & Nilsson, H. (2002). Hypoxia alters gene expression in human neuroblastoma cells toward an immature and neural crest-like phenotype, Proc Natl Acad Sci U S A 99(10): 7021-7026.

Jope, R. & Johnson, G. (2004). The glamour and gloom of glycogen synthase kinase-3, Trends Biochem Sci 29(2): 95-102.

Kim, B., Kim, S. & Kim, Y. (2004). Forskolin promotes astroglial differentiation of human central neurocytoma cells, Exp Mol Med 36(1): 52-56.

Kimura, M., Hidari, K. & Suzuki, T. (2001). Engagement of endogenous ganglioside GM1a induces tyrosine phosphorylation involved in neuron-like differentiation of PC12 cells, Glycobiology 11(4): 335-343.

Kinjo, K., Kizaki, M. & Muto, A. (2000). Arsenic trioxide (As2O3)-induced apoptosis and differentiation in retinoic acid-resistant acute promyelocytic leukemia model in hGM-CSF-producing transgenic SCID mice, Leukemia 14(3): 431-438.

Lamb, J., Ramaswamy, S. & Ford, H. (2003). A mechanism of cyclin D1 action encoded in the patterns of gene expression in human cancer, Cell 114(3): 323-334.

Leszczyniecka, M., Roberts, T. & Dent, P. (2001). Differentiation therapy of human cancer: basic science and clinical applications, Pharmacol Ther 90(2-3): 105-156.

Li, Y., Yin, W. & Wang, X. (2007). Cholera toxin induces malignant glioma cell differentiation via the PKA/CREB pathway, Proc Natl Acad Sci U S A 104(33): 13438-13443.

Lin, M., Kuo, I. & Chang, C. (2008). Involvement of hypoxia-inducing factor-1alpha-dependent plasminogen activator inhibitor-1 up-regulation in Cyr61/CCN1-induced gastric cancer cell invasion, J Biol Chem 283(23): 15807-15815.

Lu, H., Li, Y. & Shu, M. (2009). Hypoxia-inducible factor-1alpha blocks differentiation of malignant gliomas, FEBS J 276(24): 7291-7304.

Maeda, T., Watanabe, Y. & Kunitomo, H. (1994). Cloning of the pka1 gene encoding the catalytic subunit of the cAMP-dependent protein kinase in Schizosaccharomyces pombe, J Biol Chem 269(13): 9632-9637.

Masco, D., Van de Walle, M. & Spiegel, S. (1991). Interaction of ganglioside GM1 with the B subunit of cholera toxin modulates growth and differentiation of neuroblastoma N18 cells, J Neurosci 11(8): 2443-2452.

Masson, N., Hurst, H. & Lee, K. (1993). Identification of proteins that interact with CREB during differentiation of F9 embryonal carcinoma cells, Nucleic Acids Res 21(11): 1163-1169.

Maxwell, P., Wiesener, M. & Chang, G. (1999). The tumour suppressor protein VHL targets hypoxia-inducible factors for oxygen-dependent proteolysis, Nature 399(6733): 271-275.

Moeller, B., Dreher, M. & Rabbani, Z. (2005). Pleiotropic effects of HIF-1 blockade on tumor radiosensitivity, Cancer Cell 8(2): 99-110.

Moss, J. & Vaughan, M. (1979). Activation of adenylate cyclase by choleragen, Annu Rev Biochem 48: 581-600.

Nurse, P. (2000). A long twentieth century of the cell cycle and beyond, Cell 100(1): 71-78.

Ougolkov, A., Bone, N. & Fernandez-Zapico, M. (2007). Inhibition of glycogen synthase kinase-3 activity leads to epigenetic silencing of nuclear factor kappaB target genes and induction of apoptosis in chronic lymphocytic leukemia B cells, Blood 110(2): 735-742.

Ougolkov, A., Fernandez-Zapico, M. & Savoy, D. (2005). Glycogen synthase kinase-3beta participates in nuclear factor kappaB-mediated gene transcription and cell survival in pancreatic cancer cells, Cancer Res 65(6): 2076-2081.

Pouyssegur, J., Dayan, F. & Mazure, N. (2006). Hypoxia signalling in cancer and approaches to enforce tumour regression, Nature 441(7092): 437-443.

Rankin, E. & Giaccia, A. (2008). The role of hypoxia-inducible factors in tumorigenesis, Cell Death Differ 15(4): 678-685.

Rask, K., Nilsson, A. & Brannstrom, M. (2003). Wnt-signalling pathway in ovarian epithelial tumours: increased expression of beta-catenin and GSK3beta, Br J Cancer 89(7): 1298-1304.

Rong, Y., Durden, D. & Van Meir, E. (2006). 'Pseudopalisading' necrosis in glioblastoma: a familiar morphologic feature that links vascular pathology, hypoxia, and angiogenesis, J Neuropathol Exp Neurol 65(6): 529-539.

Roymans, D., Vissenberg, K. & De Jonghe, C. (2001). Phosphatidylinositol 3-kinase activity is required for the expression of glial fibrillary acidic protein upon cAMP-dependent induction of differentiation in rat C6 glioma, J Neurochem 76(2): 610-618.

Sato, K., Suematsu, A. & Nakashima, T. (2006). Regulation of osteoclast differentiation and function by the CaMK-CREB pathway, Nat Med 12(12): 1410-1416.

Schluter, C., Duchrow, M. & Wohlenberg, C. (1993). The cell proliferation-associated antigen of antibody Ki-67: a very large, ubiquitous nuclear protein with numerous repeated elements, representing a new kind of cell cycle-maintaining proteins, J Cell Biol 123(3): 513-522.

Scott, R. (1997). Differentiation, differentiation/gene therapy and cancer, Pharmacol Ther 73(1): 51-65.

Sell, S. (2004). Stem cell origin of cancer and differentiation therapy, Crit Rev Oncol Hematol 51(1): 1-28.

Semenza, G. (2002). Signal transduction to hypoxia-inducible factor 1, Biochem Pharmacol 64(5-6): 993-998.

Semenza, G. (2003). Targeting HIF-1 for cancer therapy, Nat Rev Cancer 3(10): 721-732.

Shachaf, C., Kopelman, A. & Arvanitis, C. (2004). MYC inactivation uncovers pluripotent differentiation and tumour dormancy in hepatocellular cancer, Nature 431(7012): 1112-1117.

Shen, Z., Chen, G. & Ni, J. (1997). Use of arsenic trioxide (As2O3) in the treatment of acute promyelocytic leukemia (APL): II. Clinical efficacy and pharmacokinetics in relapsed patients, Blood 89(9): 3354-3360.

Sherr, C. & Roberts, J. (1999). CDK inhibitors: positive and negative regulators of G1-phase progression, Genes Dev 13(12): 1501-1512.

Shu, M., Zhou, Y. & Zhu, W. (2011). Activation of a pro-survival pathway IL-6 / JAK2 / STAT3 contributes to glial fibrillary acidic protein induction during the cholera toxin-induced differentiation of C6 malignant glioma cells, Mol Oncol 219: 1-8.

Takanaga, H., Yoshitake, T. & Hara, S. (2004). cAMP-induced astrocytic differentiation of C6 glioma cells is mediated by autocrine interleukin-6, J Biol Chem 279(15): 15441-15447.

Van Kolen, K. & Slegers, H. (2004). P2Y12 receptor stimulation inhibits beta-adrenergic receptor-induced differentiation by reversing the cyclic AMP-dependent inhibition of protein kinase B, J Neurochem 89(2): 442-453.

Walsh, D. & Van Patten, S. (1994). Multiple pathway signal transduction by the cAMP-dependent protein kinase, FASEB J 8(15): 1227-1236.

Wang, Z. & Chen, Z. (2000). Differentiation and apoptosis induction therapy in acute promyelocytic leukaemia, Lancet Oncol 1: 101-106.

Woodgett, J. (1991). cDNA cloning and properties of glycogen synthase kinase-3, Methods Enzymol 200: 564-577.

Yang, M., Wu, M. & Chiou, S. (2008). Direct regulation of TWIST by HIF-1alpha promotes metastasis, Nat Cell Biol 10(3): 295-305.

Yiu, G. & He, Z. (2006). Glial inhibition of CNS axon regeneration, Nat Rev Neurosci 7(8): 617-627.

6

DNA Double-Strand Breaks Repair and Signaling of Human Gliomas and Normal Brain Cells in Response to Radiation: Potential Impact of the ATM- and BRCA1- Dependent Pathways

Adeline Granzotto[1], Zuzana Bencokova[1], Guillaume Vogin[1], Clément Devic[1], Aurélie Joubert[1,2], Jacques Balosso[1,3] and Nicolas Foray[1]
[1]*Inserm, CR-U1052, Centre de Recherche en Cancérologie de Lyon*
[2]*Société Magelis, Cadenet*
[3]*Département de Radiothérapie, CHU de Grenoble*
France

1. Introduction

Deriving from glial, astrocyte, or dendrocyte cells, gliomas are the most frequent tumors of central nervous system. Unfortunately, most of gliomas are refractory to standard radiotherapy treatments. The median survival for patients bearing grade IV gliomas (glioblastomas) does not exceed one year even after both aggressive surgery and radiotherapy treatment (Behin et al., 2003). A standard of 60 Gy delivered in 30 fractions during six weeks remains the best radiotherapy modality against gliomas (Behin et al., 2003). This last conclusion raises the possibility that human gliomas might be generally more radioresistant than other tumor tissues. However, there is no consensus in literature about a specific radioresistance of human gliomas. Besides, the complexity of the molecular and cellular features of radiation response and the difficulty to define reliable endpoints to account for radiosensitivity whatever the tissue type may have limited the extent of some reports. In addition, three specific features of radiobiology of gliomas can be also evoked:

- cellular *in vitro* endpoints like clonogenic survival seem to be less appropriate to predict gliomas radiocurability than that of other tumour types (Taghian et al., 1992, 1993);
- animal models extensively used in glioma research may not reflect specificities of human gliomas and may bias in anti-glioma strategies (Holland, 2001);
- DNA repair capacity of gliomas is poorly documented and most of the investigations about genes mutations concern actors of proliferation rather than upstream DNA repair proteins (Zhu & Parada, 2002).

In 2004, our group obtained the most protracted survival of rats bearing radioresistant rodent gliomas by using synchrotron X-rays combined with *intracerebral* cisplatin injection. Such so-called PAT-plat treatment triggers the photoactivation of platinum atoms and produces some additional DNA double-strand breaks (DSBs) at the vicinity of cisplatin-induced DNA adducts (Biston et al., 2004). The severity of PAT-Plat-induced DSBs was shown to be due to the inhibition of the major DSB repair pathway in mammalians, namely

the non-homologous end-joining (NHEJ) process (Biston et al., 2004; Corde et al., 2003). NHEJ is required for cell viability and its inhibition has been shown to be systematically linked to radiosensitivity. This DSB repair pathway is dependent on the ATM kinase activity that may be considered as the major DNA-breaking stress signaling pathway in mammalians. The inhibition of NHEJ may be rescued by other repair pathways, like the RAD51- and/or MRE11-dependent recombination process (Dudas and Chovanec, 2004; Joubert et al., 2008). Interestingly, these last two recombination pathways were shown to require a functional BRCA1 protein, a tumor suppressor whose mutations are responsible for inherited breast cancers (Scully et al., 1997). BRCA1 is a phosphorylation substrate of ATM kinase and also required for a normal response to radiation and to alkylating agents. Consequently, tumors showing impaired BRCA1 were supposed to be sensitive to the PAT-Plat effect described above and to a number of chemotherapy drugs like cisplatin (Bhattacharyya et al., 2000; Corde et al., 2003).
In the particular case of preclinical anti-glioma radio-chemotherapy trials, the most extensively used modalities are based on syngenic rat models subjected to intracranial inoculation of non-imunogenic cell lines. This is notably the case of the C6, 9L, F98 rodent glioma cell lines. However, that all these rat glioma models are induced by N-nitrosmethylurea (NMU) or Ethylnitrosourea (ENU) -mediated mutagenesis ; which may condition their response to stress (Table 1). Since the choice of rodent glioma models is mainly motivated to date by the existence of previous raw data in the lab, their proliferation capacity in culture and/or in animals and their non-immunogenic properties, it may introduce some biases in data interpretation.

Cell line	Tumour type	Mutagen	P53 status	p16/CDKn2a/ Ink4	BRCA1 localisation after X-rays	Depositor
C6	Gliosarcoma	MNU, repetitive dose	Wild type	*Mutated*	Cytoplasm	(Benda et al., 1968)
9L	Gliosarcoma	MNU, repetitive dose	*Mutated*	*Wild type*	Nuclear	(Benda et al., 1968)
F98	Anaplastic glioma	ENU, single dose	Mutated	*Mutated*	Weak	(Wechsler et al., 1972)

Table 1. Origin and biological features of the major rodent glioma cell lines

In 2008, to evaluate the impact of the choice of a rat glioma models in a study dealing with radio- or chemotherapy, cell death pathways, cell cycle arrests, DNA repair and stress signalling were examined in response to radiation and cisplatin in C6, 9L and F98 models (Bencokova et al., 2008). Rodent glioma models showed a large spectrum of cellular radiation response. Surprisingly, BRCA1 was found to be functionally impaired in C6 and F98 favouring genomic instability, tumour heterogeneity and tolerance of unrepaired DNA damage. Furthermore, since BRCA1 acts as a tumor suppressor in a number of malignancies, our findings raise also the question of the implication of BRCA1 in brain tumors formation (Bencokova et al., 2008).

The importance of DSB repair and signaling proteins in the radiation response prompted us to investigate the radiobiological features of a number of human brain tumors, notably the activity of the NHEJ and the BRCA1-dependent pathways, in order to propose molecular assays to predict the response of gliomas to anti-cancer treatments. Some recent conceptual and technical advances in the DSB repair field have motivated such approach: 1) the importance of the potential interplay existing between the two major DSB repair pathways, NHEJ and recombination that may condition the final response to radiation (Joubert et al., 2008); 2) the existence of a temporal hierarchy between ATM- and BRCA1-dependent phosphorylation events occurring after irradiation and conditioning cell cycle arrests and cell death pathways (Foray et al., 2003); 3) the fact that immunofluorescence permits to date the quantification of the DSB induced by radiation inside each cell nucleus via biomarkers that are specific to one particular step of DSB repair and signaling. This is notably the case of γ-H2AX that is the sensor of DSB managed by NHEJ and may serve as a marker of NHEJ activity (Joubert et al., 2008; Rothkamm & Lobrich, 2003). In 2011, by having accumulated a number of immunofluorescence data in response to 2 Gy X-rays in about 200 human normal and tumor cell lines, we propose a molecular model of radiation response in which the nucleo-shuttling of active ATM forms stimulates NHEJ and inhibits exacerbated nuclease activity of MRE11 responsible for genomic instability. BRCA1 is one of the major ATM phosphorylation substrate involved in this model (Granzotto et al., 2011, submitted) (Fig. 1). Hence, in this work, we have systematically examined the γ-H2AX, ATM and BRCA1 response of 13 human glioma cell lines and 6 normal brain tissues to X-rays.

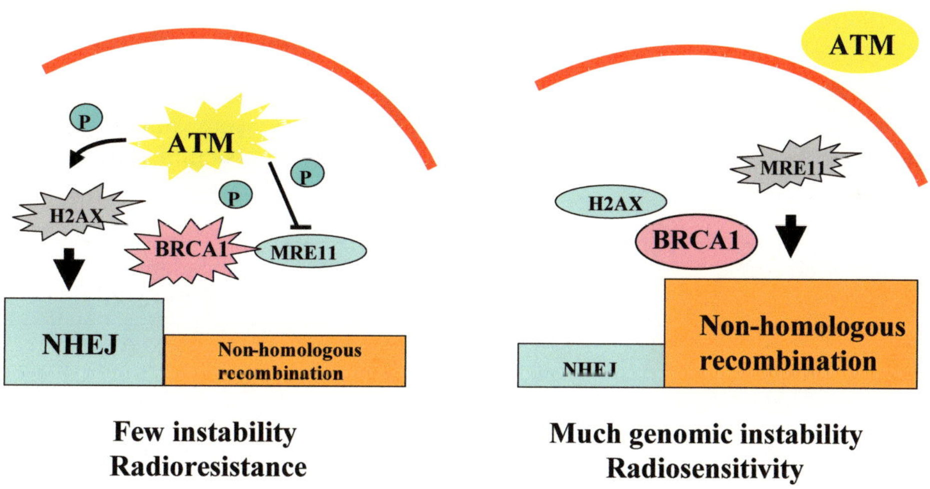

Fig. 1. Model for describing the radiation-induced ATM nucleo-shuttling

2. Materials and methods

2.1 Cell lines

Human glioma cell lines detailed in Table 2 are provided from adult donors and are purchased by commercial collections such as ATCC. They were routinely cultured as monolayers with Dulbecco's modified Eagle's minimum medium (DMEM) (Gibco-Invitrogen-France, Cergy-Pontoise, France), supplemented with 20% fetal calf serum and antibiotics.

Cell line	Tumour type	Donor age	BRCA1 functional status
SW1783 (HTB 13)	Glioblastoma astrocytoma	68	nd
U87MG (HTB 14)	Glioblastoma astrocytoma	44	+
U118MG (HTB 15)	Glioblastoma astrocytoma	50	-
U138MG (HTB 16)	Glioblastoma astrocytoma	47	-
U373MG (HTB17)	Glioblastoma astrocytoma	nd	+/-
LN229	Glioblastoma $PTEN^{+/+}$	60	+/-
CCF-STTG1	Astrocytoma	68	-
MO59J	Glioblastoma	33	+
U251	Glioblastoma $PTEN^{-/-}$	nd	nd
T98G	Glioblastoma multiforme	61	-
GHD	Glioblastoma	nd	nd
CB193	Glioblastoma	nd	-
SF767	Glioblastoma multiforme	nd	nd

Table 2. Human glioma cell lines used in this study and their BRCA1 functional status

Normal human brain cells detailed in Table 3 are provided from fetal brain and purchased by Sciencell Research Laboratories (Carlsbad, CA, USA). They were routinely cultured as monolayers with medium, serum and growth complement recommended by Science Research Laboratories.

Cell line	Cell type and brain localization	Sciencell Reference
HA	Astrocytes - cortex	#1800
HAc	Astrocytes - cerebellum	#1810
Hsc	Schwann cells	#1700
Hah	Astrocytes - hippocampal	#1830
HMC	Meningeal cells	#1400
Hasp	Astrocytes – spinal cord	#1820

Table 3. Human normal cell lines used in this study and their origin

2.2 Irradiation

An orthovoltage X-ray clinical irradiator was used to perform all the irradiations. It is described elsewhere (Joubert et al., 2005). The dose-rate was approximately 1.234 $Gy.min^{-1}$.

All the experiments were performed on cells at plateau phase of growth to avoid any bias due to cell cycle.

2.3 Immunoblottings

Preparation of nuclear extracts, immunoblotting were performed using protocols published elsewhere (Foray et al., 2003). Anti-*pBRCA1*^{ser1423} (Upstate Biotechnology-Euromedex) and anti-*BRCA1* antibodies (Santa Cruz, CA, USA) were used at 1:1000 dilution.

2.4 Immunofluorescence

Immunofluorescence protocol was described elsewhere (Foray et al., 2003). Cells were fixed in paraformaldehyde and permeabilized for 5 min at 4°C. Anti-*γ-H2AX*^{ser139} antibody was purchased from Upstate Biotechnology-Euromedex, Mundolsheim, France) and used at 1:800. Anti-*pATM*^{ser1981} (Abcam, Cambridge, UK), anti-*pBRCA1*^{ser1423} (Upstate Biotechnology-Euromedex) and anti-*BRCA1* antibodies (Santa Cruz, Tebu-Bio, Le Perray, France) were used at 1:100 dilution. Incubations with anti-mouse TRITC or with anti-rabbit FITC secondary antibodies (Sigma-Aldrich) (dilution at 1:100) were performed at 37°C in 2% BSA for 20 min. Nuclei were counterstained by 4,6-Diamidino-2-phenylindole (DAPI) (Sigma-Aldrich) for 10 min. Coverslips were mounted in Vectashield (Abcys, Paris, France) and examined with an Olympus fluorescence microscope. Fifty nuclei per condition were analyzed. DAPI staining permitted also to indirectly evaluate yield of G_1 cells (nuclei with homogeneous DAPI staining), S cells (nuclei showing numerous γ-H2AX foci), G_2 cells (nuclei with heterogeneous DAPI staining) and metaphase (visible chromosomes) (Joubert et al., 2008). It is noteworthy that in our conditions, the ATM and DNA-PK kinases that phosphorylate the H2AX histones require some minutes post-irradiation to be fully active. Consequently, the earliest time post-irradiation was fixed at 10 min, in agreement with previous reports (Joubert et al., 2008). The quantification of foci was performed by eye-scoring and verified by semi-automatic scoring Cell^F software from Soft Imaging System GmbH (Münster, Germany) that permits to quantify nuclei and foci size.

3. Results

3.1 Glioma cell lines elicit a wide range of radiation-induced DSB repair capacity

In a previous report, we have shown that the number of unrepaired DSB assessed 24 h after 2 Gy is quantitatively correlated with intrinsic radiosensitivity reflected by clonogenic cell survival at 2 Gy (SF2) (Joubert et al., 2008). As a first step, we focused therefore on the DSB repair capacity of the human gliomas by using *anti-* γ-H2AX immunofluorescence. Glioma models described a continuous range of responses between 2 to 58% of unrepaired DSBs, corresponding to an SF2 range of 80 to 2%, respectively (Fig. 2). In agreement with previous reports, MO59J cells exhibited one of the most severe human DSB repair deficiency (Chavaudra et al., 2004; Lees-Miller et al., 1995) (Fig. 2).

By taking into account survival data available in literature (Joiner et al., 2001), our findings were in agreement with a general correlation between SF2 and unrepaired DSBs obtained from 20 human tumour cell lines (Chavaudra et al., 2004). Here, the human glioma cell lines tested describe therefore a wide range of NHEJ repair capacity and radiosensitivity that does not suggest a global tendency to radioresistance for brain tumor cells. Interestingly, the average DSB repair rate of human radioresistant skin fibroblasts appears to be systematically faster than that of the glioma cell lines tested here.

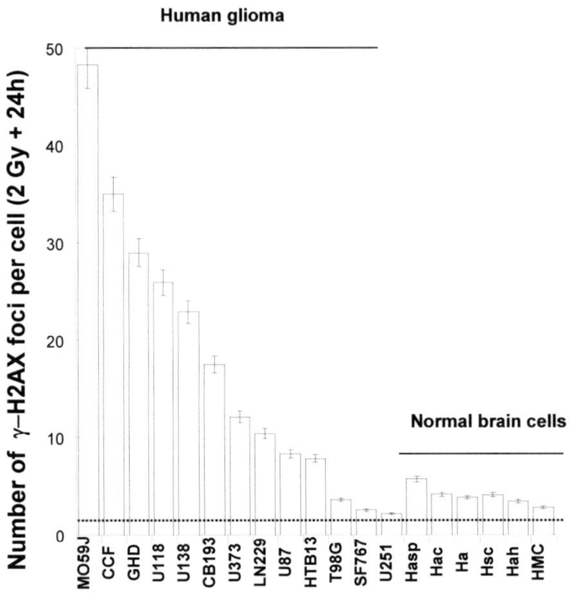

Fig. 2. Number of γ-H2AX foci assessed 24 h after 2 Gy X-rays in the indicated human tumour and normal brain cell lines. Data shown are the mean ± standard error of 3 independent replicates, at least. Dotted cell lines indicated the average corresponding value of γ-H2AX foci for radioresistant skin fibroblasts published elsewhere (Joubert et al., 2008).

3.2 Most glioma cell lines elicit impaired radiation-induced ATM kinase activity

Since phosphorylation of γ-H2AX requires the ATM kinase activity, cell lines were also subjected to immunofluorescence with antibodies against the autophosphorylated forms of ATM (pATM) (Bakkenist and Kastan, 2003). Very few pATM foci were observed constitutively, suggesting a moderate ATM kinase activity in all the glioma models (data not shown). MO59J elicited a marked delay in the radiation-induced ATM activation, likely due to its ATM mutations (Tsuchida et al., 2002). Although the other cell lines exhibited a various number of pATM foci at 10 min post-irradiation ranging from about 1 to 70 pATM foci per cell, the great majority of them show a ATM kinase activity at 10 min post-irradiation that is abnormally lower than radioresistant skin fibroblasts (Fig. 3).

3.3 Most glioma cells elicit impaired radiation-induced BRCA1 phosphorylation

Ionizing radiation cause BRCA1 phosphorylation, visible by a protein migration shift (Scully et al., 1997a,b). Among 13 glioma cell lines of the collection, 8 were subjected to anti-*BRCA1* immunoblots. Our results revealed that BRCA1 migrated at the expected size for all the cell lines. However, BRCA1 appeared differentially expressed: U138 and U373 elicited the weakest spontaneous BRCA1 expression and U87, MO59J and GHD the highest one (Fig. 4). Only 3 (MO59J, U87, GHD) among 8 irradiated cell lines showed the typical shift of BRCA1 phosphorylation, suggesting that the functional BRCA1 status is impaired in the great majority of glioma cell lines. U373 and LN229 showed a second band above BRCA1 that seemed too high to represent any BRCA1 phosphorylation signal (Fig. 4).

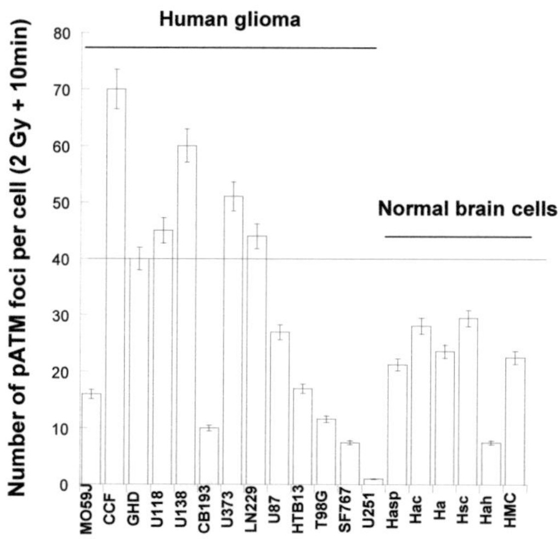

Fig. 3. Number of pATM foci assessed 10 min after 2 Gy X-rays in the indicated human tumour and normal brain cell lines. Data shown are the mean ± standard error of 3 independent replicates, at least. Dotted cell lines indicated the average corresponding value of pATM foci for radioresistant skin fibroblasts obtained in our lab (Granzotto et al., submitted).

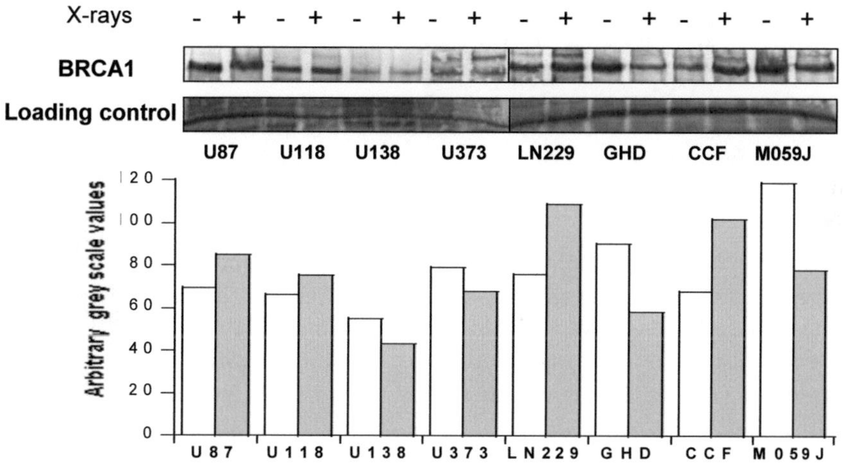

Fig. 4. Representative example of anti-*BRCA1* immunoblots of nuclear extracts from the indicated human cells exposed to 15 Gy followed by 4 h for repair. Expression of BRCA1 was quantified by grey scale analysis in arbitrary units.

In agreement with anti-*BRCA1* immunoblots, only MO59J, U87, GHD elicited radiation-induced BRCA1 foci. It is however noteworthy that some cell lines exhibit spontaneous BRCA1 foci likely due to S-G2/M phase, consistent with the findings that radiation and cell cycle triggers the phosphorylation of different BRCA1 serine residues (Bakkenist & Kastan, 2003; Gatei et al., 2000; Xu et al., 2001) (Fig. 5A). Immunofluorescence with antibodies against the phosphorylated BRCA1 Ser^{1423} ($pBRCA1^{ser1423}$) was performed, as well. Again, only MO59J, U87, GHD exhibited positive $pBRCA1^{ser1423}$ signals (Fig. 5B). Altogether, these findings suggest that BRCA1 is functionally impaired in the majority (5/8) of human glioma models in response to radiation. It must be reminded that functional BRCA1 impairments are due either to *BRCA1* mutations or to the absence of BRCA1 protein partners, like RAD51 (Scully et al., 1997a,b). Particularly, all the cell lines exhibited RAD51 foci whether spontaneously (in S/G2M) after irradiation (data not shown). Hence, BRCA1 impairments were observed in the majority of human glioma models, independently of their RAD51 activity.

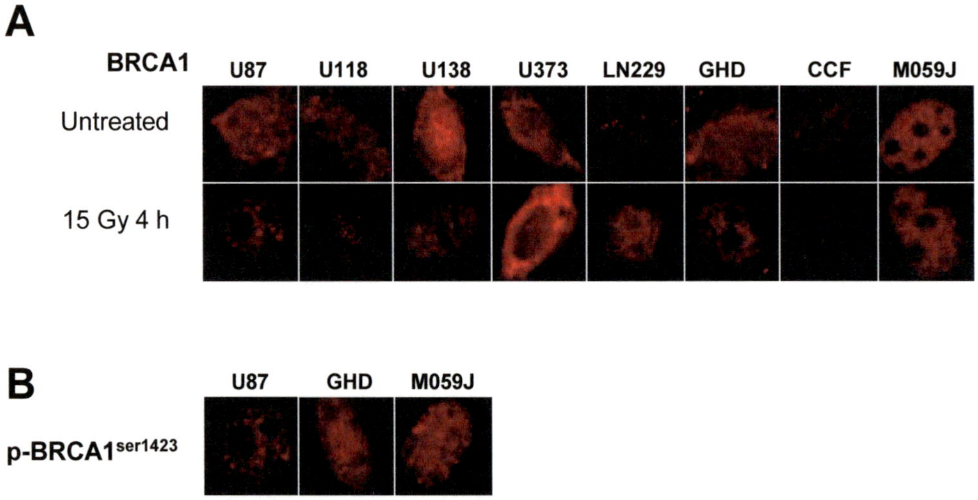

Fig. 5. A. Anti-*BRCA1* immunofluorescence applied to the indicated cell lines after 15 Gy X-rays followed by 4 h for repair. B. Representative examples of $pBRCA1^{ser1423}$ signals obtained in U87, GHD and M059J cell lines in the same conditions.

3.4 Normal brain cells elicit a wide range of radiation-induced DSB repair capacity

Human brain cells showed few residual γ-H2AX foci after 2 Gy followed by 24 h for repair, suggesting a larger radioresistance than the human glioma cell lines tested (Fig.2). However, inside the normal brain cells group, there is no significant difference between the brain localizations tested (Fig.2). Conversely, the yields of γ-H2AX foci of human astrocytes are systematically higher than radioresistant fibroblasts ($p<0.02$) (Fig. 2).

3.5 Normal brain cells elicit impaired radiation-induced ATM kinase activity

In order to investigate further the radiobiological features of human normal brain cells, we assessed the number of pATM foci 10 min post-irradiation. Normal human brain cells exhibited significantly less γ-H2AX foci 10 min post-irradiation than radioresistant fibroblasts ($p=0.01$), suggesting that ATM-dependent DSB recognition is slightly impaired in normal brain cells (Fig. 3). The measured ATM kinase activity in normal human brain cells lead to a lack of recognition of about 10 to 30 DSB at the dose of 2 Gy, corresponding to about 12.5 to 37.5% of radiation-induced DSB, respectively. Again, no significant difference was observed between the brain localizations tested.

3.6 Normal brain cells elicit impaired radiation-induced BRCA1 phosphorylation

In our attempts to investigate the functional status of BRCA1 in response to radiation, we have systematically observed a very weak BRCA1 and pBRCA1 signals in all the normal brain cells, whatever the conditions, suggesting a significant impairment of the functional status of this protein (data not shown). It is noteworthy that even in the rare normal brain cells observed in S or G2/M phase, the yield of BRCA1 foci was negligible.

3.7 Intercomparisons between human glioma and normal brain cells

In order to compare glioma and normal brain cells data, we plotted, for all the cell lines tested, the number of γ-H2AX foci per cell assessed 24 h post-irradiation (that is an indicator of radiosensitivity) against the number of pATM foci assessed 10 min post-irradiation (that is an indicator of the early ATM kinase activity in response to radiation) (Fig. 6).

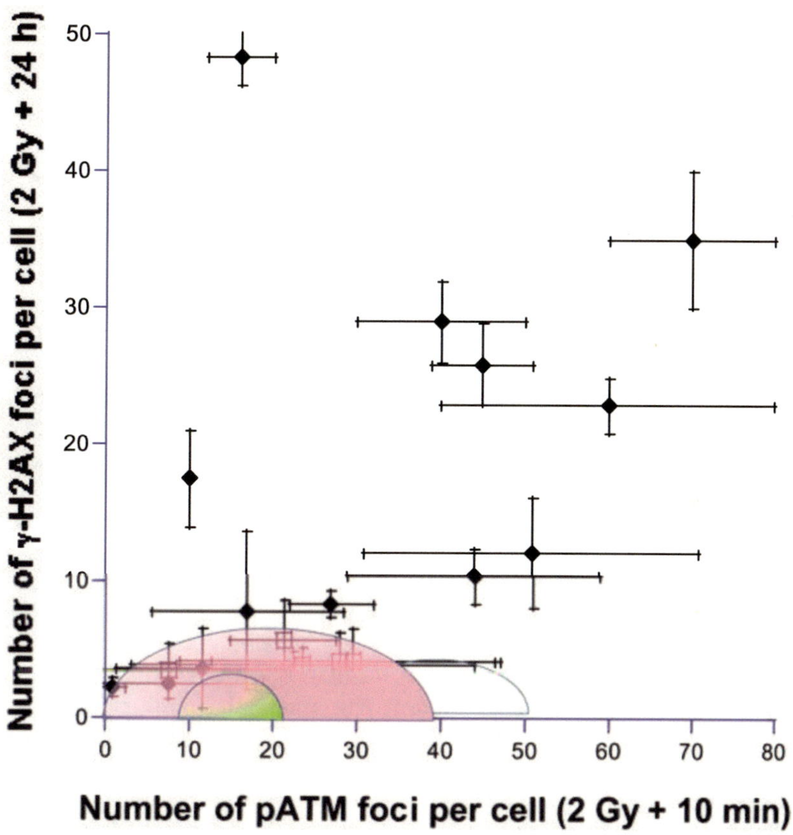

Fig. 6. Number of residual γ-H2AX foci per cell as a function of the corresponding number of pATM foci per cell for all the human glioma (closed losanges) and normal brain cells (open squares) described in this report. All the foci data are shown in Fig. 1 and 2 as histogram. Each plot is represented by the mean ± standard error of 3 independent replicates, at least. Blue and pink confidence zones correspond to the values from human primary fibroblasts belonging to the radiosensitivity group I and II, respectively (see Discussion). Green confidence zone corresponds to values from the C6, 9L and F98 rodent glioma cells.

The fig. 6 clearly shows that the normal brain cells tested here are more DSB repair deficient with a lower ATM kinase activity than the most radioresistant skin fibroblasts. Conversely, the normal brain cells may belong to a group of cells characterized by a moderate but significant radiosensitivity associated with genomic instability. With regard to the glioma cells, they covered all the range of DSB repair and ATM kinase activity, likely due to their intrinsic instability. Interestingly, the γ-H2AX and pATM values from the C6, 9L and F98 rodent glioma cells correspond to a very restricted genetic conditions that are not representative of human glioma.

4. Discussion

4.1 New advances in DSB repair models

As evoked in the Introduction chapter, it has been demonstrated that radiation-induced DSB can be determined from the number of nuclear foci formed by the phosphorylation of the variant histone H2AX and easily quantifiable using immunofluorescence (Rothkamm & Lobrich, 2003). Although successfully tested in hyper-radiosensitive cells and presented as powerful predictive assay, some preliminary data showed us that *γ-H2*AX immunofluorescence does not necessarily predict the whole range of human radiosensitivity. Recently, unlike the majority of studies focusing on mutations of one single gene, we have deliberately chosen to extend our investigations to the largest spectrum of radiosensitivity possible with human cells, independently of gene mutations. The relationship between cellular radiosensitivity and DSB repair data was examined in a collection of 40 non-transformed human fibroblasts representing at least 8 different genetic syndromes (Joubert et al., 2008). The systematic application of the most extensively used molecular assays, namely immunofluorescence, PFGE and plasmid assays allowed us to propose a quantitative correlation between molecular and cellular radiosensitivity that is relevant for all mammalian cells: survival fraction at 2 Gy (SF2) was found to be inversely proportional to the amount of unrepaired DSB, whatever the genes mutations and the assays applied.

Form this correlation, a classification of genetic diseases associated with cellular radiosensitivity in 3 groups was also proposed in our recent study (Joubert et al., 2008): group I: radioresistance; group II: moderate radiosensitivity and high cancer proneness; group III: hyper-radiosensitivity. Obviously, the definition of these three groups tentatively proposed is provisional and is conditioned to the extension of additional cell lines in our systematic study of human radiosensitivity. A number of other biomarkers and tissue types have to be investigated to better document the molecular and cellular bases of this classification: this is notably the case of ATM, BRCA1, DNA-PK, 53BP1 and NBS1 proteins, all involved in the radiation response and of brain, breast, prostate tissues, all involved in the most frequent cancers.

Our results show that human glioma may exhibit a very wide range of radiosensitivity and may be characterized by impaired radiation-induced ATM kinase activity and BRCA1 phosphorylation. Normal brain cells share with gliomas these last two features. Conversely, can these results suggest that impaired ATM kinase activity and BRCA1 phosphorylation are specific to brain cells, whether normal or not?

4.2 Role of ATM in the radiation response of the brain

Ataxia telangiectasia (AT) is caused by homozygous ATM mutations and is a rare autosomal dominant syndrome associated with the highest radiosensitivity in humans (McKinnon,

1987). AT is a neurodegenerative disease. The prominent neurological sign of AT is an inexorable loss of cerebellar function, cerebellar atrophy, especially in vermal regions and loss of Purkinje cells (Lavin, 2008; McKinnon, 1987; Taylor et al., 1994). The role of ATM in brain cells and the dramatic consequences of its deletion or inhibition is well-documented but studies mianly concern rodent models. For example, it has been shown recently that cell populations in the Atm-/- central nervous system may be radioresistant (Gosink et al., 1999). To define specific radiosensitivities of neural populations, Gosink et al. (1999) have analyzed Atm-/- astrocytes and showed that Atm-/- astrocytes exhibit premature senescence, express constitutively high levels of p21, and have impaired p53 stabilization. However, in contrast to radiosensitive Atm-/- fibroblasts and radioresistant Atm-/- neurons, radiosensitivity of Atm-/- astrocytes was similar to wild-type astrocytes (Gosink et al., 1999).
By contrast, studies about the role of ATM on normal brain cells are more rare but also dominated by rodent models. For example, Soares et al. (1998) have shown that Atm expression during mouse development was highest in the embryonic mouse nervous system, where it was predominantly associated with regions undergoing mitosis. During the period of Purkinje cell neurogenesis, Atm was highly expressed in the area containing Purkinje cell precursors. However, in the postnatal cerebellum, Atm expression in Purkinje cells was very low, while expression in proliferating granule neurons was high. The only region of the adult nervous system that exhibited elevated Atm expression were the postmitotic sensory neurons of the dorsal root ganglia (Soares et al., 1998). Their data suggest an early developmental requirement for ATM in the cerebellum, and other regions of the central nervous system, but a global decrease of ATM expression.
Here, our data suggest that cytoplasmic ATM kinase activity in human brain cells is endogenously lower than in fibroblasts. According to our molecular model described in Fig. 1, normal brain cells may be a bit more radiosensitive to primary fibroblasts but overall more proned to radiation-induced genomic instability. Hence, while human glioma cells may exhibit a wide range of X-rays response, the fact that normal brain cells surrounding tumors may be radiosensitive should lead to cautiousness about the clinical transfer of anti-glioma radiotherapies.

4.3 Response of brain to radiation and gliomagenesis : Importance of BRCA1

BRCA1 is a phosphorylation substrate of ATM. Hence, if ATM kinase is naturally less active in normal brain cells, it is logical to observe impaired BRCA1 phosphorylation in normal brain cells. BRCA1 is an interesting protein in carcinogenesis because of its involvement in both breast cancers and DNA repair (Foray et al., 1999; Huen et al., 2010). Furthermore, its role is very important in chemotherapy since this protein is required for a normal response to alkylating agents (Bhattacharyya et al., 2000; Corde et al., 2003). However, up to date, nothing has really related BRCA1 to brain tumors. In 2008, our systematic radiobiological analysis of pointed out the possibility that BRCA1 may be not functional in rodent glioma models whose majority was induced by nitrosourea treatment. Interestingly, a paper published in 2003 presented ENU mutagenesis as an interesting tool to produce knockout rats, and especially BRCA1 and BRCA2 mutants (Zan et al., 2003). Hence, BRCA1 impairments in rodent glioma models may not have the same origin than those observed in human gliomas. This remark raises therefore the question of the relevance of the use of chemo-induced tumours in preclinical trials. This question is inasmuch important as Fig.6 shows that radiobiological features of rodent glioma models are not representative of those of human gliomas.

There were considerable advances in the investigations on gliomas-specific molecular markers. However, the great majority of them generally focus on actors of proliferation. A number of loss of heterozygosity have been reported in gliomas but there is still no consensus for any specific molecular signature (Bredel et al., 2005; Zhu & Parada, 2002). Very few concerned p53 and BRCA1. Loss of p53 and activation of growth factor receptor tyrosine kinase signalling pathway initiates tumour formation whereas disruption of RB pathway contributes to the progression of tumour development (Bredel et al., 2005; Zhu & Parada, 2002). However, the great majority of targeted proteins that act in the proliferation process, are partners of BRCA1 but are mainly *gatekeepers* than *caretakers* like BRCA1. This is notably the case of the p16/Cdkn2a/Ink4a whose homozygous deletions have been observed in C6 and F98 but not in 9L rodent glioma models (Bencokova et al., 2008). The p16/Cdkn2a/Ink4a protein belongs to the BRCA1-dependent cascade of stress-induced events, was shown to co-precipitate with BRCA1, and phosphorylate it at serine 1497 in response to cell cycle progression and DNA damage (Ruffner et al., 1999). Recently, it appears that BRCA1-negative cells show high p16/Cdkn2a/Ink4a cyclin-dependent kinase activity and that are 2- to 4-fold more sensitive to CDK inhibitors (Deans et al., 2004). Hence, the p16/Cdkn2a/Ink4a deletions found in C6 and F98 but not in 9L, together with our findings that BRCA1 is functionally impaired in C6 and F98 but not in 9L, suggest a model in which ATM- and p16/Cdkn2a/Ink4a-dependent may interplay with BRCA1.
To date, two major models of glioblastomas formation are proposed: glioma generation would be mediated either by genomic instability and uncontrolled differentiation or by rapid transformation of some pre-existing neural stem cells (Zhu & Parada, 2002). BRCA1 impairments are rather consistent with a glioma generation facilitated by genomic instability. Impaired BRCA1 may notably contribute to the lack of control of tyrosine kinase pathways that exacerbate cellular proliferation (Foray et al., 2002). Our findings raised the question of the implication of this protein in the tumorigenicity of brain tumours as well. Such assumption is supported by the fact that BRCA1 tumor suppressor activity is not necessarily restricted to inherited breast and/or ovarian cancer (Rosen et al., 2005). Notably, adenovirus experiments pointed out the potential role of BRCA1 in lung and colon malignancies (Marot et al., 2006). Our data suggest therefore that, in addition to an endogenously low ATM kinase activity that would be specific to brain cells and may lead to a reduced BRCA1 function, gliomagenesis may be facilitated by mutations in proteins partners of a complex including BRCA1.

5. Conclusions

Radiobiological investigations on extensively used rodent models have revealed that nitrosourea-directed mutagenesis may select particular mutations of BRCA1 genes that can be at the origin of the glioma formation. This BRCA1 mutation and impairment has some consequences on the radiation response but overall on the chemo-response of rodent glioma. Hence, rodent glioma models may not be representative of the human glioma models. Once the role of BRCA1 has been pointed out, the observation that radiation-induced phosphorylation of BRCA1 is also impaired in the majority of human glioma models provides clues that :

- this tumour suppressor gene may be involved in gliomagenesis
- upstream partner proteins like ATM may be involved in gliomagenesis, as well
- downstream partner poteines like p16 or p53 may be indirectly used a glioma markers.

In parallel, human normal brain cells appeared impaired in the radiation-induced ATM kinase activity, suggesting an endogenous specificity of brain cells by comparison to other tissues like skin. Since a lower ATM kinase activity and/or expression logically lead to impaired BRCA1 phosphorylation, our data suggest that brain may be more sensitive to tumour formation than other tissue for stress requiring the ATM and BRCA1-dependent pathways (Fig.7).
Our results may also provide interesting elements for anti-glioma strategies. Indeed, since BRCA1 is required for the response to alkylating agents, radio-chemotherapy with platinated agents may be one of the approaches compatible with our findings. Obviously, further molecular and cellular investigations with a larger number of cell lines may consolidate this working hypothesis.

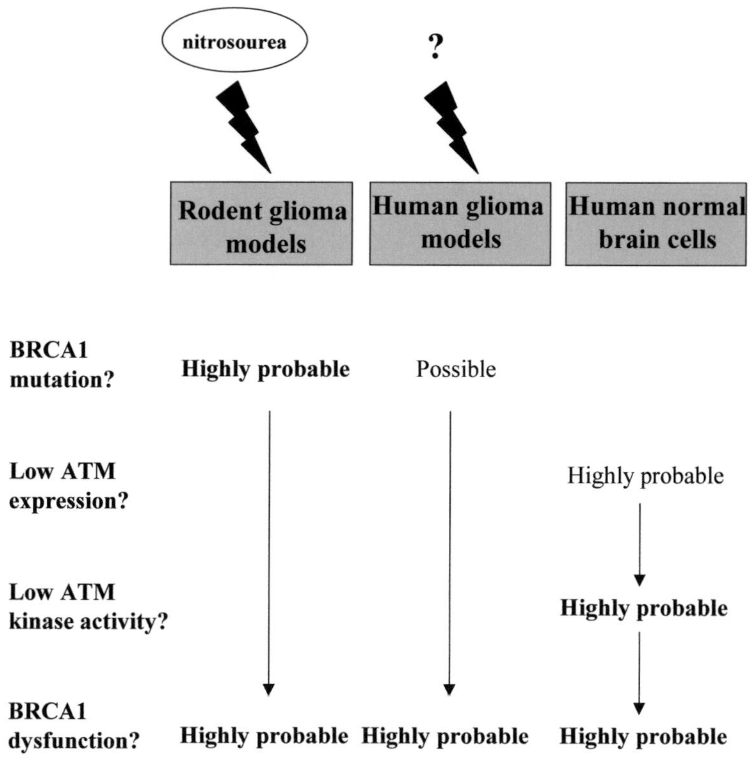

Fig. 7. Schematic recapitulation of our observation. Bold expressions represent the first experimental observations.

6. Acknowledgments

We would like to thank Drs E.P Malaise and V. Favaudon for fruitful discussions. Z.B. is a PhD fellowship of Roche-France. This work was also supported by the Institut National du Cancer (INCA) (GRRAAL Project), the Association Pour la Recherche sur l'Ataxie-Telangiectasie (APRAT), the Association pour la Recherche contre le Cancer (ARC), the Electricité de France, the Ligue contre le Cancer (Comité de la Savoie), the ETOILE hadrontherapy project and the Region Rhone-Alpes.

7. References

Bakkenist, C. J. and Kastan, M. B. (2003). DNA damage activates ATM through intermolecular autophosphorylation and dimer dissociation. *Nature* 421, 499-506.

Behin, A., Hoang-Xuan, K., Carpentier, A. F. and Delattre, J. Y. (2003). Primary brain tumours in adults. *Lancet* 361, 323-31.

Bencokova, Z., Pauron, L., Devic, C., Joubert, A., Gastaldo, J., Massart, C., Balosso, J. and Foray, N. (2008). Molecular and cellular response of the most extensively used rodent glioma models to radiation and/or cisplatin. *J Neurooncol* 86, 13-21.

Benda, P., Lightbody, J., Sato, G., Levine, L. and Sweet, W. (1968). Differentiated rat glial cell strain in tissue culture. *Science* 161, 370-1.

Bhattacharyya, A., Ear, U. S., Koller, B. H., Weichselbaum, R. R. and Bishop, D. K. (2000). The breast cancer susceptibility gene BRCA1 is required for subnuclear assembly of Rad51 and survival following treatment with the DNA cross-linking agent cisplatin. *J Biol Chem* 275, 23899-903.

Biston, M. C., Joubert, A., Adam, J. F., Elleaume, H., Bohic, S., Charvet, A. M., Esteve, F., Foray, N. and Balosso, J. (2004). Cure of Fisher rats bearing radioresistant F98 glioma treated with cis-platinum and irradiated with monochromatic synchrotron X-rays. *Cancer Res* 64, 2317-23.

Bredel, M., Bredel, C., Juric, D., Harsh, G. R., Vogel, H., Recht, L. D. and Sikic, B. I. (2005). High-resolution genome-wide mapping of genetic alterations in human glial brain tumors. *Cancer Res* 65, 4088-96.

Chavaudra, N., Bourhis, J. and Foray, N. (2004). Quantified relationship between cellular radiosensitivity, DNA repair defects and chromatin relaxation: a study of 19 human tumour cell lines from different origin. *Radiother Oncol* 73, 373-82.

Corde, S., Balosso, J., Elleaume, H., Renier, M., Joubert, A., Biston, M. C., Adam, J. F., Charvet, A. M., Brochard, T., Le Bas, J. F. et al. (2003). Synchrotron photoactivation of cisplatin elicits an extra number of DNA breaks that stimulate RAD51-mediated repair pathways. *Cancer Res* 63, 3221-7.

Deans, A. J., Simpson, K. J., Trivett, M. K., Brown, M. A. and McArthur, G. A. (2004). Brca1 inactivation induces p27(Kip1)-dependent cell cycle arrest and delayed development in the mouse mammary gland. *Oncogene* 23, 6136-45.

Dudas, A. and Chovanec, M. (2004). DNA double-strand break repair by homologous recombination. *Mutat Res* 566, 131-67.

Foray, N., Marot, D., Gabriel, A., Randrianarison, V., Carr, A. M., Perricaudet, M., Ashworth, A. and Jeggo, P. (2003). A subset of ATM- and ATR-dependent phosphorylation events requires the BRCA1 protein. *Embo J* 22, 2860-71.

Foray, N., Marot, D., Randrianarison, V., Venezia, N. D., Picard, D., Perricaudet, M., Favaudon, V. and Jeggo, P. (2002). Constitutive association of BRCA1 and c-Abl and its ATM-dependent disruption after irradiation. *Mol Cell Biol* 22, 4020-32.

Foray, N., Randrianarison, V., Marot, D., Perricaudet, M., Lenoir, G. and Feunteun, J. (1999). Gamma-rays-induced death of human cells carrying mutations of BRCA1 or BRCA2. *Oncogene* 18, 7334-42.

Gatei, M., Young, D., Cerosaletti, K. M., Desai-Mehta, A., Spring, K., Kozlov, S., Lavin, M. F., Gatti, R. A., Concannon, P. and Khanna, K. (2000). ATM-dependent phosphorylation of nibrin in response to radiation exposure. *Nat Genet* 25, 115-9.

Gosink, E. C., Chong, M. J. and McKinnon, P. J. (1999). Ataxia telangiectasia mutated deficiency affects astrocyte growth but not radiosensitivity. *Cancer Res* 59, 5294-8.

Granzotto, A., Joubert, A., Viau, M., Devic, C., Maalouf, M., Thomas, C., Vogin, G., Malek, K., Colin, C., Balosso, J. et al. (2011). Individual response to ionising radiation: what predictive assay(s) to choose? *Comptes Rendus de l'Académie des Sciences,* in press.

Holland, E. C. (2001). Brain tumor animal models: importance and progress. *Curr Opin Oncol* 13, 143-7.

Huen, M. S., Sy, S. M. and Chen, J. (2010). BRCA1 and its toolbox for the maintenance of genome integrity. *Nat Rev Mol Cell Biol* 11, 138-48.

Joiner, M. C., Marples, B., Lambin, P., Short, S. C. and Turesson, I. (2001). Low-dose hypersensitivity: current status and possible mechanisms. *Int J Radiat Oncol Biol Phys* 49, 379-89.

Joubert, A., Biston, M. C., Boudou, C., Ravanat, J. L., Brochard, T., Charvet, A. M., Esteve, F., Balosso, J. and Foray, N. (2005). Irradiation in presence of iodinated contrast agent results in radiosensitization of endothelial cells: consequences for computed tomography therapy. *Int J Radiat Oncol Biol Phys* 62, 1486-96.

Joubert, A., Gamo, K., Bencokova, Z., Gastaldo, J., Rénier, W., Chavaudra, N., Favaudon, V., Arlett, C. and Foray, N. (2008). DNA double-strand break repair defects in syndromes associated with acute radiation response: at least two different assays to predict intrinsic radiosensitivity? *International Journal of Radiation Biology* 84, 1-19.

Lavin, M. F. (2008). Ataxia-telangiectasia: from a rare disorder to a paradigm for cell signalling and cancer. *Nat Rev Mol Cell Biol* 9, 759-69.

Lees-Miller, S. P., Godbout, R., Chan, D. W., Weinfeld, M., Day, R. S., 3rd, Barron, G. M. and Allalunis-Turner, J. (1995). Absence of p350 subunit of DNA-activated protein kinase from a radiosensitive human cell line. *Science* 267, 1183-5.

Marot, D., Opolon, P., Brailly-Tabard, S., Elie, N., Randrianarison, V., Connault, E., Foray, N., Feunteun, J. and Perricaudet, M. (2006). The tumor suppressor activity induced by adenovirus-mediated BRCA1 overexpression is not restricted to breast cancers. *Gene Ther* 13, 235-44.

McKinnon, P. J. (1987). Ataxia-telangiectasia: an inherited disorder of ionizing-radiation sensitivity in man. Progress in the elucidation of the underlying biochemical defect. *Hum Genet* 75, 197-208.

Rosen, E. M., Fan, S. and Isaacs, C. (2005). BRCA1 in hormonal carcinogenesis: basic and clinical research. *Endocr Relat Cancer* 12, 533-48.

Rothkamm, K. and Lobrich, M. (2003). Evidence for a lack of DNA double-strand break repair in human cells exposed to very low x-ray doses. *Proc Natl Acad Sci U S A* 100, 5057-62.

Ruffner, H., Jiang, W., Craig, A. G., Hunter, T. and Verma, I. M. (1999). BRCA1 is phosphorylated at serine 1497 in vivo at a cyclin-dependent kinase 2 phosphorylation site. *Mol Cell Biol* 19, 4843-54.

Scully, R., Chen, J., Ochs, R. L., Keegan, K., Hoekstra, M., Feunteun, J. and Livingston, D. M. (1997a). Dynamic changes of BRCA1 subnuclear location and phosphorylation state are initiated by DNA damage. *Cell* 90, 425-35.

Scully, R., Chen, J., Plug, A., Xiao, Y., Weaver, D., Feunteun, J., Ashley, T. and Livingston, D. M. (1997b). Association of BRCA1 with Rad51 in mitotic and meiotic cells. *Cell* 88, 265-75.

Soares, H. D., Morgan, J. I. and McKinnon, P. J. (1998). Atm expression patterns suggest a contribution from the peripheral nervous system to the phenotype of ataxia-telangiectasia. *Neuroscience* 86, 1045-54.

Taghian, A., Ramsay, J., Allalunis-Turner, J., Budach, W., Gioioso, D., Pardo, F., Okunieff, P., Bleehen, N., Urtasun, R. and Suit, H. (1993). Intrinsic radiation sensitivity may not be the major determinant of the poor clinical outcome of glioblastoma multiforme. *Int J Radiat Oncol Biol Phys* 25, 243-9.

Taghian, A., Suit, H., Pardo, F., Gioioso, D., Tomkinson, K., DuBois, W. and Gerweck, L. (1992). In vitro intrinsic radiation sensitivity of glioblastoma multiforme. *Int J Radiat Oncol Biol Phys* 23, 55-62.

Taylor, A. M., Byrd, P. J., McConville, C. M. and Thacker, S. (1994). Genetic and cellular features of ataxia telangiectasia. *Int J Radiat Biol* 65, 65-70.

Tsuchida, R., Yamada, T., Takagi, M., Shimada, A., Ishioka, C., Katsuki, Y., Igarashi, T., Chessa, L., Delia, D., Teraoka, H. et al. (2002). Detection of ATM gene mutation in human glioma cell line M059J by a rapid frameshift/stop codon assay in yeast. *Radiat Res* 158, 195-201.

Wechsler, W., Ramadan, M. A. and Gieseler, A. (1972). Isogenic transplantation of ethylnitrosourea-induced tumors of the central and peripheral nervous system in two different inbred rat strains. *Naturwissenschaften* 59, 474.

Xu, B., Kim, S. and Kastan, M. B. (2001). Involvement of Brca1 in S-phase and G(2)-phase checkpoints after ionizing irradiation. *Mol Cell Biol* 21, 3445-50.

Zan, Y., Haag, J. D., Chen, K. S., Shepel, L. A., Wigington, D., Wang, Y. R., Hu, R., Lopez-Guajardo, C. C., Brose, H. L., Porter, K. I. et al. (2003). Production of knockout rats using ENU mutagenesis and a yeast-based screening assay. *Nat Biotechnol* 21, 645-51.

Zhu, Y. and Parada, L. F. (2002). The molecular and genetic basis of neurological tumours. *Nat Rev Cancer* 2, 616-26.

7

Glioma Proteomics: Methods and Current Perspective

Kumaravel Somasundaram,
Mamatha B Nijaguna and Durairaj Mohan Kumar
Department of Microbiology and Cell Biology
Indian Institute of Science, Bangalore
India

1. Introduction

The Glioblastoma (WHO grade IV astrocytoma) is the most common and malignant primary adult brain cancer. The present standard treatment appears to be maximal safe resection of the tumor followed by irradiation and temozolomide adjuvant chemotherapy. Despite advances in treatment modalities, the median survival is very poor. In addition, recent molecular and genetic profiling studies using various genomic technologies have identified several markers and unique signatures as prognostic and predictive factors of GBM. However, none of them are translated into clinics. Thus with a requirement of additional more potent markers, proteomics appears to be more promising in particular for reasons like transcript levels does not correlate with protein levels due to variety of reasons like differences in translation efficiency, protein stability and miRNA regulation. The conventional methods like 2-dimensional gel electrophoresis have been in use for nearly last few decades. However, our ability to identify the proteins through mass spectrometry created renewed interest in proteomics. It is anticipated that the technological advancements happening in proteomics like gel free high throughput quantitative methods is going to revolutionize the biomarker discovery for classification, prognosis, monitoring treatment response and novel targets for better treatment besides understanding of glioma biology.

2. Why proteomics is essential?

The foundation stone for our understanding that cancer is a genetic disease and it arises due to changes in genes or gene activity was laid down by the field of tumor virology (Javier and Butel, 2008). Throughout the last century, the field of tumor virology has discovered groundbreaking findings that helped us to understand the causes of cancer. In the new era of genomics, the techniques like DNA microarray technology, where one can detect changes in the expression of several thousand genes simultaneously, further accelerated the process of our understanding of cancer. This helped us in developing molecular markers and gene signatures leading to improved and more accurate diagnosis, tumor grading and alternate therapeutic methods including targeted therapies. However, the detection of genes or their expression by itself does not reflect the dynamics of various processes in the cell.

Proteomics is the study of all the proteins expressed by a given cell, tissue, or organism at a given time and under specific conditions. Since the proteins are the functional units of the cell, the development of cancer is directly influenced by the protein synthesis, level and their interaction with other molecules. It is now understood that cancer development and progression is largely due to aberrant signaling pathways in which the entire network of proteins play a major role, the proteomics becomes vital to the further advancement of our understanding of various cellular processes. Genomics based studies are not sufficient in our desire towards complete understanding of cancer. For example, the analysis of mRNA level does not necessarily reflect the protein content in the cell always. While the formation of mRNA by transcription is the first and an important step in gene expression, protein level is controlled by other steps like translation and stability of mRNA and protein. Multiple proteins can be formed from a gene due to alternate splicing. It is predicted that a human gene on an average can encode three or more proteins (Wilkins *et al.*, 1996). Proteins are also subjected to post-translational modifications which play a major role in regulating their functions by altering their localization, interactions and turnover. It is estimated that the proteins can undergo as many as 200 different kinds of modifications (Krishna and Wold, 1993). Protein function is also regulated by their localization and interaction with other proteins. By using proteomic approach, it is possible to identify the changes in protein modifications, subcellular localization and protein-protein interactions for many proteins expressed in a cell. Proteomics also help in annotation of genome as predicting genes from genomic data by using bioinformatics algorithm is not always accurate. An integration of genomic data with proteomic studies is needed to achieve complete annotation of the genome.

3. Proteomic methods

3.1 Detection methods

Conventionally, the protein identification was done by carrying out Edman degradation, a chemical method used for the sequencing of amino acids from the N-terminal end of a peptide (Edman, 1949). The limitations of this method are that it is very exhaustive, time consuming and requires more protein sample. Mass spectrometers traditionally used for measuring the mass of small molecules became an important and indispensible tool in protein identification since the introduction of *M*atrix-*A*ssisted *L*aser *D*esorption/*I*onization (MALDI) methodology (Karas and Hillenkamp, 1988).

3.1.1 Mass spectrometer

Mass spectrometer comprises three principle components: ionization source, analyzer, and detector. Ionization source can be either MALDI or *E*lectrospray *I*onization (ESI). In MALDI, the analyte is co-crystallized with matrix, which imparts laser energy on analyte and thus helps in its ionization. The ions generated in MALDI are singly charged. In ESI, the analytes in aqueous phase are introduced through a fine capillary needle into a high voltage chamber, wherein solvent evaporates leaving behind analytes as multiply charged ions. The generated ions are then separated based on their mass/charge (m/z) ratio by analyzer.

Different types of analyzers are *T*ime *O*f *F*light (TOF), quadrupole and *F*ourier *T*ransform *I*on Cyclotron *R*esonance (FT-ICR). The TOF analyzer is commonly used in MALDI based mass spectrometry. In TOF analyzer, an electric field accelerates the ions in a vacuum tube and allows to drift towards the detector. Since all the ions posses similar charge, their kinetic energy will be identical. Thus, the ions are separated merely based on their masses. The ion with least mass will reach the detector first. In quadrupole mass analyzer, a radio frequency (RF) field is created between four parallel metal rods through which ions passes. The paths of ions are either stabilized or destabilized selectively by superimposing oscillating electrical fields such that ions in a certain range of m/z ratio are allowed to reach the detector at any given time. Thus, quadrupole mass analyzer acts as a mass-selective filter. In FT-ICR, the charged ions experience movement in a fixed magnetic field which is known as ion cyclotron resonance wherein the frequency of an ion's cycling is determined by its mass to charge ratio. These ions are excited by radio frequency (RF) signal which produces image current measurable by the detector.

The final component of MS is a detector, which is either an electron multiplier. When the ions hit the surface of the detector, the current signal thus produced is recorded and is represented as mass spectrum.

3.1.2 Protein identification using peptide mass finger printing (PMF) and tandem MS

Most often in proteomics, the protein identification is achieved by MALDI-TOF MS analysis. Typically, the protein is digested with trypsin and the resulting peptide mixture is analyzed on MALDI, which generates a spectrum with peaks representing singly charged masses of peptides. The list of peptide masses are searched against tryptic peptides generated *in silico* from a database of protein (Pappin *et al.*, 1993) or translated nucleic acid sequences (James *et al.*, 1994) to confirm the protein identity. This process is called as peptide mass finger printing. However, if protein sample contains more than one protein, it may result in complex spectra that are less successfully handled by existing algorithms and software. Spectral peaks corresponding to peptides with known possible modifications can be successfully matched to database peptide sequences if the possibility of the modification is specified by the user. However unanticipated modifications will lead to incorrect identification of the protein. In such cases, tandem MS (MS/MS) provides the most powerful tool to unambiguously detect protein identity and modification.

3.2 Separation methods

3.2.1 Gel based separation methods

2-dimensional gel electrophoresis (2DE) is probably the first introduced proteomic technique and being widely used for a large scale separation and identification of protein(s). It was first described and demonstrated by O' Farrell (O' Farrell, 1975). In 1977, Anderson and coworkers applied 2DE to separate the plasma proteins (Anderson and Anderson, 1977). Since then 2DE technique has been enormously used to profile the proteome of many organisms, organelles, cell lines and biological fluids. This technique separates proteins based on two independent properties of the proteins. In the first step, isoelectric focusing (IEF), the proteins are separated according to their isoelectric point. In the second step, proteins are separated based on their molecular weight in sodium dodecyl sulphate polyacrylamide gel electrophoresis (SDS-PAGE). The protein spots are visualized by coomasie blue staining or silver staining and the digital images of the gels can be analyzed through software to obtain the quantitative information of the protein spots. The protein spot of interest is excised, destained and subjected to tryptic digestion. The tryptic peptides are analyzed in MS to acquire the *P*eptide *M*ass *F*ingerprint (PMF). The peaks in a PMF correspond to peptides derived from protein spot excised on a 2D gel. The peptide mass values are searched against the appropriate database to confirm the identity of the protein spot. But the conventional 2DE based separation and visualization techniques often lack reproducibility in proteome separation and sensitivity to detect low abundant proteins.

In order to improve the conventional 2DE in this respect, Differential gel electrophoresis (DIGE) was introduced (Unlu *et al.*, 1997). In DIGE, the two different samples are first labeled with fluorescent dyes (Cy3 and Cy5), then mixed together and subjected to DE on a single gel. The gel is subsequently scanned at different wavelengths to generate the images corresponding to different samples used in the experiment. This provides two advantages in protein identification: first, the fluorescent labeling is very sensitive and hence it can detect even very less abundant proteins; second, the control (Cy3) and test (Cy5) samples are separated on a single gel thereby eliminating the gel-to-gel variation and artifacts. Therefore, any variation seen between two differentially labeled samples is mostly due to actual biological differences. After the fluorescent images are generated for software based analysis, the gel is counter stained with coomassie or silver stain, the spot of interest is subjected to MS to confirm its identity. But, most often, the spots seen by fluorescent stain is not visualized by the conventional staining methods. Therefore, the protein spot(s) of interest for identification is preferably taken from a preparatory gel run independently. When more number of control and test samples are to be analyzed by DIGE, generally a common pool consisting equal amounts of all samples is made and labeled with Cy2 dye. This Cy2 labeled pool is run along with control (Cy3) and test (Cy5) in every gel as internal standard which helps in normalizing variation between gels.

3.2.2 Non-gel based separation methods

3.2.2.1 Lable free methods

Despite the advancements in 2DE, it is no longer effective in situations like identification of proteins with low abundance, high hydrophobicity, extreme pI and molecular weight. To overcome these problems, in-solution separation or *L*iquid *C*hromatography (LC) method was coupled with ESI-MS based identification of proteins. In LC based proteomics, complex mixture of proteins are first digested to peptides by proteases, separated by one or more dimensions of LC and subjected to tandem MS analysis. The protein identification is achieved based on one or more identified peptide sequences. The separation and analysis of tryptic peptides rather than the protein is termed as bottom-up approach. To achieve the efficient separation of peptides, the combination of multi-dimensional chromatography has been in use and this technique is popularly called as *Mu*lti*d*imensional *P*rotein *I*dentification *T*echnology (MudPit) (Washburn *et al.*, 2001). MudPit is a most common two-dimensional LC separation which combines *S*trong *C*ation E*x*change (SCX) chromatography with reverse phase (RP). The fractions separated by RP are directly injected into online ESI-MS or on MALDI target plate for analysis by MS/MS.

3.2.2.2 Labeling methods

The combination of protein labeling approaches with LC-based separation coupled to ESI-MS has greatly facilitated the large scale identification and quantification of the proteins. Such a combined approach is called as quantitative proteomics. The different labeling techniques include *S*table *I*sotope *L*abeling of *A*mino acids in *C*ell culture (SILAC), *I*sotope *C*oded *A*ffinity *T*ag (ICAT), *I*sobaric *T*ag for *R*elative and *A*bsolute *Q*uantification of peptides (iTRAQ) and Proteolytic ^{18}O labeling. These techniques differentially label the proteins of two (or more) conditions; this is achieved by metabolic incorporation of isotopically distinct amino acids in live cells (SILAC), through chemical labeling of proteins with isotopically distinct tags bound to –SH groups (ICAT) or isobaric amine specific tags bound to amino groups (iTRAQ) (**Figure.1**).

3.2.2.2.1 SILAC

SILAC involves growing cells under two different conditions (Control Vs Test): one in medium containing 'light' amino acid and other in 'heavy' amino acid containing medium (Ong *et al.*, 2002). Heavy amino acid containing ^{2}H instead of H, or ^{13}C instead of ^{12}C or ^{15}N instead of ^{14}N is used. Incorporation of a heavy amino acid into a peptide results in a known mass shift compared with peptide containing light amino acid. For example, a six carbon containing amino acid like arginine when labeled with ^{13}C isotope can differentiate a given peptide derived from two different conditions by 6 Da mass difference. The protein samples of control and test conditions are mixed in equal proportion, subjected to trypsin digestion, which selectively cleaves at the carboxyl side of arginine or lysine. The resulting peptide mixture is analyzed by LC-MS to generate a MS spectrum wherein each peptide appears as a pair with expected mass difference. The relative abundance of a peptide is obtained by comparing the intensities of peptides within a pair (**Figure.1A**).

3.2.2.2.2 ICAT

In 1999 Aebersold and co-workers (Gygi *et al.*, 1999) introduced the ICAT method for relative quantitation of protein abundance. ICAT reagent contains three moieties: biotin tag to isolate the ICAT labeled peptides, a linker with either eight hydrogen or eight deuterium giving an isotope mass difference of 8 Da and cysteine reactive malemide group. In this technique, the complex protein mixtures from two different conditions (Control Vs Test) are labeled using heavy and light ICAT reagent such that one condition contains hydrogen whereas other contains deuterium giving rise to 8 Da mass difference. The labeled protein samples from two different conditions are mixed equally and subjected to proteolytic digestion, thus obtained mixture of peptides are affinity purified using avidin column to enrich the labeled peptides. The peptides are analysed by LC-MS to obtain the relative abundance of a given protein (**Figure.1B**).

3.2.2.2.3 iTRAQ

In iTRAQ, the peptides derived from different protein samples are labelled with iTRAQ tags. The tag is covalently linked to N-terminal amine group/side chain amine groups of peptides. The tag is of 145 Da and consists of three moieties, N-hydroxy succinimide (NHS) ester for reaction with primary amine groups on peptides, balance moiety (carbonyl group) and reporter moiety. The reporter moiety may have varying mass like 114, 115, 116 and 117 Da and hence four different conditions (4-plex) can be analysed and relative quantification obtained simultaneously (Ross et al., 2004). The peptides from different conditions are labeled with iTRAQ tags which differ in their reporter ions, pooled, fractionated in nano-LC and analysed by tandem mass spectrometry. Due to isobaric mass of iTRAQ tags, the peptides appear as single peaks in MS scan. When the iTRAQ-peptides are analysed on MS/MS, the tagged peptides dissociates into peptide sequence, a neutral balance moiety and reporter ions. The protein identification is achieved by searching the peptide sequence against the database(s). The relative abundance of protein is estimated by the relative peak intensity of the liberated reporter ions (**Figure.1C**).

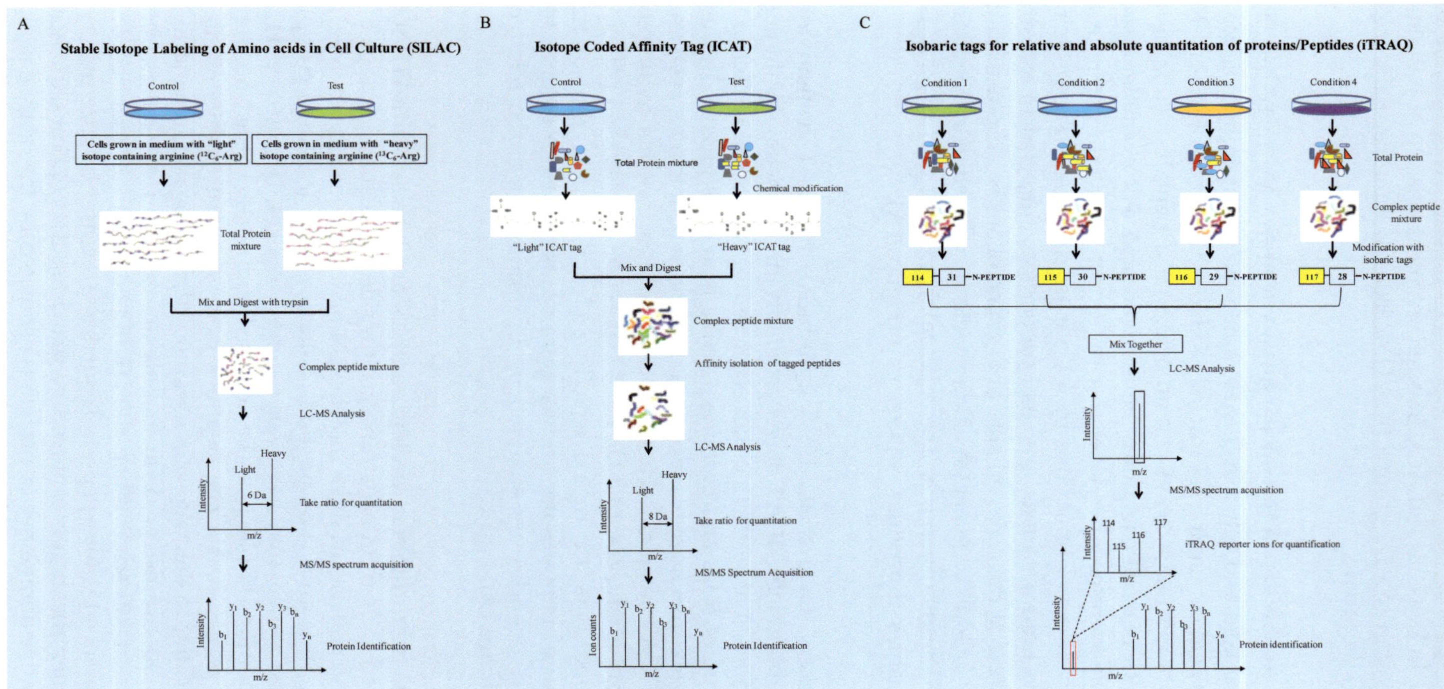

Fig. 1. A. Peptide quantitation using SILAC method. Cells are grown in "light" and "heavy" arginine containing medium, total protein mixtures are combined and digested with trypsin. The resulting peptide mixture is subjected LC/MS, where in light and heavy amino acid containing peptides appear as a pair of peaks. The ratio between the light and heavy isotope containing peptides provide the relative abundance of the peptide. Tandem mass spectometry is performed to confirm the protein identity. B. Peptide quantitation using ICAT method. Total protein mixtures from two different conditions are differently labeled with "light" and "heavy" ICAT tags. The samples are combined in equal proportion, digested with trypsin and ICAT tagged peptides are enriched by affinity isolation. Then the tagged peptides appear as pair of peaks in LC-MS analysis and the relative abundance of the peptide is estimated by taking the ratio of relative intensity between "light" and "heavy" peptides. Protein identification is achieved by tandem mass spectometry. C. Peptide quantitation using iTRAQ method. Total protein mixture from different conditions are digested and modified with isobaric tags on the N-terminus of all peptides. All tagged to peptide groups are mixed together and subjected to LC-MS/MS analysis. After fragmentation and peptide identification, the low mass region of the MS/MS spectrum displays the reporter ions liberated by the fragmentation of the isobaric tag. The ratio of reporter ions in the MS/MS spectrum provides relative abundance of the peptide in each condition.

3.3 Other proteomic methods

We describe here briefly about other techniques available for proteomic analysis. More detailed information can be obtained from elsewhere (Angenendt *et al.*, 2006; Diamandis, 2003; Haab, 2005; Kim *et al.*, 2009; Petricoin *et al.*, 2002). A relatively new proteomic technique that is suitable for high-throughput profiling is *S*urface *E*nhanced *L*aser *D*esorption/*I*onization-*T*ime-*O*f-*F*light (SELDI-TOF) which combines affinity chromatography on a modified surface (surface-enhanced) with MALDI-TOF. Protein chips with different chromatographic surfaces either chemically modified like hydrophobic, hydrophilic, cationic, anionic and metal ion or biochemically modified like antibody-antigen, receptor-ligand and DNA-protein are used to fractionate proteins from complex protein mixtures. In the next step, an energy adsorbing matrix is layered over the protein chip and a spectrum will be obtained following laser desorption/ionization. While SELDI is capable of producing protein spectra that can discriminate tumor from normal controls, it does not provide the identity of the protein markers involved. SELDI based proteomic approach involves a pattern discovery phase wherein a discriminatory peak pattern is identified and pattern matching phase in which the identified pattern is validated.
A powerful chip-based proteomic technique which does not utilize mass spectrometry is antibody and protein arrays. Antibody array essentially utilizes antibodies, which are covalently immobilized onto a solid surface like glass slide to capture labeled antigens. In contrast, the protein array contains proteins of interest arrayed on a flat surface. The main use of protein array is to detect autoantibodies seen in conditions like autoimmune disorders and cancer. Since the main hurdle in development of protein array is expression and purification of proteins, alternate techniques like chemical synthesis, cell-free DNA expression or cell-free in situ expression of PCR products are being developed (Angenendt *et al.*, 2006). A modification of antibody arrays is bead arrays wherein antibodies are immobilized to spherical particles containing integrated reporter fluorescent dyes. Since the reporter dye encodes the identity of capture agent attached to the bead, a multiplex assay format is produced by mixing beads with different reporter dyes and capture agents. Because of higher sample throughput, bead arrays are particularly suitable for screening large number of samples.

4. Application of proteomics in glioma

Histological methods relying on microscopic description of glioma helped us not only classification and also making therapeutic decisions (Brat *et al.*, 2008). Subjectivity and inter-observer variations in histopathology may lead to compromise in making choices in therapeutic modalities (Brat *et al.*, 2008). In the last two decades, genomics in the form of various high throughput techniques helped us enormously not only in increasing our understanding of glioma biology but also resulted in the identification of several gene or gene signatures for diagnosis, grading and glioma therapy. These findings have not been translated into clinic and hence the patient outcome remains low. With requirement of better validated robust markers, proteomics appears to be promising in making the lead. We have summarized important discoveries in glioma research using various proteomic methods.

4.1 Glioma tumor tissue and cell line based studies

Using 2DE, Iwadate et al analyzed 85 tissue samples (52 GBM, 13 AA, 10 DA and 10 normal brain samples), and identified 57 protein spots which could be used to differentiate tumors from normal brain tissue (Iwadate *et al.*, 2004). Out of the differentially regulated protein spots, the identity was found for 5 spots by MALDI-TOF and were categorized into various biological functions like signal transduction related proteins, molecular chaperones, transcription and translation regulators, cell cycle-mediating proteins, extracellular matrix-related proteins, and cell adhesion molecules. High levels expression of four proteins-VREB1, GRP78, RhoA and Rac1 and lower expression of enolase in grade IV tumors compared to lower grade tumors was also confirmed by immunohistochemistry. In another attempt to identify differentially expressed proteins between astrocytoma grades, 10 grade II and 10 grade IV samples were analyzed by 2DE followed by mass spectrometry, which resulted in the identification of 15 differentially expressed proteins (Odreman *et al.*, 2005). These findings were subsequently validated by western blotting and immunohistochemcial staining. The proteins more highly expressed in glioblastoma multiforme were peroxiredoxin 1 and 6, the transcription factor BTF3, and R-B-crystallin, whereas protein disulfide isomerase A3, the catalytic subunit of the cAMP-dependent protein kinase, and the glial fibrillary acidic protein were increased in low-grade astrocytomas. Hiratsuka et al used six non tumoral samples and five glioma samples (one grade II, two grade III and two grade IV) for 2DE and MALDI-TOF spectrometry investigation and identified 11 upregulated proteins and 4 down regulated proteins in glioma compared to normal samples (Hiratsuka *et al.*, 2003). Northern blotting confirmed the glioma downregulation of SIRT2. Further, overexpression of SIRT2 resulted in perturbation of microtubule network and reduced colony formation suggesting SIRT2 may act as tumor suppressor in glioma. Ngo *et al.*, used a 2D-DIGE based proteomic approach to identify differences in protein expression between two glioma cells which differ in their chromosome 1p status (Ngo *et al.*, 2007). The rational for this study is that 1p+/- anaplastic oligodendroglioma patients respond better to chemotherapeutic agents like procarbazine, 1-(2-chloroethyl)-3-cyclohexyl-l-nitrosourea, and vincristine. Comparison of A172 (1p+/-) and U251 (1p+/+) glioma cell lines identified 9 spots as differentially regulated proteins, out of which the identity was found by MALDI-TOF/TOF MS for 18 proteins which included three proteins α-enolase, stathmin and DJ-1 encoded by 1p region. Further analysis revealed that decreased stathmin, a microtubule associated protein, was found to be associated with loss of heterozygosity, increased recurrence-free survival in anaplastic ologidendroglioma patients. Expression of stathmin was also found to correlate inversely with overall survival of nitrsourea treated mice carrying xenograft tumors. On mechanistic front, this group identified an increased mitotic arrest in cells with less stathmin expression upon nitrosoureas treatment as potential reason for improved patient outcome with 1p+/- anaplastic oligodendroglioma tumors.

In an effort to identify proteins that could affect sensitivity of glioma cells to chemotherapy, Puchades et al., analysed the protein profiles by 2DE of control U87 glioma cells or infected with p53 adenovirus or treated with SN38, a topoisomearse 1 inhibitor either alone or in combination. Of many proteins modulated by this treatment, they found galectin1 to be down regulated by p53 which is further enhanced by SN38 treatment. Further investigation revealed a high level expression of galectin 1 in glioma cell lines and down regulation of galectin 1 sensitized glioma cells to chemotherapy suggesting that galectin 1 could be a potential therapeutic target (Puchades *et al.*, 2007). Another interesting review work compared systematically many independent glioma proteomic studies and identified 10 proteins- PHB, Hsp20, serum albumin, epidermal growth factor receptor (EGFR), EA-15, RhoGDI, APOA1, GFAP, HSP70 and PDIA3 to be differentially expressed in gliomas (Deighton *et al.*, 2010)

4.2 Serum and CSF based studies

Using combination of 2DE and MALDI-TOF MS, Kumar *et al.*, analyzed 14 GBM and 6 normal control sera and identified haptoglobin (Hp) α2 chain as an up regulated serum protein in GBM patients (Kumar *et al.* 2010). GBM-specific upregulation was confirmed by ELISA based quantitation of haptoglobin (Hp) in the serum of 99 GBM patients as against lower grades (49 grade III/AA; 26 grade II/DA) and 26 normal individuals. Further validation done using RT-qPCR on an independent set of tumor and normal brain samples and immunohistochemcial staining on a subset of above samples showed an increasing levels of Hp transcript and protein respectively with tumor grade and were highest in GBM. Further investigation revealed that overexpression of Hp either by stable integration of Hp cDNA or exogenous addition of purified Hp to immortalized astrocytes resulted in increased cell migration. Conversely, RNAi-mediated silencing of Hp in glioma cells decreased cell migration. Mouse melanoma and human glioma cells over expressing Hp showed increased tumor growth with decreased mice survival in mouse xenograft model. SELDI-TOF analysis of serum samples coupled with artificial neural network (ANN) algorithm followed by discriminant analysis identified a fifteen peak pattern which can classify low grade (I/II) from high grade (III/IV) tumors with an accuracy of 85.7% (Liu *et al.*, 2005). Petrik *et al.*, compared the SELDI-TOF mass spectra derived from 200 serum samples that comprised of 58 control subjects and 36 patients with grade II astrocytoma, 15 with anaplastic astrocytoma, and 91 with glioblastoma and identified a peak with size of 2.740 kDa showing decreasing intensity with increasing astrocytoma grade (Petrik *et al.*, 2008). The peak was subsequently identified by tandem MS as B-chain of α2-Heremans-Schmid glycoprotein (AHSG). This finding was validated by measuring the serum AHSG levels using turbidimetry in an independent set of serum samples. More interestingly, multivariate Cox proportional hazards model identified serum AHSG levels were to be an independent predictor of patient survival with normal levels being associated with prolonged survival. Analysis of cerebrospinal fluid samples from 60 patients comprising 47 brain tumors and 13 nontumor controls by two independent proteomic techniques, 2DE and cleavable ICAT, found an exclusive presence of attractin in grade III and IV astrocytoma (Khwaja *et al.*, 2006). High-grade specific upregulation of attractin in CSF was validated by western blotting and immunohistochemistry in an independent set of samples. Analysis of tumor samples demonstrated the source of high levels seen in CSF as tumors. Finally, this study showed the attractin from CSF could induce glioma cell migration suggesting the importance of attractin in high invasive nature of high-grade gliomas. Others studies where proteomic approaches were used in analysis of serum and CSF of glioma patients are reviewed recently (Niclou *et al.*, 2010; Somasundaram *et al.*, 2009).

5. Conclusions

Proteomics is certain to become part of important discoveries in glioma as it has already become an integral part of glioma research. Although glioma proteomics research have not yielded any breakthrough findings close to becoming an application in clinics, the great advances in the proteomic technology in the form of more powerful and sensitive mass spectrometers, quantitative proteomic methods like SILAC, ICAT, iTRAQ, and improvements in data analysis in the form of sophisticated databases and bioinformatic software likely to hasten the biomarker discovery in the years to come. While gel based separation techniques like 2DE or 2D-DIGE will continue to be in use, the label free or labeled quantitative MS methods will take the center stage. Further, serum biomarker discovery field is where proteomic platform is likely to play a major role. However, one major drawback of current proteomic studies is that most of them are of low throughput studies having utilized small number of samples. This obviously requires extensive validation perhaps using other techniques like ELISA or tissue microarray in large number of samples. Prospective validation studies are also needed to confirm the clinical benefit to the patients.

6. Acknowledgements

This study was supported by a grant from DBT, Government of India. Infrastructural support by funding from ICMR (Center for Advanced studies in Molecular Medicine), DBT, DST (FIST) and UGC to department of MCB, Indian Institute of Science is acknowledged. MBN and DMK gratefully acknowledge senior research fellowship from IISc and CSIR respectively.

7. References

Anderson L, Anderson NG (1977). High resolution two-dimensional electrophoresis of human plasma proteins. *Proc. Natl. Acad. Sci. U S A*.74: 5421–25.

O'Farrell PH (1975). High resolution two-dimensional electrophoresis of proteins. *J. Biol. Chem*.250: 4007–21.

Angenendt P, Kreutzberger J, Glokler J, Hoheisel JD (2006). Generation of high density protein microarrays by cell-free in situ expression of unpurified PCR products. *Mol Cell Proteomics* 5: 1658-66.

Brat DJ, Prayson RA, Ryken TC, Olson JJ (2008). Diagnosis of malignant glioma: role of neuropathology. *J Neurooncol* 89: 87-311.

Deighton RF, McGregor R, Kemp J, McCulloch J, Whittle IR (2010) Glioma pathophysiology: insights emerging from proteomics. *Brain Pathol* 0: 691-703.

Diamandis EP (2003). Point: Proteomic patterns in biological fluids: do they represent the future of cancer diagnostics? *Clin Chem* 49: 1272-5.

Edman P (1949). A method for the determination of amino acid sequence in peptides. *Arch Biochem* 2: 475.

Gygi SP, Rist B, Gerber SA, Turecek F, Gelb MH, Aebersold R (1999). Quantitative analysis of complex protein mixtures using isotope-coded affinity tags. *Nat Biotechnol* 17: 994-9.

Haab BB (2005). Antibody arrays in cancer research. *Mol Cell Proteomics* 4: 377-83.

Hiratsuka M, Inoue T, Toda T, Kimura N, Shirayoshi Y, Kamitani H *et al* (2003). Proteomics-based identification of differentially expressed genes in human gliomas: down-regulation of SIRT2 gene. *Biochem Biophys Res Commun* 309: 558-66.

Iwadate Y, Sakaida T, Hiwasa T, Nagai Y, Ishikura H, Takiguchi M *et al* (2004). Molecular classification and survival prediction in human gliomas based on proteome analysis. *Cancer Res* 64: 496-501.

James P, Quadroni M, Carafoli E, Gonnet G (1994). Protein identification in DNA databases by peptide mass fingerprinting. *Protein Sci* 3: 1347-50.

Javier RT, Butel JS (2008). The history of tumor virology. *Cancer Res* 68: 7693-706.

Karas M, Hillenkamp F (1988). Laser desorption ionization of proteins with molecular masses exceeding 10,000 daltons. *Anal Chem* 60: 299-301.

Khwaja FW, Duke-Cohan JS, Brat DJ, Van Meir EG (2006). Attractin is elevated in the cerebrospinal fluid of patients with malignant astrocytoma and mediates glioma cell migration. *Clin Cancer Res* 12: 6331-6.

Kim BK, Lee JW, Park PJ, Shin YS, Lee WY, Lee KA *et al* (2009). The multiplex bead array approach to identifying serum biomarkers associated with breast cancer. *Breast Cancer Res* 11: R22.

Krishna RG, Wold F (1993). Post-translational modification of proteins. *Adv Enzymol Relat Areas Mol Biol* 67: 65-98.

Kumar DM, Thota B, Shinde SV, Prasanna KV, Hegde AS, Arivazhagan A *et al* Proteomic identification of haptoglobin alpha2 as a glioblastoma serum biomarker: implications in cancer cell migration and tumor growth. *J Proteome Res* 9: 5557-67.

Liu J, Zheng S, Yu JK, Zhang JM, Chen Z (2005). Serum protein fingerprinting coupled with artificial neural network distinguishes glioma from healthy population or brain benign tumor. *J Zhejiang Univ Sci B* 6: 4-10.

Ngo TT, Peng T, Liang XJ, Akeju O, Pastorino S, Zhang W *et al* (2007). The 1p-encoded protein stathmin and resistance of malignant gliomas to nitrosoureas. *J Natl Cancer Inst* 99: 639-52.

Niclou SP, Fack F, Rajcevic U (2010). Glioma proteomics: status and perspectives. *J Proteomics* 73: 1823-38.

Odreman F, Vindigni M, Gonzales ML, Niccolini B, Candiano G, Zanotti B *et al* (2005). Proteomic studies on low- and high-grade human brain astrocytomas. *J Proteome Res* 4: 698-708.

Ong SE, Blagoev B, Kratchmarova I, Kristensen DB, Steen H, Pandey A *et al* (2002). Stable isotope labeling by amino acids in cell culture, SILAC, as a simple and accurate approach to expression proteomics. *Mol Cell Proteomics* 1: 376-86.

Pappin DJ, Hojrup P, Bleasby AJ (1993). Rapid identification of proteins by peptide-mass fingerprinting. *Curr Biol* 3: 327-32.

Petricoin EF, Ardekani AM, Hitt BA, Levine PJ, Fusaro VA, Steinberg SM *et al* (2002). Use of proteomic patterns in serum to identify ovarian cancer. *Lancet* 359: 572-7.

Petrik V, Saadoun S, Loosemore A, Hobbs J, Opstad KS, Sheldon J *et al* (2008). Serum alpha - HS glycoprotein predicts survival in patients with glioblastoma. *Clin Chem* 54: 713-22.

Puchades M, Nilsson CL, Emmett MR, Aldape KD, Ji Y, Lang FF *et al* (2007). Proteomic investigation of glioblastoma cell lines treated with wild-type p53 and cytotoxic chemotherapy demonstrates an association between galectin-1 and p53 expression. *J Proteome Res* 6: 869-75.

Somasundaram K, Nijaguna MB, Kumar DM (2009). Serum proteomics of glioma: methods and applications. *Expert Rev Mol Diagn* 9: 695-707.

Unlu M, Morgan ME, Minden JS (1997). Difference gel electrophoresis: a single gel method for detecting changes in protein extracts. *Electrophoresis* 18: 071-7.

Washburn MP, Wolters D, Yates JR, 3rd (2001). Large-scale analysis of the yeast proteome by multidimensional protein identification technology. *Nat Biotechnol* 19: 42-7.

Wilkins MR, Sanchez JC, Williams KL, Hochstrasser DF (1996). Current challenges and future applications for protein maps and post-translational vector maps in proteome projects. *Electrophoresis* 17: 830-8.

8

Evolvement of Molecular Biomarkers in Targeted Therapy of Malignant Gliomas

Erica Hlavin Bell*, Mersiha Hadziahmetovic* and Arnab Chakravarti
Department of Radiation Oncology
The Ohio State University
U.S.A.

1. Introduction

Gliomas account for almost half of all diagnosed adult brain tumors (Siker et al., 2006). Glioblastoma multiforme (GBM), the most aggressive type of glioma, is also the most common primary malignant brain tumor. Even though tremendous effort has been made to treat high grade gliomas, the prognosis for patients with malignant gliomas remains poor. The dismal prognosis of patients with glioblastoma is in part caused by the resistance of these tumors to both chemotherapy and radiation. Furthermore, high grade gliomas often diffusely infiltrate into neighboring brain tissue, thus complicating treatment and commonly preventing a cure for the disease. Treatment modalities containing chemotherapy often have high levels of toxicity and depending on the drug have to be locally injected as crossing the blood-brain barrier is an impediment for certain drug therapies. The addition of temozolomide (TMZ) to the standard of care treatment for GBM in 2005 circumvented the aforementioned problems as it is taken orally, crosses the blood-brain barrier, and has a relatively low toxicity profile. However, the average life expectancy of patients treated with the addition of temozolomide increased by only a couple of months. Therefore, more effective treatment strategies are critically needed for the treatment of gliomas. In recent years, the research efforts in identifying molecular biomarkers for tumor subtypes have exponentially increased. These biomarkers can help serve a diagnostic role by helping classify grade or subtype, as well as a predictive role in determining the expected response to a specific treatment, and/or a prognostic role in estimating the natural course of the disease. Furthermore, gaining a better understanding of the molecular mechanisms involved in gliomagenesis, migration, and tumor resistance is essential for identifying novel tumor targets to overcome the poor prognosis of patients harboring gliomas. Additionally, characterizing the best treatment(s) for each grade and molecular subtype of gliomas will enable clinicians to increase efficacy of therapies for patients. The ability to categorize tumors based on molecular biomarkers for each glioma grade will further enhance the effectiveness of treatments by broadening the therapeutic window between normal and malignant tissues. In this chapter, molecular mechanisms (see Figure 1) and genetic alterations underlying the etiology of gliomas, corresponding molecular biomarkers (see

* These authors contributed equally to this manuscript.

Table 1) within the discussed pathways, and novel targeted therapies currently being investigated (see Table 2) are reviewed in detail.

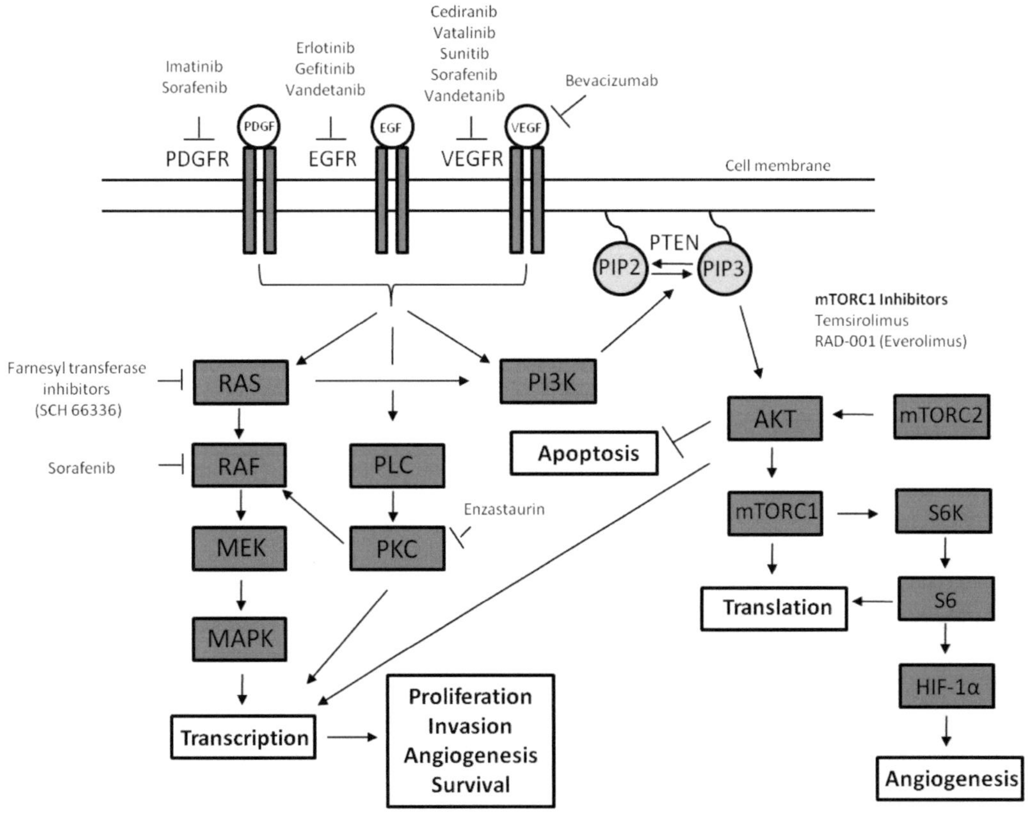

Fig. 1. Growth Factor Signaling Pathways in Malignant Gliomas and Corresponding Targeted Therapies

2. Molecular mechanisms contributing to gliomas, corresponding molecular biomarkers, and relevant targeted therapies

2.1 LOH of 1p/19q

Loss of heterozygosity (LOH) of chromosomes 1p and 19q is the most common genetic alteration in oligodendroglioma tumors (Gladson et al., 2010). This hallmark alteration is detected in 40-90% of oligodendrogliomas (Cairncross & Jenkins, 2008; Gladson et al., 2010; Jansen et al., 2010; Riemenschneider et al., 2010) and can be readily detected by fluorescent *in situ* hybridization (FISH) or southern blotting in the pathology lab. Therefore, loss of 1p/19q is used as a diagnostic marker of oligodendrogliomas. Co-deletion of 1p/19q is also found in 20-30% of mixed glial tumors (Aldape et al., 2007) and <10% of diffuse astrocytic gliomas (including GBMs) (Riemenschneider et al., 2010) . Although the regions of chromosomes 1p and 19q have been mapped, the actual tumor suppressor genes whose loss is involved in the promotion of growth in oligodendroglioma tumors are yet to be identified.

Interestingly, LOH at these loci confers a favorable response to chemotherapy, radiation, and survival (Nutt, 2005; Gladson et al., 2010). Exactly how the unidentified genes on chromosomes 1p and 19q contribute to a more favorable therapeutic response remains to be determined. Initially, the favorable response was first observed in a large percentage (approximately two-thirds) of patients with anaplastic oligodendrogliomas (grade III) that had a sustained response to chemotherapy. In 1998, Cairncross and colleagues first identified that coincident loss of chromosomal arms 1p and 19q confers chemotherapeutic sensitivity, prolonged recurrence-free and overall survival in patients with anaplastic oligodendroglioma (AO) treated with combination of procarbazine, lomustine and vincristine (PCV) chemotherapy (Cairncross et al., 1998). Following this discovery, interest in the use of chemotherapy for patients with oligodendroglial or mixed gliomas (oligoastrocytoma) was the impetus behind several clinical trials that corroborated these findings. In a series of 162 patients with either pure or mixed glioma, Smith et al. showed that the combined loss of 1p and 19q is a statistically significant predictor of prolonged survival in patients with pure oligodendroglioma, independent of tumor grade (Smith et al., 2000). No such association was demonstrated in patients with astrocytic neoplasms. All patients with the co-deletion were alive after a median follow-up of 67.5 months, as opposed to 73% of those without the combined deletion. In this study, loss of 1p or 19q in isolation was not a significant predictor of overall survival in any of the subtypes examined, but patients with pure oligodendroglioma did demonstrate a trend ($p = 0.15$) toward better survival if their tumors exhibited loss of 1p or loss of 19q. In another series, 50 patients with anaplastic oligodendroglioma were treated with a chemotherapeutic regimen (PCV in 48 patients) as the main initial adjuvant therapy, and patients with combined deletion of 1p and 19q had marked and durable responses to chemotherapy, resulting in longer overall survival, with or without postoperative radiation therapy (Ino et al., 2001). Patients with chromosome 1p alterations also responded superiorly to chemotherapy, but had shorter duration of response and patient survival. Tumors lacking 1p loss, but having a *TP53* gene mutation, responded to chemotherapy but recurred quickly. The group that fared the worst included tumors with intact 1p and wild-type *TP53*; these were poorly responsive, aggressive tumors that were clinically similar to glioblastomas. Loss of 1p has also been shown to increase radiation sensitivity (Bauman et al., 2000). Within the subset of patients with anaplastic oligodendroglioma who have the 1p/19q co-deletion, those with polysomy of chromosomes 1 and 19 were found to have an earlier recurrence than those without polysomy (Snuderl et al., 2009). Hirose and colleagues classified microdissected tissue from 140 patients with WHO grade II-III supratentorial gliomas based on whole genome profile, and reaffirmed that patients with 1p/19q deletion show long progression-free survival, while loss of 10q in association with gain of 7p appeared to predict poor outcome (Hirose et al., 2011).

Loss of both 1p and 19q has also been shown to increase sensitivity to temozolomide (TMZ), a monofunctional alkylating agent (Kouwenhoven et al., 2006). Due to a more favorable toxicity profile of TMZ compared with PCV, Radiation Therapy Oncology Group (RTOG) conducted a phase II trial of pre-irradiation and concurrent TMZ in patients with newly diagnosed anaplastic or mixed oligoastrocytoma. The objective response rate was 58% (32% complete response), and rate of progression during the pre-RT TMZ was only 10%, as compared to 20% in historical control with PCV (Vogelbaum et al., 2009). All patients with codeletion of 1p/19q and/or O6-methyl guanine DNA methyltransferase gene (MGMT) promoter methylation were free from progression at 6 months. Whether a chemotherapy-only regimen is sufficient to provide long-term control in patients with 1p/19q co-deleted anaplastic oligodendroglioma or mixed oligoastrocytoma without the use of concurrent or serial radiotherapy remains to be determined. European Organisation for Research and Treatment of Cancer (EORTC) is currently conducting CATNON, a Phase III intergroup trial on concurrent and adjuvant TMZ chemotherapy in patients with non-1p/19q deleted anaplastic glioma. The objectives of this trial are to assess whether RT concurrent with daily TMZ improves OS as compared to no daily TMZ in this patient population, and whether adjuvant TMZ improves overall survival as compared to no adjuvant TMZ.

Due to the overall increased survival of patients with co-deletions it is thought that LOH of 1p and 19q might be a prognostic marker of increased survival rather than a predictive marker of specific therapies. Nevertheless, this classification remains to be determined although there are retrospective data that demonstrated absence of increased survival without treatment, a result that suggests that 1p/19q co-deletion is a predictive marker of favorable response to many treatment regimens since it is not treatment specific (Riemenschneider et al., 2010).

Furthermore, there are common alterations that are found with 1p/19q co-deletion, such as isocitrate dehydrogenase 1 (IDH1) and IDH2 mutations (Yan et al., 2009). LOH of 1p/19q also has been shown to be mutually exclusive of *TP53* mutations, 10q deletion, and amplification of epidermal growth factor receptor (EGFR) (Nutt, 2005). Surprisingly, the location of the tumor site also appears to be associated with 1p/19q co-deletions (Jansen et al., 2010). In glioblastoma, deletions involving 1p and 19q are uncommon, but have been identified in a small percentage and appear to predict shortened survival (Smith et al., 2000). At the present time in the clinic, determining 1p/19q status is part of the standard of care for patients with oligodendroglial tumors, to help guide choice and sequencing of therapy. This information often serves as useful information when clinicians are determining the course of therapy based on the knowledge that patients with oligodendrogliomas that harbor co-deletions of chromosomes 1p and 19q will likely survive longer and be more responsive to a broad range of treatments.

2.2 Cell cycle regulation

2.2.1 p53

TP53 is the gene that encodes the important tumor suppressor protein, p53. In 1989, further karyotypic and LOH analysis defined the location of a tumor suppressor on chromosome 17, and the *TP53* tumor suppressor gene was later identified to be responsible for alterations in GBM at this locus (Van Meir et al., 2010). p53 is often referred to as the "guardian of the genome" as it is involved in a multitude of critical processes that regulate normal cell function, such as cell cycle control, DNA damage response, cell death, differentiation, and inhibition of angiogenesis (Fischer & Aldape, 2010). It is a critical factor in the G1/S checkpoint whereby activated p53 can signal increased levels of p21, a CDK2 inhibitor, resulting in cell cycle arrest (Van Meir et al., 2010). In the absence of p53, the cell cycle can become unregulated and lead to uncontrolled proliferation resulting in tumorigenesis. p53 prevents excess proliferation from triggering apoptosis because p53 also regulates the apoptosis response by controlling pro-apoptotic proteins, such as Bax and Fas (Fischer & Aldape, 2010; Van Meir et al., 2010).

Low grade astrocytomas often possess inactivating mutations of the tumor suppressor gene, *TP53*. Therefore it is thought that p53 mutations are a hallmark of low-grade gliomas and consequently also occur in secondary GBM that arise from lower grade gliomas (Noda et al., 2009). Loss of p53 is observed in grade II astrocytomas (35-60%), grade III astrocytomas (~50%), primary GBM (~30%), and secondary GBM (~60-65%) (Sulman et al., 2009; Bourne & Schiff, 2010; Gladson et al., 2010). Additionally, p53 mutations are found in ~44% of grade II oligoastrocytoma and ~13% of oligodendroglioma cases (Bourne & Schiff, 2010). Overexpression of p53 has also been observed in ~50% of GBM cases (Kim et al., 2010). Interestingly, tumors that harbor 1p/19q co-deletions do not contain p53 mutations (Noda et al., 2009; Fischer & Aldape, 2010). MDM2, a negative regulator of p53, has also been reported to be amplified or mutated in anaplastic astrocytoma (AA) (13-43%) and in glioblastoma (~10-27%) (Gladson et al., 2010; Kim et al., 2010). Currently, p53 is not thought to be predictive or prognostic (Tabatabai et al., 2010). However, it does have a role in the diagnostic setting as it can help distinguish tumor grade.

2.2.2 Rb/P16INK4A/CDK4

Rb, also known as the retinoblastoma protein, is a tumor suppressor that is the central protein responsible for antiproliferative signaling. Rb blocks proliferation by binding and inhibiting the E2F transcription factors, which are necessary for the G1 to S phase transition and DNA replication (Fischer & Aldape, 2010; Van Meir et al., 2010). Furthermore, Rb is normally inactivated by cyclin D1 and CDK4/CDK6 complexes in order for DNA synthesis to proceed. p16, which is located on chromosome 19, is an additional regulator of this pathway as it negatively regulates CDK4 and CDK6 and therefore also functions as a tumor suppressor (Fischer & Aldape, 2010; Van Meir et al., 2010).

Inhibition of the Rb pathway is common in high grade gliomas, and tumors usually only harbor a single altered component of the pathway (Fischer & Aldape, 2010). Tumor progression to anaplastic astrocytomas is typically characterized by common mutations in this pathway, such as p16 or Rb mutations and amplification or overexpression of CDK4 (Noda et al., 2009; Fischer & Aldape, 2010). Loss of the Rb gene and mutation occur in approximately 30% and 13-25% of grade II and III astrocytomas, respectively (Gladson et al., 2010). Additionally, deletions or mutations of the Rb gene occur in 40% of secondary GBM cases (Gladson et al., 2010). The frequency of Rb mutations in all high grade-gliomas is common and is estimated to occur in approximately 25% of all cases (Fischer & Aldape, 2010). Deletion or mutation of p16INK4A as a consequence of loss of chromosome 9p or hypermethylation occurs in approximately 12-62.5% of anaplastic astrocytoma cases (Gladson et al., 2010). p16 loss has also been reported in 20-57% of GBM cases (Sulman et al., 2009; Kim et al., 2010).

Interestingly, since cyclins and cyclin-dependent kinase (CDK) inhibitors are subject to proteosomal degradation, cell cycle regulation can be modified through proteasome inhibitors. Bortezomib, a proteasome inhibitor, has been shown to induce cell death in cultured glioma cell lines by decreasing levels of CDK2, CDK4, and E2F4 subsequently leading to apoptosis in cultured glioma cell lines (Fischer & Aldape, 2010). Although alterations of the Rb pathway are very common in gliomas, it remains to be determined how these hallmark mutations will translate into a clinically meaningful target. However, a recent study did demonstrate that p16 mutations were strong prognostic indicators of OS in GBM patients treated with TMZ (Ang et al., 2010). Recently, two Phase I trials using bortezomib with and without concurrent temozolomide and radiotherapy for glioblastoma have been reported, and found the combination to be well-tolerated and safe (Kubicek et al., 2009; Phuphanich et al., 2010).

2.3 Proliferation, invasion, and angiogenesis pathways

2.3.1 IDH

Isocitrate dehydrogenase (IDH), is an enzyme that catalyzes the conversion of isocitrate into α-ketoglutarate within the citric acid cycle. IDH1 and IDH2 are involved in a variety of metabolic processes such as signal transduction, lipid synthesis, oxidative stress, and oxidative respiration (Riemenschneider et al., 2010). IDH mutations were initially identified to be associated with gliomas in 2008 when a genome-wide mutational analysis was conducted in GBM (Riemenschneider et al., 2010; Yen et al., 2010). IDH1 and IDH2 mutations were also found in lower grade gliomas in addition to glioblastomas, making IDH the first discovery of somatic genetic alterations in metabolic enzymes in gliomas (Yen et al., 2010). In low grade brain tumors, IDH mutations are common genetic alterations of gliomas arising from the astrocytic and oligodendroglial lineage. These mutations are also identified in secondary GBMs from a lower grade origin (Fischer & Aldape, 2010; Jansen et al., 2010). IDH1 and IDH2 mutations are currently used as diagnostic markers for diffuse WHO grade II and III gliomas as well as secondary GBMs (Jansen et al., 2010; Riemenschneider et al., 2010). IDH1 and IDH2 mutations are often identified concomitantly with 1p/19q co-deletions or p53 mutations (Jansen et al., 2010; Riemenschneider et al., 2010). Mutations in the IDH1 gene were identified in approximately 80% of diffuse astrocytomas and 85% of secondary glioblastomas. In contrast, only 5% of primary glioblastomas carry an IDH mutation (Yan et al., 2009; Fischer & Aldape, 2010).

It remains to be determined how these alterations cause tumorigenesis, although the metabolic role of IDH has been recently examined in the context of oncogenesis. IDH1 mutations are thought to lead to increased formation of 2-hydroxyglutarate (2HG) through a gain of function mutation (Jansen et al., 2010; Riemenschneider et al., 2010; Yen et al., 2010). There is evidence that D-2HG can exert a direct inhibitory effect on adenosine 5′ triphosphate synthase, which interrupts mitochrondrial processes and gives rise to selective pressure to promote metabolic adaptation and a shift towards aerobic glycoysis. This metabolic shift could confer a growth advantage in an increased proliferative state, such as in tumor progression (Yen et al., 2010). Additionally, another possible tumorigenic role of 2HG is its involvement in hypoxia-inducible factor 1 alpha (HIF1α) degradation, thus IDH mutations are thought to lead to increased levels of HIF1α which can facilitate tumor growth (Jansen et al., 2010; Riemenschneider et al., 2010; Yen et al., 2010). Other hypotheses on the role of IDH mutations in gliomagenesis that are being explored are its possible involvement in angiogenesis, glucose transport, glycolysis, and inhibition of apoptosis (Riemenschneider et al., 2010; Yen et al., 2010). Therefore, 2HG has been implicated in tumorigenesis, and is thought to be a potential therapeutic target, a serum biomarker for cancers harboring IDH1 and IDH2 mutations, and a potential response biomarker. Interestingly, there is evidence that D-2HG may be visualized via magnetic resonance spectroscopy, which in theory could make it possible to perform non-invasive detection of tumors with IDH mutations to help diagnose and guide therapy before surgery (Yen et al., 2010).

Patients that harbor IDH mutations appear to have a prognostic advantage compared with patients without IDH mutations for all gliomas (Jansen et al., 2010; Riemenschneider et al.,

2010). Specifically, somatic mutations were present in 18 of 149 (12%) GBMs and seemed to correlate with increased survival, as the overall survival was 31 months in patients with IDH mutations compared to 15 months in those without IDH mutations (Jansen et al., 2010). Although IDH is a useful diagnostic and prognostic tool, it currently does not appear to be able to predict responsiveness to a particular type of therapy (Riemenschneider et al., 2010). More clinical trials examining IDH mutations need to be performed to determine its role as a predictive molecular biomarker.

2.3.2 PDGFR

Platelet-derived growth factor (PDGF) plays an important role in cell proliferation, cell migration, and angiogenesis. Thus, PDGF receptor (PDGFR) is classified as producing a pro-proliferative signal and both the level of PDGF and PDGFRs is important in angiogenesis and tumor growth in gliomas (Noda et al., 2009; Gladson et al., 2010). Amplification of PDGFRα occurs in approximately 7% of oligodendroglial tumors (Gladson et al., 2010). Astrocytic tumors commonly (3-33%) exhibit amplification of the PDGFRα and/or PDGFRβ genes and of the genes encoding their ligands (Gladson et al., 2010). Also, PDGFRα and PDGFRβ amplification occurs in approximately 20-29% of primary GBM and 60% of secondary GBM. Due to its frequency, amplification of PDGF appears to be a key regulator of gliomagenesis, specifically overexpression of PDGFRβ was shown to initiate gliomagenesis when expressed in the neural stem progenitor cell (Gladson et al., 2010). Amplification of PDGFR has also been associated with patient outcome, thus suggesting it could serve as a prognostic biomarker (Toedt et al., 2011). Imatinib is an orally administered tyrosine kinase inhibitor (TKI) of PDGFR, c-abl and c-kit, and is currently being tested in clinical trials to assess its efficacy in malignant gliomas. A multicenter phase II study evaluating imatinib plus hydroxyurea in 231 patients with recurrent glioblastoma did not demonstrate a clinically meaningful anti-tumor activity (Reardon et al., 2009). Precisely, progression-free survival at 6 months and median overall survival were 10.6% and 26.0 weeks, respectively. A Phase II trial has been initiated by Supko et al. that will test the efficacy of tandutinib, a PDGFRβ inhibitor, in patients with recurrent GBM (Supko, 2009).

2.3.3 EGFR/NFKBIA

PDGFR is not the only common growth factor receptor involved in gliomagenesis. Epidermal growth factor receptor (EGFR) also promotes a pro-proliferative signal, and is another common molecular hallmark of glioblastoma (Fischer & Aldape, 2010). In 1984, extra copies of chromosome 7 were identified in malignant gliomas, which resulted in EGFR amplification/overexpression (Van Meir et al., 2010). EGFR promotes cell proliferation, invasion and angiogenesis, induces resistance to apoptosis, and may mediate radiation resistance (Sulman et al., 2009; Gladson et al., 2010). EGFR amplification at 7p12 is the most commonly amplified and overexpressed gene in primary GBM (30-70%) (Fischer & Aldape, 2010; Gladson et al., 2010; Kim et al., 2010; Riemenschneider et al., 2010). Additionally, EGFRvIII is the most prominent mutated receptor tyrosine kinase receptor in GBM (Noda et al., 2009; Riemenschneider et al., 2010). This mutation occurs in ~50% of GBM cases that overexpress EGFR (Riemenschneider et al., 2010). EGFRvIII arises from loss of exons 2 and 7 which leads to loss of the ligand binding domain, thereby promoting constitutive activation of EGFR and the PI3K/AKT pathway (Noda et al., 2009; Jansen et al., 2010). Both EGFR and PDGFR coordinate with integrins and other cell adhesion receptors. In glioma tissue, an increase in growth factors as well as receptors is typically observed (Gladson et al., 2010). EGFR also contributes to invasion as evidenced by the observation that GBMs harboring constitutively active EGFRvIII receptors display a more invasive phenotype than those with wild-type EGFR (Fischer & Aldape, 2010). One of the main molecular distinctions between primary and secondary GBMs is that primary GBMs tend to have EGFR amplifications (~30-70%), whereas secondary GBMs that arise from lower grade gliomas tend to not have EGFR alterations (~5-8%) (Noda et al., 2009; Sulman et al., 2009; Fischer & Aldape, 2010; Kim et al., 2010). In addition, EGFR amplifications occur in approximately 15% of grade III anaplastic astrocytomas (Sulman et al., 2009; Gladson et al., 2010).

One example of targeted therapy is the inhibition of EGFR tyrosine kinase (TKI). Several studies using EGFR TKIs have shown some anti-tumor activity in patients with glioblastoma. EGFR overexpression has been demonstrated in malignant gliomas, and is associated with anti-apoptotic tendency conferred by activated signaling pathways, tumor survival, and proliferation (Nicholas et al., 2006). Surprisingly, the activity did not correlate with the level of EGFR overexpression. Gefinitib and erlotinib are examples of EGFR TKIs that inactivate the downstream signaling pathways, and have been tested in the recurrent GBM setting (Perez-Soler, 2004). However, clinical studies utilizing EGFR inhibitor monotherapy have shown only marginal results for patients with recurrent glioblastoma (Rich et al., 2004; Prados et al., 2009; van den Bent et al., 2009). When used in combination with ionizing radiation, however, the EGFR inhibitors have been shown to augment the anti-proliferative and pro-apoptotic activity induced by ionizing radiation in several human cancer cell lines, as well as in mice bearing human colon cancer xenografts, as demonstrated by Bianco and colleagues (Bianco et al., 2002).

RTOG conducted a phase I/II study (0211) utilizing gefitinib with radiotherapy in patients with newly diagnosed GBM, and compared with historical studies, the combined therapy did not improve survival (Chakravarti, 2006). Prados and colleagues performed a phase II study of combining erlotinib with RT and TMZ in patients with newly-diagnosed GBM, and demonstrated a 5-month improvement in the median survival with this approach (19.3 months *versus* 14.1 months in the combined historical control studies) (Prados et al., 2009). In this study, a strong positive correlation between MGMT promoter methylation and survival was re-demonstrated. However, other studies utilizing a similar approach of combined targeted and conventional therapy showed inferior outcomes and high treatment-related toxicity and death rate (Brown et al., 2008; Peereboom et al., 2010).

The efficacy of EGFR inhibitors remains controversial for newly diagnosed glioblastoma, although some patients have been reported to respond dramatically to EGFR inhibitors. To reconcile the disparity between EGFR overexpression in glioblastomas (up to 50% tumors) with only 10-20% of GBM patients that have a response to EGFR TKIs, biological markers to predict treatment response have been reported, and these can potentially be used to identify the patients that will derive survival benefit from the addition of an EGFR inhibitor (Mellinghoff et al., 2005). Specifically, co-expression of EGFR deletion mutant variant III (EGFRvIII) and the tumor-suppressor protein PTEN was significantly associated with a clinical response to EGFR TKI. In a recent phase II multicenter trial of EGFRvIII-targeted vaccination in 18 patients with glioblastoma who received the standard therapy of gross total resection followed by RT and concurrent TMZ, the 6-month PFS after vaccination was 67%, and median overall survival was 26 months (Sampson et al., 2010). The development of specific antibody or delayed-type hypersensitivity to EGFRvIII had a significant effect on OS. When these patients recurred, 82% had lost EGFRvIII expression.

Resistance to these EGFR inhibitors is thought to be due to other mutations downstream of EGFR, such as PTEN inactivation (Noda et al., 2009). Another potential problem with this type of targeted therapy is that EGFR activates several downstream pathways that might act in parallel to drive oncogenesis. In addition, patients with GBM treated with TMZ that had EGFR amplification, maintenance of PTEN, and wild-type p53 and p16 were strong prognostic indicators of overall survival (Ang et al., 2010). Furthermore, coexpression of normal PTEN and mutant EGFRvIII, combined with lower levels of AKT and overexpressed EGFR have been identified as predictive markers of radiation response (Fischer & Aldape, 2010). Although the predictive and prognostic use of EGFR remains to be completely defined, it does appear that there is some correlation with survival and treatment response (Tabatabai et al., 2010). In addition, the high percentage of GBM cases with EGFR overexpression and EGFR mutations strengthens the possibility that targeted therapy of EGFR may be a useful treatment for gliomas.

Due to high frequency of amplification and activating mutations of EGFR in gliomas, the deletion of NFKBIA, an inhibitor of the EGFR-signaling pathway, was hypothesized to be an additional putative molecular biomarker of gliomas as well. A recent study examined 790 human GBM cases for deletions, mutations, or expression of NFKBIA and EGFR (Bredel et al., 2010). The molecular data was then correlated to outcome data in 570 patients. The results showed that NFKBIA is often deleted, but not mutated in glioblastomas. Most deletions occurred in nonclassical subtypes of GBM and were inversely correlated with EGFR alterations. Importantly, deletion and decreased expression levels of NFKBIA were associated with decreased survival and displayed similar outcomes to patients with EGFR amplifications (Bredel et al., 2010).

2.3.4 VEGF

The formation of new blood vessels (angiogenesis) is one of the major steps in progression of malignant gliomas. Angiogenesis is controlled through many factors, such as vascular endothelial growth factor (VEGF) which is controlled by the transcription factor HIF1α, EGF and PDGF (Deighton et al., 2010; Fischer & Aldape, 2010). VEGF is considered to be the driving factor of angiogenesis in astrocytic gliomas. It has been identified in grade II astrocytoma (36.8%), grade III astrocytoma (66.7%) and in glioblastomas (64.1%) (Oehring et al., 1999). Additionally, a strong correlation between VEGF expression and survival was identified indicating VEGF as a possible prognostic factor in patients with gliomas (Oehring et al., 1999).

One class of targeted therapy includes antiangiogenic agents that target VEGF. Glioblastoma has long been recognized as a highly angiogenic tumor (Ahluwalia & Gladson, 2010). Bevacizumab, a humanized monoclonal antibody that recognizes and blocks VEGF, was approved by the Food and Drug Administration (FDA) as a second-line or salvage treatment of glioblastoma. Recent studies of recurrent glioblastoma have shown that bevacizumab improved response rate and progression-free survival, but specific adverse effects have also been reported, such as intracranial hemorrhage, gastrointestinal perforation, and thromboembolic complications (Vredenburgh, 2010; Friedman, 2009). In one study of 73 patients with recurrent high-grade gliomas who already received a VEGFR TKI (cediranib, sorafenib, pazopanib, or sunitinib), bevacizumab salvage therapy conferred 21% radiologic partial response rate; 12.5% patients were alive and progression-free at six months, and median overall survivial was 5.2 months (range 1.3-28.9+ months) after bevacizumab (Scott et al., 2010).

To evaluate its effect in the up-front setting, Lai et al. conducted a phase II study of bevacizumab plus TMZ during and after RT for patients with newly diagnosed glioblastoma (Lai et al., 2011). They reported a median overall survival and progression-free survival of 19.6 and 13.6 months, respectively. The authors concluded that the addition of bevacizumab improved progression-free survival, but not overall survival, compared with their historical studies. Currently, RTOG is conducting a Phase III double-blind placebo-controlled trial of conventional concurrent chemoradiation and adjuvant TMZ plus bevacizumab versus conventional concurrent chemoradiation and adjuvant TMZ in patients with newly diagnosed GBM. Results are awaited, as this study will determine the efficacy of adding bevacizumab to the current standard treatment of GBM.

Sathornsumetee and colleagues recently reported results of a Phase II trial with bevacizumab and erlotinib, an EGFR inhibitor, in patients with recurrent high grade gliomas (both GBM and anaplastic astrocytoma (AA)). In this trial, the progression-free survival at six months (PFS-6) was 28% for patients with GBM and 44% for patients with AA. Median overall survival was 42 and 71 weeks for patients with GBM and AA, respectively (Sathornsumetee et al., 2010).

In another study evaluating the efficacy of adding sorafenib, an oral VEGFR TKI, to maintenance TMZ following the standard radiotherapy and TMZ in the first-line treatment of 47 patients with GBM, the addition of sorafenib did not appear to improve the efficacy of the standard therapy (Hainsworth et al., 2010). However, 40% patients in this study did not receive any maintenance sorafenib due to early disease progression, lending credence to the hypothesis that the administration of angiogenesis inhibitors concurrently with RT and TMZ may optimize the opportunity to improve therapy. The aforementioned RTOG Phase III trial will help answer this question.

Cilengitide, one of the other anti-angiogenic drugs, inhibits $\alpha v\beta 3$ and $\alpha v\beta 5$ integrin receptors, resulting in apoptosis of glioblastoma cells (Taga et al., 2002). Cilengitide monotherapy for recurrent glioblastoma has a modest effect and confers an approximate 6-month progression-free survival of 15% (Reardon et al., 2008). Currently, Stupp and colleagues are conducting randomized studies of RT plus TMZ with or without cilengitide for newly diagnosed glioblastoma. The Phase I/IIa study of cilengitide and temozolomide with concomitant radiotherapy followed by cilengitide and temozolomide maintenance therapy in 52 patients with newly diagnosed glioblastoma demonstrated promising activity in patients with MGMT promoter methylation. Specifically, 6- and 12-month progression-free survival rates were 69% and 33%, while the 12- and 24-month overall survival rates were 68% and 35% for all patients. The PFS and OS benefit was most pronounced in patients with MGMT promoter methylation (13.4 and 23.2 months versus 2.4 and 13.1 months) (Stupp et al., 2010).

2.4 Signal transduction pathways

Alterations of signaling molecules in gliomas are often involved in gliomagenesis. These signaling molecules act downstream of the cell surface growth factors and cell adhesion receptors to amplify and propagate growth and proinvasion signals. Examples of these signaling molecules include: tyrosine kinase FAK, src family tyrosine kinases, RAS, PI3K, and PTEN. PI3K and PTEN are molecules that regulate glioma cell survival and proliferation. Normally, PI3K promotes proliferation and survival, where as PTEN negatively regulates this process. Many glioblastomas have dysregulation of signaling cascades downstream of the growth factor, such as PTEN mutations and mutations within the PI3K/AKT pathway (Jansen et al., 2010).

2.4.1 PI3K/AKT/PTEN pathway

PTEN (phosphatase and tensin homolog) is a tumor suppressor gene, a negative regulator of the P13K/AKT pathway, and a known inhibitor of angiogenesis. It was first identified as a tumor suppressor located on chromosome 10 in 1997 (Van Meir et al., 2010). PTEN codes for a protein that preferentially dephosphorylates the phosphoinositide substrate, PIP3, and once PTEN is lost PIP3 levels accumulate and lead to constitutive P13K signaling and AKT activation (Maehama & Dixon, 1998). Thus, it is not surprising that loss of PTEN is associated with poor prognosis (Ermoian et al., 2002; Ang et al., 2010; Gladson et al., 2010).
PTEN mutations are common in ~8% of oligodendrogliomas and there is evidence that the presence of this mutation in patients is associated with poor prognosis (Sasaki et al., 2001). Downregulation of this gene has also been found in 50% of grade II and grade III oligodendrogliomas, which appears to be a consequence of promoter methylation (Wiencke et al., 2007; Bourne & Schiff, 2010). In grade II and III astrocytomas, PTEN promoter methylation occurs in ~43-67% of cases (Wiencke et al., 2007; Bourne & Schiff, 2010). In glioblastoma, PTEN is deleted due to LOH of chromosome 10q in ~50-70% of primary cases and ~54-63% secondary cases as well as mutated in ~14-47% of primary cases (Fujisawa et al., 2000; Ohgaki et al., 2004). Methylation of the PTEN promoter in glioblastoma (9%) has also been observed (Wiencke et al., 2007). In many cases loss of PTEN (50% of high grade gliomas) results in unregulated PI3K signaling, AKT activation, and upregulation of mTOR (mammalian target of rapamycin) signaling, which increases protein translation through activation of S6 kinase 1 (S6K1) and eIF4E-binding protein 1 (4E-BP1) (Fischer & Aldape, 2010; Zoncu et al., 2011). mTOR signaling is also known to play a role in hypoxic adaptation of tumors (Van Meir et al., 2010).
Currently, PTEN is thought to be a prognostic molecular marker as patients with loss of PTEN have decreased survival. Based on preclinical evidence that loss of PTEN activates the mTOR pathway, and thereby sensitizes tumors to the inhibition of mTOR, a proof-of-concept Phase I trial utilizing neoadjuvant rapamycin in patients with recurrent GBM showed dramatic anticancer activity in half of the patients (7/14) (Cloughesy et al., 2008). However, rapamycin treatment led to AKT activation in 7/14 patients, implying inadequate inhibition of the mTOR complex 2 (mTORC2). In a Phase II trial utilizing CCI-779, a dihydroxylmethyl propionic acid ester of sirolimus that targets the mTORC pathway, there was no evidence of efficacy in patients with recurrent GBM, as only 1/43 patients was progression-free at 6 months (Chang et al., 2005). North Central Cancer Treatment Group Study (NCCTG) conducted a Phase II trial of once-weekly intravenous temsirolimus, an mTORC1 inhibitor, in 63 patients with recurrent GBM, improving radiographic response in 36% of patients, as well as conferring a significantly longer time to progression in responders (5.4 months versus 1.9 months) (Galanis et al., 2005). In a more recent Phase I trial by NCCTG, the combination of everolimus, an mTORC1 inhibitor, with chemoradiotherapy in 18 patients with newly diagnosed GBM showed that the combination was reasonably well-tolerated, and Phase II dose established (Sarkaria et al., 2010). To date, no clinical trials combining inhibition of both the mTORC1 and mTORC2 have been reported.
In recent years, PTEN status has also been examined as a predictive factor for efficiency of certain targeted therapies, such as poly (ADP-ribose) polymerase (PARP) inhibitors (Dedes et al., 2010; McEllin et al., 2010). It is now known that PTEN is important for maintaining the levels of key proteins involved in homologous recombination, such as Rad51B, Rad51C and Rad51D (Shen et al., 2007). McEllin and colleagues demonstrated that PTEN-null astrocytes had decreased transcript levels of these proteins, consistent with deficiency in homologous

recombination in PTEN-null cells. In their experiments, PTEN-null astrocytes were significantly more sensitive to PARP inhibitor compared with PTEN-proficient cells (McEllin et al., 2010). Data from clinical trials utilizing PARP inhibitors in patients with recurrent or newly diagnosed GBM are awaited.

Mutations of PTEN are not the only molecular markers of gliomas in the PI3K pathway. PI3K signaling is an important mediator of cell growth and proliferation, thus its activation is frequent and associated with poor prognosis in glioma patients (Fischer & Aldape, 2010). Multiple growth factors, such as EGFR, exert their oncogenic effects through activation of PI3K/AKT pathway, which is constitutively activated in up to 70% of GBM due to PTEN loss (Kreisl et al., 2009). An additional study looking at 84 cases in GBM identified pAKT overexpression and PI3K overexpression in 16% and 6% of the cases, respectively (Kim et al., 2010). Downstream of AKT is the serine/threonine kinase, mammalian target of rapamycin (mTOR), which regulates protein biosynthesis, ribosome biogenesis, and the transcription of essential genes (Fischer & Aldape, 2010; McBride et al., 2010). As noted above, inhibitors of mammalian target of rapamycin (mTOR) have been shown to decrease PI3K/AKT activation, and combined mTOR and EGFR inhibition has demonstrated synergy in GBM xenografts (Goudar et al., 2005). In a pilot study of everolimus, an mTOR inhibitor, and gefitinib, an EGFR inhibitor, in the treatment of 22 patients with recurrent GBM, 36% of patients had stable disease and 14% a partial response (PR) (Kreisl et al., 2009). Although disease control was short lived (median progression-free survival (PFS) 2.6 months), the patients with PR all had intact PTEN, and AKT activation was observed in 80% of tumors in which PTEN was lost. In another Phase II study with erlotinib, an EGFR TKI, and sirolimus, an mTOR inhibitor, in 32 patients with recurrent GBM, were also well-tolerated, but had negligible activity among unselected patients. Precisely, no patients achieved either a complete or partial response, and the estimated 6-month progression-free survival for all patients was 3.1%, but somewhat better for patients not on enzyme-inducing antiepileptic drugs (Reardon et al., 2010). Of all tumor markers tested (EGFR, EGFRvIII, PTEN, pAKT and pS6), only pAKT expression achieved borderline significance in association with PFS. Coexpression of EGFR vIII with intact PTEN has been shown to predict sensitivity to EGFR inhibitor monotherapy (Mellinghoff et al., 2005). Activation of the PI3K/mTOR pathway occurs in most adult low grade gliomas, too (McBride et al., 2010). In a recent study, methylation of PTEN, expression of phospho-PRAS40 and phospho-S6 all correlated with decreased survival which suggests that these molecular alterations can be used as prognostic markers for both high and low grade gliomas. Phospho-S6 is a downstream mediator of mTOR, whereas PRAS40 is phosphorylated by AKT and inhibits negative regulation of mTOR thereby further increasing PI3K/AKT signaling (McBride et al., 2010).

In summary, PTEN may be a possible predictive biomarker of glioma response to specific therapies, in addition to its role as a prognostic marker due to its association with aggressive tumor phenotypes and survival. Since upregulation of the P13K/mTOR pathway through a variety of mechanisms predicts overall decreased survival, the use of selective PI3K, AKT, or mTOR inhibitors in the treatment of gliomas appears to be a valid therapeutic target to combat gliomagenesis.

2.4.2 RAS/MAPK pathway

The MAPK pathway, an additional important signal transduction pathway involved in gliomagenesis, is initiated through integrins or receptor tyrosine kinase (RTK) receptors. Growth factors can bind to these RTKs, such as TGF-β, and stimulate the downstream activation of RAS and phosphorylation of MAPK (mitogen-activated protein kinase) by MEK. Phosphorylated MAPK then signals the activation of nuclear transcription factors, such as genes involved in cell cycle progression (Fischer & Aldape, 2010). MAPK signaling is also involved in apoptosis, cell differentiation, and cell migration (Sulman et al., 2009). RAS is often activated in gliomas, however it does not usually contain mutations, but rather an unregulated RTK or integrin activation (Fischer & Aldape, 2010). Specifically, the rate limiting step of RAS activation is farnesylation, which explains the use of farnesyltransferase inhibitors in gliomas. Two separate farnesyl transferase inhibitors, tipifarnib and lonafarnib, have led to mixed results in clinical trials. A Phase II trial with pre-radiation tipifarnib (R115777) in patients with newly diagnosed GBM with residual enhancing disease on postoperative MR imaging showed that there were no tumor responses, and the study was stopped early due to progression of disease in 12 (48%) patients (Lustig et al., 2008). In a Phase II study by North American Brain Tumor Consortium, tipifarnib in patients with recurrent malignant glioma showed modest evidence of activity. Precisely, 12% of GBM patients had progression-free survival more than 6 months (Cloughesy et al., 2006).

In terms of biomarkers, MAPK proteins appear to be both predictive and prognostic molecular biomarkers. Phosphorylated MAPK was found to be inversely correlated with survival, as well as associated with increased radiation resistance (Pelloski et al., 2006). Additionally, upregulation of the MAPK pathway can occur through the proto-oncogene BRAF. Abnormal activation of BRAF, most commonly by gene duplication and fusion, has recently been identified as the characteristic genetic aberration in pilocytic astrocytomas. It occurs in ~60-80% of pilocytic astrocytoma cases (Riemenschneider et al., 2010).

2.5 DNA repair

2.5.1 MGMT

DNA repair response is a critical factor that greatly influences the effectiveness of the majority of chemotherapy agents and radiation. O6-methyl guanine DNA methyltransferase gene (MGMT) is located at chromosome 10q26 and encodes a DNA repair protein that removes the alkyl groups from the O6 position of guanine, which are commonly produced by chemotherapeutic alkylating agents. MGMT is one of the principal enzymes involved in DNA repair, and it is irreversibly inactivated upon removing alkyl groups from the O6 position of guanine. *De novo* synthesis of MGMT is required to replenish the enzyme, and the MGMT promoter needs to be functional if DNA repair is to take place. The MGMT promoter is downregulated by hypermethylation of a CpG island in a 5' region of the gene (Gerson, 2004). Once hypermethylated, the promoter downregulates MGMT and thereby hampers this enzyme's ability to repair DNA damage induced by alkylating agents such as temozolomide. Methylation status of the MGMT promoter, as well as its association with other genetic parameters, has become a major focus of biological marker research. Gliomas often possess decreased MGMT expression levels, which are thought to be primarily due to increased MGMT promoter methylation as previously mentioned. A correlation between MGMT promoter methylation and response of malignant gliomas to alkylating chemotherapy has been observed (Riemenschneider et al., 2010). MGMT hypermethylation has been identified in 11% of grade II astrocytoma, 27% of oligoastrocytoma, and 62% of oligodendroglioma cases (Bourne & Schiff, 2010). In addition, DNA hypermethylation was found in 36% of primary GBM and 75% of secondary GBM cases (Gladson et al., 2010). The heretofore reported frequencies of MGMT promoter methylation vary widely. In the EORTC-NCIC cohort, 45% of assessable cases had MGMT promoter methylation. In a series of 102 patients with various grades and gliomas subtypes, Jha and colleagues found the presence of MGMT promoter methylation in 67.6% cases (79% in Grade II gliomas, 71% in Grade III gliomas, and 57% in GBM), suggesting an inverse relationship between methylation status and tumor grade (Jha et al., 2010). Purely oligodendroglial tumors showed the highest percentage of cases with MGMT promoter methylation (84%), compared with 63.5% in astrocytic tumors. The methylation status of MGMT promoter was not shown to be significantly associated with 1p/19q loss of heterozygosity, nor was there significant association of promoter methylation with EGFR amplification or *TP53* mutation.

Genetic /Protein Alteration	Normal Gene Function	Putative Biomarker Status
1p/19q co-deletion	unknown, involved in gliomagenesis	diagnostic, prognostic, predictive
p53/MDM2/p14ARF	cell cycle arrest, apoptosis, genomic stability	p53-diagnostic
Rb/p16/CDK4	regulates cell cycle progression	p16-prognostic
IDH	citric acid cycle (cell metabolism)	diagnostic, prognostic
PDGFR	cell proliferation signaling	prognostic
EGFR	cell proliferation signaling	diagnostic, prognostic, predictive
VEGF	angiogenesis	prognostic
PTEN	negative regulator of PI3K/AKT activation	prognostic, predictive
PI3K/AKT	cell proliferation, survival	prognostic
MAPK	signaling pathway involved in gene expression, cell cycle, apoptosis, cell differentiation and migration	prognostic, predictive
MGMT	DNA repair enzyme	prognostic, predictive

Table 1. Common Alterations in Malignant Gliomas and their Putative Biomarker Status

In the landmark EORTC/NCIC study by Stupp and colleagues, 573 patients with newly-diagnosed GBM, 84% of which were surgically debulked, were randomized to receive RT alone (60 Gy in 30 fractions) or RT plus continuous daily TMZ (75 mg/m^2 BSA from the first to the last day of RT), followed by six cycles of adjuvant TMZ (150-200 mg/m^2 BSA for 5 days during each 28-day cycle). At a median follow-up of 28 months, the median survival was 14.6 months with RT plus TMZ versus 12.1 months with RT alone, rendering the hazard

TARGETS	AGENTS	PATIENT	PHASE	RESULTS	REFERENCE
Growth factor ligands					
VEGF	BEV + RT + TMZ → TMZ + BEV	New Dx	II	OS 19.6 months, PFS 13.6 months versus 21.1 and 7.6 months in control cohort, and versus 14.6 and 6.9 months in EORTC cohort.	Lai
VEGF	BEV + RT + TMZ → TMZ + BEV	New Dx	III	mPFS 17mo (vs 7 mo without BEV). mOS not reached (17 mo without BEV).	Gruber
VEGF	BEV + Irinotecan	Recurrent	II	PFS-6 37%	Gilbert
VEGF	BEV + Fotemustine	Recurrent	II	Overall response 35%. mTTP 2.6 mo. 15/31 FFP (2-8 mo)	Soffietti
VEGF	BEV q 3 weeks	Recurrent	II	PFS-6 32%, mPFS 3.9 mo, mOS 6.6 mo. 0% CR, 25% PR, 50% SD.	Raizer
VEGF, Vascularity	BEV + Fosbretabulin	Recurrent	I	Pilot study outline only reported.	Altaha
TGF-β 2	Trabedersen	Recurrent	IIb	AA: OS-24mo 83% with lower dose. GBM: mOS 17.4 mo. Phase III started.	Bogdahn
Growth factor receptors					
pan-VEGFR	Cediranib + RT+ TMZ	New Dx	Ib	MTD reached. 6/6 pts alive at 156 days median follow up. Phase II underway.	Chi
pan-VEGFR	Vatalanib + RT + TMZ	New Dx	I/II	MTD reached. Phase II discontinued due to industry decision not to further develop agent.	Brandes
pan-VEGFR	Cediranib	Recurrent	II	56.7% radiologic response, PFS-6 25.8%, manageable toxicity. Biomarkers associated with response and survival.	Batchelor
VEGFR-2	CT-322	Recurrent	II	MTD reached. Clinically active. PFS-6 with CT-322 alone 21.4%, with CT-322 plus irinotecan 57.1%	Schiff
VEGFR	RT + TMZ → TMZ + Sorafenib	New Dx		Median PFS 6 months; PFS-1 year 16%. Median OS 12 months. 40% patients did not receive maintenance sorafenib.	Hainsworth
VEGFR	Sunitinib + Irinotecan	Recurrent	I	MTD reached. 73% SD.	Friedman
VEGFR	Sunitinib	Recurrent	II	mTTP 1.6 mo, mOS 3.8 mo.	Neyns
PDGFR-β	Tandutinib	Recurrent	I	MTD achieved. Phase II initiated.	Supko
Intracellular effectors					
PKC-β and PI3K/Akt pathway	Enzastaurin vs Lomustine	Recurrent	III	n=266; OS 6.6 vs 7.1 months, median PFS 1.5 vs 1.6 months. No superior efficacy compared with lomustine, but better hematologic toxicity.	Wick
PKC-β and PI3K/Akt pathway	Enzastaurin + RT + TMZ	New Dx	II	24/60 PD. OS, PFS will be reported.	Butowski
mTOR	Temsirolimus + RT + TMZ	New Dx	I	MTD established. Increased risk of opportunistic infections.	Sarkaria
mTOR	RAD001 + TMZ (maintenance)	New Dx	I	MTD reached.	Mason
bcl-2	R-(-)-gossypol	Recurrent	II	OS pending. 1/43 PR. 7/43 SD.	Fiveash
VEGFR, PDGFR, *RAF*	TMZ + Sorafenib (maintenance)	New Dx	II	CR 1%, PR 11%, SD 49%, PD 31%. mPFS 6 mo. mOS 16 mo.	Lamar
RAS (Farnesyl transferase)	SCH 66336 + TMZ	Recurrent	I	MTD reached. 2 PR, 14 SD, 11 PD	Desjardins
VEGF, Histone De-acetylase	Vorinostat + BEV + Irinitecan	Recurrent	I	Currently enrolling at the Dose Level 3 vorinostat, with planned follow-up Phase II trial.	Chinnaiyan
PARP-1	BSI-201	New Dx	I	MTD not reached with TMZ, encouraging safety profile.	Blakeley
Multitargeted kinase inhibitors					
VEGF, EGFR	BEV + Erlotinib	Recurrent	II	PFS-6 28% (GBM) and 44% (AA); median OS 42 weeks (GBM) and 71 weeks (AA).	Sathornsumetee
VEGFR, EGFR	Vandetanib + RT+ TMZ	New Dx	I	MTD reached. DLTs included GI hemorrhage, GI perforation and cytopenias. Phase II under way.	Drappatz
VEGFR, EGFR	Vandetanib + Etoposide	Recurrent	I	MTD not reached. "Patients remaining stable on study."	Herndon
VEGFR, EGFR, PDGFR	Vandetanib + Imatinib + Hydroxyurea	Recurrent	I	MTD reached. 1/16 PR, 15/16 SD for at least 4 weeks.	Kirkpatrick
VEGFR-2, EGFR	Vandetanib	Recurrent	I/II	MTD reached; median PFS6 1.8 mo, median OS 7.4 mo	Mcnicol
VEGFR, EGFR	BEV + Cetuximab + Irinotecan	Recurrent	II	Radiographic response 34%, PFS-6 30%. 3/32 patients with DVT. Efficacy not superior compared with Bev + Irinotecan alone.	Hasselbalch
EGFR, mTOR	Erlotinib + Temsirolimus	Recurrent	I/II	MTD reached. No PR, 30% SD. PFS-6 12.5%	Chang
EGFR, mTOR	Erlotinib + Sirolimus	Recurrent	II	47% with SD, no patients with PR or CR. PFS-6 3.1%. PFS better for patinets not on EIAEDs (p=0.03).	Reardon
EGFR, VEGFR	Erlotinib + Sorafenib	Recurrent	I/II	MTD reached. Outcome data pending.	Prados
VEGFR, mTOR	Sorafenib + Temsirolimus	Recurrent	I/II	MTD reached. PFS-6 0%.	Wen
MET, RET, VEGFR2	XL184	Recurrent	II	38% had > 50% tumor reduction (PR), 35% between +24% and -49% enhancement, 27% > 25% PD.	De Groot
MET, RET, VEGFR2	XL184	Progressive	II	PFS6 21%; ORR 21% (AAT naive) vs 8% (prior AAT); mean duration of response 5.9 months.	Wen
VEGFR, PDGFR, *KIT*, EGFR, HER-2	Pazopanib + Lapatinib	Recurrent	I/II	MTD reached. Ph I: 3% PR, 18% SD. Ph II: 1/2 PR, 1/2 CR.	Frentzas
Miscellaneous					
Integrins	Cilentide + RT + TMZ → RT + TMZ	New Dx	I/IIa	PFS-6 69%, PFS-12 33%, OS-12 68%, OS-12 35%. PFS and OS longer if MGMT promoter methylated.	Stupp
Selective Inegrin	Cilengitide	Recurrent	IIa	OS at all time points significantly higher with 2 gr dose vs 0.5 gr dose	Fink
LDL receptor-related protein	ANG1005	Recurrent	I	MTD Reached; SD in 56% pts. Median time to progression in responders 23.9 weeks	Drappatz
CDK/TRKA	PHA-848125	Recurrent	I	MTD reached; transaminase elevation dose-limiting.	Benouaich-Amiel

Table 1. Recent clinical trials with targeted therapy. OS - overall survivial. PFS - progression free survival. MTD - maximum tolerated dose. SD - stable disease. PR - partial response. CR - complete response. GBM - glioblastoma. AA - anaplastic astrocytoma. RT - radiation therapy. TMZ - temozolomide. BEV – bevacizumab. (Bogdahn, 2009; Chang, 2009; Soffietti, 2009; Batchelor et al., 2010; Brandes et al., 2010; Drappatz et al., 2010; Hainsworth et al., 2010; Hasselbalch et al., 2010; Reardon et al., 2010; Sarkaria et al., 2010; Sathornsumetee et al., 2010; Stupp et al., 2010; Wick et al., 2010; Lai et al., 2011; Altaha, June 2010; Benouaich-Amiel, June 2010; Blakeley, June 2010; Chinnaiyan, June 2010; Drappatz, June 2010; Fink, June 2010; Mcnicol, June 2010; Schiff, June 2010; Wen,

June 2010; Butowski, May 2009; Chi, May 2009; De Groot, May 2009; Desjardins, May 2009; Fiveash, May 2009; Frentzas, May 2009; Friedman, May 2009; Gilbert, May 2009; Gruber, May 2009; Herndon, May 2009; Kirkpatrick, May 2009; Lamar, May 2009; Mason, May 2009; Neyns, May 2009; Prados, May 2009; Raizer, May 2009; Supko, May 2009; Wen, May 2009)

ratio (HR) for death 0.63 in the combined modality group. Moreover, the two-year overall survival (OS-2) was 26.5% with RT+TMZ and 10.4% with RT alone (Stupp et al., 2005). The 5-year analysis showed that OS-5 was 9.8% with RT and TMZ, versus 1.9% with RT alone (Stupp et al., 2009). In this trial, patients whose tumor had a methylated MGMT gene promoter had improved survival (median 21.7 *versus* 12.7 months, OS-2 46% *versus* 13.8%) relative to those with an unmethylated *MGMT* promoter, and the methylation status was the strongest predictor for outcome and benefit from TMZ chemotherapy (Hegi et al., 2005). Another study analyzing 125 patients with GBM showed that MGMT promoter methylation was associated with improved median overall survival (61 weeks vs. 42 weeks) (Ang et al., 2010). These studies suggest that MGMT promoter methylation status could possibly be used as a strong predictive marker of response to chemotherapeutic alkylating agents. Furthermore, it is thought that the benefit of MGMT promoter hypermethylation only applies to chemotherapy. However, one study suggested that decreased MGMT confers sensitivity to radiation alone, as well (Rivera et al., 2010). However, this remains controversial as it is thought that this observation is due to the overall prognostic value of MGMT and is independent of the treatment type (Riemenschneider et al., 2010).

Given the increased prevalence of MGMT promoter methylation in lower grade tumors, the effectiveness of adjuvant monotherapy with TMZ has been tested in a trial setting, with reported response rates of up to 52%. Kesari and colleagues conducted a phase II study of protracted daily TMZ (75 $mg/m^2/d$ for 49 consecutive days of each cycle, followed by 28 days off between cycles, until evidence of progression or unacceptable toxicity for a maximum of six cycles) in 44 patients with newly diagnosed low-grade glioma. After a median follow-up of 39.4 months, 21 patients progressed with an overall median progression-free survival of 38 months (Kesari et al., 2009). Patients with methylated MGMT promoter had a significantly longer overall survival (100% alive at analysis, *versus* 29 months with unmethylated promoter), as did patients with single or co-deleted 1p or 19q. The efficacy of protracted TMZ for the treatment of low grade gliomas was also shown in another series with 25 patients, with a response rate of 52%, and a relatively well-tolerated toxicity profile (Pouratian et al., 2007).

An even more pressing clinical challenge is improving the chemotherapy response in GBM patients without the MGMT promoter methylation. Optimizing the adjuvant chemotherapy regimen is one potential strategy to improve patient outcomes, given the inverse relationship between the level of tumoral MGMT and chemosensitivity. A randomized Phase II trial of adjuvant dose-dense (150 mg/m^2 days 1 to 7 and 15 to 21) or metronomic (50 mg/m^2 continuous daily) TMZ showed that the former approach conferred a 1 year survival of 80%, median survival 17.1 months and PFS-6 months of 56% (Clarke et al., 2009). Specifically, in the unmethylated MGMT subset, the median survival was 15.4 months, which was superior to the 12.7 months reported for the patients with unmethylated MGMT in the EORTC/NCIC trial. The dose-dense TMZ schedule suggests that the more effective inhibition of MGMT may be most beneficial to GBM patients with unmethylated MGMT promoter.

In patients that do not have suppressed levels of MGMT, O6-benzylguanine can be used as a MGMT-inactivating agent. This treatment has shown synergistic effects in combination with TMZ and RT in several pre-clinical models (Wedge et al., 1997; Noda et al., 2009). However, GBMs often have decreased concentrations of MGMT, which could make these tumors more susceptible to TMZ (Jansen et al., 2010). Decreased MGMT appears to serve a prognostic role in GBM, as a recent study showed that 46% of patients with MGMT-methylated tumors were alive at 2 years *versus* 23% of unmethylated patients when treated with RT plus TMZ (Jansen et al., 2010). MGMT promoter methylation as a biomarker in grade II gliomas remains controversial. However, for grade III gliomas MGMT promoter hypermethylation appears to be a positive prognostic marker and for grade IV it is believed to be a prognostic as well as a predictive marker for alkylating agent chemotherapy (Riemenschneider et al., 2010; Tabatabai et al., 2010). Furthermore, it is believed that the predictive power of MGMT is only for chemotherapy, although this remains a controversial topic as discussed before (Riemenschneider et al., 2010). Moreover, MGMT promoter methylation has been shown to be closely linked to pseudoprogression (Nutt, 2005; Riemenschneider et al., 2010). Although MGMT can be useful as a marker of survival, the current standard of care for GBM does not require knowing MGMT status; however, it may help distinguish between pseudoprogression and true progression (Nutt, 2005; Riemenschneider et al., 2010) as well as possibly determining if a MGMT-specific inhibitor should be combined with the current standard treatment modality.

2.6 Other pathways

2.6.1 Glutamatergic system

The glutamatergic system has been found to play a key role in the proliferation, survival and migration of gliomas (Ishiuchi et al., 2007; De Groot et al., 2008). Glioma cells release glutamate in concentrations that are toxic to surrounding neurons and glia (Takano et al., 2001). However, the glutamate reuptake is reduced due to downregulation of glutamate transporters (EAAT2/GLT-1) (Ye et al., 1999). In a phase II trial with talampanel, an oral noncompetitive antagonist of α-amino-3-hydroxy-5-methyl-4-isoxazolepropionic acid (AMPA) glutamate receptor and standard RT + TMZ in patients with newly diagnosed glioblastoma, a median survival of 18.3 months was reached in all patients. In patients 70 years or younger, the median survival was 20.3 months. The two year survival was also superior compared with EORTC RT + TMZ data (41.7% vs 26.5%, respectively) (Grossman et al., 2009).

2.6.2 Epigenetic regulation

Histone deacetylases (HDAC) are enzymes that affect acetylation status of histones, as well as that of cell cycle regulatory proteins (Arts et al., 2003). Histone deacetylation leads to tight coiling of chromatin and silencing of expression of various genes, including those implicated in the regulation of cell survival, tumor cell differentiation, cell cycle arrest and apoptosis (Jones & Baylin, 2002). North Central Cancer Treatment Group (NCCTG) conducted a Phase II trial of vorinostat, a small-molecule inhibitor of human HDAC1, 2, 3, 6 and 8 that crosses the blood-brain barrier, in 66 patients with recurrent glioblastoma (Galanis et al., 2009). The agent was administered at a dose of 200 mg twice a day for 14 days every 3 weeks, and was well tolerated. The 6-month PFS was 15.2%, with median time to progression of 1.9 months and median survival of 5.7 months. However, in patients who were progression-free at 6 months, the duration of disease stability ranged from 6.8 to 28+ months, suggesting that there is a patient sub-population that can derive definite clinical benefit from this therapy. Incorporation of vorinostat in the current standard of care with RT + TMZ will be tested by the NCCTG/North American Brain Tumor Coalition in a phase I/II trial.

3. Conclusion

As we learn more about cellular pathways and effectors involved in gliomagenesis, there will likely be a paradigm shift from the uniform standard-of-care treatment for all patients to a more individualized treatment based on molecular biomarkers. The aforementioned novel targeting therapies add to our armamentarium both as single agents and in combination with radiation, chemotherapy, and other targeted molecular agents. Ultimately, this will enable us to devise a more effective treatment strategy by tackling the underpinnings of resistance of malignant gliomas. As our knowledge increases, the challenge before the scientific and clinical community will be to identify the key targets and formulate therapy accordingly. Foregoing the "kitchen sink" approach will lessen the harm done to patients, as the aforementioned clinical trials show that targeted therapies may cause serious toxicities.

Although most studies mentioned are phase I or II, with a relatively short follow-up time, several of these agents warrant testing in a larger and randomized setting to truly discern their efficacy and safety, with the overarching hope of improving our patients' prognosis. The most recent update from Stupp and colleagues regarding integrin inhibition with addition of cilengitide to standard chemoradiotherapy shows promise to potentially become the new standard-of-care for patients with GBM, suggesting that the most effective strategy is to target both the extracellular (*e.g.,* integrin) and intracellular effectors. Moreover, just as the methylation status of the MGMT promoter did, greater characterization of gene expression by epigenetic regulation may help us elucidate additional mechanisms of resistance or sensitivity to therapy.

In summary, gaining a better understanding of the molecular brain tumor population(s) that benefit from each targeted therapy will lead to more effective personalized therapy. It is hoped that a more targeted therapeutic approach will overcome the current limitations in the treatment of patients with malignant gliomas and result in a better prognosis for patients with brain tumors.

4. Acknowledgements

E. Hlavin Bell and M. Hadziahmetovic contributed equally to this chapter. We thank the Department of Radiation Oncology at the James Cancer Hospital and Richard Solove Research Institute at The Ohio State University. E. Hlavin Bell was funded by the Barbara Hughes Fellowship.

5. References

Ahluwalia, M. S. & C. L. Gladson (2010). Progress on antiangiogenic therapy for patients with malignant glioma. *J Oncol,* Vol. 2010, No., 689018, ISBN 1687-8469

Aldape, K., P. C. Burger, et al. (2007). Clinicopathologic aspects of 1p/19q loss and the diagnosis of oligodendroglioma. *Arch Pathol Lab Med,* Vol. 131, No. 2, (Feb), 242-251, ISBN 1543-2165

Altaha (June 2010). A pilot study of fosbretabulin with bevacizumab in recurrent high-grade gliomas. ASCO Annual Meeting,28:15s, San Diego, California

Ang, C., M. C. Guiot, et al. (2010). Clinical significance of molecular biomarkers in glioblastoma. *Can J Neurol Sci,* Vol. 37, No. 5, (Sep), 625-630, ISBN 0317-1671

Arts, J., S. de Schepper, et al. (2003). Histone deacetylase inhibitors: from chromatin remodeling to experimental cancer therapeutics. *Curr Med Chem,* Vol. 10, No. 22, (Nov), 2343-2350

Batchelor, T. T., D. G. Duda, et al. (2010). Phase II study of cediranib, an oral pan-vascular endothelial growth factor receptor tyrosine kinase inhibitor, in patients with recurrent glioblastoma. *J Clin Oncol,* Vol. 28, No. 17, (Jun 10), 2817-2823, ISBN 1527-7755

Bauman, G. S., Y. Ino, et al. (2000). Allelic loss of chromosome 1p and radiotherapy plus chemotherapy in patients with oligodendrogliomas. *Int J Radiat Oncol Biol Phys,* Vol. 48, No. 3, (Oct 1), 825-830, ISBN 0360-3016

Benouaich-Amiel, A. (June 2010). Phase I study of the oral CDK-TRKA inhibitor PHA-848125 in recurrent malignant glioma (MG). ASCO Annual Meeting,28:15s, San Diego, California

Bianco, C., G. Tortora, et al. (2002). Enhancement of antitumor activity of ionizing radiation by combined treatment with the selective epidermal growth factor receptor-tyrosine kinase inhibitor ZD1839 (Iressa). *Clin Cancer Res,* Vol. 8, No. 10, (Oct), 3250-3258, ISBN 1078-0432

Blakeley, J. O. (June 2010). Poly (ADP-ribose) polymerase-1 (PARP1) inhibitor BSI-201 in combination with temozolomide (TMZ) in malignant glioma. J Clin Oncol,28:15s, San Diego, California

Bogdahn, U. (2009). Randomized, active-controlled phase IIb study with trabedersen (AP 12009) in recurrent or refractory high-grade glioma patients: basis for phase III endpoints. ASCO Annual Meeting,27:15s, Orlando, Florida

Bourne, T. D. & D. Schiff (2010). Update on molecular findings, management and outcome in low-grade gliomas. *Nat Rev Neurol,* Vol. 6, No. 12, (Dec), 695-701, ISBN 1759-4766

Brandes, A. A., R. Stupp, et al. (2010). EORTC study 26041-22041: phase I/II study on concomitant and adjuvant temozolomide (TMZ) and radiotherapy (RT) with PTK787/ZK222584 (PTK/ZK) in newly diagnosed glioblastoma. *Eur J Cancer,* Vol. 46, No. 2, (Jan), 348-354, ISBN 1879-0852

Bredel, M., D. M. Scholtens, et al. (2010). NFKBIA Deletion in Glioblastomas. *N Engl J Med,* Vol., No., (Dec 22), ISBN 1533-4406

Brown, P. D., S. Krishnan, et al. (2008). Phase I/II trial of erlotinib and temozolomide with radiation therapy in the treatment of newly diagnosed glioblastoma multiforme: North Central Cancer Treatment Group Study N0177. *J Clin Oncol,* Vol. 26, No. 34, (Dec 1), 5603-5609, ISBN 1527-7755

Butowski, N. (May 2009). Phase II and pharmacogenomics study of enzastaurin plus temozolomide and radiation therapy in patients with glioblastoma multiforme or gliosarcoma. ASCO Annual Meeting,27:15s, Orlando, Florida

Cairncross, G. & R. Jenkins (2008). Gliomas with 1p/19q codeletion: a.k.a. oligodendroglioma. *Cancer J,* Vol. 14, No. 6, (Nov-Dec), 352-357, ISBN 1528-9117

Cairncross, J. G., K. Ueki, et al. (1998). Specific genetic predictors of chemotherapeutic response and survival in patients with anaplastic oligodendrogliomas. *J Natl Cancer Inst,* Vol. 90, No. 19, (Oct 7), 1473-1479, ISBN 0027-8874

Chakravarti, A. (2006). An update of phase II results from RTOG 0211: a phase I/II study of gefitinib with radiotherapy in newly diagnosed glioblastoma. ASCO Annual Meeting,24:18s, Atlanta, Georgia

Chang, S. M. (2009). Phase I/II study of erlotinib and temsirolimus for patients with recurrent malignant gliomas (MG) (NABTC 04-02). ASCO Annual Meeting,27:15s, Orlando, Florida

Chang, S. M., P. Wen, et al. (2005). Phase II study of CCI-779 in patients with recurrent glioblastoma multiforme. *Invest New Drugs,* Vol. 23, No. 4, (Aug), 357-361, ISBN 0167-6997

Chi, A. S. (May 2009). Phase Ib study of cediranib in combination with daily temozolomide and radiation in patients with newly diagnosed glioblastoma. ASCO Annual Meeting,27:15s, Orlando, Florida

Chinnaiyan, P. (June 2010). A phase I trial of vorinostat in combination with bevacizumab and irinotecan in recurrent glioblastoma. ASCO Annual Meeting,28:15s, San Diego, California

Clarke, J. L., F. M. Iwamoto, et al. (2009). Randomized phase II trial of chemoradiotherapy followed by either dose-dense or metronomic temozolomide for newly diagnosed glioblastoma. *J Clin Oncol,* Vol. 27, No. 23, (Aug 10), 3861-3867, ISBN 1527-7755

Cloughesy, T. F., P. Y. Wen, et al. (2006). Phase II trial of tipifarnib in patients with recurrent malignant glioma either receiving or not receiving enzyme-inducing antiepileptic drugs: a North American Brain Tumor Consortium Study. *J Clin Oncol,* Vol. 24, No. 22, (Aug 1), 3651-3656, ISBN 1527-7755

Cloughesy, T. F., K. Yoshimoto, et al. (2008). Antitumor activity of rapamycin in a Phase I trial for patients with recurrent PTEN-deficient glioblastoma. *PLoS Med,* Vol. 5, No. 1, (Jan 22), e8, ISBN 1549-1676

De Groot, J. F. (May 2009). A phase II study of XL184 in patients (pts) with progressive glioblastoma multiforme (GBM) in first or second relapse. ASCO Annual Meeting,27:15s, Orlando, Florida

De Groot, J. F., Y. Piao, et al. (2008). Knockdown of GluR1 expression by RNA interference inhibits glioma proliferation. *J Neurooncol,* Vol. 88, No. 2, (Jun), 121-133, ISBN 0167-594X

Dedes, K. J., D. Wetterskog, et al. (2010). PTEN deficiency in endometrioid endometrial adenocarcinomas predicts sensitivity to PARP inhibitors. *Sci Transl Med,* Vol. 2, No. 53, (Oct 13), 53ra75, ISBN 1946-6242

Deighton, R. F., R. McGregor, et al. (2010). Glioma pathophysiology: insights emerging from proteomics. *Brain Pathol,* Vol. 20, No. 4, (Jul), 691-703, ISBN 1750-3639

Desjardins, A. (May 2009). Phase I trial combining SCH 66336 to temozolomide (TMZ) for patients with grade 3 or 4 malignant gliomas (MG). ASCO Annual Meeting,27:15s, Orlando, Florida

Drappatz, J. (June 2010). ANG1005: Results of a phase I study in patients with recurrent malignant glioma. ASCO Annual Meeting,28:15s, San Diego, California

Drappatz, J., A. D. Norden, et al. (2010). Phase I study of vandetanib with radiotherapy and temozolomide for newly diagnosed glioblastoma. *Int J Radiat Oncol Biol Phys,* Vol. 78, No. 1, (Sep 1), 85-90, ISBN 1879-355X

Ermoian, R. P., C. S. Furniss, et al. (2002). Dysregulation of PTEN and protein kinase B is associated with glioma histology and patient survival. *Clin Cancer Res,* Vol. 8, No. 5, (May), 1100-1106, ISBN 1078-0432

Fink, K. (June 2010). Long-term effects of cilengitide, a novel integrin inhibitor, in recurrent glioblastoma: A randomized phase IIa study. ASCO Annual Meeting,28:15s, San Diego, California

Fischer, I. & K. Aldape (2010). Molecular tools: biology, prognosis, and therapeutic triage. *Neuroimaging Clin N Am,* Vol. 20, No. 3, (Aug), 273-282, ISBN 1557-9867

Fiveash, J. B. (May 2009). NABTT-0702: A phase II study of R-(-)gossypol (AT-101) in recurrent glioblastoma multiforme (GBM). ASCO Annual Meeting,27:15s, Orlando, Florida

Frentzas (May 2009). Pazopanib and lapatinib in patients with relapsed malignant glioma: results of a phase I/II study. ASCO Annual Meeting,27:15s, Orlando, Florida

Friedman, H. S. (May 2009). A phase I study of sunitinib plus irinotecan in the treatment of patients with recurrent malignant glioma. ASCO Annual Meeting,27:15s, Orlando, Florida

Fujisawa, H., R. M. Reis, et al. (2000). Loss of heterozygosity on chromosome 10 is more extensive in primary (de novo) than in secondary glioblastomas. *Lab Invest,* Vol. 80, No. 1, (Jan), 65-72, ISBN 0023-6837

Galanis, E., J. C. Buckner, et al. (2005). Phase II trial of temsirolimus (CCI-779) in recurrent glioblastoma multiforme: a North Central Cancer Treatment Group Study. *J Clin Oncol,* Vol. 23, No. 23, (Aug 10), 5294-5304, ISBN 0732-183X

Galanis, E., K. A. Jaeckle, et al. (2009). Phase II trial of vorinostat in recurrent glioblastoma multiforme: a north central cancer treatment group study. *J Clin Oncol,* Vol. 27, No. 12, (Apr 20), 2052-2058, ISBN 1527-7755

Gerson, S. L. (2004). MGMT: its role in cancer aetiology and cancer therapeutics. *Nat Rev Cancer,* Vol. 4, No. 4, (Apr), 296-307, ISBN 1474-175X

Gilbert, M. R. (May 2009). RTOG 0625: A phase II study of bevacizumab with irinotecan in recurrent glioblastoma (GBM). ASCO Annual Meeting,27:15s, Orlando, Florida

Gladson, C. L., R. A. Prayson, et al. (2010). The pathobiology of glioma tumors. *Annu Rev Pathol,* Vol. 5, No., 33-50, ISBN 1553-4014

Goudar, R. K., Q. Shi, et al. (2005). Combination therapy of inhibitors of epidermal growth factor receptor/vascular endothelial growth factor receptor 2 (AEE788) and the mammalian target of rapamycin (RAD001) offers improved glioblastoma tumor growth inhibition. *Mol Cancer Ther,* Vol. 4, No. 1, (Jan), 101-112, ISBN 1535-7163

Grossman, S. A., X. Ye, et al. (2009). Talampanel with standard radiation and temozolomide in patients with newly diagnosed glioblastoma: a multicenter phase II trial. *J Clin Oncol,* Vol. 27, No. 25, (Sep 1), 4155-4161, ISBN 1527-7755

Gruber, M. L. (May 2009). Bevacizumab in combination with radiotherapy plus concomitant and ajuvant temozolomide for newly diagnosed glioblastoma: update progression-free survival, overall survival, and toxicity. ASCO Annual Meeting,27:15s, Orlando, Florida

Hainsworth, J. D., T. Ervin, et al. (2010). Concurrent radiotherapy and temozolomide followed by temozolomide and sorafenib in the first-line treatment of patients with glioblastoma multiforme. *Cancer,* Vol. 116, No. 15, (Aug 1), 3663-3669, ISBN 0008-543X

Hasselbalch, B., U. Lassen, et al. (2010). Cetuximab, bevacizumab, and irinotecan for patients with primary glioblastoma and progression after radiation therapy and temozolomide: a phase II trial. *Neuro Oncol,* Vol. 12, No. 5, (May), 508-516, ISBN 1523-5866

Hegi, M. E., A. C. Diserens, et al. (2005). MGMT gene silencing and benefit from temozolomide in glioblastoma. *N Engl J Med,* Vol. 352, No. 10, (Mar 10), 997-1003, ISBN 1533-4406

Herndon, J. (May 2009). Phase I trial of vendetanib and oral etoposide for recurrent malignant gliomas. ASCO Annual Meeting,27:15s, Orlando, Florida

Hirose, Y., H. Sasaki, et al. (2011). Whole genome analysis from microdissected tissue revealed adult supratentorial grade II-III gliomas are divided into clinically relevant subgroups by genetic profile. *Neurosurgery,* Vol., No., (Feb 23), ISBN 1524-4040

Ino, Y., R. A. Betensky, et al. (2001). Molecular subtypes of anaplastic oligodendroglioma: implications for patient management at diagnosis. *Clin Cancer Res,* Vol. 7, No. 4, (Apr), 839-845, ISBN 1078-0432

Ishiuchi, S., Y. Yoshida, et al. (2007). Ca2+-permeable AMPA receptors regulate growth of human glioblastoma via Akt activation. *J Neurosci,* Vol. 27, No. 30, (Jul 25), 7987-8001, ISBN 1529-2401

Jansen, M., S. Yip, et al. (2010). Molecular pathology in adult gliomas: diagnostic, prognostic, and predictive markers. *Lancet Neurol,* Vol. 9, No. 7, (Jul), 717-726, ISBN 1474-4465

Jha, P., V. Suri, et al. (2010). O6-methylguanine DNA methyltransferase gene promoter methylation status in gliomas and its correlation with other molecular alterations: first Indian report with review of challenges for use in customized treatment. *Neurosurgery,* Vol. 67, No. 6, (Dec), 1681-1691, ISBN 1524-4040

Jones, P. A. & S. B. Baylin (2002). The fundamental role of epigenetic events in cancer. *Nat Rev Genet,* Vol. 3, No. 6, (Jun), 415-428, ISBN 1471-0056

Kesari, S., D. Schiff, et al. (2009). Phase II study of protracted daily temozolomide for low-grade gliomas in adults. *Clin Cancer Res,* Vol. 15, No. 1, (Jan 1), 330-337, ISBN 1078-0432

Kim, B., J. K. Myung, et al. (2010). The clinicopathologic values of the molecules associated with the main pathogenesis of the glioblastoma. *J Neurol Sci,* Vol. 294, No. 1-2, (Jul 15), 112-118, ISBN 1878-5883

Kirkpatrick (May 2009). Phase I study of vandetanib, imatinib mesylate, and hydroxyurea for recurrent malignant glioma. ASCO Annual Meeting,27:15s, Orlando, Florida

Kouwenhoven, M. C., J. M. Kros, et al. (2006). 1p/19q loss within oligodendroglioma is predictive for response to first line temozolomide but not to salvage treatment. *Eur J Cancer,* Vol. 42, No. 15, (Oct), 2499-2503, ISBN 0959-8049

Kreisl, T. N., A. B. Lassman, et al. (2009). A pilot study of everolimus and gefitinib in the treatment of recurrent glioblastoma (GBM). *J Neurooncol,* Vol. 92, No. 1, (Mar), 99-105, ISBN 0167-594X

Kubicek, G. J., M. Werner-Wasik, et al. (2009). Phase I trial using proteasome inhibitor bortezomib and concurrent temozolomide and radiotherapy for central nervous system malignancies. *Int J Radiat Oncol Biol Phys,* Vol. 74, No. 2, (Jun 1), 433-439, ISBN 1879-355X

Lai, A., A. Tran, et al. (2011). Phase II study of bevacizumab plus temozolomide during and after radiation therapy for patients with newly diagnosed glioblastoma multiforme. *J Clin Oncol,* Vol. 29, No. 2, (Jan 10), 142-148, ISBN 1527-7755

Lamar, R. E. (May 2009). Phase II trial of radiation therapy/temozolomide followed by temozolomide/sorafenib in the first-line treatment of glioblastoma multiforme. ASCO Annual Meeting,27:15s, Orlando, Florida

Lustig, R., T. Mikkelsen, et al. (2008). Phase II preradiation R115777 (tipifarnib) in newly diagnosed GBM with residual enhancing disease. *Neuro Oncol,* Vol. 10, No. 6, (Dec), 1004-1009, ISBN 1522-8517

Maehama, T. & J. E. Dixon (1998). The tumor suppressor, PTEN/MMAC1, dephosphorylates the lipid second messenger, phosphatidylinositol 3,4,5-trisphosphate. *J Biol Chem,* Vol. 273, No. 22, (May 29), 13375-13378, ISBN 0021-9258

Mason, W. P. (May 2009). A phase I study of temozolomide (TMZ) and RAD001 in patients (pts) with glioblastoma multiforme (GBM). ASCO Annual Meeting,27:15s, Orlando, Florida

McBride, S. M., D. A. Perez, et al. (2010). Activation of PI3K/mTOR pathway occurs in most adult low-grade gliomas and predicts patient survival. *J Neurooncol,* Vol. 97, No. 1, (Mar), 33-40, ISBN 1573-7373

McEllin, B., C. V. Camacho, et al. (2010). PTEN loss compromises homologous recombination repair in astrocytes: implications for glioblastoma therapy with temozolomide or poly(ADP-ribose) polymerase inhibitors. *Cancer Res,* Vol. 70, No. 13, (Jul 1), 5457-5464, ISBN 1538-7445

Mcnicol, K. A. (June 2010). Phase I/II study of vandetanib for patients with recurrent malignant gliomas. ASCO Annual Meeting,28:15s, San Diego, California

Mellinghoff, I. K., M. Y. Wang, et al. (2005). Molecular determinants of the response of glioblastomas to EGFR kinase inhibitors. *N Engl J Med,* Vol. 353, No. 19, (Nov 10), 2012-2024, ISBN 1533-4406

Neyns, B. (May 2009). Phase II trial of sunitinib malate in patients with temozolomide refractory recurrent high-grade glioma. ASCO Annual Meeting,27:15s, Orlando, Florida

Nicholas, M. K., R. V. Lukas, et al. (2006). Epidermal growth factor receptor - mediated signal transduction in the development and therapy of gliomas. *Clin Cancer Res,* Vol. 12, No. 24, (Dec 15), 7261-7270, ISBN 1078-0432

Noda, S. E., A. El-Jawahri, et al. (2009). Molecular advances of brain tumors in radiation oncology. *Semin Radiat Oncol,* Vol. 19, No. 3, (Jul), 171-178, ISBN 1532-9461

Nutt, C. L. (2005). Molecular genetics of oligodendrogliomas: a model for improved clinical management in the field of neurooncology. *Neurosurg Focus,* Vol. 19, No. 5, (Nov), E2, ISBN 1092-0684

Oehring, R. D., M. Miletic, et al. (1999). Vascular endothelial growth factor (VEGF) in astrocytic gliomas--a prognostic factor? *J Neurooncol,* Vol. 45, No. 2, 117-125, ISBN 0167-594X

Ohgaki, H., P. Dessen, et al. (2004). Genetic pathways to glioblastoma: a population-based study. *Cancer Res,* Vol. 64, No. 19, (Oct 1), 6892-6899, ISBN 0008-5472

Peereboom, D. M., D. R. Shepard, et al. (2010). Phase II trial of erlotinib with temozolomide and radiation in patients with newly diagnosed glioblastoma multiforme. *J Neurooncol,* Vol. 98, No. 1, (May), 93-99, ISBN 1573-7373

Pelloski, C. E., E. Lin, et al. (2006). Prognostic associations of activated mitogen-activated protein kinase and Akt pathways in glioblastoma. *Clin Cancer Res,* Vol. 12, No. 13, (Jul 1), 3935-3941, ISBN 1078-0432

Perez-Soler, R. (2004). HER1/EGFR targeting: refining the strategy. *Oncologist,* Vol. 9, No. 1, 58-67, ISBN 1083-7159

Phuphanich, S., J. G. Supko, et al. (2010). Phase 1 clinical trial of bortezomib in adults with recurrent malignant glioma. *J Neurooncol,* Vol. 100, No. 1, (Oct), 95-103, ISBN 1573-7373

Pouratian, N., J. Gasco, et al. (2007). Toxicity and efficacy of protracted low dose temozolomide for the treatment of low grade gliomas. *J Neurooncol,* Vol. 82, No. 3, (May), 281-288, ISBN 0167-594X

Prados, M. (May 2009). Phase I/II study of sorefenib and erlotinib for patients with recurrent glioblastoma (GBM) (NABTC 05-02). ASCO Annual Meeting,27:15s, Orlando, Florida

Prados, M. D., S. M. Chang, et al. (2009). Phase II study of erlotinib plus temozolomide during and after radiation therapy in patients with newly diagnosed glioblastoma multiforme or gliosarcoma. *J Clin Oncol,* Vol. 27, No. 4, (Feb 1), 579-584, ISBN 1527-7755

Raizer, J. J. (May 2009). A phase II trial of single-agent bevacizumab given every 3 weeks for recurrent malignant gliomas. ASCO Annual Meeting,27:15s, Orlando, Florida

Reardon, D. A., A. Desjardins, et al. (2010). Phase 2 trial of erlotinib plus sirolimus in adults with recurrent glioblastoma. *J Neurooncol,* Vol. 96, No. 2, (Jan), 219-230, ISBN 1573-7373

Reardon, D. A., G. Dresemann, et al. (2009). Multicentre phase II studies evaluating imatinib plus hydroxyurea in patients with progressive glioblastoma. *Br J Cancer,* Vol. 101, No. 12, (Dec 15), 1995-2004, ISBN 1532-1827

Reardon, D. A., K. L. Fink, et al. (2008). Randomized phase II study of cilengitide, an integrin-targeting arginine-glycine-aspartic acid peptide, in recurrent glioblastoma multiforme. *J Clin Oncol,* Vol. 26, No. 34, (Dec 1), 5610-5617, ISBN 1527-7755

Rich, J. N., D. A. Reardon, et al. (2004). Phase II trial of gefitinib in recurrent glioblastoma. *J Clin Oncol,* Vol. 22, No. 1, (Jan 1), 133-142, ISBN 0732-183X

Riemenschneider, M. J., J. W. Jeuken, et al. (2010). Molecular diagnostics of gliomas: state of the art. *Acta Neuropathol,* Vol. 120, No. 5, (Nov), 567-584, ISBN 1432-0533

Rivera, A. L., C. E. Pelloski, et al. (2010). MGMT promoter methylation is predictive of response to radiotherapy and prognostic in the absence of adjuvant alkylating chemotherapy for glioblastoma. *Neuro Oncol,* Vol. 12, No. 2, (Feb), 116-121, ISBN 1523-5866

Sampson, J. H., A. B. Heimberger, et al. (2010). Immunologic escape after prolonged progression-free survival with epidermal growth factor receptor variant III peptide vaccination in patients with newly diagnosed glioblastoma. *J Clin Oncol,* Vol. 28, No. 31, (Nov 1), 4722-4729, ISBN 1527-7755

Sarkaria, J. N., E. Galanis, et al. (2010). North Central Cancer Treatment Group Phase I Trial N057K of Everolimus (RAD001) and Temozolomide in Combination with Radiation Therapy in Patients with Newly Diagnosed Glioblastoma Multiforme. *Int J Radiat Oncol Biol Phys,* Vol., No., (Sep 22), ISBN 1879-355X

Sasaki, H., M. C. Zlatescu, et al. (2001). PTEN is a target of chromosome 10q loss in anaplastic oligodendrogliomas and PTEN alterations are associated with poor prognosis. *Am J Pathol,* Vol. 159, No. 1, (Jul), 359-367, ISBN 0002-9440

Sathornsumetee, S., A. Desjardins, et al. (2010). Phase II trial of bevacizumab and erlotinib in patients with recurrent malignant glioma. *Neuro Oncol,* Vol. 12, No. 12, (Dec), 1300-1310, ISBN 1523-5866

Schiff, D. (June 2010). Phase II study of CT-322, a targeted biologic inhibitor of VEGFR-2 based on a domain of human fibronectin, in recurrent glioblastoma (rGBM). ASCO Annual Meeting,28:15s, San Diego, California

Scott, B. J., E. C. Quant, et al. (2010). Bevacizumab salvage therapy following progression in high-grade glioma patients treated with VEGF receptor tyrosine kinase inhibitors. *Neuro Oncol,* Vol. 12, No. 6, (Jun), 603-607, ISBN 1523-5866

Shen, W. H., A. S. Balajee, et al. (2007). Essential role for nuclear PTEN in maintaining chromosomal integrity. *Cell,* Vol. 128, No. 1, (Jan 12), 157-170, ISBN 0092-8674

Siker, M. L., A. Chakravarti, et al. (2006). Should concomitant and adjuvant treatment with temozolomide be used as standard therapy in patients with anaplastic glioma? *Crit Rev Oncol Hematol,* Vol. 60, No. 2, (Nov), 99-111, ISBN 1040-8428

Smith, J. S., A. Perry, et al. (2000). Alterations of chromosome arms 1p and 19q as predictors of survival in oligodendrogliomas, astrocytomas, and mixed oligoastrocytomas. *J Clin Oncol,* Vol. 18, No. 3, (Feb), 636-645, ISBN 0732-183X

Snuderl, M., A. F. Eichler, et al. (2009). Polysomy for chromosomes 1 and 19 predicts earlier recurrence in anaplastic oligodendrogliomas with concurrent 1p/19q loss. *Clin Cancer Res,* Vol. 15, No. 20, (Oct 15), 6430-6437, ISBN 1078-0432

Soffietti, R. (2009). Phase II study of bevacizumab and nitrosourea in patients with recurrent malignant glioma: a multicenter Italian study. ASCO Annual Meeting,27:15s, Orlando, Florida

Stupp, R., M. E. Hegi, et al. (2009). Effects of radiotherapy with concomitant and adjuvant temozolomide versus radiotherapy alone on survival in glioblastoma in a randomised phase III study: 5-year analysis of the EORTC-NCIC trial. *Lancet Oncol,* Vol. 10, No. 5, (May), 459-466, ISBN 1474-5488

Stupp, R., M. E. Hegi, et al. (2010). Phase I/IIa study of cilengitide and temozolomide with concomitant radiotherapy followed by cilengitide and temozolomide maintenance therapy in patients with newly diagnosed glioblastoma. *J Clin Oncol,* Vol. 28, No. 16, (Jun 1), 2712-2718, ISBN 1527-7755

Stupp, R., W. P. Mason, et al. (2005). Radiotherapy plus concomitant and adjuvant temozolomide for glioblastoma. *N Engl J Med,* Vol. 352, No. 10, (Mar 10), 987-996, ISBN 1533-4406

Sulman, E. P., M. Guerrero, et al. (2009). Beyond grade: molecular pathology of malignant gliomas. *Semin Radiat Oncol,* Vol. 19, No. 3, (Jul), 142-149, ISBN 1532-9461

Supko, J. G. (May 2009). Feasibility and phase I trial of tandatunib in patients with recurrent glioblastoma. ASCO Annual Meeting,27:15s, Orlando, Florida

Tabatabai, G., R. Stupp, et al. (2010). Molecular diagnostics of gliomas: the clinical perspective. *Acta Neuropathol,* Vol. 120, No. 5, (Nov), 585-592, ISBN 1432-0533

Taga, T., A. Suzuki, et al. (2002). alpha v-Integrin antagonist EMD 121974 induces apoptosis in brain tumor cells growing on vitronectin and tenascin. *Int J Cancer,* Vol. 98, No. 5, (Apr 10), 690-697, ISBN 0020-7136

Takano, T., J. H. Lin, et al. (2001). Glutamate release promotes growth of malignant gliomas. *Nat Med,* Vol. 7, No. 9, (Sep), 1010-1015, ISBN 1078-8956

Toedt, G., S. Barbus, et al. (2011). Molecular signatures classify astrocytic gliomas by IDH1 mutation status. *Int J Cancer,* Vol. 128, No. 5, (Mar 1), 1095-1103, ISBN 1097-0215

van den Bent, M. J., A. A. Brandes, et al. (2009). Randomized phase II trial of erlotinib versus temozolomide or carmustine in recurrent glioblastoma: EORTC brain tumor group study 26034. *J Clin Oncol,* Vol. 27, No. 8, (Mar 10), 1268-1274, ISBN 1527-7755

Van Meir, E. G., C. G. Hadjipanayis, et al. (2010). Exciting new advances in neuro-oncology: the avenue to a cure for malignant glioma. *CA Cancer J Clin,* Vol. 60, No. 3, (May-Jun), 166-193, ISBN 1542-4863

Vogelbaum, M. A., B. Berkey, et al. (2009). Phase II trial of preirradiation and concurrent temozolomide in patients with newly diagnosed anaplastic oligodendrogliomas and mixed anaplastic oligoastrocytomas: RTOG BR0131. *Neuro Oncol,* Vol. 11, No. 2, (Apr), 167-175, ISBN 1522-8517

Vredenburgh, J. (2010). Bevacizumab (BEV) in combination with temozolomide (TMZ) and radiation therapy (XRT) followed by BEV, TMZ, and irinotecan for newly diagnosed glioblastoma multiforme (GBM). ASCO Annual Meeting,28:15s, San Diego, California

Wedge, S. R., J. K. Porteous, et al. (1997). In vitro evaluation of temozolomide combined with X-irradiation. *Anticancer Drugs,* Vol. 8, No. 1, (Jan), 92-97, ISBN 0959-4973

Wen, P. Y. (June 2010). Phase II study of XL184 (BMS 907351), an inhibitor of MET, VEGFR2, and RET, in patients with progressive glioblastoma (GB). ASCO Annual Meeting,28:15s, San Diego, California

Wen, P. Y. (May 2009). Phase I/II study of sorafenib and temsirolimus for patients with recurrent glioblastoma (GBM) (NABTC 05-02). ASCO Annual Meeting,27:15s, Orlando, Florida

Wick, W., V. K. Puduvalli, et al. (2010). Phase III study of enzastaurin compared with lomustine in the treatment of recurrent intracranial glioblastoma. *J Clin Oncol,* Vol. 28, No. 7, (Mar 1), 1168-1174, ISBN 1527-7755

Wiencke, J. K., S. Zheng, et al. (2007). Methylation of the PTEN promoter defines low-grade gliomas and secondary glioblastoma. *Neuro Oncol,* Vol. 9, No. 3, (Jul), 271-279, ISBN 1522-8517

Yan, H., D. W. Parsons, et al. (2009). IDH1 and IDH2 mutations in gliomas. *N Engl J Med,* Vol. 360, No. 8, (Feb 19), 765-773, ISBN 1533-4406

Ye, Z. C., J. D. Rothstein, et al. (1999). Compromised glutamate transport in human glioma cells: reduction-mislocalization of sodium-dependent glutamate transporters and enhanced activity of cystine-glutamate exchange. *J Neurosci,* Vol. 19, No. 24, (Dec 15), 10767-10777, ISBN 1529-2401

Yen, K. E., M. A. Bittinger, et al. (2010). Cancer-associated IDH mutations: biomarker and therapeutic opportunities. *Oncogene,* Vol. 29, No. 49, (Dec 9), 6409-6417, ISBN 1476-5594

Zoncu, R., A. Efeyan, et al. (2011). mTOR: from growth signal integration to cancer, diabetes and ageing. *Nat Rev Mol Cell Biol,* Vol. 12, No. 1, (Jan), 21-35, ISBN 1471-0080

Part 2

Chemotherapy and Other Therapeutic Strategies

Glioblastoma: Current Chemotherapeutic Status and Need for New Targets and Approaches

Aditi Jain[1], James CK Lai[1,2], Golam MI Chowdhury[3,4], Kevin Behar[3,4] and Alok Bhushan[1,2]
[1]*Department of Biomedical and Pharmaceutical Sciences College of Pharmacy and ISU Biomedical Institute, Idaho State University*
[2]*Mountain States Tumor and Medical Research Institute, Boise, ID*
[3]*Magnetic Resonance Research Center*
[4]*Department of Psychiatry, Yale University School of Medicine, New Haven, CT USA*

1. Introduction

Glioblastoma is the most aggressive, invasive and malignant type of glioma : a tumor which arises from the glial cells in the brain (Wrensch et al., 2002). Glioblastoma represents 54% of all the gliomas and 18% of all brain tumors (CBTRUS, 2011). It is the frequently occurring brain tumor in humans. Patients with glioblastoma usually survive 12-15 months or less after diagnosis. (Krex et al., 2007; Chandana et al., 2008).

Because prognosis for patients with glioblastoma is abysmal and current therapies for the disease are ineffective, this review critically evaluates the current chemotherapeutic status of glioblastoma and highlights the need for new therapeutic targets and approaches. The ultimate goal is to improve the outcome of glioblastoma patients.

2. Glioblastoma biology

The incidence of glioblastoma peaks with increasing age and affects adults of ages 50 to 70 (Wrensch et al., 2002). Multiple genetic mutations, upregulation or amplification of genes contribute to glioblastoma carcinogenesis. Depending on the aberrant signaling pathways involved, glioblastoma can develop either as a primary or a secondary tumor (Kleihues & Ohgaki , 1999; Ohgaki & Kleihues, 2007). Primary glioblastoma (representing >60% of all glioblastoma cases) frequently occurs in adults/older patients as a single step transformation with no clinical background. Genetic changes in primary glioblastoma include Epidermal Growth Factor Receptor overexpression (50-60%), mutations in PTEN (30%) and amplification of mdm2 gene. Secondary glioblastoma arises from a slowly progressing low grade astrocytoma or anaplastic astrocytoma to a malignant glioblastoma and affects the young population. Secondary glioblastoma patients survive longer than those with primary glioblastoma multiforme: genetic hallmark of the former group includes Tp53 inactivation (>60%) and overexpression of PDGF ligand and/or receptor. Primary and secondary glioblastomas share similar morphologies, rendering them indistinguishable (Kleihues & Ohgaki , 1999; Ohgaki & Kleihues, 2007).

3.Current therapies

3.1 Carmustine

Carmustine (BCNU) was the first tested and approved drug for treating glioblastoma: it showed modest improvement in patient survival in 1960s (Levin, 1999). Belonging to the class of nitrosoureas, it alkylates the *O6*-guanine position in the DNA and cross-links the DNA, thereby inhibiting cancer growth (Reithmeier et al., 2010). Carmustine is a lipophilic drug and crosses the blood-brain barrier (Louis et al, 2007). After being approved by FDA in 1977, it has been the mainstay of adjuvant therapy for glioblastoma (Salvati et al., 2009). When glioblastoma patients were treated with carmustine after radiation therapy, their survival improved (Brandes et al., 2004). Many still ongoing preclinical and clinical studies have also tested carmustine in combination with other chemotherapeutic drugs (Silvani et al., 2009; Reardon et al., 2004). In 2009, a study comparing temozolomide and carmustine in glioblastoma indicated that carmustine was more toxic than temozolomide alone though both had comparable efficacy (Vinjamuri et al., 2009). Combination therapies with receptor tyrosine kinase inhibitors like genistein, tryphostin and carmustine were synergisitic (Liang & Ullyatt 1998; Khoshyomn et al., 2002). Despite its use as a mainstay therapy, the survival rates of patients on carmustine alone are quite low. Short half-life, chemo-resistance, high systemic toxicity, and difficult delivery to target site, limits carmustine's effectiveness in treating glioblastoma (Johannessen et al., 2008).

3.2 Gliadel wafers

Gliadel wafers are biodegradable polymers loaded with carmustine, approved for treating recurrent glioblastoma (Panigrahi et al., 2011; Aoki et al., 2007). After glioblastoma is surgically removed, the wafers are implanted in its cavity. As the polymer is degraded, it releases the drug slowly (Panigrahi et al., 2011). In 1995, gliadel wafers showed promises because of their local action and high doses of loaded drug delivered to the target site with few off-target effects (Brem et al., 1995). Gliadel-treated patients showed median survival of 7.2 months compared to 5.4 months in the placebo group. In 2003, a randomized, placebo-controlled, multicenter, multi-national, double-blind phase 3 trial demonstrated a higher survival to risk ratio in glioblastoma patients treated with gliadel wafers, with a median survival rate of 13.9 months compared to 11.6 months in placebo controls (Westphal et al., 2003). An ongoing study adopts a multimodality approach of using gliadel wafers with other chemotherapies in glioma patients who have undergone surgery (McGirt et al., 2009). Gliadel wafer with temozolomide increased the median survival of patients with newly diagnosed glioblastoma to 21 months (McGirt et al., 2009). Although beneficial, the use of gliadel wafers for intracranial treatment of glioblastoma is complicated by edema, seizures, post-operative infections, and hydrocephalus (Gallego et al., 2007; Weber & Goebel, 2005): the complications versus benefits merits re-evaluation.

3.3 Cisplatin

In 1965, Barnet Rosenberg *et al* discovered inhibition of E. coli cell division by a platinum compound (i.e., cisplatin) formed in electrolysis of platinum electrodes (Rosenberg et al, 1965). Cisplatin was soon employed as an anticancer agent (Rosenberg et al, 1969; Williams, J.M.A Whitehouse, 1979). Cisplatin is a platinum complex with two chloride atoms and two amine groups positioned in a *cis* configuration. Once inside the body, the two chloride atoms are displaced by water molecules, the resulting hydrated complex crosslinks with

DNA strands, triggering programmed cell death (C.J. Williams, J.M.A Whitehouse, 1979). In 1980's cisplatin's efficacy on brain tumor was evaluated (Stewart et al, 1982). Although combination therapy of cisplatin with carmustine and radiation therapy was successful, patients on cisplatin therapy (with or without carmustine) developed ocular and orbital toxicities (Miller et al., 1985). Numerous other clinical trials evaluating the effectiveness of cisplatin chemotherapy in glioblastoma have demonstrated few benefits. Combination of cisplatin with temozolomide, etoposide, thalidomide, or tyrosine kinase inhibitors as a treatment option for glioblastoma have also been studied but have not significantly increased patient survival (Silvani et al., 2004; Lassen et al., 1999; Murphy et al., 2007; Nagane et al., 2007). Additionally, a phase three trial of cisplatin and carmustine administered concurrently with radiation therapy did not have significant improved outcome as compared to carmustine alone and radiation therapy (Buckner et al., 2006).

3.4 Temodar

A drug of interest since 1990, temozolomide constitutes the first line chemotherapy for treating glioblastoma following surgery and radiation (Villano et al., 2009). It is an oral alkylating agent that adds a methyl group to the O6 position of guanine residue of the DNA: the resulting methylated adduct induces apoptosis (Villano et al., 2009; Malcolm et al., 2002; Roos et al., 2007). Being lipid soluble, temzolomide shows good bioavailability and readily crosses the blood-brain barrier. In 2005, a breakthrough study demonstrated a regimen of radiation therapy followed by adjuvant and concomitant temozolomide treatment prolonged survival of glioblastoma patients compared to patients treated with radiation alone (Stupp et al., 2005). Since then it has become a standard therapy for glioblastoma with or without modifications. Combination chemotherapies of temozolomide and other drugs are in various phases of clinical trials but none showed benefits compared to temozolomide treatment alone (Ren et al., 2009). One of the major drawbacks of temozolomide therapy is recurrence of glioblastoma. The lesion produced in the DNA by temozolomide could be corrected by the repair enzyme O6 methyl guanine DNA methyl transferase, encoded by the MGMT gene (Sarkaria et al., 2008). Response rates to temozolomide therapy depend on the transferase activity and cancers with high levels of MGMT activity gradually acquire resistance to temozolomide (Nagane et al., 2007). The promoter methylation status of MGMT governs a drug's efficacy towards the tumor. Patients with an increased % of MGMT methylation respond more favorably to temozolomide treatment (Hegi et al., 2008). Drugs mimicking this enzyme are being tested in combination with temozolomide to prevent MGMT actions. One such drug is O6 benzylguanine, which acts as a pseudo-substrate to MGMT enzyme (Kaina et al., 2010; Dolan & Pegg, 1997). However, due to its dose-related hematologic toxicity, its use in combination with alkylating agents is still under investigation (Dolan & Pegg, 1997; Quinn et al., 2009). A recent study showed that patients with unmethylated MGMT tumors benefitted from the combination of interferon β and temozolomide, as compared to patients who received temozolomide alone, highlighting the role of interferon β and also suggesting that methylation status of MGMT is not a sole parameter controlling treatment outcome (Motomura et al., 2011). Tumor resistance to temozolomide as with other alkylating agents is a common phenomenon seen in patients with glioblastoma. Apart from MGMT, many studies have shown that resistance to temozolomide is mutlifactorial (Sarkaria et al., 2008). Strategies to overcome this resistance have been analyzed in order to improve temozolomide's activity against glioma and other cancers (Sarkaria et al., 2008; Tentori & Graziani , 2002). With greater understanding of diverse mechanisms responsible for imparting resistance to cancer cells and the role played by growth factor receptors in glioblastoma tumorigenesis, new therapies in combination with temozolomide are being evaluated. Such combination therapies include use of protein tyrosine/serine-threonine kinase inhibitors and temozolomide (Chaponis et al., 2011; Guillard et al., 2009; Peereboom et al., 2010). Though some studies demonstrated beneficial effects, others have reported greater toxicity. Thus, as a promising drug for treating glioblastoma, temozolomide only modestly enhances patient survival. There is a need to find other small molecules with efficacy and safety profiles superior to those of current therapies to be targeted to glioblastoma therapy.

4. Potential drug targets and new therapies

4.1 Epidermal growth factor receptor (EGFR) and cellular signaling pathways

EGFR plays a critical role in cancer progression and invasion. Present in all germ layers, EGFR is activated by several ligands including EGF. Binding of EGF results in homodimerization and/or heterodimerization with other members of the EGFR family (HER2, HER3 and HER4), leading to tyrosine phosphorylation of its cytoplasmic domain. This activation initiates a series of signaling pathways resulting in cell division. In cancer cells, mutations or amplification of EGFR leads to uncontrolled cell proliferation (Yarden, 2001). Activation of EGFR leads to activation of downstream elements such as phosphatidylinositol-3 kinase (PI3K), which converts phosphatidylinositol diphosphate (PIP_2) to phosphatidylinositol triphosphate (PIP_3). Protein kinase B or AKT binds the PIP3 with the pleckstrin homology (PH) domain, resulting in phosphorylation of AKT at threonine 308 and serine 473 sites. Phosphorylated AKT leads to cell growth, motility and proliferation by activating several downstream signaling pathways (Chakravarti et al., 2004).

PTEN/MMAC/TEP-1, (Phosphatase and tensin homologue deleted on chromosome ten/mutated in multiple advanced cancer/Transforming growth factor β regulated and epithelial cell enriched phosphatase) a tumor suppressor gene located on chromosome 10 is mutated in gliomas. PTEN dephosphorylates PIP3 to PIP2 in the PI3 kinase pathway and acts as a negative regulator of this pathway (Cheng & Nicosia, 2001). Continuous activation of PI3K/Akt pathway is associated with malignant transformation of cells. Activation of PI3K pathway and mutations in PTEN occur frequently in GBM tumors when compared to non-GBM tumors (Chakravarti et al., 2004).Mammalian target of rapamycin (mTOR) is a serine/threonine kinase known to function downstream of PI3K/Akt pathway. Akt activates mTOR through inhibition of TSC1/2 complex and activation of Ras homologue-enriched in brain (Rheb). mTOR regulates translation initiation through two pathways - eukaryotic translation initiation factor (eIF4E) binding proteins (4EBP1) and ribosomal p70 S6 kinase (p70S6K) (Hay & Sonenberg, 2004).Inhibition of signaling pathways generated by activation of EGFR are important targets to develop new drugs for the treatment of glioblastoma because EGFR is amplified and overexpressed in such tumors (Lo, 2010; Penar et al., 1997).

4.2 PLCγ1

Phospholipase C gamma one (PLCγ1) is an enzyme important in cell signaling. In its phosphorylated active form, it cleaves the membrane phospholipid, phosphatidylinositol 4,

5 biphosphate (PIP2) to diacylglycerol (DAG) and inositol triphosphate (IP3). IP3 increases intracellular calcium stores. DAG together with calcium activates protein kinase C which further participates in signal transduction pathways (Kim et al., 2000). Growth factor receptor activation is an important mediator of PLCγ1 phosphorylation and functioning. Overexpression of epidermal growth factor receptors (EGFR) in glioblastoma multiforme (GBM) promotes PLCγ1 activation (Chen et al., 1994; Yang et al., 1994; Wahl et al., 1992). Many functions attributed to PLCγ1 activation include proliferation, differentiation, cell motility and invasion of tumor cells (Jones et al., 2005; Wells & Grandis, 2003). Furthermore, PLCγ1 is associated with breast cancer metastasis and is highly expressed in breast cancer tissues (Arteaga et al., 1991). Activation of PLCγ1 by tyrosine kinase receptors mediates actin cytoskeleton rearrangement, through release of actin modifying proteins gelsolin, profilin, myosin type I (Chen et al., 1996). In the resting state, these proteins are bound to PIP2 and participate in cell motility only when they are released during hydrolysis of PIP2 by PLCγ1. Thus, this mechanism defines the role played by the enzyme in cell motility and invasion (Chen et al., 1996). Molecular inhibition of PLCγ1 is associated with decreased invasion in gliomas, prostate, breast and bladder carcinomas (Turner et al., 1997; Katterle et al., 2004; Khoshyomn et al., 1999). A chemical inhibitor of PLCγ1, U73122 inhibits invasion of glioblastoma cells into co-cultured fetal rat brain aggregates (Khoshyomn et al., 1999). During invasion, tumor cells undergo a series of steps to proliferate and thrive locally (Tysnes & Mahesparan, 2001). Thus, these functional considerations of the role of PLCγ1 in glioblastoma proliferation and invasion strongly suggest PLCγ1 could be a drug target.

4.4 Invasion

The characteristic feature of glioblastoma, which makes it a lethal disease, is its propensity to invade surrounding normal brain tissues (Giese et al., 2003). Unlike other cancers, glioblastoma does not metastasize to distinct organs but infiltrates peritumoral regions (Giese et al., 2003; Nakada et al., 2007). Glioblastoma patients show poor survival because of the inability of current therapies to control the aggressively invasive glioblastoma, which is spurred on by autocrine and paracrine factors released from the tumor and its microenvironment, respectively (Hoelzinger et al., 2007). Overexpression and activity of the epidermal growth factor receptors in almost all glioblastomas is responsible for signaling pathways leading to invasion (Guillamo et al., 2009). These signals help the cancer cells to detach from the bulk of the tumor and adhere to the extracellular matrix components of other cells. The latter process follows only when the tumor invades through the matrix to the surrounding brain parenchyma. Thus, during invasion, a family of proteases known as the matrix metalloproteases and urokinase plasminogen activator receptor system play an active role (VanMeter et al., 2001; Mohanam et al., 2001). Being soluble zinc-dependent enzymes and secreted as inactive zymogens (pro-MMPs) (Visee & Nagase, 2003), matrix metalloproteases (MMPs) cleave the basement membrane and extracellular matrix components like collagen, fibronectin, laminin, and vitronectin. They help in tissue remodeling, angiogenesis, and metastasis (VanMeter et al., 2001). Out of the 24 members in the MMP family, only two forms are overexpressed in glibolastoma and their expression correlates with the degree of malignancy and poor survival rate (Deryugina et al., 1997; Choe et al., 2002). These two forms are MMP-2 (72 kDa type IV collagenase or gelatinase A) and MMP-9 (92 kDa type IV collagenase or gelatinase B) and differ from other members in their substrate preference. Some metalloproteases are not secreted but are expressed on the surface of tumor cells. MT1-MMP (membrane bound matrix metalloprotease-1) is one such protease which is upregulated in glioblastomas. A major role of MT1-MMP is in the cleavage of pro-MMPs to active MMPs at the cell surface. Together with MMP-2, and MMP-9, MT1-MMP imparts an invasive phenotype to glioblastoma multiforme (Fillmore et al., 2001; Nakada et al., 2001). Urokinase plasminogen activator and receptor (uPA/uPAR) system is important in cancer cell migration and invasion (D'Alessio & Blasi, 2009; Duffy, 2004). Once this system is activated, it converts the inactive plasminogen to the active plasmin. Plasmin degrades the extracellular matrix components (D'Alessio & Blasi, 2009). Increased expression of uPAR on the surface of glioblastoma correlates with poor prognosis. In contrast with normal brain tissue, high grade gliomas (i.e., glioblastoma) exhibit increased activity of the uPA/uPAR system (Mohanam et al., 1998; MacDonald et al., 1998). This system can also activate cell proliferation pathways by interacting with other proteins like vitronectin and integrins (Sidenius & Blasi, 2003).Many studies and clinical trials are now focusing on anti-invasive chemotherapies as a treatment option for glibolastoma. Apart from synthetic derivatives, natural compounds in soy, curcumin can also inhibit glioblastoma invasion *in vitro* (Puli et al., 2006; Senft et al., 2010). Their activity *in vivo* warrants further research. Since a vast signaling network is aberrant in glioblastoma, therapies directed toward a single target cannot be expected to lead to positive outcomes. For example, one clinical trial showed marimastat to be ineffective in increasing survival of patients post-radiosurgery (Levin et al., 2006). Consequently, combination therapies targeting invasion and other pathways in glioblatoma are still ongoing.

4.5 Angiogenesis

Angiogenesis, the process of formation of new blood vessels from existing blood capillaries, is one major contributor to glioblastoma multiforme carcinogenesis and helps the tumor cells to flourish (Tate & Aghi, 2009). To maintain the demand of food, nutrients, and oxygen, tumor cells recruit new blood vessels from those already present (Folkman, 1971; Tate & Aghi, 2009). Likewise, malignant gliomas are highly vascularised and have an angiogenic phenotype (Jain et al., 2007). Angiogenesis takes place with the over-expression of angiogenic factors or when the angiogenic imbalance strikes. One growth factor involved is vascular endothelial growth factor (VEGF), which promotes formation of endothelium in normal cells (Kargiotis et al., 2006). In glioblastoma, VEGF-a, a pro-angiogenic factor from the VEGF family, plays a crucial role in angiogenesis. VEGF-a is secreted in large amounts by glioblastoma cells and can elicit responses like extracellular matrix degradation, endothelial cell proliferation, and expression of other angiogenic factors such as urokinase type plasminogen activator, plasminogen activator inhibitor-1 and matrix metalloproteases (Plate et al., 1992). Secreted VEGF stimulates angiogenesis by binding to specific tyrosine kinase VEGF receptors on endothelial cells of blood vessels surrounding the tumor and initiates proliferation of endothelial cells, thereby ensuring the metabolic demands of the growing tumor are adequately met. There are other pro-angiogenic factors like angiopoetins, IL-8, hepatocyte growth factors, endothelins that are expressed by glioblastoma cells when the "angiogenic switch" is turned on: all these factors have functions similar to that of VEGF in promoting angiogenesis (Argyriou et al., 2009). Some new treatment strategies for GBM include targeting VEGF/VEGF receptors (VEGFR) by monoclonal antibody or VEGFR traps, respectively (Beal et al., 2011). Approved by FDA in 2009 for treating recurrent glioblastoma, bevacizumab (Avastin) is a humanized monoclonal antibody against VEGF-a (Beal et al., 2011). Bevacizumab decreases tumor blood vessel density and remodels tumor vasculature in a neuroblastoma xenograft model (Dickson et al., 2007). The National Cancer Comprehensive Network recommends bevacizumab with or without other chemotherapy in case of glioblastoma recurrence (National Comprehensive Cancer Network clinical practice guidelines in oncology-central nervous system cancers. v.1.2010). Combination chemotherapy of bevacizumab with irinotecan shows favorable results in phase 2 trials of recurrent malignant glioma (Vredenburgh et al., 2007). Clinical trials are on-going for using bevacizumab in new cases of glioblastoma (Lai et al, 2010). Inclusion of anti-angiogenic therapies to cancer treatment is favorable, because they facilitate increased penetration of conventional chemotherapies and show better response rates (Jain, 2001). Other than bevacizumab, anti-angiogenic agents in various phases of clinical trials include cediranib, cilengitide, and aflibercept (Batchelor et al., 2010; Reardon et al., 2008; Wachsberger et al., 2007). Though favorable responses and anti-tumor effects occur with combination of various anti-angiogenic agents in different cancer models, efficacy of bevacizumab monotherapy in increasing glioblastoma patient survival has not transpired. Emergence of an invasive phenotype while angiogenesis is being targeted in glioblastoma constitutes a major limitation of anti-angiogenic monotherapies (Lamszus et al., 2003; Verhoeff et al., 2009; Keunen et al., 2011). Thus, improved therapies need to be developed to target glioblastoma.

4.6 Metabolism

Metabolic and other functional roles of astrocytes under physiological conditions: In mammalian nervous system, neurons and astrocytes are intimately and functionally interrelated: astrocytes play key roles in neurotransmitter and substrate cycling in conjunction with neurons (Chowdhury et al., 2007; Hertz et al., 2007). Moreover, astrocytes protect neurons against various pathophysiological assaults (e.g., oxidative stress, ammonia toxicity) (Dukhande et al., 2006; Wong et al., 2010). However, to what extent these physiological roles are still assumed by astrocytes once they are transformed into astrocytomas has not been elucidated. Nevertheless, recent new evidence suggests that cancer cells, and to a lesser known extent astrocytomas too, exhibit metabolic adaptation and other phenotypic alterations that allow them to survive, proliferate, and invade into their surrounding space occupied by normal cells/tissues (Bhardwaj et al., 2010; Lino & Merlo, 2009; Ordys et al., 2010; Semenza, 2011; Stegh et al., 2008).

Metabolic adaptation and/or reprogramming in cancer cells in general and astrocytoma/glioblastoma in particular: As early as the 1920's, Otto Warburg and his associates were the first to note that cancer cells appear to depend on glycolysis for energy production and survival even though oxygen is not in short supply. (Warburg et al., 1927). Warburg's extensive investigation into the metabolic characteristics of multiple types of cancer cells prompted him to hypothesize that cancer cells reply on glycolysis for energy supply because their mitochondrial oxidative metabolism is dysfunctional (Warburg, 1956). His hypothesis has been neglected for some 80 years until the recent resurgence of interests in "the role metabolic reprogramming in cancer progression" (Semenza, 2011). The recent "renaissance of the Warburg Hypothesis" (Warburg et al., 1927, Warburg, 1956) has stimulated a new era in elucidating the aggressive nature of many malignant tumors (including glioblastoma) and their purported dependence on glycolysis for energy and survival (Bhardwaj et al., 2010; Lino & Merlo, 2009; Ordys et al., 2010; Semenza, 2011; Stegh et al., 2008). While numerous studies have documented mutations in mitochondrial DNA (mtDNA) in a variety of cancers (Czarnecka & Bartnik, 2009) can thus tentatively provide a mechanistic connection to dysfunctional mitochondrial oxidative metabolism as predicted by the Warburg hypothesis, other recent evidence suggests this aspect of the Warburg hypothesis requires critical re-appraisal (Bayley & Devilee, 2010; Dang et al., 2011; Frezza et al., 2011; Ordys et al., 2010; Srivastava & Moraes, 2009).

The aspect of the Warburg hypothesis emphasizing dysfunctional mitochondrial oxidative metabolism in cancer cells deserves a critical re-appraisal because recent studies on cancer cell metabolism have uncovered new mechanistic roles for mTOR and p53. These mechanistic roles are new additions to the already established role of mTOR in tumor development and progression and the fact that in over 50% of the cancer types, p53, a tumor-suppressor, is mutated and their p53 mutation is associated with either decreased apoptosis and/or enhanced proliferation potential in those cancers. Earlier, we have already discussed the importance of these two phenotypic characteristics of glioblastoma.

mTOR complex 1 (mTORC1) is aberrantly activated in many human cancers thereby positioning it to modulate on metabolic changes common to cancer cells (Yecies & Manning, 2011). Furthermore, recent characterization of the metabolism of cancer cells reveals that, mTORC1 activation is adequate to promote an increase in glucose uptake, glycolysis, and lipid synthesis in addition to the pentose phosphate shunt pathway (Ramanathan & Schreiber, 2009; Yecies & Manning, 2011). Because these are all metabolic phenotypes of cancers, mTORC1 has emerged as a central relay for various oncogenic signaling pathways and their convergence in regulating metabolism in cancer cells (Yecies & Manning, 2011). The finding that mTOR functions as a positive regulator of hypoxia-inducible factor 1 (HIF-1) activation by hypoxia (Hudson et al., 2002) highlights the importance of mTOR in regulating signals that lead mammalian cells, especially cancer cells, to adapt to oxygen- and nutrient-poor environments. Furthermore, mTOR is known to exert a direct control of mitochondria (Ramanathan & Schreiber, 2009). Thus, these new mechanistic roles of mTOR strengthen the notion we have discussed earlier that mTOR exhibits good potential as a target for new anti-cancer drug discovery. There has been increasing evidence demonstrating that p53 can regulate multiple metabolic pathways. p53 contributes to the regulation of glycolysis, oxidative phosphorylation, glutamine catabolism, synthesis of nucleotides, fatty acid oxidation, insulin sensitivity, mitochondrial integrity, antioxidant response, autophagy, and mTOR signaling (Maddocks & Vousden, 2011). Inactivation of p53 in cancer cells promotes the Warburg effect as p53 suppresses glycolysis and promotes oxidative phosphorylation. However, there are some known but complex cross-talks between the signaling pathways regulated by mTOR and p53 (Maddocks & Vousden, 2011): nevertheless, whether the interactions between mTOR and p53 signaling favor glioblastoma cell growth and proliferation remains to be fully elucidated.

Some recent cancer cell metabolism studies have further challenged the reliance of cancer cells on glycolysis for energy production and lipid synthesis: in fact, such studies have argued that glycolysis alone is inadequate to maintain the metabolic needs of growing and actively dividing cancer cells (Dang et al., 2011; Maddocks & Vousden, 2011; Shanware et al., 2011). Thus, many researchers have re-discovered the importance of glutamine in meeting the inadequacy of glycolysis to fuel growth and proliferation of many cancer types including gliomas (Dang et al., 2011; Maddocks & Vousden, 2011; Shanware et al., 2011). In this context, as alluded to above, neuroscientists have long recognized the importance of glutamine in astrocytic metabolism and astrocytes-neurons metabolic and neurotransmitter cycling (Chowdhury et al., 2007; McKenna, 2007). Consequently, these recent interests in the role of glutamine in cancer cell metabolism call into question the need to better appreciate the metabolic and neurotransmitter cycling roles of glutamine in glioblastomas. Because these roles in glioblastomas are poorly understood, these knowledge gaps prompted us to consider the appropriate techniques and approaches to allow the acquisition of this knowledge. Indeed, the recent rapid advances in magnetic resonance imaging (MRI) and nuclear magnetic resonance (NMR) spectroscopy provide exciting new possibilities in this area of research and development.

Technological advances that can be exploited to diagnose and/or treat glioblastoma:MRI and other imaging techniques in diagnosing glioblastoma: Recent advances in magnetic resonance imaging (MRI) and related imaging techniques have opened new possibilities in the differential and more accurate clinical assessment of brain tumors including glioblastomas (Cha, 2009; Lemort et al., 2007; Wang & Lam, 2008). Historically, uses of MRI in the diagnosis of brain tumors were initially focused on neuromorphological demonstration, confirmation, and localization of brain tumors. However, the rapid advances of MRI, functional MRI, and magnetic resonance spectroscopy (MRS) spectroscopy in the last decade have allowed the diagnostic imaging of neurotumors combining the use of physiology-based imaging methods that complement the more traditional morphology-based imaging protocols. For example, "High-resolution spectroscopic imaging may contribute to pre-therapeutic grading and characterization of gliomas, as can diffusion techniques. The latter also hold promise in predicting survival in malignant supratentorial astrocytoma and could help to define areas for biopsy. Both methods can differentiate recurrent tumour from radiation injury. Perfusion-weighted magnetic resonance techniques offer potential markers of tumour angiogenesis and capillary permeability, and correlate well with vascular endothelial growth factor expression in grade II and grade III tumours. Functional magnetic resonance imaging can assess whether surgical treatment is feasible and select patients for intraoperative cortical stimulation" (Lemont et al., 2007).

Recently, use of the nanoparticles in the diagnosis and detection of cancers, including glioblastomas, has gained much impetus because of putative enhancement involving their applications in MRI (Bhushan et al., 2010; Cole et al., 2011). The advances in development of newer cancer imaging and therapies based on metallic nanoparticles may help in early detection of cancer and thus contribute to decreasing deaths due to cancer. Various cancer imaging and therapies based on use of metallic nanoparticles are at different stages of preclinical and clinical development. Nanoparticles composed of iron oxide nanoparticles, zinc oxide nanoparticles, gold nanoparticles, silver nanoparticles, and cerium oxide nanoparticles have tremendous potentials to be developed as novel diagnostic and therapeutic agents in cancer (Bhushan et al., 2010; Jain 2010). Furthermore, enhanced cancer biomarker and genetic mutation detection techniques would help in identifying individuals at high risk for developing cancer. In this context, multi-functional metallic nanoparticles show exciting therapeutic potentials and these are currently under development for cancer therapy to be clinically applied in the near future. Metallic nanoparticles can be engineered to enhance the efficacy of current diagnostic and imaging techniques in cancer (Bhushan et al., 2010). Clearly, with the explosive advances in the design and applications of new metallic nanoparticles, this application area in cancer diagnosis and assessment shows exciting new potentials.

Technological advances that can be exploited to treat glioblastoma: As already alluded to above, the recent "renaissance of the Warburg Hypothesis" has stimulated much research into cancer cell metabolism (Bhardwaj et al., 2010; Lino & Merlo, 2009; Ordys et al., 2010; Semenza, 2011; Stegh et al., 2008). Indeed, the presumed dependence of cancer cells on glycolysis for cancer cell growth and proliferation has prompted much new investigation into exploring the glycolytic pathway as a new target for anti-cancer drug discovery (Bhardwaj et al., 2010; Chatterji et al., 2007; Chatterji et al., 2009; Lai et al., 2008; Lino & Merlo, 2009). We have demonstrated that two glycolytic enzyme inhibitors, 3-bromopyruvate and iodoacetate, showed efficacy in lowering the survival of pancreatic cancer (Bhardwaj et al., 2010) and glioblastoma U87 (Chatterji et al., 2007; Chatterji et al., 2009; Lai et al., 2008) cells. Thus, our studies strongly suggest that glycolytic enzyme inhibitors exhibit proof-of-concept potential in discovering new anti-cancer drugs (Bhardwaj et al., 2010; Chatterji et al., 2007; Chatterji et al., 2009; Lai et al., 2008). Consistent with our findings (Bhardwaj et al., 2010; Chatterji et al., 2007; Chatterji et al., 2009; Lai et al., 2008) are the results of human clinical trials employing 2-deoxyglucose (2-DG) in combination therapy with radiation for treatment of glioma (Prasanna et al., 2009). An inhibitor of glucose transport and glycolysis, 2-DG reportedly enhances the effects of radiation in inducing glioma cell death (Prasanna et al., 2009). Thus, the glycolytic pathway in glioblastoma constitutes an excellent target for further anti-cancer drug discovery studies. Nevertheless, because the prognosis of patients diagnosed with glioblastoma is abysmal, there is an urgent need to more fully elucidate the metabolic phenotype of glioblastomas along with exploring glycolysis as a target for discovering new anti-cancer drugs.

Magnetic resonance spectroscopy to elucidate metabolic adaptations/alterations in glioblastoma: High lactate accumulation, despite adequate oxygen availability, is a metabolic pattern commonly associated with malignant transformation of the uncontrolled dividing cell. This metabolic phenotype, termed aerobic glycolysis and historically known as the Warburg effect, is characterized by high glycolytic rates and reduced mitochondrial oxidation (Bhardwaj et al., 2010; Lino & Merlo, 2009; Ordys et al., 2010; Semenza, 2011; Stegh et al., 2008), features that favor cell survival in the hypoxic microenvironments found in tumors. This phenotype also favors the routing of key metabolic intermediates away from oxidative metabolism and toward anabolic processes required by rapidly dividing cells (McFate et al., 2008). However, the mechanistic relationship between altered glucose metabolism and malignancy remains poorly understood due to prior lack of appropriate techniques to study such phenomena. MRS has become a major tool in the non-invasive characterization of brain tumor metabolism *in vivo* and *in vitro*. A highly versatile technique, MRS allows measurements of the concentrations of many neurochemicals, including the kinetics of single enzyme-catalyzed reactions such as LDH (Xu et al., 2007) or creatine kinase (Smith et al., 1997), as well as the rates of entire metabolic pathways, such as the TCA cycle and the glutamate/glutamine neurotransmitter cycle (Sibson et al., 2001; de Graaf et al., 2003). MRS is commonly employed with several stable (non-radioactive) isotopes of biological importance such as ^{1}H, ^{13}C, ^{15}N, and ^{31}P, allowing investigation of many aspects of cellular metabolism. Of these nuclei, only ^{1}H and ^{31}P exist at ~100% natural abundance, thus requiring no specific enrichment prior to their measurement. Because ^{13}C exists at low natural abundance (~1.1%), selective enrichment of ^{13}C in appropriate substrates allow its use as a metabolic tracer. The high chemical specificity of ^{13}C MRS, which can distinguish ^{13}C isotope incorporation into not only different molecules, but also specific carbon positions within the same compound, allows the fate of the ^{13}C label into and through multiple metabolic pathways to be followed (Zwingmann and Leibfritz, 2003). Until recently the low sensitivity of ^{13}C detection (and correspondingly large detection volume) has precluded its use for *in vivo* imaging of tumors, although with the advent of Dynamic Nuclear Polarization (DNP) and hyperpolarized biomarkers of tumor metabolism (see below), direct ^{13}C detection could become a major tool in tumor staging and response to targeted therapies.

As discussed above, brain tumors such as gliomas produce increased amounts of lactate, which can be measured by ^{1}H MRS (Kaibara et al., 1998; Herholz et al., 1992; Terpstra et al., 1998; McKnight, 2004). Glucose production of lactate through glycolysis, whether produced anaerobically (hypoxia) or aerobically, can be determined from the change in lactate concentration verses time in a series of sequentially acquired ^{1}H or ^{13}C NMR spectra. Lactate can be measured either without isotopic labeling (e.g., by differencing of ^{1}H spectra or by use of selective lactate-editing techniques), or with ^{13}C isotopic enrichment of the precursor glucose pool, and both approaches have their specific advantages depending on the desired information. With ^{13}C isotopic enrichment additional MRS techniques can be employed, such as direct ^{13}C detection with ^{1}H-decoupling to enhance sensitivity and resolution, or direct ^{1}H detection with ^{13}C-editing to differentiate ^{13}C-labeled from unlabeled proton resonances, so-called heteronuclear ^{1}H-[^{13}C] MRS. Because the heteronuclear ^{13}C-edited ^{1}H differencing technique (Fitzpatrick et al., 1990) permits both labeled and unlabeled species to be measured from a single set of acquired spectra, the fractional enrichment of lactate-C3 reflects the sum of the pathways contributing carbon atoms (both ^{13}C and ^{12}C) to the C3 position of lactate.

The use of heteronuclear ^{1}H-[^{13}C] MRS to characterize the C6 glioma metabolic phenotype (high glycolysis and low oxidation) was elegantly demonstrated for the rat brain *in vivo by* Terpstra et al., (1998). These authors found that the glioma metabolized glucose to lactate increased lactate turnover and reduced oxidative metabolism of glucose by the reduced incorporation of ^{13}C label in glutamate, which is a measure of TCA cycle flux. ^{1}H and $^{1}H/^{13}C$ heteronuclear MRS methods have also been used to study glioma biopsies *ex vitro* (Barton et al., 1999; Martínez-Bisbal et al., 2004) and glial-derived tumor cell lines in vitro (Portais et al., 1993; Serkova et al., 1996; Lehtimäki et al., 2003). In ongoing studies in our laboratory, we incubated cultured human glioblastoma U87 cells with [1,6-$^{13}C_2$]glucose as a tracer and measured the metabolite profiles in extracts of these cells using ^{1}H-[^{13}C] MRS (Fig. 1). The extract spectra revealed high levels of lactate, with lower levels of glutamate and alanine, as well as other substances not yet identified. Inspection of ^{13}C labeled metabolites revealed substantial turnover of lactate-C3 (percentage enrichment, ~31%) compared to a lower enrichment in glutamate-C4 (~14%), consistent with a more glycolytic (and less oxidative) metabolic phenotype. The high glycolytic and low oxidative rates displayed by gliomas suggest these pathways as potential therapeutic targets, as emphasized in several reports (Mathupala et al., 2010).

More recently, the introduction of hyperpolarized MRS, which increases the detection sensitivity of an NMR-active nucleus up to 10,000 times, has generated intense excitement in the possibility of imaging low concentration metabolites. Special techniques are employed to achieve hyperpolarization, although the lifetime is brief, decaying according to the spin-lattice relaxation time. Thus, ^{13}C in carbonyl groups, which exhibit long T1's (many tens of seconds) can be suitable employed as metabolic probes. Particularly promising as a biomarker of tumor metabolism has been the development of hyperpolarized ^{13}C-labeled substrates such as [1-^{13}C]pyruvate (Kurhanewicz et al., 2011). Tumors express high amounts of LDH, which catalyzes a rapid exchange between pyruvate and lactate. The rapid appearance of hyperpolarized [1-^{13}C]lactate can thus serve as an indirect measure of LDH activity and tumorgenicity. Additional metabolic products are seen, such as [1-^{13}C]alanine, resulting from alanine transaminase, and $H^{13}CO_3$, arising through decarboxylation by pyruvate dehydrogenase and subsequent hydration by carbonic anhydrase. Reduced $H^{13}CO_3$ reflecting reduced TCA cycle flux can also be used as a biomarker of tumor mitochondrial metabolism (Terpstra et al., 1998). The method was recently applied to the study of human glioblastoma xenografts in rats (Park et al., 2010) and glioblastoma cells and murine xenografts *in vitro* and *in vivo* to follow the effects of an inhibitor (and anticancer agent) of phosphotidylinositol-3-kinase on tumor growth (Ward et al, 2010). For studies of brain tumors, hyperpolarized molecules such as [1-^{13}C]pyruvate and other substrates may prove particularly useful because the blood-brain-barrier, which normally restricts the passage of substrates, is disturbed during tumor growth, allowing for faster uptake and more time for metabolism prior to the decay of polarization.

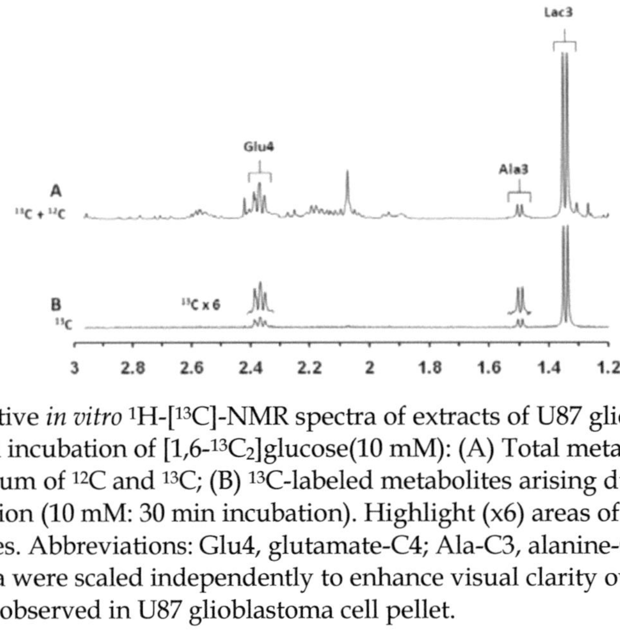

Fig. 1. Representative *in vitro* ^{1}H-[^{13}C]-NMR spectra of extracts of U87 glioblastoma cell pellet after 30 min incubation of [1,6-$^{13}C_2$]glucose(10 mM): (A) Total metabolite intensity representing the sum of ^{12}C and ^{13}C; (B) ^{13}C-labeled metabolites arising during [1,6-$^{13}C_2$]glucose infusion (10 mM: 30 min incubation). Highlight (x6) areas of Glu and Ala ^{13}C-labeled metabolites. Abbreviations: Glu4, glutamate-C4; Ala-C3, alanine-C3 and Lac3, lactate-C3. Spectra were scaled independently to enhance visual clarity owing to the lower amino acid levels observed in U87 glioblastoma cell pellet.

4.7 MicroRNA approach

Gene expression can be regulated by microRNAs. MicroRNAs are 19-25 nucleotides long and are capable of inhibiting translation and mRNA degradation thereby blocking protein production. microRNAs are named by numbers and the number reflects the sequence when they are identified. The next microRNA discovered will be the next number. Also mature microRNAs are named as miR whereas the primary transcript is named as mir. They influence multiple processes in several diseases including cancer (Mendell, 2005). In cancer, their effects are found in invasion, migration and metastasis (Nana-Sinkam & Croce, 2011). They play roles as oncogenes and tumor suppressor genes in several cancer types. Each miRNA can affect several genes and each gene can be regulated by several microRNAs. The relationship between the target RNA and microRNA in regulating many pathological states is emerging (Perron et al., 2007). Thus, it is timely to investigate the impact of microRNAs in glioblastoma invasion and migration and apply this knowledge in mapping cancer therapeutic strategies. An emerging role of microRNA in resistance may be attributed to its effect on MDR. MicroRNAs mR-27a, miR-451 and miR-138 are known to impact response to chemotherapeutic drugs in several cancers including esophageal, breast, and ovarian cancers and leukemia (Hing et al., 2010; Li et al., 2010; Zhao et al., 2010; Kovalchuk et al., 2008). P-glycoprotein is present in the blood-brain barrier and may be regulated by miR-27a and miR451 (Zhu et al., 2008). In glioblastoma, 10 different miRNA were identified and shown to be predictor of prognosis (Srinivasan et al., 2011). In addition, miR-10b (Gabriely et al., 2011) has been implicated in progression of gliomas. MiR-101 that regulates PcG protein EZH2, a histone methyltransferase, may play a role in glioblastoma progression (Smits et al, 2010). Other microRNA's implicated in glioblastoma progression are listed in Table 1.

4.8 Isoflavones

Micronutrients may be employed as chemopreventive agents: they may be employed to suppress or reverse carcinogenesis, thereby preventing the development of cancer. "Micronutrients include any dietary substance, essential or non-essential that are present in small amounts and brings about a physiological effect" (Greenwald et al., 2002). Example of micronutrients include, but are not limited to, vitamins, minerals, soy phytoestrogens, and other phytochemicals (Russo et al., 2005). Isoflavones are phytoestrogen compounds highly enriched in soy and exhibit anticancer properties. Epidemiological studies have demonstrated that Asian population consuming diets rich in isoflavones show lower incidences of hormone-related cancers (Lee et al., 1991). Genistein (4', 5, 7-trihydroxyisoflavone) and biochanin A (4'-methoxy, 5, 7-dihydroxy isoflavone) are natural isoflavonoid phytoestrogens and are found in soy and subterranean clover, respectively (Persky & Van Horn, 1995). Genistein is a well studied chemopreventive agent (Taylor et al., 2009; Sarkar & Li, 2002). Genistein exerts its anti-cancer properties via several mechanisms: inhibition of tyrosine phosphorylation, weak estrogenic and anti-estrogenic properties, as an anti-oxidant, inhibition of topoisomerase II, inhibition of angiogenesis, and induction of cell differentiation in breast cancer cells (Barnes & Peterson, 1995; Fotsis et al., 1993; Messina et al., 1994). Genistein also competes with ATP for binding to the tyrosine kinase domain, thereby inhibiting tyrosine kinase-mediated signaling processes (Chen et al., 2003). Our work in an *in vitro* co-culture model showed genistein inhibits glioblastoma invasion by inhibiting EGFR tyrosine kinase activity (Penar et al., 1997; Penar et al., 1998). Biochanin A has inhibitory potential on lung tumor development in mice induced by benzo(a)pyrene (Lee et al., 1991). Both genistein and biochanin A inhibit serum- and EGF-stimulated growth of human prostate cancer cells (Peterson & Barnes, 1993; Hempstcok et al., 1998). Biochanin A also inhibits the incidence and growth of xenograft tumors in athymic mice subsequent to injection of prostate cancer cells (LNCap) into the mice (Rice et al., 2002). We have demonstrated that both genistein and biochanin A inhibit invasion of glioblastoma cells by lowering the expression and activity of matrix-degrading enzymes (Puli et al., 2006). Soy isoflavones appear to be safe and effective in pre-clinical studies but clinical trials supporting their efficacy are still required (Virk-Baker et al., 2010).

MICRO RNA	FUNCTIONAL EFFECTS	REFERENCES
miR-7	EGFR, Akt pathway	Kefas et al., 2008
miR-10b	Resistance, Invasion	Ujifuku et al., 2010; Sasayama et al., 2009
miR-21	Apoptosis, EGFR, Tumor suppressor, MMP, Resistance	Shi et al., 2010; Ren et al., 2010; Zhou et al., 2010; Li et al., 2009; Conti et al., 2009; Chen et al., 2008; Papagiannakopoulos et al., 2008; Gabriely et al., 2008; corsten et al., 2007; Chan et al., 2005
miR-34a	Oncogenes	Li et al., 2009; Li et al., 2009
miR-93	Angiogenesis, tumor growth	Fang et al., 2011
miR-124a	Migration, Invasion	Fowler et al., 2011; Silber et al., 2008
miR125a	Invasion	Cortez et al., 2010
miR-128	Oncogenes, Stem cell renewal factor	Godlewski et al., 2008
miR-137	Differentiation	Silber et al., 2008
miR-146b-5p	EGFR, Migration, Invasion	Fowler et al., 2011; Xia et al., 2009
miR-153	Apoptosis	Xu et al., 2010; Xu et al., 2011
miR-181	Resistance	Slaby et al., 2010
miR-181a	Radiosensitivity	Chen et al., 2010
miR-181b	Proliferation	Conti et al., 2009
miR-195	Resistance	Ujifuku et al., 2010
miR-196	Prognosis	Guan et al., 2010
miR-221/222	P27(kip) survivin, radiosensitivity, PUMA	Wang et al., 2011; Zhang CZ et al., 2010; Zhang C et al., 2009; Lorimer, 2009; Zhang et al., 2009; Conti et al., 2009; Lukiw et al., 2009; Gillies & Lorimer, 2007
miR-326	Pyurvate kinase M2	Kefas et al., 2010
miR-328	ABCG2 expression, resistance	Li et al., 2010
miR-451	Tumor suppressor, proliferation, migration, resistance, metabolic stress	Nan et al,2010; Godlewski et al., 2010; Godlewski et al., 2010; Gal et al., 2008
miR-455-3p	Resistance	Ujifuku et al., 2010

Table 1. MicroRNA implicated in Glioblastoma Progression and Treatment

4.9 Implications of targeting the blood-brain barrier in developing novel approaches

Targeting drugs that cross the blood-brain barrier (BBB) to reach the extracellular/interstitial space (ECS) in brain post formidable challenges because the capillary endothelial cells are lined with intercellular tight junctions that restrict transfer of molecules from blood to the ECS (Lino & Merlo, 2009; Patel et al., 2009; Redzic, 2011). Moreover, the capillary endothelium on the brain side is completely surrounded or wrapped by astroglial end feet (Patel et al., 2009; Redzic, 2011). Several strategies have been proposed to deal with the restrictions of the BBB. Such strategies include: chemically modified delivery systems; biologically assisted delivery systems; disruption of the BBB; use of molecular Trojan horses such as peptidomimetic monoclonal antibodies; and particulate drug carrier systems (Juillerat-Jeanneret , 2008; Patel et al., 2009). Nevertheless, among these strategies, which are particularly suitable for delivering drugs to target glioblastomas remain to be definitively ascertained. Glioblastomas are cancer cells that exhibit diverse genotypic and phenotypic characteristics that allow them to adapt to their microenvironment so as to facilitate their proliferation and invasion into the surrounding normal brain tissue (see Lino & Merlo, 2009 and references therein). Consequently, further research is needed to combine a realistic assessment of their genotypic and phenotypic characteristics and how they adapt to their intracerebral niche along with selecting the appropriate strategy to target the desired efficacious chemotherapeutic agent to such gliomas. For example, on the one hand, around low-grade gliomas, the BBB is intact and usually restrictive to drug penetration; on the other hand, around high-grade, more malignant gliomas, the BBB becomes leaky as a result of the tumors actively secreting proteases and other factors that can actively degrade the tight junctions between the endothelial cells at their vicinity (Lino & Merlo, 2009). However, as the tumor grows aggressively, an increasing pressure in the ECS is being built up, ultimately leading to capillary and venous collapse. Consequently, any strategizing in optimizing the delivery of chemotherapeutic agents to the gliomas will have to consider the physiological and/or pathophysiological status of the capillaries that deliver oxygen and nutrients to the gliomas.

5. Conclusions

Several new approaches have been developed to treat glioblastomas during the last two decades. However, these approaches have not resulted in lowering the mortality and morbidity of patients suffering from this disease. The reason for this therapeutic inadequacy is that we are dealing with a tumor with highly malignant character and that the presence of the blood-brain barrier precludes easy access for drugs to target to the tumor. We have discussed the progress in understanding the aggressive phenotypic characteristics of glioblastomas and identified multiple drug targets (including key cell signaling and invasive processes) for treatment of this devastating disease. We have also emphasized the importance and the need to fully elucidate metabolic adaptive characteristics of glioblastoma employing the versatile new techniques involving nuclear magnetic resonance spectroscopy and imaging. Additionally, we have highlighted the use of new technologies whereby the restrictions of the blood-brain barrier to drug targeting can be circumvented. We included a brief review of some new roles of micro-RNAs in glioblastoma progression and treatment and showed their potential in mapping new strategies in treating glioblastomas. Ultimately, a successful strategy in treating glioblastomas leading to improved patient outcome and survival necessarily involves a combination of drug targets based on a deeper appreciation of the metabolic adaptations of glioblastomas.

6. References

Akiyama, T., Ishida, J., Nakagawa, S., Ogawara, H., Watanabe, S., Itoh, N., Shibuya, M.,& Fukami, Y. (1987). Genistein, a specific inhibitor of tyrosine-specific protein kinases. *J Biol Chem*, Vol. 262, No.12, pp. 5592-5595.

Andronesi OC, Blekas KD, Mintzopoulos D, Astrakas L, Black PM, Tzika AA. (2008). Molecular classification of brain tumor biopsies using solid-state magic angle spinning proton magnetic resonance spectroscopy and robust classifiers. *Int J Oncol*, Vol. 33, No.5, pp.1017-1025.

Aoki ,T., Hashimoto, N., Matsutani, M. (2007). Management of glioblastoma. *Expert Opin Pharmacother*, Vol. 8, No. 18, pp. 3133-46.

Argyriou, AA., Giannopoulou, E., Kalofonos, HP. (2009). Angiogenesis and anti-angiogenic molecularly targeted therapies in malignant gliomas.*Oncology*, Vol. 77, No.1, pp. 1-11.

Arteaga, CL., Johnson, MD., Todderud, G., Coffey, RJ., Carpenter, G., & Page, DL. (1991). Elevated content of the tyrosine kinase substrate phospholiase C-gamma 1 in primary human breast carcinomas. *Proc Natl Acad Sci U S A*, Vol. 88, No. 23, pp. 10435-10439.

Asadi-Moghaddam, K., Chiocca, EA., & Lawler, SE. (2010). Potential role of miRNAs and their inhibitors in glioma treatment. Expert Rev Anticancer Ther, Vol.10, No.11, pp. 1753-1762.

Balmaceda C, Critchell D, Mao X, Cheung K, Pannullo S, DeLaPaz RL, Shungu DC. (2006). Multisection ^{1}H magnetic resonance spectroscopic imaging assessment of glioma response to chemotherapy. *J Neurooncol*, Vol. 76, No.2, pp. 185-191.

Barnes, S., & Peterson, TG. (1995). Biochemical targets of the isoflavone genistein in tumor cell lines. *Proc Soc Exp Biol Med*, Vol. 208, No. 1, pp. 103-8.

Barton SJ, Howe FA, Tomlins AM, Cudlip SA, Nicholson JK, Bell BA, Griffiths JR.(1999) . Comparison of *in vivo* ^{1}H MRS of human brain tumours with ^{1}H HR-MAS spectroscopy of intact biopsy samples *in vitro*. *MAGMA*, Vol. 8, No.2, pp.121-128.

Batchelor, TT., Duda, DG., di Tomaso, E., Ancukiewicz, M., Plotkin, SR., Gerstner, E., Eichler, AF., Drappatz, J., Hochberg, FH., Benner, T., Louis, DN., Cohen, KS., Chea, H., Exarhopoulos, A., Loeffler, JS., Moses, MA., Ivy, P., Sorensen, AG., Wen, PY.,& Jain, RK. (2010). Phase II study of cediranib, an oral pan-vascular endothelial growth factor receptor tyrosine kinase inhibitor, in patients with recurrent glioblastoma. *J Clin Oncol*, Vol.28, No.17, pp. 2817-23.

Bayley, JP. & Devilee, P. (2010). Warburg tumors and the mechanisms of mitochondrial tumor suppressor genes. Barking up the right tree? *Current Opinion in Genetics & Development* , Vol. 20 , pp. 324-329.

Beal, K., Abrey, LE., & Gutin, PH. (2011). Antiangiogenic agents in the treatment of recurrent or newly diagnosed glioblastoma: analysis of single-agent and combined modality approaches. *Radiat Oncol*, Vol. 6, pp. 2.

Bhardwaj, V., Rizvi, N., Lai, MB., Lai, JCK., & Bhushan, A .(2010). Glycolytic enzyme inhibitors affect pancreatic cancer survival by modulating its signaling and energetics. *Anticancer Res*, Vol. 30, No.3, pp. 743-749.

Bhushan, A., Patil, PP., Leung, SW., & Lai, JCK. (2011). Metallic Nanoparticles in Cancer Imaging and Therapy (in press)

Brandes, AA., Tosoni, A., Amistà, P., Nicolardi, L., Grosso, D., Berti, F., & Ermani, M. (2004). How effective is BCNU in recurrent glioblastoma in the modern era? A phase II trial. *Neurology*, Vol. 63, No. 7, pp. 1281-1284.

Brem, H., Piantadosi, S., Burger, PC., Walker, M., Selker, R., Vick, NA., Black, K., Sisti, M., Brem, S., & Mohr, G. (1995). Placebo-controlled trial of safety and efficacy of intraoperative controlled delivery by biodegradable polymers of chemotherapy for recurrent Gliomas. *Lancet*, Vol. 345, No. 8956, pp. 1008-1012.

Buckner, JC., Ballman, KV., Michalak, JC., Burton, GV., Cascino, TL., Schomberg, PJ., Hawkins, RB., Scheithauer, BW., Sandler, HM., Marks, RS., &O'Fallon, JR. North Central Cancer Treatment Group 93-72-52; Southwest Oncology Group 9503 Trials. Phase III trial of carmustine and cisplatin compared with carmustine alone and standard radiation therapy or accelerated radiation therapy in patients with glioblastoma multiforme: North Central Cancer Treatment Group 93-72-52 and Southwest Oncology Group 9503 Trials. *J Clin Oncol*, Vol. 24, No. 24, pp. 3871-9.

CBTRUS (2011). CBTRUS Statistical report: Primary Brain and Central Nervous System Tumors Diagnosed in the Unites States in 2004-2007. Central Brain Tumor Registry of the United States, Hinsdale, IL. www.cbtrus.org

Cha, S. (2009). Neuroimaging in neuro-oncology. *Neurotherapeutics*, Vol. 6 , pp. 465-477.

Chakravarti ,A., Zhai, G., Suzuki, Y.,& Sarkesh, S. (2004) . The prognostic significance of phosphotidylinositol 3-kinase pathway activation in human gliomas. *Journal of Clinical Oncology*, Vol. 22, No.10, pp. 1926-1933.

Chan, JA., Krichevsky, AM., Kosik, KS. (2005). MicroRNA-21 is an antiapoptotic factor in human glioblastoma cells. *Cancer Res*, Vol .65, No.14, pp. 6029-6033.

Chandana, SR., Movva, S., Arora, M., & Singh, T. (2008). Primary brain tumors in adults. Am Fam Physician, Vol. 77, No. 10, pp. 1423-30.

Chaponis, D., Barnes, JW., Dellagatta, JL., Kesari, S., Fast, E., Sauvageot, C., Panagrahy, D., Greene, ER., Ramakrishna, N., Wen, PY., Kung, AL., Stiles, C., & Kieran, MW. (2011). Lonafarnib (SCH66336) improves the activity of temozolomide and radiation for orthotopic malignant gliomas. *J Neurooncol* .[Epub ahead of print].

Chatterji, T., Dukhande, VV., Bhushan, A., & Lai, JCK. (2009). Glucose Withdrawal Results in Resistance to Cytotoxic Effect of Glycolytic Enzyme Inhibitors in U87 Glioblastoma Cells. Proceedings *of 100th Annual Meeting, American Association for Cancer Research*, Denver, CO, April 2009, Vol. 50, p. 828.

Chatterji, T., Rizvi, N., Isaac, AO., Lai, MB., Dukhande, VV., Bhushan, A., & Lai, JCK. (2007). Metabolic Inhibitors Differentially Alter Astrocytoma and Neuroblastoma Cell Survival and Metabolism. *Annual Meeting, Society for Neuroscience*, San Diego, CA November 2007, (in Abstracts Volume).

Chen, G., Zhu, W., Shi, D., Lv, L., Zhang, C., Liu, P.,& Hu, W. (2010). MicroRNA-181a sensitizes human malignant glioma U87MG cells to radiation by targeting Bcl-2. *Oncol Rep.*, Vol. 23, No. 4, pp. 997-1003.

Chen, P., Murphy-Ullrich, JE., & Wells, A. (1996). A role for gelsolin in actuating epidermal growth factor receptor mediated cell motility. *J Cell Biol,* Vol. 134, No. 3, pp. 689-98.

Chen, P., Xie, H., Sekar, MC., Gupta, K.,& Wells, A. (1994). Epidermal growth factor receptor-mediated cell motility: phospholipase C activity is required, but mitogen-activated protein kinase activity is not sufficient for induced cell movement. *J Cell Biol,* Vol. 127, pp. 847-857.

Chen, WF., Huang, MH., Tzang, CH., Yang, M., & Wong, MS. (2003). Inhibitory actions of genistein in human breast cancer (MCF-7) cells. *Biochim Biophys Acta,* Vol. 1638, No.2, pp. 187-96.

Chen, Y., Liu, W., Chao, T., Zhang, Y., Yan, X., Gong, Y., Qiang, B., Yuan, J., Sun, M., & Peng, X. (2008). MicroRNA-21 down-regulates the expression of tumor suppressor PDCD4 in human glioblastoma cell T98G. *Cancer Lett,* Vol.272, No.2, pp. 197-205.

Cheng, JQ., & Nicosia, SV. (2001). AKT signal transduction pathway in oncogenesis. Schwab D, editor. *Encylopedia reference of cancer,* Berlin (Germany): Springer, p. 35-37.

Choe, G., Park, JK., Jouben-Steele, L., Kremen, TJ., Liau, LM., Vinters, HV., Cloughesy, TF., & Mischel, PS. (2002). Active matrix metalloproteinase 9 expression is associated with primary glioblastoma subtype. *Clin Cancer Res,* Vol. 8, No.9, pp. 2894-901.

Chowdhury, GM., Gupta, M., Gibson, KM., Patel, AB.,& Behar, KL. (2007a). Altered cerebral glucose and acetate metabolism in succinic semialdehyde dehydrogenase-deficient mice: evidence for glial dysfunction and reduced glutamate/glutamine cycling. *J Neurochem,* Vol. 103, pp. 2077-2091.

Chowdhury, GM., Patel, AB., Mason, GF., Rothman, DL.,& Behar, KL. (2007b). Glutamatergic and GABAergic neurotransmitter cycling and energy metabolism in rat cerebral cortex during postnatal development. *J Cereb Blood Flow Metab,* Vol.27, No. 12, pp. 1895-907.

Chowdhury, GMI., Banasr, M., de Graaf, RA., Rothman, DL., Behar, KL., & Sanacora, G. (2008). Chronic riluzole treatment increases glucose metabolism in rat prefrontal cortex and hippocampus. *J Cereb Blood Flow Metab,* Vol. 28, pp. 1892-1897.

Chowdhury, GMI., Lai, JCK., & Leung, SW.(2008). Nanotoxicity Studies of the CNS: Potential Application of Magnetic Resonance Spectroscopy Methods. *12th World Multi-Conference on Systemics, Cybernetics and Informatics/14th International Conference on Information Systems Analysis and Synthesis,* VOL II, PROCEEDINGS Pages: 1-5.

Cole AJ, Yang VC, David AE. (2011). Cancer theranostics: the rise of targeted magnetic nanoparticles. *Trends Biotechnol.* 2011 Apr 11. [Epub ahead of print]

Conti, A., Aguennouz, M., La Torre, D., Tomasello, C., Cardali, S., Angileri, FF., Maio, F., Cama, A., Germanò, A., Vita, G., Tomasello, F. (2009). miR-21 and 221 upregulation and miR-181b downregulation in human grade II-IV astrocytic tumors. J Neurooncol, Vol. 93, No.3, pp. 325-32.

Corsten, MF., Miranda, R., Kasmieh, R., Krichevsky, AM., Weissleder, R., & Shah, K. (2007). MicroRNA-21 knockdown disrupts glioma growth in vivo and displays synergistic cytotoxicity with neural precursor cell delivered S-TRAIL in human gliomas. *Cancer Res,* Vol. 67, No.19, pp. 8994-9000.

Cortez, MA., Nicoloso, MS., Shimizu, M., Rossi, S., Gopisetty, G., Molina, JR., Carlotti, C Jr., Tirapelli, D., Neder, L., Brassesco, MS., Scrideli, CA., Tone, LG., Georgescu, MM., Zhang, W., Puduvalli, V., & Calin, GA. (2010). miR-29b and miR-125a regulate podoplanin and suppress invasion in glioblastoma. *Genes Chromosomes Cancer,* Vol. 49, No.11, pp. 981-990.

Czarnecka, A., & Bartnik, E. (2009). Mitochondrial DNA mutations in tumors. In: *Cellular Respiration and Carcinogenesis,* Apte, SP., & Sarangarajan, R. (eds.), pp. 119-130, Humana Press, New York, NY.

D'Alessio, S., & Blasi, F. (2009). The urokinase receptor as an entertainer of signal transduction. Front Biosci, Vol. 14, pp. 4575-87.

Dang, CV., Hamaker, M., Sun, P., Le, A. & Gao, P. (2011). Therapeutic targeting of cancer cell metabolism. *Journal of Molecular Medicine,* Vol. 89, pp. 205-212.

Darkes, Malcolm JM., Plosker, Greg L., & Jarvis, B. (2002).Temozolomide:A Review of its Use in the Treatment of Malignant Gliomas,Malignant Melanoma and Other Advanced Cancers. *Am J Cancer,* Vol. 1, No. 1, pp. 55-80.

De Graaf, RA., Mason, GF., Patel, AB.,Behar, KL., & Rothman, DL. *(2003). In* vivo ^{1}H-[^{13}C]-NMR spectroscopy of cerebral metabolism. *NMR Biomed,* Vol. 16, pp. 339–357

Deryugina, EI., Bourdon, MA., Luo, GX., Reisfeld, RA., & Strongin, A. (1997). Matrix metalloproteinase-2 activation modulates glioma cell migration. *J Cell Sci,* Vol. 110, No. 19, pp. 2473-82.

Dickson, PV., Hamner, JB., Sims, TL., Fraga, CH., Ng, CY., Rajasekeran, S., Hagedorn, NL., McCarville, MB., Stewart, CF., Davidoff, AM. (2007). Bevacizumab-induced transient remodeling of the vasculature in neuroblastoma xenografts results in improved delivery and efficacy of systemically administered chemotherapy. *Clin Cancer Res,* Vol.13, No.13, pp. 3942–3950.

Dolan, ME.,& Pegg, AE. (1997). O6-benzylguanine and its role in chemotherapy. Clin Cancer Res, Vol. 3, No. 6, pp. 837-47.

Duffy, MJ. (2004). The Urokinase Plasminogen Activator System: Role in Malignancy. *Current Pharmaceutical Design,* Vol. 10, pp. 39-49.

Dukhande, VV., Malthankar-Phatak, GH., Hugus, JJ., Daniels, CK., & Lai, JCK. (2006). Manganese Induced Neurotoxicity is Differentially Enhanced by Glutathione Depletion in Astrocytoma and Neuroblastoma Cells. *Neurochem. Res,* Vol. 31, No.11, pp. 1349-1357.

Fang, L., Deng, Z., Shatseva, T., Yan,g J., Peng, C., Du, WW., Yee, AJ., An,g LC., He, C., Shan, SW., & Yang BB. (2011). MicroRNA miR-93 promotes tumor growth and angiogenesis by targeting integrin-β8. *Oncogene,* Vol. 30, No. 7, pp. 806-821.

Fillmore, HL., VanMeter, TE., & Broaddus, WC. (2001). Membrane-type matrix metalloproteinases (MT-MMPs): expression and function during glioma invasion. *J Neurooncol,* Vol. 53, No. 2, pp. 187-202.

Fotsis, T., Pepper, M., Adlercreutz, H., Fleischmann, G., Hase, T., Montesano, R., & Schweigerer. L. (1993). Genistein, a dietary-derived inhibitor of in vitro angiogenesis. *Proc Natl Acad Sci U S A,* Vol. 90, No.7, pp. 2690-2694.

Fowler, A., Thomson, D., Giles, K., Maleki, S., Mreich, E., Wheeler, H., Leedman, P., Biggs, M., Cook, R., Little, N., Robinson, B.,& McDonald K. (2011). miR-124a is frequently down-regulated in glioblastoma and is involved in migration and invasion. *Eur J Cancer,* Vol. 47, No. 6, pp. 953-963.

Fitzpatrick SM, Hetherington HP, Behar KL, Shulman RG .(1990). The flux from glucose to glutamate in the rat brain *in vivo* as determined by ^{1}H-observed, ^{13}C-edited NMR spectroscopy. *J Cereb Blood Flow Metab,* Vol. 10, No. 2, pp.170-179.

Frezza, C., Pollard, PJ., & Gottlieb, E. (2011). Inborn and acquired metabolic defects in cancer. *Journal of Molecular Medicine,* Vol. 89, pp. 213-220.

Gabriely, G., Wurdinger, T., Kesari, S., Esau, CC., Burchard, J., Linsley, PS., & Krichevsky, AM. (2008). MicroRNA 21 promotes glioma invasion by targeting matrix metalloproteinase regulators. *Mol Cell Biol,* Vol. 28. No.17, pp. 5369-5380.

Gabriely, G., Yi, M., Narayan, RS., Niers, JM., Wurdinger, T., Imitola, J., Ligon, KL., Kesari, S., Esau, C., Stephens, RM., Tannous, BA., & Krichevsky, AM. (2011). Human glioma growth is controlled by microRNA-10b. *Cancer Res.* ePub Apr 11.

Gal, H., Pandi, G., Kanner, AA., Ram, Z., Lithwick-Yanai, G., Amariglio, N., Rechavi, G., & Givol, D. (2008). MIR-451 and Imatinib mesylate inhibit tumor growth of Glioblastoma stem cells. *Biochem Biophys Res Commun,* Vol. 376, No.1, pp. 86-90.

Gallego, JM., Barcia, JA., Barcia-Mariño, C. (2007). Fatal outcome related to carmustine implants in glioblastoma multiforme. *Acta Neurochir (Wien),* Vol. 149, No. 3, pp. 261-265.

Giese, A., Bjerkvig, R., Berens, ME.,& Westphal, M. (2003). Cost of migration: invasion of malignant gliomas and implications for treatment. . *J Clin Oncol,* Vol. 21. No. 8, pp. 1624-36.

Gillies, JK., & Lorimer, IA. (2007). Regulation of p27Kip1 by miRNA 221/222 in glioblastoma. *Cell Cycle,* Vol.6. No.16, pp. 2005-2009.

Godlewski, J., Bronisz, A., Nowicki, MO., Chiocca, EA.,& Lawler, S. (2010). microRNA-451: A conditional switch controlling glioma cell proliferation and migration. Cell Cycle. Vol. 9, No. 14, pp. 2742-2748.

Godlewski, J., Nowicki, MO., Bronisz, A., Nuovo, G., Palatini, J., De Lay, M., Van Brocklyn, J., Ostrowski, MC., Chiocca, EA., Lawler, SE. (2010). MicroRNA-451 regulates LKB1/AMPK signaling and allows adaptation to metabolic stress in glioma cells. *Mol Cell,* Vol. 37, No.5, pp. 620-632.

Godlewski, J., Nowicki, MO., Bronisz, A., Williams, S., Otsuki, A., Nuovo, G., Raychaudhury, A., Newton, HB., Chiocca, EA.,& Lawler, S. (2008). Targeting of the Bmi-1 oncogene/stem cell renewal factor by microRNA-128 inhibits glioma proliferation and self-renewal. *Cancer Res,* Vol. 68, No.22, pp. 9125-9130.

Greenwald, P. (2002). Cancer prevention clinical trials. *J Clin Oncol, Vol.* 20, No.18, pp. 14S-22S.

Greenwald, P., Milner, JA., Anderson, DE., & McDonald, SS. (2002). Micronutrients in cancer chemoprevention. *Cancer Metastasis Rev.,* Vol. 21, No. 3-4, pp. 217-30.

Griffin JL, Lehtimäki KK, Valonen PK, Gröhn OH, Kettunen MI, Ylä-Herttuala S, Pitkänen A, Nicholson JK, Kauppinen RA .(2003). Assignment of ^{1}H nuclear magnetic resonance visible polyunsaturated fatty acids in BT4C gliomas undergoing ganciclovir-thymidine kinase gene therapy-induced programmed cell death. *Cancer Res,* Vol. 63, No.12, pp.3195-3201.

Grossman, SA., Ye, X., Piantadosi, S., Desideri. S., Nabors, LB., Rosenfeld, M., & Fisher, J. (2010). Survival of patients with newly diagnosed glioblastoma treated with radiation and temozolomide in research studies in the United States. *Clin Cancer Res,* Vol. 16, No. 8, pp. 2443–2449.

Guan, Y., Mizoguchi, M., Yoshimoto, K., Hata, N., Shono, T., Suzuki, SO., Araki, Y., Kuga, D., Nakamizo, A., Amano, T., Ma, X., Hayashi, K.,& Sasaki, T. (2010). MiRNA-196 is upregulated in glioblastoma but not in anaplastic astrocytoma and has prognostic significance. *Clin. Cancer Res.,* Vol. 16, No. 16, pp. 4289-4297.

Guillamo, JS., de Boüard, S., Valable, S., Marteau, L., Leuraud, P., Marie, Y., Poupon, MF., Parienti, JJ., Raymond, E., & Peschanski, M.(2009). Molecular Mechanisms Underlying Effects of Epidermal Growth Factor Receptor Inhibition on Invasion, Proliferation, and Angiogenesis in Experimental Glioma. *Clin Cancer Res,* Vol.15, pp. 3697-3704.

Guillard, S., Clarke, PA., Te Poele, R., Mohri, Z., Bjerke, L., Valenti, M., Raynaud,F., Eccles, SA., & Workman, P.(2009). Molecular pharmacology of phosphatidylinositol 3-kinase inhibition in human glioma. *Cell Cycle,* Vol. 8, No. 3, pp. 443-53.

Hay, N., & Sonenberg, N.(2004) . Upstream and downstream of mTOR. *Genes Dev,* Vol.18, pp. 1926-1945.

Hegi, ME., Liu, L., Herman, JG., Stupp, R., Wick, W., Weller, M., Mehta, MP.,& Gilbert ,MR. (2008). Correlation of O6-Methylguanine Methyltransferase (MGMT) Promoter Methylation With Clinical Outcomes in Glioblastoma and Clinical Strategies to Modulate MGMT Activity. *Journal of Clinical Oncology,* Vol. 26, No. 25, pp. 4189-4199.

Hempstock, J., Kavanagh, JP., & George, NJ. (1998). Growth inhibition of prostate cell lines in vitro by phyto-oestrogens. *Br J Urol,* Vol.82, NO.4, pp. 560-563.

Hertz L, Peng L, Dienel GA .(2007). Energy metabolism in astrocytes: high rate of oxidative metabolism and spatiotemporal dependence on glycolysis/glycogenolysis. *J Cereb Blood Flow Metab,* Vol. 27, pp. 219-249.

Hoelzinger, DB., Demuth, T., & Berens, ME. (2007). Autocrine Factors That Sustain Glioma Invasion and Paracrine Biology in the Brain Microenvironment. *J Natl Cancer Inst ,* Vol. 99, No. 21, pp. 1583-1593.

Hong L., Han Y., Zhang H., Li M., Gong T., Sun L., Wu K., Zhao, Q., & Fan, D. (2010). The prognostic and chemotherapeutic value of miR-296 in esophageal squamous cell carcinoma. *Ann Surg.,* Vol. 251, No. 6, pp. 1056-1063.

Hudson, CC., Liu, M., Chiang, GG., Otterness, DM., Loomis, DC., Kaper, F., Giaccia, AJ., & Abraham, RT. (2002). Regulation of hypoxia-inducible factor 1α expression and function by the mammalian target of rapamycin. *Mol Cell Biol,* Vol. 22, pp. 7004-7014.

Hu S, Lustig M, Balakrishnan A, Larson PE, Bok R, Kurhanewicz J, Nelson SJ, Goga A, Pauly JM, and Vigneron DB .(2010). 3D compressed sensing for highly accelerated hyperpolarized ^{13}C MRSI with *in vivo* applications to transgenic mouse models of cancer. *Magn Reson Med,* Vol. 63, No.2, pp. 312–321.

Jain KK.(2010). Advances in the field of nanooncology. *BMC Med,* Vol.8, pp.83.

Jain, RK.(2001). Normalizing tumor vasculature with anti-angiogenic therapy: a new paradigm for combination therapy. *Nat Med,* Vol. 7, No.9, pp. 987-989.

Jain, RK., di Tomaso, E., Duda, DG., Loeffler, JS., Sorensen, AG.,& Batchelor, TT. (2007). Angiogenesis in brain tumours. *Nat Rev Neurosci, Vol.*8, No.8, pp. 610-622.

Johannessen,TC., Bjerkvig, R., & Tysnes, BB.(2008). DNA repair and cancer stem-like cells--potential partners in glioma drug resistance? *Cancer Treat Rev*, Vol. 34, No.6, pp. 558-567.

Jones, NP., Peak, J., Brader, S., Eccles, SA., & Katan, M.(2005). PLCgamma1 is essential for early events in integrin signalling required for cell motility. J Cell Sci, Vol. 118, No. 12, pp. 2695-2706.

Juillerat-Jeanneret, L. (2008). The targeted delivery of cancer drugs across the blood-brain barrier: chemical modifications of drugs or drug-nanoparticles? *Drug Discov Today*, Vol. 13, pp. 1099-1106.

Kaina, B., Margison, GP., & Christmann, M. (2010). Targeting O^6-methylguanine-DNA methyltransferase with specific inhibitors as a strategy in cancer therapy. *Cell Mol Life Sci*, Vol. 67, No. 21, pp. 3663-3681.

Kargiotis, O., Rao, JS.,& Kyritsis, AP. (2006). Mechanisms of angiogenesis in gliomas. *J Neurooncol*, Vol.78, No.3, pp. 281-293.

Katakowski, M., Zheng, X., Jiang, F., Rogers, T., Szalad, A.,& Chopp , M. (2010). MiR-146b-5p suppresses EGFR expression and reduces in vitro migration and invasion of glioma. *Cancer Invest*, Vol. 28, No. 10, pp. 1024-1030.

Katterle, Y., Brandt, BH., Dowdy, SF., Niggemann, B., Zänker, KS., & Dittmar, T. (2004). Antitumour effects of PLC-gamma1-(SH2)2-TAT fusion proteins on EGFR/c-erbB-2-positive breast cancer cells. Br J Cancer, Vol. 90, No. 1, pp. 230-235.

Kefas, B., Comeau, L., Erdle, N., Montgomery, E., Amos, S.,& Purow, B. (2010). Pyruvate kinase M2 is a target of the tumor-suppressive microRNA-326 and regulates the survival of glioma cells. *Neuro Oncol.* Vol. 12, No. 11, pp. 1102-1112.

Kefas, B., Godlewski, J., Comeau, L., Li, Y., Abounader, R., Hawkinson, M., Lee, J., Fine, H., Chiocca, EA., Lawler, S., & Purow, B. (2008). microRNA-7 inhibits the epidermal growth factor receptor and the Akt pathway and is down-regulated in glioblastoma. *Cancer Res*, Vol.68, No.10, pp. 3566-3572.

Keunen, O., Johansson, M., Oudin, A., Sanzey, M., Rahim, SA., Fack, F., Thorsen, F., Taxt, T., Bartos, M., Jirik, R., Miletic, H., Wang, J., Stieber, D., Stuhr, L., Moen, I., Rygh, CB., Bjerkvig, R.,& Niclou, SP. (2011). Anti-VEGF treatment reduces blood supply and increases tumor cell invasion in glioblastoma. *Proc Natl Acad Sci U S A*, Vol.108, No.9, pp. 3749-3754.

Khoshyomn, S., Nathan, D., Manske, GC., Osler, TM., & Penar, PL.(2002) Synergistic effect of genistein and BCNU on growth inhibition and cytotoxicity of glioblastoma cells. *J Neurooncol.*, Vol. 57, No.3, pp. 193-200.

Khoshyomn, S., Penar, PL., Rossi, J., Wells, A., Abramson, DL., & Bhushan, A. (1999). Inhibition of phospholipase C-gamma1 activation blocks glioma cell motility and invasion of fetal rat brain aggregates. Neurosurgery, Vol. 44, No.3, pp. 568-577.

Kim, MJ., Kim, E., Ryu, SH., & Suh, PG. (2000). The mechanism of phospholipase C-γ1 regulation. *Experimental and Molecular Medicine*, Vol. 32, No. 3, pp. 101-109.

Kleihues, P. & Ohgaki, H. (1999). Primary and secondary glioblastomas: from concept to clinical diagnosis. *Neuro Oncol*, Vol. 1,pp. 44-51.

Kovalchuk, O., Filkowski, J., Meservy, J., Ilnytskyy, Y., Tryndyak, VP., Chekhun, VF., & Pogribny, IP. (2008). Involvement of microRNA-451 in resistance of the MCF-7 breast cancer cells to chemotherapeutic drug doxorubicin. *Mol Cancer Ther.* , Vol. 7, No. 7, pp. 2152-2159.

Krex, D., Klink, B., Hartmann, C., von Deimling, A., Pietsch, T., Simon, M., Sabel, M., Steinbach, J.P., Heese, O., Reifenberger, G., Weller, M. & Schackert, G. (2007). Long-term survival with glioblastoma multiforme. *Brain,* Vol. 13, pp. 2596-2606.

Kurhanewicz J, Vigneron DB, Brindle K, Chekmenev EY, Comment A, Cunningham CH, Deberardinis RJ, Green GG, Leach MO, Rajan SS, Rizi RR, Ross BD, Warren WS, Malloy CR .(2011). Analysis of cancer metabolism by imaging hyperpolarized nuclei: prospects for translation to clinical research. *Neoplasia,* Vol.13, No.2, pp. 81-97.

Lai, A., Tran, A., Nghiemphu, PL., Pope, WB., Solis, OE., Selch, M., Filka, E., Yong, WH., Mischel, PS., Liau, LM., Phuphanich, S., Black, K., Peak, S., Green, RM., Spier, CE., Kolevska, T., Polikoff, J., Fehrenbacher, L., Elashoff, R.,& Cloughesy, T. (2011). Phase II study of bevacizumab plus temozolomide during and after radiation therapy for patients with newly diagnosed glioblastoma multiforme. *J Clin Oncol,* Vol. 29, No.2, pp. 142-148.

Lai, JCK., Bhardwaj, V., Chatterji, T., Rizvi, N., Isaac ,AO., Lai, MB., Johnson, T., Leung, SW., Daniels, CC., & Bhushan, A .(2008). Inhibitors of Glycolytic Enzymes: Induction of Cancer Cell Death & Alteration in Cell Signaling. *In Advances in Cancer Research in Idaho Symposium, organized by Idaho Cancer Research Association in association with the 50th Annual Meeting of the Idaho Academy of Science,* College of Western Idaho, Nampa, ID March 2008, in Program & Abstracts, p. 12.

Lamszus, K., Kunkel, P.,& Westphal, M. (2003). Invasion as limitation to anti-angiogenic glioma therapy. *Acta Neurochir Suppl,* Vol.88, pp. 169-177.

Lassen, U,. Kristjansen, PE., Wagner, A., Kosteljanetz, M.,& Poulsen, HS.(1999). Treatment of newly diagnosed glioblastoma multiforme with carmustine, cisplatin and etoposide followed by radiotherapy. A phase II study. *J Neurooncol,* Vol. 43, No.2, pp. 161-166.

Lawler, S., & Chiocca, EA. (2009). Emerging functions of microRNAs in glioblastoma. J Neurooncol, Vol.92, No.3, pp. 297-306

Lebon, V., Petersen, KF., Cline, GW., Shen, J., Mason, GF., Dufour, S., Behar, KL., Shulman, GI.,& Rothman, DL. (2002). Astroglial contribution to brain energy metabolism in humans revealed by ^{13}C nuclear magnetic resonance spectroscopy: elucidation of the dominant pathway for neurotransmitter glutamate repletion and measurement of astrocytic oxidative metabolism. *J Neurosci,* Vol. 22, pp. 1523–1531.

Lee, HP., Gourley, L., Duffy, SW., Esteve. J., Lee, J., & Day, NE. (1991). Dietary effects on breast-cancer risk in Singapore. *Lancet,* Vol. 337, No.8751 , pp. 1197-200.

Lee, YS., Seo, JS., Chung, HT., & Jang, JJ.(1991). Inhibitory effects of biochanin A on mouse lung tumor induced by benzo(a)pyrene. *J Korean Med Sci,* Vol. 6, No. 4, pp. 325-328.

Lehtimäki KK, Valonen PK, Griffin JL, Väisänen TH, Gröhn OH, Kettunen MI, Vepsäläinen J, Ylä-Herttuala S, Nicholson J, Kauppinen RA .(2003). Metabolite changes in BT4C rat gliomas undergoing ganciclovir-thymidine kinase gene therapy-induced programmed cell death as studied by ^{1}H NMR spectroscopy *in vivo, ex vivo,* and *in vitro. J Biol Chem,* Vol. 278, No.46, pp.45915-45923.

Lemort, M., Canizares-Perez, AC., Van der Stappen, A., & Kampouridis, S. (2007). Progress in magnetic imaging of brain tumors. Curr Opin Oncol, pp. 616-622.

Levin, VA. (1999). Chemotherapy for brain tumors of astrocytic and oligodendroglial lineage: the past decade and where we are heading. *Neuro Oncol*, Vol. 1, No.1, pp. 69-80.

Levin, VA., Phuphanich, S., Yung, WK., Forsyth, PA., Maestro, RD., Perry, JR., Fuller, GN., & Baillet, M. (2006). Randomized, double-blind, placebo-controlled trial of marimastat in glioblastoma multiforme patients following surgery and irradiation. J Neurooncol, Vol. 78, No. 3, pp. 295-302.

Li, WQ., Li, YM., Tao, BB., Lu ,YC., Hu, GH., Liu, HM., He, J., Xu, Y.,& Yu, HY. (2010). Downregulation of ABCG2 expression in glioblastoma cancer stem cells with miRNA-328 may decrease their chemoresistance. *Med Sci Monit,* Vol. 16, No. 10, pp. HY27-30.

Li, Y., Guessous, F., Zhang, Y., Dipierro, C., Kefas, B., Johnson, E., Marcinkiewicz, L., Jiang, J., Yang, Y., Schmittgen, TD., Lopes, B., Schiff, D., Purow, B., & Abounader, R.(2009). MicroRNA-34a inhibits glioblastoma growth by targeting multiple oncogenes. *Cancer Res, Vol.* 69, No.19, pp. 7569-7576.

Li, Y., Li, W., Yang, Y., Lu, Y., He, C., Hu, G., Liu, H., Chen, J., He, J., Yu, H. (2009). MicroRNA-21 targets LRRFIP1 and contributes to VM-26 resistance in glioblastoma multiforme. *Brain Res*, Vol. 1286, pp. 13-18.

Li, ZM, Hu, S., Xiao, L., Wang, J., Cai, J., Yu, LL.,& Wang, ZH. (2010). Expression of microRNA 27a and its correlation with drug resistance in human ovarian cancer A2780/Taxol cells. *Zhonghua Fu Chan Ke Za Zhi.*, Vol. 45, No. 5, pp. 372-375.

Liang, BC., & Ullyatt, E. (1998). Chemosensitization of glioblastoma cells to bis-dichloroethyl-nitrosourea with tyrphostin AG17. Clin Cancer Res., Vol. 4, No. 3, pp. 773-781.

Lino, M., & Merlo, A. (2009). Translating biology into clinic: the case of glioblastoma. *Current Opinion Cell Biol*, Vol. 21, pp. 311-316.

Lo, HW. (2010). EGFR-targeted therapy in malignant glioma: novel aspects and mechanisms of drug resistance. *Curr Mol Pharmacol*, Vol. 3, No.1, pp. 37-52.

Lorimer, IA. (2009). Regulation of p27Kip1 by miRNA 221/222 in glioblastoma. *Cell Cycle*, Vol. 8, No. 17, pp. 2685.

Lukiw, WJ., Cui, JG., Li, YY., & Culicchia, F. (2009). Up-regulation of micro-RNA-221 (miRNA-221; chr Xp11.3) and caspase-3 accompanies down-regulation of the survivin-1 homolog BIRC1 (NAIP) in glioblastoma multiforme (GBM). *J Neurooncol*, Vol. 91, No.1, pp. 27-32.

MacDonald, TJ., DeClerck, YA., & Laug, WE. (1998). Urokinase induces receptor mediated brain tumor cell migration and invasion. *Neurooncol,* Vol. 40, No.3, pp.215-226.

Maddocks, ODK., & Vousden, KH. (2011). Metabolic regulation by p53. *J Mol Med,* Vol. 89, pp. 237-245.

Malthankar-Phatak, GH., Patel, AB., Xia, Y., Hong, S., Chowdhury, GM., Behar, KL., Orina, IA.,& Lai, JC.(2008). Effects of continuous hypoxia on energy metabolism in cultured cerebro-cortical neurons. *Brain Res*, Vol. 1229, pp. 147-154.

Martínez-Bisbal MC, Martí-Bonmatí L, Piquer J, Revert A, Ferrer P, Llácer JL, Piotto M, Assemat O, Celda B. (2004). ^{1}H and ^{13}C HR-MAS spectroscopy of intact biopsy samples *ex vivo* and *in vivo* ¹H MRS study of human high grade gliomas. *NMR Biomed,* Vol.17, No.4, pp.191-205.

Mathupala SP, Ko YH, Pedersen PL. (2010). The pivotal roles of mitochondria in cancer: Warburg and beyond and encouraging prospects for effective therapies. *Biochim Biophys Acta.* 1797(6-7), pp. 1225-1230.

McGirt, MJ., Than, KD., Weingart, JD., Chaichana, KL., Attenello, FJ., Olivi, A. (2009). Gliadel (BCNU) wafer plus concomitant temozolomide therapy after primary resection of glioblastoma multiforme. *J Neurosurg,* Vol. 110, pp. 583-588.

McKnight TR.(2004). Proton magnetic resonance spectroscopic evaluation of brain tumor metabolism. *Semin Oncol,* Vol. 31, No.5, pp.605-617.

Mendell, JT. (2005). MicroRNAs: critical regulators of development, cellular physiology and malignancy. *Cell Cycle,* Vol.4, No.9, pp. 1179-1184.

Messina, MJ., Persky, V., Setchell, KD.,& Barnes, S. (1994). Soy intake and cancer risk: a review of the in vitro and in vivo data. *Nutr Cancer,* Vol. 21, No.2, pp. 113-131.

Miller, DF., Bay, JW., Lederman, RJ., Purvis, JD., Rogers, LR., Tomsak, RL. (1985). Ocular and orbital toxicity following intracarotid injection of BCNU (carmustine) and cisplatinum for malignant gliomas. *Ophthalmology,* Vol. 92, No.3, pp. 402-406.

Mohanam, S., Gladson, CL., Rao, CN., & Rao, JS. (1999). Biological significance of the expression of urokinase-type plasminogen activator receptors (uPARs) in brain tumors. *Front Biosci,* Vol. 15, No. 4, pp. D178-87.

Motomura, K., Natsume, A., Kishida, Y., Higashi, H., Kondo, Y., Nakasu, Y., Abe, T., Namba, H., Wakai, K.,& Wakabayashi, T. (2011). Benefits of Interferon-b and Temozolomide Combination Therapy for Newly Diagnosed Primary Glioblastoma With the Unmethylated MGMT Promoter. A Multicenter Study. *Cancer,* Vol. 117, No.8, pp. 1721-1730.

Murphy, S., Davey, RA., Gu, XQ., Haywood, MC., McCann, LA., Mather, LE., & Boyle, FM.(2007). Enhancement of cisplatin efficacy by thalidomide in a 9L rat gliosarcoma model. *J Neurooncol,* Vol. 85, No.2, pp. 181-189.

Nagane, M., Kobayashi, K., Ohnishi, A., Shimizu, S., & Shiokawa, Y. (2007). Prognostic significance of O6-methylguanine-DNA methyltransferase protein expression in patients with recurrent glioblastoma treated with temozolomide. . *Jpn J Clin Oncol,* Vol. 37, No. 12, pp. 897-906.

Nagane, M., Narita, Y., Mishima, K., Levitzki, A., Burgess, AW., Cavenee, WK.,& Huang, HJ.(2001). Human glioblastoma xenografts overexpressing a tumor-specific mutant epidermal growth factor receptor sensitized to cisplatin by the AG1478 tyrosine kinase inhibitor. *J Neurosurg,* Vol.95, No. 3, pp. 472-479.

Nakada, M., Kita, D., Futami, K., Yamashita, J., Fujimoto, N., Sato, H., & Okada, Y. (2001). Roles of membrane type 1 matrix metalloproteinase and tissue inhibitor of metalloproteinases 2 in invasion and dissemination of human malignant glioma. *J Neurosurg,* Vol. 94, No. 3, pp. 464-473.

Nakada, M., Nakada, S., Demuth, T., Tran, NL., Hoelzinger, DB., & Berens, ME. (2007). Molecular targets of glioma invasion. *Cell Mol Life Sci,* Vol. 64, No. 4, pp. 458-478.

Nan, Y., Han, L., Zhang, A., Wang, G., Jia, Z., Yang, Y., Yue, X., Pu, P., Zhong, Y., Kang, C. (2010). MiRNA-451 plays a role as tumor suppressor in human glioma cells. *Brain Res.,* Vol. 1359, pp.14-21.

Nana-Sinkam, SP., & Croce, CM. (2011). MicroRNAs as therapeutic targets in cancer. *Transl Res., Vol.* 157, No.4, pp. 216-225.

National Comprehensive Cancer Network clinical practice guidelines in oncology-central nervous system cancers. v.1.2010. http://www.nccn.org/professionals/physician_gls/PDF/cns.pdf

Ohgaki, H., & Kleihues, P. (2007). Genetic pathways to primary and secondary glioblastoma. *Am J Pathol*, Vol. 170, No. 5, pp. 1445-1453.

Ordys, BB., Launay, S., Deighton, RF., McCulloch, J., & Whittle, IR. (2010). The role of mitochondria in glioma pathophysiology. *Mol Neurobiol*, Vol. 42, pp. 64-75.

Panigrahi , M., Das, PK., & Parikh, PM. (2011). Brain tumor and Gliadel wafer treatment. *Indian J Cancer*, Vol. 48, No. 1, pp. 11-17.

Papagiannakopoulos, T., Shapiro, A., & Kosik, KS. (2008). MicroRNA-21 targets a network of key tumor-suppressive pathways in glioblastoma cells. *Cancer Res*, Vol.68, No.19, pp. 8164-8172.

Park I, Larson PE, Zierhut ML, Hu S, Bok R, Ozawa T, Kurhanewicz J, Vigneron DB, Vandenberg SR, James CD, Nelson SJ. (2010). Hyperpolarized ^{13}C magnetic resonance metabolic imaging: application to brain tumors. *Neuro Oncol*, Vol.12, No.2, pp.133-144.

Patel AB, de Graaf RA, Mason GF, Rothman DL, Shulman RG, Behar KL (2005) The contribution of GABA to glutamate/glutamine cycling and energy metabolism in the rat cortex *in vivo*. *Proc Natl Acad Sci USA*, Vol. 102, No.15, pp.5588-5593.

Patel, MM., Goyal, BR., Bhadada, SV., Bhatt, JS., & Amin, AF. (2009). Getting into the brain. Approaches to enhance brain drug delivery. *CNS Drugs*, Vol. 23, pp. 35-58.

Peereboom, DM., Shepard, DR., Ahluwalia, MS., Brewer, CJ., Agarwal, N., Stevens, GH., Suh, JH., Toms, SA., Vogelbaum, MA., Weil, RJ., Elson, P., &Barnett, GH.(2010). Phase II trial of erlotinib with temozolomide and radiation in patients with newly diagnosed glioblastoma multiforme. *J Neurooncol*, Vol. 98, No. 1, pp. 93-9.

Penar, PL., Khoshyomn, S., Bhushan, A.,& Tritton, TR. (1997). Inhibition of epidermal growth factor receptor-associated tyrosine kinase blocks glioblastoma invasion of the brain. *Neurosurgery*, Vol.40, No.1, pp. 141-151.

Penar, PL., Khoshyomn, S., Bhushan, A.,& Tritton, TR. (1998). Inhibition of glioma invasion of fetal brain aggregates. *In Vivo*, Vol. 12, No.1, pp. 75-84.

Perron MP., Boissonneault V., Gobeil LA., Ouellet , DL., & Provost, P. (2007). Regulatory RNAs: future perspectives in diagnosis, prognosis, and individualized therapy. *Methods Mol Biol.*, Vol. 361, pp. 311-26.

Persky, V., & Van Horn, L. (1995). Epidemiology of soy and cancer: perspectives and directions. *J Nutr*, Vol. 125, No. 3, pp. 709S-712S.

Peterson, G.,& Barnes. S. (1993). Genistein and biochanin A inhibit the growth of human prostate cancer cells but not epidermal growth factor receptor tyrosine autophosphorylation. *Prostate*, Vol. 22, No.4, pp. 335-345.

Petroff, OA., Errante, LD., Rothman, DL., Kim, JH.,& Spencer, DD. (2002). Glutamate-glutamine cycling in the epileptic human hippocampus. *Epilepsia*, Vol. 43, pp. 703-10.

Plate, KH., Breier, G., Weich, HA., & Risau, W. (1992). Vascular endothelial growth factor is a potential tumour angiogenesis factor in human gliomas in vivo. *Nature,* Vol. 359,pp. 845-848.

Portais JC, Schuster R, Merle M, Canioni P .(1993) . Metabolic flux determination in C6 glioma cells using carbon-13 distribution upon [1-^{13}C]glucose incubation. *Eur J Biochem,* Vol. 217, No.1, pp.457-468.

Prasanna, VK., Venkataramana, NK., Dwarakanath, BS., & Santhosh, V. (2009). Differential responses of tumors and normal brain to the combined treatment of 2-DG and radiation in glioablastoma. J Cancer Res Ther, Vol. 5, No. 1, pp. S44-S47.

Puli S, Lai JC, Bhushan A: Inhibition of matrix degrading enzymes and invasion in human glioblastoma (U87MG) cells by isoflavones. J Neurooncol 79(2):135-42, 2006.

Quinn, JA. (2009). Phase II trial of temozolomide plus o6-benzylguanine in adults with recurrent, temozolomide-resistant malignant glioma. J Clin Oncol, Vol. 27, No. 8, pp. 1262-1267.

Rae, C., Moussa, Cel-H., Griffin, JL., Bubb, WA., Wallis, T.,& Balcar, VJ. (2005). Group I and II metabotropic glutamate receptors alter brain cortical metabolic and glutamate/glutamine cycle activity: a ^{13}C NMR spectroscopy and metabolomic study. *J Neurochem,* Vol. 02, pp. 405- 416.

Ramanathan, A., & Schreiber, SL. (2009). Direct control of mitochondrial function by mTOR. *Proc Natl Acad Sci,* Vol. 106, pp. 22229-22232.

Reardon, DA., Fink, KL., Mikkelsen, T., Cloughesy, TF., O'Neill, A., Plotkin, S., Glantz, M., Ravin, P., Raizer, JJ., Rich, KM., Schiff, D., Shapiro, WR., Burdette-Radoux, S., Dropcho, EJ., Wittemer, SM., Nippgen, J., Picard, M.,& Nabors, LB. (2008). Randomized phase II study of cilengitide, an integrin-targeting arginine-glycine-aspartic acid peptide, in recurrent glioblastoma multiforme. *J Clin Oncol,* Vol. 26, No. 34, pp. 5610-5617.

Reardon, DA., Quinn, JA., Rich, JN., Gururangan, S., Vredenburgh, J., Sampson, JH., Provenzale, JM., Walker, A., Badruddoja, M., Tourt-Uhlig, S., Herndon, JE 2nd., Dowell, JM., Affronti, ML., Jackson, S., Allen, D., Ziegler, K., Silverman, S., Bohlin, C., Friedman, AH., Bigner, DD., & Friedman, HS. (2004). Phase 2 trial of BCNU plus irinotecan in adults with malignant glioma. *Neuro Oncol,* Vol. 6, No.2, pp. 134-144.

Redzic, Z. (2011). Molecular biology of the blood-brain and the blood-cerebrospinal fluid barriers: similarities and differences. *Fluids and Barriers of the CNS,* Vol. 8, No. 3, pp. 1-25.

Reithmeier, T., Graf, E., Piroth, T., Trippel, M., Pinsker, MO., & Nikkhah, G.(2010). BCNU for recurrent glioblastoma multiforme: efficacy, toxicity and prognostic factors. *BMC Cancer* , Vol. 10, No. 30, pp. 1-8.

Ren, H., Tan, X., Dong, Y., Giese, A., Chou, TC., Rainov, N., & Yang, B. (2009). Differential Effect of Imatinib and Synergism of Combination Treatment with Chemotherapeutic Agents in Malignant Glioma Cells. *Basic & Clinical Pharmacology & Toxicology,* Vol. 104, pp. 241–252.

Ren, Y., Zhou, X., Mei, M., Yuan, XB., Han, L., Wang, GX., Jia, ZF., Xu, P., Pu, PY., Kang, CS. (2010) MicroRNA-21 inhibitor sensitizes human glioblastoma cells U251 (PTEN-mutant) and LN229 (PTEN-wild type) to taxol. *BMC Cancer.,* Vol. 10, No. 27.

Rice, L., Samedi, VG., Medrano, TA., Sweeney, CA., Baker, HV., Stenstrom, A., Furman, J., & Shiverick, KT. (2002). Mechanisms of the growth inhibitory effects of the isoflavonoid biochanin A on LNCaP cells and xenografts. *Prostate*, Vol. 52, No.3, pp. 201-212.

Roos, WP., Batista, LF., Naumann, SC., Wick, W., Weller, M., Menck, CF.,& Kaina B. (2007). Apoptosis in malignant glioma cells triggered by the temozolomide-induced DNA lesion O6-methylguanine. *Oncogene*, Vol. 26, pp. 186–197.

Rosenberg, B., Van Camp, L., & Krigas, T. (1965). Inhibition of cell division in Escherichia coli by electrolysis products from a platinum electrode. Nature , Vol. 205, No.4972, pp. 698–699.

Rosenberg, B., Vancamp, L., Trosko, JE., & Mansour, VH. (1969). Platinum Compounds: a New Class of Potent Antitumour Agents. Nature , Vol. 222, No. 5191, pp. 385–386.

Russo, M., Tedesco, I., Iacomino, G., Palumbo, R., Galano, G., & Russo, GL. (2005). Dietary Phytochemicals in Chemoprevention of Cancer. Current Medicinal Chemistry - Immunology, Endocrine & Metabolic Agents, Vol, 5, No, 1, pp. 61-72.

Salvati , M., D'Elia, A., Formichella, AI., & Frati, A. (2009). Insights into pharmacotherapy of malignant glioma in adults. *Expert Opin Pharmacother*, Vol. 10, No. 14, pp. 2279-90.

Sarkar, FH., Li, Y. (2002). Mechanisms of cancer chemoprevention by soy isoflavone genistein. *Cancer Metastasis Rev*, Vol. 21, No.3-4, pp. 265-80.

Sarkaria, JN., Kitange, GJ., James, CD., Plummer, R., Calvert, H., Weller, M., Wick, W. (2008). Mechanisms of Chemoresistance to Alkylating Agents in Malignant Glioma. *Clin Cancer Res*, Vol. 14, No.10, pp. 2900-2908.

Sasayama, T., Nishihara, M., Kondoh, T., Hosoda, K., & Kohmura, E. (2009). MicroRNA-10b is overexpressed in malignant glioma and associated with tumor invasive factors, uPAR and RhoC. *Int J Cancer*, Vol.125, No.6, pp. 1407-1413.

Semenza, GL. (2011). A return to cancer metabolism. *Journal of Molecular Medicine*, Vol. 89, pp. 203-204.

Senft, C., Polacin, M., Priester, M., Seifert, V., Kögel, D., & Weissenberger, J. (2010). The nontoxic natural compound Curcumin exerts anti-proliferative, anti-migratory, and anti-invasive properties against malignant gliomas.*BMC Cancer*, Vol. 10, No. 491, pp. 1-8.

Serkova N, Brand A, Christians U, Leibfritz D .(1996). Evaluation of the effects of immunosuppressants on neuronal and glial cells *in vitro* by multinuclear magnetic resonance spectroscopy. Biochim Biophys Acta, Vol. 1314. No. 1-2, pp. 93-104.

Shi, L., Chen, J., Yang, J., Pan, T., Zhang, S.,& Wang, Z.(2010). MiR-21 protected human glioblastoma U87MG cells from chemotherapeutic drug temozolomide induced apoptosis by decreasing Bax/Bcl-2 ratio and caspase-3 activity. *Brain Res.*, Vol. 1352, pp. 255-264.

Sibson, NR., Mason, GF., Shen, J., Cline, GW., Herskovits, AZ., Wall, JE., Behar, KL., Rothman , DL., & Shulman, RG.(2001). *In vivo* ^{13}C NMR measurement of neurotransmitter glutamate cycling, anaplerosis and TCA cycle flux in rat brain during [2-^{13}C]glucose infusion. *J Neurochem* , Vol. 76, pp. 975–989.

Sidenius, N., & Blasi, F. (2003). The urokinase plasminogen activator system in cancer: recent advances and implication for prognosis and therapy. Cancer Metastasis Rev, Vol. 22, No. 2-3, pp. 205-222.

Silber, J., Lim, DA., Petritsch, C., Persson, AI., Maunakea, AK., Yu, M., Vandenberg, SR., Ginzinger, DG., James, CD., Costello, JF., Bergers, G., Weiss, WA., Alvarez-Buylla, A., & Hodgson, JG. (2008). miR-124 and miR-137 inhibit proliferation of glioblastoma multiforme cells and induce differentiation of brain tumor stem cells. *BMC Med.* 2008, Vol.6, pp. 14.

Silvani, A., Eoli, M,. Salmaggi, A., Lamperti, E., Maccagnano, E., Broggi, G., & Boiardi, A. (2004). Phase II trial of cisplatin plus temozolomide, in recurrent and progressive malignant glioma patients.*J Neurooncol*, Vol. 66, No. 1-2, pp. 203-208.

Silvani, A., Gaviani, P., Lamperti, EA., Eoli, M., Falcone, C., Dimeco, F., Milanesi, IM., Erbetta, A., Boiardi, A., Fariselli, L.,& Salmaggi, A. (2009). Cisplatinum and BCNU chemotherapy in primary glioblastoma patients. *J Neurooncol*, Vol. 94, No. 1, pp. 57-62.

Slaby, O., Lakomy, R., Fadrus, P., Hrstka, R., Kren, L., Lzicarova, E., Smrcka, M., Svoboda, M., Dolezalova, H., Novakova, J., Valik, D., Vyzula, R., & Michalek, J. (2010). MicroRNA-181 family predicts response to concomitant chemoradiotherapy with temozolomide in glioblastoma patients. *Neoplasma*, Vol. 57, No. 3, pp. 264-269.

Smith CD, Landrum W, Carney JM, Landfield PW, Avison MJ .(1997). Brain creatine kinase with aging in F-344 rats: analysis by saturation transfer magnetic resonance spectroscopy. *Neurobiol Aging*, Vol. 18, No.6, pp. 617-622.

Smits, M., Nilsson, J., Mir, SE., van der Stoop, PM., Hulleman, E., Niers, JM., de Witt Hamer, PC., Marquez, VE., Cloos, J., Krichevsky, AM., Noske, DP., Tannous, BA.,& Würdinger, T. (2010). miR-101 is down-regulated in glioblastoma resulting in EZH2-induced proliferation, migration, and angiogenesis. *Oncotarget.*, Vol. 1, No. 8, pp. 710-720.

Srinivasan, S., Patric, IR.,& Somasundaram, KA. (2011). Ten-microRNA Expression Signature Predicts Survival in Glioblastoma. *PLoS One.*, Vol. 6, No. 3, e17438.

Srivastava, S., & Moraes, CT. (2009).Cellular adaptations to oxidative phosphorylation defects in cancer. In: *Cellular Respiration and Carcinogenesis*, Apte, SP., & Sarangarajan, R. (eds.), pp. 55-72, Humana Press, New York, NY.

Stegh, AH., Chin, L., Louis , DN., & DePinho, RA. (2008). What drives intense apoptosis resistance and propensity for necrosis in glioblastoma? A role for Bcl2L12 as a multifunctional cell death regulator. *Cell Cycle*, Vol. 7, No.18, pp. 2833-2839.

Stewart, DJ., Wallace, S., Feun, L., Leavens, M., Young, SE., Handel ,S., Mavligit, G., & Benjamin, RS. (1982). A phase I study of intracarotid artery infusion of cis-Diamminedichloroplatinum(II) in patients with recurrent malignant intracerebral tumors. *Cancer Res*, Vol. 42, No. 5, pp. 2059-2062.

Stupp, R., Mason, WP., van den Bent, MJ., Weller, M., Fisher, B., Taphoorn, MJ. , Brandes, AA., Marosi, C., Bogdahn, U., Curschmann, J., Janzer, RC., Ludwin, SK., Gorlia, T., Allgeier, A., Lacombe, D., Cairncross, JG., Eisenhauer, E., & Mirimanoff, RO. (2005). Radiotherapy plus concomitant and adjuvant temozolomide for glioblastoma. *N. Engl. J. Med*, Vol. 352, pp. 987–996.

Tate, MC., & Aghi, MK. (2009). Biology of angiogenesis and invasion in glioma. *Neurotherapeutics*, Vol. 6, No.3, pp. 447-457.

Taylor, CK., Levy, RM., Elliott, JC., & Burnett, BP. (2009). The effect of genistein aglycone on cancer and cancer risk: a review of in vitro, preclinical, and clinical studies. *Nutr Rev,* Vol. 67, No.7, pp. 398-415.

Tentori, L., & Graziani, G. (2002). Pharmacological Strategies to Increase the Antitumor Activity of Methylating Agents. *Current Medicinal Chemistry,* Vol. 9, pp. 1285-1301.

Terpstra M, Gruetter R, High WB, Mescher M, DelaBarre L, Merkle H, Garwood M .(1998). Lactate turnover in rat glioma measured by *in vivo* nuclear magnetic resonance spectroscopy. *Cancer Res,* Vol. 58, No.22, pp.5083-5088.

Turner, T., Epps-Fung, MV., Kassis, J., & Wells, A. (1997). Molecular inhibition of phospholipase Cγ signaling abrogates DU-145 prostate tumor cell invasion. Clin Cancer Res, Vol. 3, No. (12 Pt 1), pp. 2275-2282.

Tysnes, BB., & Mahesparan, R. (2001). Biological mechanisms of glioma invasion and potential therapeutic targets. *Journal of Neuro-Oncology,* Vol. 53, pp. 129–147.

Ujifuku, K., Mitsutake, N., Takakura, S., Matsuse, M., Saenko, V., Suzuki, K., Hayashi, K., Matsuo, T., Kamada, K., Nagata, I.,& Yamashita, S. (2010). miR-195, miR-455-3p and miR-10a(*) are implicated in acquired temozolomide resistance in glioblastoma multiforme cells. *Cancer Lett.,* Vol. 296, No. 2, pp. 241-248.

VanMeter ,TE., Rooprai, HK., Kibble, MM., Fillmore, HL., Broaddus, WC., & Pilkington, GJ. (2001). The role of matrix metalloproteinase genes in glioma invasion:co-dependent and interactive proteolysis. *J Neurooncol,* Vol. 53, No.2, pp. 213-235.

Verhoeff, JJ., van Tellingen, O., Claes, A., Stalpers, LJ., van Linde, ME., Richel, DJ., Leenders, WP.,& van Furth, WR. (2009). Concerns about anti-angiogenic treatment in patients with glioblastoma multiforme. *BMC Cancer,* Vol.9, pp. 444.

Villano, JL., Seery, TE., & Bressler, LR. (2009). Temozolomide in malignant gliomas: current use and future targets. *Cancer Chemother Pharmacol,* Vol. 64, pp. 647–655.

Vinjamuri, M., Adumala, RR., Altaha, R., Hobbs, GR., & Crowell, EB Jr. (2009). Comparative analysis of temozolomide (TMZ) versus 1,3-bis (2-chloroethyl)-1 nitrosourea (BCNU) in newly diagnosed glioblastoma multiforme (GBM) patients. *J Neurooncol, Vol.* 91, No. 2, pp.221-225.

Virk-Baker, MK., Nagy, TR., & Barnes, S. (2010). Role of phytoestrogens in cancer therapy. *Planta Med,* Vol. 76, No.11, pp. 1132-1142.

Visse, R.,& Nagase, H. (2003). Matrix metalloproteinases and tissue inhibitors of metalloproteinases: structure, function, and biochemistry. *Circ Res,* Vol. 92, No. 8, pp. 827-839.

Vredenburgh, JJ., Desjardins, A., Herndon, JE II., Dowell, JM., Reardon, DA., Quinn, JA., Rich, JN., Sathornsumetee, S., Gururangan, S., Wagner, M., Bigner, DD., Friedman, AH., & Friedman, HS. (2007). Phase II trial of bevacizumab and irinotecan in recurrent malignant glioma. *Clin Cancer Res,* Vol.13, No.4, pp.1253–1259.

Wachsberger, PR., Burd, R., Cardi, C., Thakur, M., Daskalakis, C., Holash, J., Yancopoulos, GD.,& Dicker, AP.(2007). VEGF trap in combination with radiotherapy improves tumor control in u87 glioblastoma. *Int J Radiat Oncol Biol Phys,* Vol. 67, No.5, pp. 1526-1537.

Wahl, MI., Jones, GA., Nishibe, S., Rhee, SG., & Carpenter, G. (1992). Growth factor stimulation of phospholipase C-gamma 1 activity. Comparative properties of control and activated enzymes. J Biol Chem, Vol. 267, No. 15, pp. 10447-10456.

Wang, X., Han, L., Zhang, A., Wang, G., Jia, Z., Yang, Y., Yue, X., Pu, P., Shen, C., Kang, C. (2011). Adenovirus-mediated shRNAs for co-repression of miR-221 and miR-222 expression and function in glioblastoma cells. *Oncol Rep,* Vol. 25, No. 1, 97-105.

Wang, YX., & Lam, WWM .(2008). Characterisation of brain disorders and evaluation of therapy by functional and molecular magnetic resonance techniques. *Hong Kong Med J,* Vol. 14, pp. 469-478.

Warburg, O. (1956). On the origin of cancer cells. *Science,* Vol. 123, pp. 309-314.

Warburg, O., Wind, F., & Negelein, E. (1927). The metabolism of tumors in the body. *Journal of General Physiology,* Vol. 8 , pp. 519-530.

Ward CS, Venkatesh HS, Chaumeil MM, Brandes AH, Vancriekinge M, Dafni H, Sukumar S, Nelson SJ, Vigneron DB, Kurhanewicz J, James CD, Haas-Kogan DA, Ronen SM .(2010). Noninvasive detection of target modulation following phosphatidylinositol 3-kinase inhibition using hyperpolarized ^{13}C magnetic resonance spectroscopy. *Cancer Res,* Vol. 70, No.4, pp.1296-1305.

Weber, EL., Goebel, EA. (2005). Cerebral edema associated with Gliadel wafers: two case studies. *Neuro-Oncol,* Vol. 7, pp. 84–89.

Wells, A., & Grandis, JR. (2003). Phospholipase C-gamma1 in tumor progression. Clin Exp Metastasis, Vol. 20, No. 4, pp. 285-290.

Wen, PY., & Kesari, S. (2008). Malignant gliomas in adults. *N Engl J Med,* Vol. 359, No.5, pp. 492–507.

Westphal ,M., Hilt, DC., Bortey, E., Delavault, P., Olivares, R., Warnke, PC., Whittle, IR., Jääskeläinen, J.,& Ram, Z. (2003). A phase 3 trial of local chemotherapy with biodegradable carmustine (BCNU) wafers (Gliadel wafers) in patients with primary malignant glioma. *Neuro Oncol,* Vol.5, No.2, pp. 79-88.

Williams, CJ., & Whitehouse, JMA.(1979). Cis-platinum: a new anticancer agent. *British Medical Journal,* Vol. 1, pp. 1689-1691.

Wong, YYW., Jaiswal, AR., Bhushan, A., Leung, SW., & Lai, JCK. (2010). Further Elucidation of Neuroprotective Properties of Astrocytoma (Astrocytes-like) Cells. *Journal of the Idaho Academy of Science,* Vol. 46, No. 1, pp. 52-57.

Wrensch, M., Minn, Y., Chew, T., Bondy, M., & Berger, MS. (2002). Epidemiology of primary brain tumors: Current concepts and review of the literature. *Neuro-oncology,* Vol. 4, No. 4, pp. 278- 299.

Xia, H., Qi, Y., Ng, SS., Chen, X., Li, D., Chen, S., Ge, R., Jiang, S., Li, G., Chen, Y., He, ML., Kung, HF., Lai, L., & Lin, MC. (2009). microRNA-146b inhibits glioma cell migration and invasion by targeting MMPs. *Brain Res,* Vol. 1269, pp. 158-165.

Xu, J., Liao, X., Lu, N., Liu, W.,& Wong, CW. (2011). Chromatin-modifying drugs induce miRNA-153 expression to suppress Irs-2 in glioblastoma cell lines. *Int J Cancer.* (Epub ahead of print).

Xu, J., Liao, X., Wong, C. (2010). Downregulations of B-cell lymphoma 2 and myeloid cell leukemia sequence 1 by microRNA 153 induce apoptosis in a glioblastoma cell line DBTRG-05MG. *Int J Cancer,* Vol. 126, No.4, pp. 1029-1035.

Xu S, Yang J, Shen J.(2007). In vivo ^{13}C saturation transfer effect of the lactate dehydrogenase reaction. *Magn Reson Med,* Vol. 57, No.2, pp. 258-264.

Yarden, Y. (2001). The EGFR family and its ligands in human cancer. signalling mechanisms and therapeutic opportunities. Eur J Cancer., Vol.37, No. 4, pp. S3-8.

Yecies, JL., & Manning, BD. (2011). mTOR links oncogenic signaling to tumor cell metabolism. *J Mol Med,* Vol. 89, pp. 221-228.

Zhang, C., Kang, C., You, Y., Pu, P., Yang, W., Zhao, P., Wang, G., Zhang, A., Jia, Z., Han, L., & Jiang, H. (2009). Co-suppression of miR-221/222 cluster suppresses human glioma cell growth by targeting p27kip1 in vitro and in vivo. *Int J Oncol,* Vol. 34, No. 6, pp. 1653-1660.

Zhang, C., Wang, G., Kang, C., Du, Y., & Pu, P. (2009). Up-regulation of p27 (kip1) by miR-221/222 antisense oligonucleotides enhances the radiosensitivity of U251 glioblastoma. *Zhonghua Yi Xue Yi Chuan Xue Za Zhi,* Vol. 26, No. 6, pp. 634-638.

Zhang, CZ., Zhang, JX., Zhang, AL., Shi, ZD., Han, L., Jia, ZF., Yang, WD., Wang, GX., Jiang, T., You, YP., Pu, PY., Cheng, JQ.,& Kang CS. (2010). MiR-221 and miR-222 target PUMA to induce cell survival in glioblastoma. *Mol Cancer.* ,Vol. 9, pp. 229.

Zhao, X., Yang, L., Hu, J., & Ruan, J. (2010). miR-138 might reverse multidrug resistance of leukemia cells. *Leuk Res.*, Vol. 34, No. 8, pp. 1078-1082.

Zhou, X., Ren, Y., Moore, L., Mei, M., You, Y., Xu, P., Wang, B., Wang, G., Jia, Z., Pu, P., Zhang, W., & Kang, C. (2010). Downregulation of miR-21 inhibits EGFR pathway and suppresses the growth of human glioblastoma cells independent of PTEN status. *Lab Invest.* Vol. 90, No. 2, pp. 144-155.

Zhu, H., Wu, H., Liu, X., Evans, BR., Medina, DJ., Liu, CG., & Yang, JM. (2008). Role of MicroRNA miR-27a and miR-451 in the regulation of MDR1/P-glycoprotein expression in human cancer cells. *Biochem Pharmacol.,* Vol. 76, No.5, pp. 582-588.

Zhu, Y., & Parada, LF. (2002). Molecular biology and genetics of neurologic tumors. *Nature Reviews Cancer*, Vol. 2, No.8, pp. 616-626.

Zwingmann, C., & Leibfritz, D. (2003). Regulation of glial metabolism studied by ^{13}C-NMR. *NMR Biomed,* Vol. 16, pp. 370-99.

10

Chemotherapy of Medulloblastoma in Children

Dezső Schuler, Péter Hauser and Miklós Garami
2ndDepartment of Paediatrics, Faculty of Medicine
Semmelweis University, Budapest
Hungary

1. Introduction

Medulloblastoma is one of the most common childhood tumour of the central nervous system. During the past years several researchers dealt with its aetiology, pathology and therapy: surgical-, radio- and chemotherapy. The objective of the present chapter is to review the chemotherapy and we shall present our results and the few clinical data about the targeted therapy.

2. Incidence

Tumours of the central nervous system (CNS) are the second most common childhood malignant diseases after hematological malignancies. The incidence is similar in the different developed countries: in Europe is 29.9/million (1978-1997), in USA 30.7/million (1992-2006). However, the highest incidence is registered in Hungary and the Scandinavian countries. In Hungary the incidence was 37.41/million between 1999 and 2008 and 43.9/million in 2009. The cause of this high incidence in Hungary is unknown (Gupta & Banerjee et al, 2004; Hauser et al., 2003; Kaderali et al., 2009; McNeil et al., 2002; Peris-Bonet et al., 2006; Pizzo & Poplack, 2011). Astrocytomas and medulloblastoma are the most frequent among childhood CNS tumours.

3. Prognostic factors

The prognostic factors are especially important in risk group assignment of brain tumours, because the increased intensity of treatment in high risk cases has much more side effects, than the therapy of the average risk patients.

The most frequently used prognostic factors in the past were: the size of the tumour, the metastases including the tumour cells in the spinal fluid 2 weeks after the surgery (Chang (T_{1-4}; M_{0-3}) (Laurent et al., 1985) and the extent of the surgical intervention (Albright et al., 1996). Later the age and the histology of tumour were also introduced (Ellison, 2010; Giangaspero et al., 2006; Packer et al., 1994). According to several publications residual tumour mass greater than 1.5 cm^2 after the surgical intervention, the presence of metastases, age younger than 3 years are unfavourable prognostic factors (Albright et al., 1996; Chang et al., 1969; Eberhart et al., 2002; Jenkin et al., 2000; Klesse & Bowers, 2010) The histology of the tumours (desmoplastic/nodular, classic, large cell/anaplastic) is an important, independent prognostic factor too, which was proved by Rutkowski et al. in a study of 260 young children (Rutkowski et al, 2010).

Several biological factors have prognostic value (ERBB2, TP53, PDGFRA, TRKC, CDK6, α and β-catenin). The prognostic role of the aberrantly expressed miRNAs is yet under investigation (Birks et al., 2011). However, the most reliable and independent prognostic factor is microarray gene expression profile (Aihara et al., 2010; Fernandez-T et al., 2004; Pizzo & Poplack, 2010; Rutkowski et al., 2010; Tabori et al., 2010). Four distinct groups were established by Northcott (Northcott et al., 2010): Wnt, Shh, C and D. Wnt and Shh was previously described as the wingless type and sonic hedgehoge pathway involvement in the tumorproliferation (Wechsler-Reya & Scott, 2001). In Group C and D a clear molecular pathway involvement could not be clearly identified. The new classification does not follow the classical pathological classification (as classic, desmoplastic, large cell/anaplastic subtypes) and it shows some association with age and metastatis production. The separation of these groups by immunohistochemical analysis only was a great step toward the everyday practice in using this classification as prognostic factor. Group Wnt, Shh, C, D are characterized by the presence of CTNNB1, GLI1, NPR3 and KCNA1 proteins. Wnt and Shh groups seem to need less intensive therapy with outstanding survival and less side effects.
Most centres use the following prognostic factors: the young age (<3 years) residual tumour after surgery, the metastases, the histology and in some centres the MYCC/MYCN amplification and the expression of ERBB2 (Pizzo & Poplack, 2010; Rutkowski et al., 2010; Takei et al., 2009).

4. Therapy

The therapy of the malignant tumours is surgical, radio- and chemotherapy, similarly to other childhood tumours. In brain tumours the most important is the surgical therapy and is curative if it is radical ablation and no metastases are found. However, the surgical therapy is hindered by the localisation of the tumour and the difficulty in differentiating the tumour from the normal tissues.
The radiotherapy of medulloblastoma is an important and effective part of therapy. However its use is limited by the irreversible damage caused in children, which is specially serious in young children and infants causing serious neurocognitive damage (Fouladi et al., 2005; Mulhern et al., 2004). Hence it should be avoided in children less than 3 years old in spite of their lower survival rate (Johnston et al., 2009). It is remarkable, that the increased intensity of the chemotherapy enabled the decrease of the craniospinal radiation dose in the average risk cases without the worsening the survival to 23.4Gy along an unchanged focus-dose (55.8Gy) which decreased significantly the late side-effects (Mulhern et al., 1998; Packer et al., 1999, 2006).

4.1 Chemotherapy

It is difficult to compare the different studies to select the optimal treatment protocol due to the non-uniform prognostic factors, the lack of reliable - centrally checked - patho-histological and molecular diagnostics and the often low number of patients and duration of observation. Hoff (von Hoff et al., 2009) and collaborators published the results of a 10 years long follow up. In their patient-group 12% of relapse occurred five years or more after the end of therapy.
An important obstacle of the chemotherapy is the blood-brain barrier despite the fact that the tumour breaks through the barrier when growing. There were several trials for increasing the possibility of passing the barrier but without any provable result. (Kobrinsky et al., 1999; Prados et al., 2003)

The additive curative effect of chemotherapy after surgery and radiotherapy was proved by a prospective, multicentric, randomised trial in 1990 (Evans et al., 1990; Tait et al., 1990). In the beginning vincristine and the nitrosoureas were applied, which are still used in several protocols for the treatment of medulloblastoma. However, the usefulness of vincristine was recently challenged because vincristine could not be detected in the spinal fluid in measurable concentration after 1,5 mg/m^2 i.v. bolus injection. Later more and more chemotherapeutic drug combinations have been used. The key agents are the nitrosoureas (lomustine, carmustine), cyclophosphamide, vincristine and the later used cisplatin, carboplatin, and etoposide (Mueller & Chang, 2009). Some protocols apply ifosfamide alternating with cyclophosphamide (Park et al., 2010). The application of methotrexate is limited not only because of its potential side effects, but also because it can be used only before radiotherapy, however, some protocols described rather good results in cases when no irradiation was done (Bleyer, 1981; Chi et al., 2004; Fossati-Bellani et al., 1990; Rutkowski et al., 2005). The alkylating oral drug dibromdulcitol was an excellent substance for the treatment of medulloblastomas because its favourable pharmacokinetic properties in the spinal fluid and its tolerable toxicity (Paál et al., 1994; Schuler et al., 1988, 1992). Later in spite of the good clinical results the drug became unavailable. However, this may be partially substituted by temozolomide, but there is no study yet, which proves its efficacy in medulloblastoma.

The increased arsenal of the chemotherapeutics and the higher intensity of the treatment resulted in improved survival. In cases with favourable prognosis the survival rate is already over 80%, and around 70% in cases with unfavourable prognosis (Gottardo & Gajjar, 2008). However, the toxicity of the treatment increased, too. Therefore, besides improving survival rates reducing early and late toxicity are also important. In the future a less toxic treatment is expected thanks to the development of the targeted molecular therapy based on tumour-biological knowledge.

The most important criteria are:

1. the optimal timing of the chemotherapy
2. the most effective combination of cytostatics
3. sufficient intensity and length of the chemotherapy
4. a tolerable toxicity of the drugs used in the protocol.

Some trials proved that the chemotherapy given before and after the irradiation (sandwich therapy) is disadvantageous; the survival is shorter if the radiotherapy is longer than 50 days (von Hoff et al., 2009; Taylor et al., 2003). Hence the radiotherapy should be given as early after the surgery as it is possible (Bailey et al., 1995; Kortmann et al., 2000). During the radiotherapy several protocols contain the administration of vincristine (von Hoff et al., 2009; Packer et al., 1994, 1999) or in one protocol carboplatin (Jakacki et al., 2007). A preoperative chemotherapy is applied in several paediatric tumours, because it decreases the size of the tumour and facilitate the tumour removal. Hence it would be reasonable to introduce it in huge chemosensitive brain tumours, too (Schuler et al., 1993). The preoperative chemotherapy is feasible and safe in children with high risk medulloblastoma according to some pilot trials (Di Rocco et al., 1995; Grill et al., 2005; Schuler et al., 1993). However, it is not applied in the practice up to now.

In most protocols a combination of vincristine, a nitrosourea (lomustine or camustine) and a platinum compound (cisplatin or carboplatin) is used. In several protocols cyclophosphamide is used instead of nitrosourea because of the good antitumour effect and shorter bone marrow toxicity of cyclophosphamide, (von Hoff et al., 2009; Mueller & Chang, 2009; Packer et al., 1994) and in some treatment protocols etoposide is also added to this combination (Chi et al., 2004; Dhall et al., 2008; Hauser et al., 2009).

Our protocol for average risk cases begins with three intrathecal triplet (methotrexate, ara-C, prednisolone) and VECp-block (vincristine, cyclophosphamide, etoposide) after the surgery. This is followed by radiotherapy (5th - 11th week). During the radiotherapy the patients get weekly vincristine. 2 weeks after the radiotherapy chemotherapy is continued by vincristine — etoposide — cyclophosphamide/ carboplatin; vincristine — cisplatin — etoposide / BCNU blocks until the 73nd postoperative week.

In high risk cases autologous stem cell transplantation is made after the 40th postoperative week instead of maintenance therapy. If a residual tumour is present it is removed by a "second look" surgery before the transplantation.

In children less than 3 years old the therapy is similar to that in high risk cases, except that no radiotherapy is given and the stem cell transplantation is made as soon as no tumour is seen by MRI. Radiotherapy is given only, if the tumour is still present after the age of three years.

The toxicity of our protocol was tolerable; and there was no therapy related mortality. After 31 months the overall survival was 79% in the average risk patients and 63% in high risk patients.

The best therapeutic results in average risk cases were achieved by the multicentre trial HIT'91 (von Hoff et al., 2009). The overall survival in patients without metastasis was 91% after 10 years. After the removal of tumour a combination of radiotherapy and vincristine was applied, which was followed 6 weeks later by 8 cycles with lomustine (CCNU), vincristine and cisplatin. Packer et al., described a 86% survival after 3 years follow up by a similar regime (Packer et al., 1999). A 93% survival was published by Strother et al. (2001) (Strother et al., 2001) with a more aggressive therapy. They administered 4 cycles of high dose chemotherapy after surgery and radiotherapy (cyclophosphamide, cisplatin, and vincristine) followed by auto-transplantation after each cycle.

The results in high risk cases are more consistent ranging from 34 to 40% across studies (Mueller & Chang, 2009). However, Chi et al. achieved 60% overall survival after 3 years by 5 cycles of vincristine, cisplatin, etoposide, cyclophosphamide and methotrexate given after surgery followed by myeloablative chemotherapy with autologous stem cell rescue (Chi et al., 2004). The results of Gajjar et al. (Gajjar et al., 2006) was similar: 83% event free survival in average risk patients and 70% in high risk cases after 5 years.

Good survival was achieved by the COG99701 study (Jakacki et al., 2007). They administered vincristine and carboplatin during the radiotherapy in patients with metastatic medulloblastoma. 6 weeks later the patients received 6 courses of monthly cyclophosphamide and vincristine. The overall survival after 4 years was 81%.

The increased intensity of therapy resulting a longer survival has more late side effect. Hence the stratification of the tumours according to prognostic factors into average or high risk group is important.

In cases of medulloblastomas of children less than 3 years old radiotherapy should avoid. The most favourable approach after surgery is the myeloablative consolidation chemotherapy after conventional induction therapy which may result 60% overall survival after 3 years (Chi et al., 2004). The result of the intensive chemotherapy depends both on the histologic type and the presence of the residual tumour (Dhall et al., 2008). Those trials which combine the systematic and intraventricular chemotherapy had better results only among children without metastases and residual tumour (Zeltzer et al., 1999)

The survival of relapsed patients is very poor, especially in patients who had already received radiotherapy and/or auto-transplantation (Butturini et al., 2009). However, there are several trials by intensive chemotherapy and transplantations. (Park et al., 2010). The prolongation of the survival with metronomic therapy was possible in some studies. The metronomic therapy is referred to as low-dose chemotherapy or antiangiogenic chemotherapy (Kieran et al., 2005; Privitera et al., 2009; Sterba et al., 2010). Recently, the combination of the alkylating agent temozolomide with etoposide, which is a topoisomerase II inhibitor was found to be efficacious in prologing the survival in relapsed medulloblastoma. (Wang CH et al., 2009; Ruggiero A et al., 2010). However, the study of the application of the metronomic therapy for a longer time after the about 6 months long intensive and maintenance therapy in the primordial therapy of high risk cases may be justified too due to the occurrence of late relapses.

The toxicity of the previously described chemotherapeutic modalities depends on their intensity independent from the well known side effects of the radiotherapy. The most common and most serious ones are the acut myelotoxic effect and infections. Some authors describe yet anorexia, nausea, diarrhoea, pain and hypokalemia.

Better comparability of the different therapeutic modalities, improvement of results and the decrease of side effects are expected from the application of the molecular biologic procedures in the stratification and tailored therapy.

4.2 Targeted treatment

There is still not any new, successful, widely accepted therapeutic approach which can substitute or at least complement the standard treatment of medulloblastoma.

Presently, targeted treatment exists only in SHH group among the four groups described by Northcott et al. (2010). In this group tumor proliferation is attributed to the lack of inhibition of SMO protein by loss of function of inhibitory Patched protein (Ptch1) or activating mutation of SMO. SMO inhibitors, as cyclopamin, IPI-926 and the orally available GDC-0449 inhibit hedgehoge pathway. The latter went through a Phase 1 study, resulting in a 3-month long transient well-defined remission achieved in one 26-year old patient with proven Ptch1 mutation (Rudin et al., 2009).

Before the establishment of the new subgroups of medulloblastoma, there were also other molecularly targeted treatments. In some cases they were administered to some individual patients. Common feature of these treatments was the transient success, which finally turned into progression. The background of the progression could be the mutation of the targeted receptor or other involved proteins.

One of these targets were somatostatin receptors (SSTR), which were recognized in medulloblastoma cell surface in late nineties of the last century (Fruhwald et al., 2004; Guyotat et al., 2001;). Several attempts were to bind radioactive isotope to its agonist octreotide or its derivates, providing localized, targeted radiotherapy, which did not show extra survival advantage above conventional irradiation, (Beutler et al., 2005). Somatostatin analogues themselves through SSTR receptors may inhibit cell proliferation. Medulloblastoma express high amount of SSTR based on Octreoscan examination (Muller et al., 1998). Only one patient was described who received only octreotide without radioactive isotope, and was a long term survivor (Glas et al., 2008).

Receptor tirozin kinases another possible target group. There are several drugs targeting these receptors which are also expressed in a certain part of medulloblastoma (ErbB2, PDGFR). Their increased expression usually results in worse survival and increased metastatic ability (Gilbertson et al., 1995; Gilbertson & Clifford, 2003). The most experience is reported with imatinib, which proved to be effective in vitro, however, in vivo successful human experiences are still missing (Abouantoun & MacDonald, 2009). This may be partially caused by their hindered penetration through blood brain barrier.

Another possible therapeutic approach is the inhibition of histon deacetylases (HDAC). Acetylation of histones' amino terminal tails by histon acetyltransferase relaxes the chromatin for transcription, and removal of acetyl groups by HDAC repress transcription (Roth et al., 2001; de Ruijter et al., 2003). Histon hypoacetylation and inappropriate transcriptional repression are hypothesized to be a key contributor to the development of human cancers (Marks et al, 2001; Marks & Dokmanovic, 2005). HDAC inhibitors have been shown to cause pleiotropic effect on human cancer cells, including apoptosis, cell cycle arrest and differentiation (Su et al., 2011). Valproic acid (VPA), an anticonvulsive drug is one of the recently discovered HDAC inhibitors. There is one published Phase 1 study in pediatric CNS tumors, 2 patients with medulloblastoma were included (Su et al., 2011). The treatment was well-tolerated, however response was not observed among this little cohort of patients with medulloblastoma.

Another promising area in the treatment of medulloblastoma could be the administration of retinoic acid (RA). RA has been shown to have anticancer efficacy in a variety of cancers. Retinoic acid is commonly used in the treatment of certain childhood cancers. It is a drug with protean effects including cytodifferentiation, apoptosis, and inhibition of angiogenesis to name a few (Miller, 1998). RA has been shown in preclinical models to cause apoptotic cell death in medulloblastoma by promoting BMP-2 transcription (Hallahan et al., 2003). This results in production of soluble BMP-2 protein that induces p38 MAP kinase phosphorylation and ultimately apoptosis (Spiller et al., 2008). Recently a phase 3 trial has been opened to treat medulloblastoma with RA.

There are several different approaches to try to kill medulloblastoma cells by means of immunotherapy. Only some of them were introduced in small series of pediatric patients with limited success. In the last decades of the twentieth century application of lymphokine actived killer (LAK) cells directly administered intrathecally with co-administration of human recombinant IL-2 for patients with recurrent disseminated medulloblastoma was published. Some of the limited number of patients showed long term survival (Okamoto et al., 1988; Silvani et al., 1994).

Another method is the adoptive transfer of tumor-specific cytolytic T cells to the tumor bed and cerebrospinal fluid. This is an attractive strategy, but limited in its clinical application owing the paucity of defined antigens consistently expressed by medulloblastoma. So far only two in vitro animal medulloblastoma xenograft models have been published. One is targeting IL13Receptor-alpha2 by genetically modified CD8+ citotoxic T-cells expressing an IL13-zetakine chimeric immunoreceptor (Stastny et al., 2007). The other model is targeting HER2 expression, which is a feature of the malignant phenotype of medulloblastoma (Gilbertson et al., 1995). Recruiting the cellular arm of the immune response to HER2 positive tumor cells, genetically engineered HER2-specific T-cell with antigen binding property and lytic capacity were created. Adoptive transferred HER2-specific T-cells were administered in SCID mouse orthotopic medulloblastoma xenograft, which resulted in sustained regression of HER2 positive medulloblastoma, which might have resulted in a promising immunotherapeutic approach (Ahmed et al., 2007). Phase 1 study of adoptive transfer of tumor-specific cytolytic T cells exists in patients with recurrent glioblastoma multiforme and neuroblastoma.

Another immunotherapeutic method which is already investigated in human patients with recurrent medulloblastoma is based on dendritic cell-based tumor vaccination. Dendritic cells are the antigen presenting cells, which are present in central nervous system exclusively. Autologous mature dendritic cells loaded with tumor lysates derived from autologous, resected medulloblastomas were injected subcutaneously in 5 patients with medulloblastoma. Although the treatment was safe, no response was observed in any patient (Ardon et al., 2010).

Natural killer (NK) cells display the highest cytolytic activity against tumor cells, and are considered suitable candidates for adoptive immunotherapy to treat cancer patients. Castriconi et al showed that in vitro medulloblastoma cell lines express ligands for activating NK-receptors, which makes medulloblastoma highly susceptible to NK-mediated cytolysis (Castriconi et al., 2007). However, human studies using NK-cells in medulloblastoma are lacking at this moment.

5. Conclusions

The therapy of medulloblastoma has changed during the last few decades which resulted in the improvement of the long-term survival up to almost 80%. This is due to the complex chemotherapy beyond the improved surgical and radiotherapeutical techniques. After cyclophosphamide, nitrosoureas and methotrexate more effective drugs would be applied in the treatment of medulloblastoma: carboplatin, cisplatin, etoposide and ifosfamide. In resistant or relapsed cases several other drugs are used, too, as Temozolomide. The preoperative therapy in spite of the encouraging pilot studies could not become a general practice. The high dose chemotherapy with autologous stem cell rescue seems to be effective to eradicate the remained tumour cells in high risk cases. The prolongation of the chemotherapy with cytostatic drugs in low doses and/or antiproliferative agents (retinoic acid, valproic acid, antiangiogenic agents) seems to be effective to prolong the remission in incurable cases. The chemotherapy is especially important in very young children (less than 3 years old) because of the serious late side effects of radiotherapy. The targeted molecular therapy is promising, however, in spite of the several clinical studies the effectivity of molecular therapy is not proved yet in phase III. studies.

6. References

Abouantoun, TJ., & MacDonald, TJ. (2009). Imatinib blocks migration and invasion of medulloblastoma cells by concurrently inhibiting activation of platelet-derived growth factor receptor and transactivation of epidermal growth factor receptor. *Mol Cancer Ther*, 8, 5, (May 2009), 1137-47.

Ahmed, N., Ratnayake, M., Savoldo, B., Perlaky, L., Dotti, G., Wels, WS., Bhattacharjee, MB., Gilbertson, RJ., Shine, HD., Weiss, HL., Rooney, CM., Heslop, HE., & Gottschalk, S. (2007). Regression of experimental medulloblastoma following transfer of HER2-specific T cells. *Cancer Res*, 67, 12, (Jun 2007), 5957-64.

Aihara, Y., Tsuruta, T., Kawamata, T., Kanno, H., Maebayashi, K., Sakauchi, M., Wada, E., Osawa, M., Fujii, H., Kubo, O., & Hori, T. (2010). Double high-dose chemotherapy followed by autologous peripheral blood stem cell transplantation for primary disseminated medulloblastoma: a report of 3 cases. *J Pediatr Hematol Oncol*, 32, 2, (Mar 2010), e70-4.

Albright, AL., Wisoff, JH., Zeltzer, PM., Boyett, JM., Rorke, LB., & Stanley, P. (1996). Effects of medulloblastoma resections on outcome in children: a report from the Children's Cancer Group. *Neurosurgery*, 38, 2, (Feb 1996), 265-71.

Ardon, H., De Vleeschouwer, S., Van Calenbergh, F., Claes, L., Kramm, CM., Rutkowski, S., Wolff, JE., & Van Gool, SW. (2010). Adjuvant dendritic cell-based tumour vaccination for children with malignant brain tumours. *Pediatr Blood Cancer*, 54, 4, (Apr 2010). 519-25.

Bailey, CC., Gnekow, A., Wellek, S., Jones, M., Round, C., Brown, J., Phillips, A., & Neidhardt, MK. (1995). Prospective randomised trial of chemotherapy given before radiotherapy in childhood medulloblastoma. International Society of Paediatric Oncology (SIOP) and the (German) Society of Paediatric Oncology (GPO): SIOP II. *Med Pediatr Oncol*, 25, 3, (Sep 1995), 166-78.

Beutler, D., Avoledo, P., Reubi, JC., Macke, HR., Muller-Brand, J., Merlo, A., & Kühne, T. (2005). Three-year recurrence-free survival in a patient with recurrent medulloblastoma after resection, high-dose chemotherapy, and intrathecal Yttrium-90-labeled DOTA0-D-Phe1-Tyr3-octreotide radiopeptide brachytherapy. *Cancer*, 103, 4, (Feb 2005), 869-73.

Birks, DK., Barton, VN., Donson, AM., Handler, MH., Vibhakar, R., & Foreman, NK. (2011). Survey of MicroRNA expression in pediatric brain tumors. *Pediatr Blood Cancer*, 56, 2, (2011), 211-6.

Bleyer, WA. (1981). Neurologic sequelae of methotrexate and ionizing radiation: a new classification. *Cancer Treat Rep*, 65 Suppl 1, (1981), 89-98.

Butturini, AM., Jacob, M., Aguajo, J., Vander-Walde, NA., Villablanca, J., Jubran, R., Erdreich-Epstein, A., Marachelian, A., Dhall, G., & Finlay, JL. (2009). High-dose chemotherapy and autologous hematopoietic progenitor cell rescue in children with recurrent medulloblastoma and supratentorial primitive neuroectodermal tumors: the impact of prior radiotherapy on outcome. *Cancer*, 115, 13, (Jul 2009), 2956-63.

Castriconi, R., Dondero, A., Negri, F., Bellora, F., Nozza, P., Carnemolla, B., Raso, A., Moretta, L., Moretta, A., & Bottino, C. (2007). Both CD133+ and CD133- medulloblastoma cell lines express ligands for triggering NK receptors and are susceptible to NK-mediated cytotoxicity. *Eur J Immunol*, 37, 11, (Nov 2007), 3190-6.

Chang, CH., Housepian, EM., & Herbert, C. Jr. (1969). An operative staging system and a megavoltage radiotherapeutic technic for cerebellar medulloblastomas. *Radiology*, 93, 6, (Dec 1969), 1351-9.

Chi, SN., Gardner, SL., Levy, AS., Knopp, EA., Miller, DC., Wisoff, JH., Weiner, HL., & Finlay, JL. (2004). Feasibility and response to induction chemotherapy intensified with high-dose methotrexate for young children with newly diagnosed high-risk disseminated medulloblastoma. *J Clin Oncol*, 22, 24, (Dec 2004), 4881-7.

Dhall, G., Grodman, H., Ji, L., Sands, S., Gardner, S., Dunkel, IJ., McCowage, GB., Diez, B., Allen, JC., Gopalan, A., Cornelius, AS., Termuhlen, A., Abromowitch, M., Sposto, R., & Finlay, JL. (2008). Outcome of children less than three years old at diagnosis with non-metastatic medulloblastoma treated with chemotherapy on the "Head Start" I and II protocols. *Pediatr Blood Cancer*, 50, 6, (Jun 2008), 1169-75.

Eberhart, CG., Kepner, JL., Goldthwaite, PT., Kun, LE., Duffner, PK., Friedman, HS., Strother, DR., & Burger, PC. (2002). Histopathologic grading of medulloblastomas: a Pediatric Oncology Group study. *Cancer*, 94, 2, (Jan 2002), 552-60.

Ellison, DW. (2010). Childhood medulloblastoma: novel approaches to the classification of a heterogeneous disease. *Acta Neuropathol*, 120, 3, (2010), 305-16.

Evans, AE., Jenkin, RD., Sposto, R., Ortega, JA., Wilson, CB., Wara, W., Ertel, IJ., Kramer, S., Chang, CH., Leikin, SL., & Hammond, GD. (1990). The treatment of medulloblastoma. Results of a prospective randomized trial of radiation therapy with and without CCNU, vincristine, and prednisone. *J Neurosurg*, 72, 4, (Apr 1990), 572-82.

Fernandez-Teijeiro, A., Betensky, RA., Sturla, LM., Kim, JY., Tamayo, P., & Pomeroy, SL. (2004). Combining gene expression profiles and clinical parameters for risk stratification in medulloblastomas. *J Clin Oncol*, 22, 6, (Mar 2004), 994-8.

Fouladi, M., Gilger, E., Kocak, M., Wallace, D., Buchanan, G., Reeves, C., Robbins, N., Merchant, T., Kun, LE., Khan, R., Gajjar, A., & Mulhern, R. (2005). Intellectual and functional outcome of children 3 years old or younger who have CNS malignancies. *J Clin Oncol*, 23, 28, (Oct 2005), 7152-60.

Fruhwald, MC., Rickert, CH., O'Dorisio, MS., Madsen, M., Warmuth-Metz, M., Khanna, G., Paulus, W., Kühl, J., Jürgens, H., Schneider, P., & Müller, HL. (2004). Somatostatin receptor subtype 2 is expressed by supratentorial primitive neuroectodermal tumors of childhood and can be targeted for somatostatin receptor imaging. *Clin Cancer Res*, 10, 9, (May 2004), 2997-3006.

Gajjar, A., Chintagumpala, M., Ashley, D., Kellie, S., Kun, LE., Merchant, TE., Woo, S., Wheeler, G., Ahern, V., Krasin, MJ., Fouladi, M., Broniscer, A., Krance, R., Hale, GA., Stewart, CF., Dauser, R., Sanford, RA., Fuller, C., Lau, C., Boyett, JM., Wallace, D., & Gilbertson, RJ. (2006). Risk-adapted craniospinal radiotherapy followed by high-dose chemotherapy and stem-cell rescue in children with newly diagnosed medulloblastoma (St Jude Medulloblastoma-96): long-term results from a prospective, multicentre trial. *Lancet Oncol*, 7, 10, (Oct 2006), 813-20.

Giangaspero, F., Wellek, S., Masuoka, J., Gessi, M., Kleihues, P., & Ohgaki, H. (2006). Stratification of medulloblastoma on the basis of histopathological grading. *Acta Neuropathol*, 112, 1, (Jul 2006), 5-12.

Gilbertson, RJ., Pearson, AD., Perry, RH., Jaros, E., & Kelly, PJ. (1995). Prognostic significance of the c-erbB-2 oncogene product in childhood medulloblastoma. *Br J Cancer*, 71, 3, (Mar 1995), 473-7.

Gilbertson, RJ., & Clifford, SC. (2003). PDGFRB is overexpressed in metastatic medulloblastoma. *Nat Genet*, 35, 3, (Nov 2003), 197-8.

Glas, M., Hennemann, B., Hirschmann, B., Marienhagen, J., Schmidt-Wolf, I., Herrlinger, U., Bogdahn, U., & Hau, P. (2008). Complete response after treatment with a somatostatin analogue in an adult patient with recurrent medulloblastoma. *Acta Oncol*, 47, 3, (2008), 479-80.

Gottardo, NG., & Gajjar, A. (2008). Chemotherapy for malignant brain tumors of childhood. *J Child Neurol*, 23, 10, (Oct 2008), 1149-59.

Grill, J., Lellouch-Tubiana, A., Elouahdani, S., Pierre-Kahn, A., Zerah, M., Renier, D., Valteau-Couanet, D., Hartmann, O., Kalifa, C., & Sainte-Rose, C. (2005). Preoperative chemotherapy in children with high-risk medulloblastomas: a feasibility study. *J Neurosurg*, 103, 4 Suppl, (Oct 2005), 312-8.

Gupta, N., Banerjee, A., & Haas-Kogan, D. (19 March 2004). *Pediatric CNS Tumors*. (Fisrt ed.), Springer, ISBN: 3-540-00294-4, Berlin, Heidelberg, New York, Hong Kong, London, Milan, Paris, Tokyo

Guyotat, J., Champier, J., Pierre, GS., Jouvet, A., Bret, P., Brisson, C., Belin, MF., Signorelli, F., & Montange, MF. (2001). Differential expression of somatostatin receptors in medulloblastoma. *J Neurooncol*, 51, 2, (Jan 2001), 93-103.

Hallahan, AR., Pritchard, JI., Chandraratna, RA., Ellenbogen, RG., Geyer, JR., Overland, RP., Strand, AD., Tapscott, SJ., & Olson, JM. (2003). BMP-2 mediates retinoid-induced apoptosis in medulloblastoma cells through a paracrine effect. *Nat Med*, 9, (Aug 2003), 1033–1038.

Hauser, P., Jakab, Zs., Láng, O., Kondás, O., Török, S., Garami, M., Bognár, L., & Schuler, D. (2003). High incidence of brain tumors of childhood in Hungary between 1989 and 2001. *Med Pediatr Oncol*, 41, 6, (2003), 590-1.

Hauser, P., Jakab, Zs., Kiss, Cs., Szegedi, I., Bárdi, E., Bartyik, K., Ottóffy, G., Kajtár, P., Szűcs, R., Nagy, K., Cservenák, J., Masát, P., Bálint, K., Kordás, M., Bognár, L., Kocsis, B., Vízkeleti, J., Kriván, G., Kállay, K., Benyó, G., Schuler, D., & Garami, M. (2009). Előzetes eredmények a medulloblastoma/PNET kezelésében a magyar MBL2004 kezelési sémával. *Magy Belorv Arch*, 62, (2009), 196–201.

von Hoff, K., Hinkes, B., Gerber, NU., Deinlein, F., Mittler, U., Urban, C., Benesch, M., Warmuth-Metz, M., Soerensen, N., Zwiener, I., Goette, H., Schlegel, PG., Pietsch, T., Kortmann, RD., Kuehl, J., & Rutkowski, S. (2009). Long-term outcome and clinical prognostic factors in children with medulloblastoma treated in the prospective randomised multicentre trial HIT'91. *Eur J Cancer*, 45, 7, (2009), 1209-17.

Jakacki, R., Burger, P., Zhou, T., Holmes, E., Packer, R., Goldwein, J., Mehta, M., & Pollack, I. (2007.) Outcome for metastatic (M+) medulloblastoma (MB) treated with carboplatin during craniospinal radiotherapy (CSRT) followed by cyclophosphamide (CPM) and vincristine (VCR): Preliminary results of COG 99701. *J Clin Oncol*, 25, 18S, (Jun 2007), 2017.

Jenkin, D., Shabanah, MA., Shail, EA., Gray, A., Hassounah, M., Khafaga, Y., Kofide, A., Mustafa, M., & Schultz, H. (2000). Prognostic factors for medulloblastoma. *Int J Radiat Oncol Biol Phys*,47, 3, (Jun 2000), 573-84.

Johnston, DL., Keene, D., Bartels, U., Carret, AS., Crooks, B., Eisenstat, DD., Fryer, C., Lafay-Cousin, L., Larouche, V., Moghrabi, A., Wilson, B., Zelcer, S., Silva, M., Brossard, J., & Bouffet, E. (2009). Medulloblastoma in children under the age of three years: a retrospective Canadian review. *J Neurooncol*, 94, 1, (Aug 2009), 51-6.

Kaderali, Z., Lamberti-Pasculli, M., & Rutka, JT. (2009). The changing epidemiology of paediatric brain tumours: a review from the Hospital for Sick Children. *Childs Nerv Syst*, 25, 7, (Jul 2009), 787-93.

Kieran, MW., Turner, CD., Rubin, JB., Chi, SN., Zimmerman, MA., Chordas, C., Klement, G., Laforme, A., Gordon, A., Thomas, A., Neuberg, D., Browder, T., & Folkman, J. (2005). A feasibility trial of antiangiogenic (metronomic) chemotherapy in pediatric patients with recurrent or progressive cancer. *J Pediatr Hematol Oncol*. 27, 11, (Nov 2005), 573-81.

Klesse, LJ., & Bowers, DC. (2010). Childhood medulloblastoma: current status of biology and treatment. *CNS Drugs*, 24, 4, (2010), 285-301.

Kobrinsky, NL., Packer, RJ., Boyett, JM., Stanley, P., Shiminski-Maher, T., Allen, JC., Garvin, JH., Stewart, DJ., & Finlay, JL. (1999). Etoposide with or without mannitol for the treatment of recurrent or primarily unresponsive brain tumors: a Children's Cancer Group Study, CCG-9881. *J Neurooncol*, 45, 1, (1999), 47-54.

Kortmann, RD., Kühl, J., Timmermann, B., Mittler, U., Urban, C., Budach, V., Richter, E., Willich, N., Flentje, M., Berthold, F., Slavc, I., Wolff, J., Meisner, C., Wiestler, O., Sörensen, N., Warmuth-Metz, M., & Bamberg, M. (2000). Postoperative neoadjuvant chemotherapy before radiotherapy as compared to immediate radiotherapy followed by maintenance chemotherapy in the treatment of medulloblastoma in childhood: results of the German prospective randomized trial HIT '91. *Int J Radiat Oncol Biol Phys*, 46, 2, (Jan 2000), 269-79.

Laurent, JP., Chang, CH., & Cohen, ME. (1985). A classification system for primitive neuroectodermal tumors (medulloblastoma) of the posterior fossa. Cancer, 1, 56, (Oct 1985), 1807-9.

Marks, P., Rifkind, RA., Richon, VM., Breslow, R., Miller, T., & Kelly, WK. (2001). Histone deacetylases and cancer: causes and therapies. *Nat Rev Cancer*, 1, (Dec 2001), 194-202.

Marks, PA., & Dokmanovic, M. (2005). Histone deacetylase inhibitors: discovery and development as anticancer agents. *Expert Opin Investig Drugs,* 14, (Dec 2005), 1497-511.

McNeil, DE., Coté, TR., Clegg, L., & Rorke, LB. (2002). Incidence and trends in pediatric malignancies medulloblastoma/primitive neuroectodermal tumor: a SEER update. Surveillance Epidemiology and End Results. *Med Pediatr Oncol*, 39, 3, (Sep 2002), 190-4.

Miller, WH. (1998). The emerging role of retinoids and retinoic acid metabolism blocking agents in the treatment of cancer. *Cancer,* 83, (Oct 1998), 1471-1482.

Mueller, S., & Chang, S. (2009). Pediatric brain tumors: current treatment strategies and future therapeutic approaches. *Neurotherapeutics*, 6, 3, (Jul 2009), 570-86.

Mulhern, RK., Kepner, JL., Thomas, PR., Armstrong, FD., Friedman, HS., & Kun, LE. (1998). Neuropsychologic functioning of survivors of childhood medulloblastoma randomized to receive conventional or reduced-dose craniospinal irradiation: a Pediatric Oncology Group study. *J Clin Oncol*, 16, 5, (May 1998), 1723-8.

Mulhern, RK., Merchant, TE., Gajjar, A., Reddick, WE., & Kun, LE. (2004). Late neurocognitive sequelae in survivors of brain tumours in childhood. *Lancet Oncol*, 5, 7, (Jul 2004), 399-408.

Muller, HL., Fruhwald, MC., Scheubeck, M., Rendl, J., Warmuth-Metz, M., Sörensen, N., Kühl, J., & Reubi, JC. (1998). A possible role for somatostatin receptor scintigraphy in the diagnosis and follow-up of children with medulloblastoma. *J Neurooncol*, 38, 1, (May 1998), 27-40.

Northcott, PA., Korshunov, A., Witt, H., Hielscher, T., Eberhart, CG., Mack, S., Bouffet, E., Clifford, SC., Hawkins, CE., French, P., Rutka, JT., Pfister, S., & Taylor, MD. (2010). Medulloblastoma Comprises Four Distinct Molecular Variants. *J Clin Oncol.* 2010 Dec 6. [Epub ahead of print]

Okamoto, Y., Shimizu, K., Tamura, K., Miyao, Y., Yamada, M., Matsui, Y., Tsuda, N., Takimoto, H., Hayakawa, T., & Mogami, H. (1988). An adoptive immunotherapy of patients with medulloblastoma by lymphokine-activated killer cells (LAK). *Acta Neurochir (Wien)*, 94, 1-2, (1988), 47-52.

Paál, C., Erdélyi-Tóth, V., Pap, E., Csáki, C., Ferencz, T., Schuler, D., & Borsi, JD. (1994). Pharmacokinetic studies on Elobromol in children with brain tumors. *Anticancer Drugs*, 5, 5, (Oct 1994), 539-47.

Packer, RJ., Sutton, LN., Elterman, R., Lange, B., Goldwein, J., Nicholson, HS., Mulne, L., Boyett, J., D'Angio, G., Wechsler-Jentzsch, K., Reaman, G., Cohen, BH., Bruce, DA., Rorke, LB., Molloy, P., Ryan, J., LaFond, D., Evans, AE., & Schut, L. (1994). Outcome for children with medulloblastoma treated with radiation and cisplatin, CCNU, and vincristine chemotherapy. *J Neurosurg*, 81, 5, (Nov 1994), 690-8.

Packer, RJ., Goldwein, J., Nicholson, HS., Vezina, LG., Allen, JC., Ris, MD., Muraszko, K., Rorke, LB., Wara, WM., Cohen, BH., & Boyett, JM. (1999). Treatment of children with medulloblastomas with reduced-dose craniospinal radiation therapy and adjuvant chemotherapy: A Children's Cancer Group Study. *J Clin Oncol*, 17, 7, (Jul 1999), 2127-36.

Packer, RJ., Gajjar, A., Vezina, G., Rorke-Adams, L., Burger, PC., Robertson, PL., Bayer, L., LaFond, D., Donahue, BR., Marymont, MH., Muraszko, K., Langston, J., & Sposto, R. (2006). Phase III study of craniospinal radiation therapy followed by adjuvant chemotherapy for newly diagnosed average-risk medulloblastoma. *J Clin Oncol*, 24, 25, (Sep 2006), 4202-8.

Park, JE., Kang, J., Yoo, KH., Sung, KW., Koo, HH., Lim do, H., Shin, HJ., Kang, HJ., Park, KD., Shin, HY., Kim, IH., Cho, BK., Im, HJ., Seo, JJ., Park, HJ., Park, BK., & Ahn, HS. (2010). Efficacy of high-dose chemotherapy and autologous stem cell transplantation in patients with relapsed medulloblastoma: a report on the Korean Society for Pediatric Neuro-Oncology (KSPNO)-S-053 study. *J Korean Med Sci*, 25, 8, (2010), 1160-6.

Peris-Bonet, R., Martinez-Garcia, C., Lacour, B., Petrovich, S., Giner-Ripoll, B., Navajas, A., & Steliarov-Foucher, E. (2006). Childhood central nervous system tumours--incidence and survival in Europe (1978-1997): report from Automated Childhood Cancer Information System project. *European Journal of Cancer*, 42, 13, (Sept 2006), 1064-80.

Pizzo, PA., & Poplack, DG. (11 October 2010). *Principles and Practice of Pediatric Oncology* (Sixth ed.), 2011 Lippincott Williams & Wilkins, ISBN: 978-1-60547-682-7, Philadelphia, Baltimore, New York, London, Buenos Aires, Hong Kong, Sydney, Tokyo

Prados, MD., Schold, SC. Jr, Fine, HA., Jaeckle, K., Hochberg, F., Mechtler, L., Fetell, MR., Phuphanich, S., Feun, L., Janus, TJ., Ford, K., & Graney, W. (2003). A randomized, double-blind, placebo-controlled, phase 2 study of RMP-7 in combination with carboplatin administered intravenously for the treatment of recurrent malignant glioma. *Neuro Oncol*, 5, 2, (Apr 2003), 96-103.

Privitera, G., Acquaviva, G., Ettorre, GC., & Spatola, C. (2009). Antiangiogenic therapy in the treatment of recurrent medulloblastoma in the adult: case report and review of the literature. *J Oncol*, 2009, (Epub Dec 2009), 247873.

Di Rocco, C., Iannelli, A., La Marca, F., Tornesello, A., Mastrangelo, S., & Riccardi, R. (1995). Preoperative chemotherapy with carboplatin alone in high risk medulloblastoma. *Childs Nerv Syst*,11, 10, (Oct 1995), 574-8.

Roth, SY., Denu, JM., & Allis, CD. (2001). Histone acetyltransferases. Annu *Rev Biochem*, 70, (2001), 81-120.

Rudin, CM., Hann, CL., Laterra, J., Yauch, RL.,Callahan, CA., Fu, L., Holcomb, T., Stinson, J., Gould, SE., Coleman, B., LoRusso, PM., Von Hoff, DD., de Sauvage, FJ., & Low, JA.

(2009). Treatment of medulloblastoma with hedgehog pathway inhibitor GDC-0449. *N Engl J Med*, 361, 12, (Sep 2009), 1173-8.

Ruggiero, A., Rizzo, D., Attinà, G., Lazzareschi, I., Mastrangelo, S., Maurizi, P., Migliorati, R., Bertolini, P., Pastore, M., Colosimo, C., & Riccardi, R. (2010). Phase I study of temozolomide combined with oral etoposide in children with recurrent or progressive medulloblastoma. *Eur J Cancer*, 46, 16, (Nov 2010), 2943-9.

de Ruijter, AJ., van Gennip, AH., Caron, HN., Kemp, S., & van Kuilenburg, AB. (2003). Histone deacetylases (HDACs): characterization of the classical HDAC family. *Biochem J*,;370, Pt 3, (Mar 2003), 737–49.

Rutkowski, S., Bode, U., Deinlein, F., Ottensmeier, H., Warmuth-Metz, M., Soerensen, N., Graf, N., Emser, A., Pietsch, T., Wolff, JE., Kortmann, RD., & Kuehl, J. (2005). Treatment of early childhood medulloblastoma by postoperative chemotherapy alone. *N Engl J Med*, 352, 10, (Mar 2005), 978-86.

Rutkowski, S., Cohen, B., Finlay, J., Luksch, R., Ridola, V., Valteau-Couanet, D., Hara, J., Garre, ML., & Grill, J. (2010). Medulloblastoma in young children. *Pediatr Blood Cancer*, 54, 4, (Apr 2010), 635-7.

Rutkowski, S., von Hoff, K., Emser, A., Zwiener, I., Pietsch, T., Figarella-Branger, D., Giangaspero, F., Ellison, DW., Garre, ML., Biassoni, V., Grundy, RG., Finlay, JL., Dhall, G., Raquin, MA., & Grill, J. (2010). Survival and prognostic factors of early childhood medulloblastoma: an international meta-analysis. *J Clin Oncol*, 28, 33, (Nov 2010), 4961-8.

Schuler, D., Somló, P., Borsi, J., Paraicz, E., Révész, T., Kardos, G., & Koós, R. (1988). New drug combination for the treatment of relapsed brain tumors in children. *Pediatr Hematol Oncol*, 5, 2, (1988), 153-6.

Schuler, D., Somló, P., Koós, R., Kálmánchey, R., & Paraicz, E. (1992). Treatment of malignant scala posterior brain tumors in children: the chemotherapy of relapsed medulloblastoma with a dibromdulcitol containing drug regime and pharmacokinetic studies of dibromdulcitol in children. *Med Pediatr Oncol*, 20, 4, (1992), 312-4.

Schuler, D., Somló, P., Koós, R., Kálmánchey, R., & Paraicz, E. (1993). The treatment of malignant scala posterior tumors in children: II. Preliminary result of the pre- and postoperative adjuvant chemotherapy of scala posterior tumors. *Med Pediatr Oncol*, 21, 4, (1993), 274-9.

Silvani, A., Salmaggi, A., Parmiani, G., & Boiardi, A. (1994). Successful adoptive immunotherapy with lymphokine-activated killer cells in the treatment of medulloblastoma disseminated via cerebrospinal fluid: case report. *Neurosurgery*, 34, 6, (Jun 1994), 1078-80.

Spiller, SE., Ditzler, SH., Pullar, BJ., & Olson, JM. (2008). Response of preclinical medulloblastoma models to combination therapy with 13-cis retinoic acid and suberoylanilide hydroxamic acid (SAHA). *J Neurooncol*, 87, 2, (Apr 2008), 133-41.

Stastny, MJ., Brown, CE., Ruel, C., & Jensen, MC. (2007). Medulloblastomas expressing IL13Ralpha2 are targets for IL13-zetakine+ cytolytic T cells. *J Pediatr Hematol Oncol*, 29, 10, (Oct 2007), 669-77.

Sterba, J., Pavelka, Z., Andre, N., Ventruba, J., Skotakova, J., Bajciova, V., Bronisova, D., Dubska, L., & Valik, D. (2010). Second complete remission of relapsed medulloblastoma induced by metronomic chemotherapy. *Pediatr Blood Cancer*, 54, 4, (Apr 2010), 616-7.

Strother, D., Ashley, D., Kellie, SJ., Patel, A., Jones-Wallace, D., Thompson, S., Heideman, R., Benaim, E., Krance, R., Bowman, L., & Gajjar, A. (2001). Feasibility of four consecutive high-dose chemotherapy cycles with stem-cell rescue for patients with newly diagnosed medulloblastoma or supratentorial primitive neuroectodermal tumor after craniospinal radiotherapy: results of a collaborative study. *J Clin Oncol,* 19, 10, (May 2001), 2696-704.

Su, JM., Li, XN., Thompson, P., Ou, CN., Ingle, AM., Russell, H., Lau, CC., Adamson, PC., & Blaney, SM. (2011). Phase 1 study of valproic acid in pediatric patients with refractory solid or CNS tumors: a children's oncology group report. *Clin Cancer Res,* 17, 3, (Feb 2011), 589-97.

Tabori, U., Baskin, B., Shago, M., Alon, N., Taylor, MD., Ray, PN., Bouffet, E., Malkin, D., & Hawkins, C. (2010). Universal poor survival in children with medulloblastoma harboring somatic TP53 mutations. *J Clin Oncol,* 28, 8, (Mar 2010), 1345-50.

Tait, DM., Thornton-Jones, H., Bloom, HJ., Lemerle, J., & Morris-Jones, P. (1990). Adjuvant chemotherapy for medulloblastoma: the first multi-centre control trial of the International Society of Paediatric Oncology (SIOP I). *Eur J Cancer,* 26, 4, (Apr 1990), 464-9.

Takei, H., Nguyen, Y., Mehta, V., Chintagumpala, M., Dauser, RC., & Adesina, AM. (2009). Low-level copy gain versus amplification of myc oncogenes in medulloblastoma: utility in predicting prognosis and survival. Laboratory investigation. *J Neurosurg Pediatr,* 3, 1, (Jan 2009), 61-5.

Taylor, RE., Bailey, CC., Robinson, K., Weston, CL., Ellison, D., Ironside, J., Lucraft, H., Gilbertson, R., Tait, DM., Walker, DA., Pizer, BL., Imeson, J., Lashford, LS., & International Society of Paediatric Oncology, United Kingdom Children's Cancer Study Group. (2003). Results of a randomized study of preradiation chemotherapy versus radiotherapy alone for nonmetastatic medulloblastoma: The International Society of Paediatric Oncology/United Kingdom Children's Cancer Study Group PNET-3 Study. *J Clin Oncol,* 21, 8, (Apr 2003), 1581-91.

Wang, CH., Hsu, TR., Wong, TT., & Chang, KP. (2009). Efficacy of temozolomide for recurrent embryonal brain tumors in children. *Childs Nerv Syst,* 25, 5, (May 2009), 535-41.

Wechsler-Reya, R., & Scott, MP. (2001). The developmental biology of brain tumors. *Annu Rev Neurosci,* 24, (2001), 385-428.

Zeltzer, PM., Boyett, JM., Finlay, JL., Albright, AL., Rorke, LB., Milstein, JM., Allen, JC., Stevens, KR., Stanley, P., Li, H., Wisoff, JH., Geyer, JR., McGuire-Cullen, P., Stehbens, JA., Shurin, SB., & Packer, RJ. (1999). Metastasis stage, adjuvant treatment, and residual tumor are prognostic factors for medulloblastoma in children: conclusions from the Children's Cancer Group 921 randomized phase III study. *J Clin Oncol,* 17, 3, (Mar 1999), 832-45.

11

New Therapeutic Strategies for the Treatment of Brain Tumor

Rintaro Hashizume
Department of Neurological Surgery
University of California San Francisco, San Francisco
USA

1. Introduction

Despite significant advances in tumor imaging, neurosurgery, and radiotherapy, the prognosis for patients with malignant gliomas is extremely poor. The five-year survival rate for patients with glioblastoma (GBM), the most aggressive form of malignant glioma, is less than 5% after initial diagnosis (CBTRUS statistical report, 2010). Factors that contribute to the dismal prognosis associated with GBM include its infiltrative nature throughout the brain, which precludes total surgical resection and impair radiotherapy targeting, and resistance to most types of conventional cancer therapeutics. Many clinical studies using potent chemotherapeutic drugs conducted in the past decade have not demonstrated significant improvement in survival. A fundamental limitation in the treatment of brain tumors is that many systemically administered therapeutic agents do not cross the blood-brain barrier (BBB) (Abbott et al., 2010; Brightman, 1977; Huynh et al., 2006; Schlosshauer, 1993). While some small and lipophilic molecules, peptides, and protein-based agents delivered by systemic routes can reach the brain parenchyma by crossing the BBB, high doses are usually needed to achieve therapeutic levels, which can lead to substantial toxicity.

In this chapter, the application of intranasal delivery (IND), in comparison with systemic (intravascular) and/or direct invasive (intraparechymal) drug delivery, for the treatment of brain tumors is discussed.

2. The BBB: An obstacle for drug delivery to brain tumor

The brain parenchyma has both physiological and biological safeguards to prevent the entry of toxins from the bloodstream, which are collectively known as the BBB. The endothelial cells that comprise the cerebral micro-vessels are linked by tight junctions and surrounded by astrocytic processes and adjacent pericytes and a characteristic composition of the extracellular matrix. This structural arrangement prohibits most drugs from entering the brain through pericellular diffusion. Drugs that are able to diffuse through the barrier must be small (<400 Da) and lipophilic. In addition to this physiological barrier, drugs are rapidly cleared by efflux pumps such as P-glycoprotein, and a rapid turnover rate of extracellular fluid in the brain. In combination, these factors have limited the number of successful pharmacologic treatments for diseases of the brain and necessitate a closer examination of both traditional and novel methods of drug delivery (Choi et al., 2008; Eyal et al., 2009; Saunders et al., 2008).

In brain tumors such as GBM, the BBB is progressively disrupted with tumor growth by inducing large gaps between endothelial cells (Coomber et al., 1985). However, the extent of BBB disruption among individual patients, and/or among various regions within a single tumor, appears to be highly variable. BBB is most likely disrupted in the necrotic center, not at the infiltrative edge of the tumor (Gerstner & Fine, 2007). Recently, the artificially disruption of the BBB using hyper osmotic solutions has demonstrated by intra-arterial infusion of the VEGF specific antibody bevacizumab in patients with recurrent malignant glioma (Boockvar et al., 2010). However, disruption of the BBB could potentially lead to other serious complications, such as brain edema. Therefore, development of strategies to deliver targeted agents across the BBB is a critical priority.

3. Strategies for drug delivery to the brain

In the past decade a number of drug delivery strategies have been developed to overcome challenges presented by BBB. These strategies can be divided into two categories: (a) attempt to increase drug delivery of intravascularly administered drugs by manipulating either the drugs or capillary permeability, and (b) attempt to increase drug delivery by local administration.

3.1 Intravascular delivery

Several strategies have recently developed to increase the fraction of intravascular drug reaching the tumor. These include i) intra-arterial administration, ii) packaging drugs such as microcapsules and liposomes, iii) use of biologically active agents (such as bradykinin and histamine) (Greenwood, 1992), iv) use of replication-competent retroviruses to deliver oncolytic therapies (Tai & Kasahara, 2008), v) use of mesenchymal (Yong et al., 2009) or neural stem cells to deliver small molecules, antibodies, or toxic payloads (Aboody et al., 2000; Frank et al., 2009). There are also several specific transport mechanisms that have been exploited, involving the activity of several independent transporters that mediate the flux of substances important for brain function, such as carrier-mediated transporters, including the glucose and amino acid transporters (Rapoport, 1996; Tamai & Tsuji, 1996; Deeken & Loscher, 2007; Saunders et al., 2008), active efflux transporters, including P-glycoprotein and the other ATP-binding cassette (ABC) gene family members, and receptor-mediated transporters, of which transferrin receptor (TfR), insulin receptor, and low-density lipoprotein receptor (Pardridge, 2007). A further strategy has been to conjugate the therapeutic drug with a protein or a monoclonal antibody that gains access to the brain by receptor-mediated transcytosis (Pardridge, 1999). Small peptide vectors have been used to enhance brain uptake of several therapeutic drugs (Rousselle et al., 2000). These peptide-vectors cross cellular membranes safely and efficiently and have been used successfully to enhance penetration of several drugs.

The strategy of a packaging drugs and/or interfering RNAs into liposomes that more readily cross the BBB and show tumor reduction and increase in survival in mice. Liposomes are a drug carrier system consisting of a phospholipid membrane shell surrounding a hollow core used to stably encapsulate therapeutic molecules allowing increased solubility and half-life resulting in increased bioavailability. Gradual release of the drug from the liposome increases therapeutic efficacy while reducing toxicity (Gabizon,

2003). Liposomal anticancer agents have been widely used in humans and are currently approved for ovarian cancer (Tanguay, 2009) and multiple myeloma (Moreau, 2009), but remain investigational in their use for brain tumors. To increase the specificity of liposomal drugs, targeting antibodies can be attached to the surface of the liposome (Elbayoumi & Torchilin, 2009; Mamot et al., 2005). Antibody-conjugated liposomes increase the rate of liposome internalization, which increase intracellular drug concentration, thereby achieving heightened anti-tumor activity (Mamot et al., 2005). EGFR, a tyrosine kinase receptor that is over-expressed in 30-40% of high grade gliomas (Ekstrand et al., 1991). Attempts to target GBM by delivering EGFR-targeted immunoliposomes encapsulated anti-cancer agents or EGFR-specific shRNA in PEGylated liposomes bearing insulin receptor- and TfR-specific antibodies in an in vivo model has shown some promise (Mamot et al., 2005; Zhang et al., 2004). However, these antibody-based approaches have yet to translate into the clinic. Developing the right targeting antibodies to facilitate crossing of the BBB in humans, and uncovering the molecular mechanism by which the process works, remain significant impediments to clinical application.

3.2 Convection-enhanced delivery

Technology to improve direct drug delivery into the central nervous system (CNS) are currently part of intensive research, and include intraventricular or intraparenchymal injections [e.g. convection-enhanced delivery (CED)]. In particular, CED has shown promising results in both animal models and clinical trials (Huynh et al., 2006; Kawakami et al., 2004; MacKay et al., 2005; Mamot et al., 2004; Ozawa et al., 2002; Saito et al., 2006). CED is a continuous infusion that uses a convective (versus diffusive) flow to drive the therapeutic agent throughout a larger region of tissue. CED uses a slow drug infusion rate by micro infusion pump coupled with a specially designed catheter which is a 1-mm stepped design with a fused silica tubing into 24 gage needle. These optimal CED devices increase drug distribution and reduce reflux (Serwer et al., 2010) (Figure 1,2).

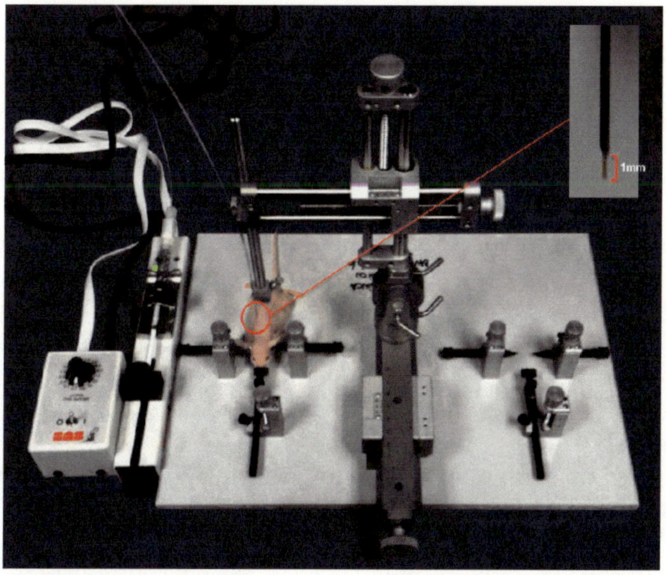

Fig. 1. CED cannula and surgical set-up.

CED is well suited for the delivery of liposomes and particulate drug carriers which have the potential to provide a sustained level of drug and to reach cellular targets with improved specificity (Murad et al., 2006; Saito et al., 2004). CED of liposomal anti-cancer agents have shown greater brain and tumor retention, and effective anti-tumor activity in GBM xenografted animals, as compared to free drugs delivery (Bidros & Vogelbaum, 2009; Noble et al., 2006; Yamashita et al., 2007). Importantly, prolonged exposure to liposomal anti-cancer agents resulted in no measurable CNS toxicity, whereas free drugs induced severe CNS toxicity.

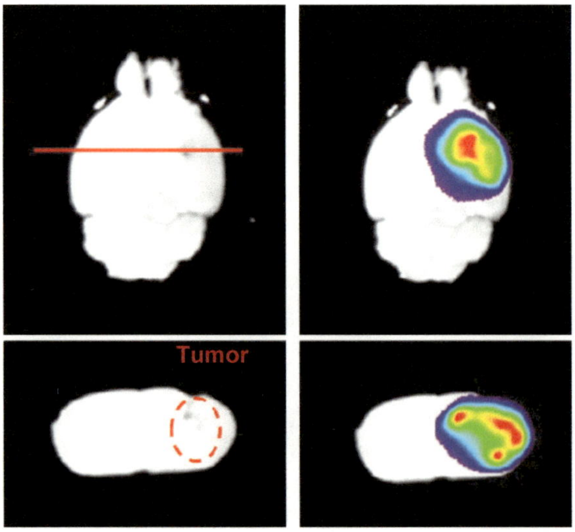

Fig. 2. Representative image of successful CED into the mice brain tumor.

CED has also been used to deliver larger particles, including purified virus and proteins. Currently, CED is being evaluated in 17 clinical trials for the delivery of small molecules, antisense oligonucleotides, and proteins (United States National Institutes of Health, 2011). However, this technique requires the use of potentially risky surgical procedures to position the catheter into the patient's brain parenchyma, and is expensive techniques. Additional limitations of these methods are inadequate CNS distribution due to reflux and leakage along with the needle tracts from the injection site and rapid turnover of the cerebrospinal fluid (CSF). The reflux and leakage through the implanted catheter leads to a measurable and significant inflammation and local edema, because drug solution infuse continuously beyond the tumor boundary into adjacent normal brain tissues (Kawakami et al., 2004; Marmot et al., 2004; Ozawa et al., 2004; Sandberg et al., 2002). Finally, CED infusions can be variable by investigators, in one study the rate of successful infusion was reported as 19% (Sampson et al., 2008).

3.3 Intranasal delivery

One technique under current investigations is to integrate a recent innovation in drug delivery to the brain, intranasal delivery (IND). IND is a practical and noninvasive method of bypassing the BBB and eliminating the surgical risk associated with direct drug administration into the brain parenchyma. It is an alternative to systemic (intravascular) and/or direct invasive (intraparechymal) drug delivery. IND relies upon the unique anatomic connections of the olfactory and trigeminal nerves from the nasal mucosa to the CNS (Dhuria et al., 2010; Thorne et al., 2004). These nerves arise in the brainstem and innervate the nasal mucosa, allowing detection of odors and other sensory stimuli (Dhanda et al., 2006; Thorne et al., 2004). Intranasally administered drugs reach the CNS and/or CSF within minutes of administration by using an extracellular route through perineural and perivascular channels, without binding to any receptor or relying upon axonal transport (Dhuria et al., 2010; Thorne et al., 2004) (Figure 3a). To administer the drugs through the nasal cavity, animals were anesthetized with 2-2.5% isoflurane and placed in an anesthesia chamber. Six μl drops of soluble form of therapeutic agents were administered with a small pipette every 2 min into alternate sides of the nasal cavity for a total of 22 min (a total volume of 66 μl). This method of administration results in consistent deposition in the olfactory epithelium without respiratory distress. Following IND, the animals remained in a supine position for 15 min in order for absorption to occur through the nasal mucosa (Figure 3b).

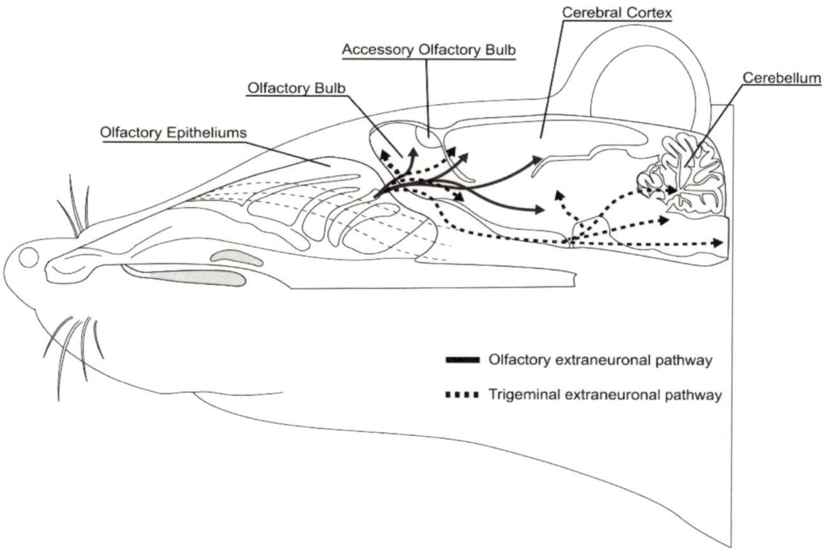

(a) Anatomical pathways of IND

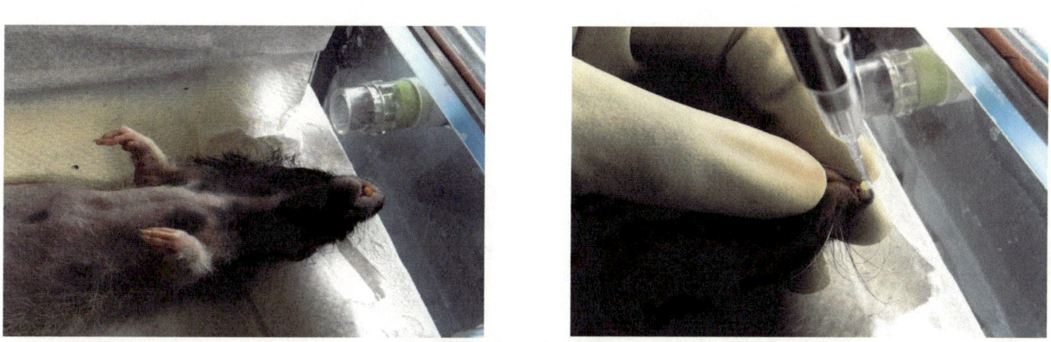

(b) IND in athymic rats

Fig. 3. (a) Anatomic and extraneuronal pathways of the olfactory and trigeminal nerves following IND (b) Demonstration of IND in an anesthetized athymic rat.

In addition to bypassing the BBB, advantages of IND are the avoidance of hepatic first-pass elimination, thereby reducing systemic side effects, and convenient self-administration for patients, a feature that would clearly aid in clinical applications, particularly in the treatment of brain tumors where repeated dosing is necessary (Dhuria et al., 2010).

Many therapeutic agents, including small molecules, growth factors, proteins, peptides, viral vectors, liposomes, nanoparticles and vaccines, have been delivered into the CNS in both animals and humans using IND for a variety of CNS disorders. Thorne *et al* reported that IGF-1 can be rapidly transported into the rat brain and upper spinal cord via the olfactory and trigeminal pathways (Thorne et al., 2004) and, IFNβ-1b can be delivered into the CNS in monkeys (Thorne et al., 2008). Furthermore, rat mesenchymal stem cells and human glioma cells have been delivered to the brain through the nasal pathway (Danielyan et al, 2009). In humans, IND with insulin improves memory in healthy adults (Banks et al., 2004; Benedict et al., 2004) and in patients with early-stage Alzheimer's disease (Reger et al., 2008) without changing the blood levels of glucose or insulin. Also, IND with the neuropeptide oxytocin has been reported to improve trust (Baumgartner et al., 2008; Kosfeld et al, 2005), social behavior (Domes et al., 2007a, 2007b; Guastella et al., 2009), and social memory (Rimmele et al., 2009), and decreased fear and anxiety (Kirsch et al., 2005; Parker et al., 2005).

In brain tumor model, many anti-cancer agents such as methotrexate (Shingaki et al., 1999; Shingaki et al., 2010), 5-fluorouracil (Sakane et al., 1999) and raltitrexed (Wang et al., 2005) have been delivered successfully to the brain using IND. Shingaki *et al* reported that intranasally delivered methotrexate reached the CSF and reduced tumor weight in rodent glioma allografts (Shingaki et al., 1999). Drug targeting of the chemotherapeutic agent raltitrexed to the brain was significantly higher following IND compared with that of intravenous administration (Wang et al., 2005). However, these chemotherapeutic agents do not discriminate between tumor and normal tissues. Thus, the application of drugs at concentrations required to kill tumor cells can also lead to toxicity in normal neural tissues. To achieve therapeutic efficacy without toxicity, the drugs need to preferentially target brain tumors while sparing normal tissue from damage.

3.3.1 Intranasal delivery of a telomerase inhibitor

Given that telomerase is expressed in essentially all cancer cells, but not in normal somatic cells (Kim et al., 1994; Phatak & Burger, 2007), the inhibition of this enzyme is an attractive therapeutic strategy for selectively targeting brain tumors while sparing normal brain tissue. The human telomerase enzyme is a specialized ribonucleoprotein reverse transcriptase containing essential RNA (hTR) and protein (hTERT) subunits. Telomerase elongates telomeres by adding the (TTAGGG)n telomeric repeats to the ends of chromosomes, protecting the chromosome ends from fusion and DNA damage recognition (Feng et al., 1995; Greider & Blackburn, 1985). During cell division in cancer cells, DNA is continuously extended or maintained by telomerase to compensate for the lost telomeric repeats resulting from the 'end-replication' problem of DNA polymerase (Levy et al., 1992; Röth et al., 2003). In the absence of telomerase activity, chromosome ends shorten with each cell division, eventually resulting in growth arrest or cell death, termed replicative senescence or crisis (Allsopp et al., 1992; Shay & Wright, 2006). Although cancer cells express telomerase, these cells typically have relatively short but stable telomere length, whereas normal cells do not express telomerase and have long, slowly shortening telomeres. These differences between cancer and normal cells make cancer cells more sensitive to telomerase inhibitors, and may allow for a substantial therapeutic window for telomerase inhibition-based treatments (Asai et al., 2003).

GRN-163, a telomerase enzyme antagonist, is a 13-mer oligonucleotide N3'→P5' thiophosphoramidate, that exhibits high RNA binding affinity for the targeted template region of hTR in a sequence-specific manner (Gryaznov et al., 2001; Herbert et al., 2002). GRN-163 has demonstrated potent inhibitory activity against human telomerase in several biochemical assays, with IC_{50} values of < 1 nM (Gryaznov et al., 2001; Herbert et al., 2002). *In vitro*, telomerase inhibition by GRN-163 induced cellular senescence and apoptosis in various human cancer cell lines (Ozawa et al., 2004; Asai et al., 2003; Herbert, 2002; Akiyama et al., 2003; Gryaznov et al., 2003; Wang et al., 2004). Although a potential limitation of oligonucleotide therapies is the bioavailability in tumor tissues (Corey, 2002), GRN-163 inhibited tumor growth in prostate cancer, multiple myeloma, lymphoma, hepatoma and glioblastoma xenografts in rodents (Ozawa et al., 2004; Asai et al., 2003; Wang et al., 2004; Hashizume et al., 2008; Djojosubroto et al., 2005). GRN-163 has been delivered successfully into the brain using IND and shown impressive oncolytic activity without harming normal brain tissue (Hashizume et al., 2008). Intranasally delivered GRN-163 exhibited favorable tumor uptake, inhibited tumor growth in human glioblastoma xenografts in rats and increased the survival of tumor-bearing animals. Following the IND of the highest possible dose of GRN-163 (0.65 µmol/µl, based on the solubility of the compound in saline solution), the compound could be detected in the cerebral hemispheres, brainstem and intracranial sections of the trigeminal nerve in naïve rats within 10 min of administration. In tumor-bearing rats, GRN-163 was detected at the edge of the tumor after 30 min, and throughout the tumor between 4 and 24 h after administration (Figure 4).

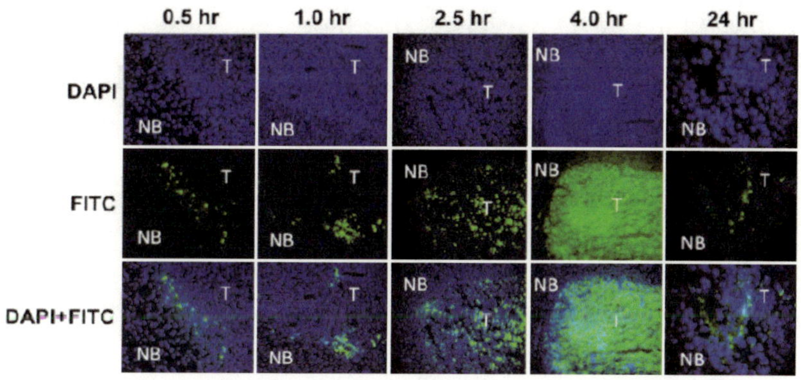

Fig. 4. Distribution of fluorescein-labeled GRN163 by IND into intracerebral tumors in athymic rats. Abbreviations: T, tumor; NB, normal brain.

Importantly, very little or no GRN-163 was found in healthy brain cells adjacent to the tumor or in any other part of the brain. This apparent selectivity may be a result of the specific binding affinity that GRN-163 exhibits for tumor cell telomerase (Herbert et al., 2002). The specificity achieved with IND appears to be superior to the results obtained using CED, which reportedly delivers drugs beyond the tumor boundary into adjacent healthy brain tissue, leading to damage to healthy sections of the brain (Kawakami et al., 2004; Mamot et al., 2004, Ozawa et al., 2004). In addition, intranasally delivered GRN-163 inhibited telomerase activity in intracranial glioblastoma xenografts in rats in a dose-dependent manner (Figure 5).

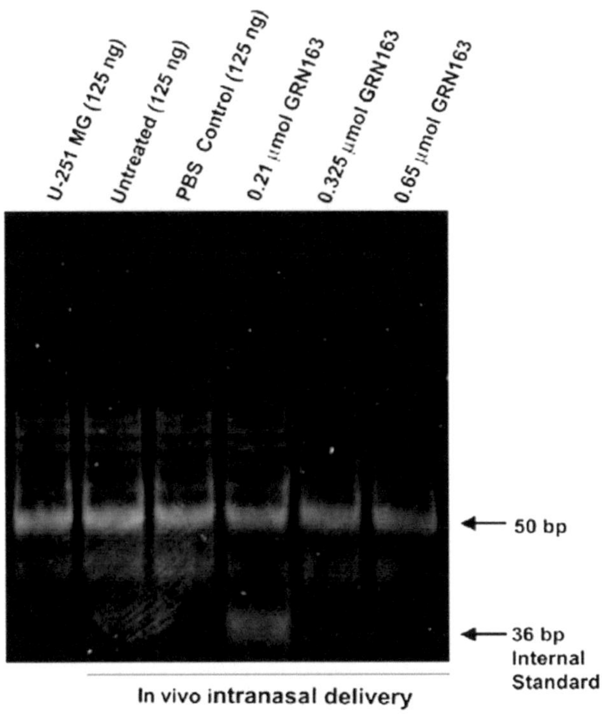

Fig. 5. Inhibition of telomerase activity by GRN163 in intracerebral GBM xenografts.

Moreover, GRN-163 (qd for 12 days) delivered intranasally at the highest solubility dose significantly prolonged the median survival from 35 days in the control group to 75.5 days in the GRN163-treated group. None of the rats that were treated with GRN-163 exhibited signs of toxicity or behavioral abnormalities during the 12-day treatment period (Figure 6).

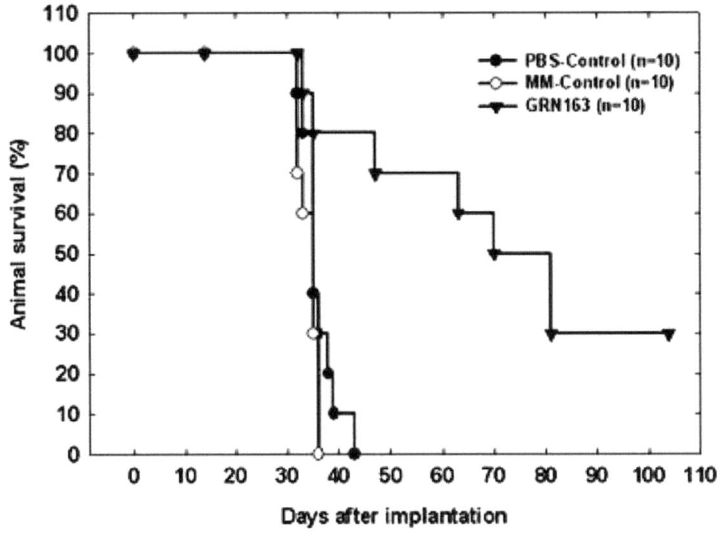

Fig. 6. Survival of rats treated with intranasal GRN163.

Because the mechanism of action of oligonucleotide-based telomerase antagonists such as GRN-163 is through the competitive inhibition of the telomerase enzyme (Gryaznov et al., 2001; Herbert et al., 2002), treated tumor cells can regain baseline telomerase activity following termination of treatment with the telomerase inhibitor. Thus, it is possible that telomerase inhibitor agents will need to be administered for an extended period of time to achieve efficacy. Hypothetically, repeated intranasal treatment is possible, and may be practical as a convenient self-administered treatment.

The lipid-modified N3'→P5' thiophosphoramidate oligonucleotide imetelstat represents the most advanced anti-telomerase therapeutic, and is a more potent derivative of GRN-163 (Herbert et al., 2005). Because of increased lipophilicity, imetelstat exhibits increased bioavailability and cellular uptake in tumors compared with nonlipidated compounds, and it is more acid-resistant than other telomerase-targeted phosphoramidate oligonucleotides (Herbert et al., 2005). Imetelstat also inhibits telomerase activity in various tumor cell lines with IC_{50} values between 3 and 300 nM in the absence of any cellular uptake enhancers (Graznov et al., 2007). In cell-based studies with GRN-163, there was generally a phenotypic lag of at least a few weeks between the onset of exposure and growth inhibition (Akiyama et al., 2003); however, with imetelstat, the addition of a 5' lipid (palmitate) moiety increased potency and resulted in a more rapid loss of telomeres (population doubling [population doubling (PD) ~ 8 for GRN-163L-treated cells and PD ~ 13 for GRN-163-treated cells] and inhibition of cell growth (Herbert et al., 2005). *In vivo* inhibition of tumor growth by imetelstat has been reported in multiple animal models (Djojosubroto et al., 2005; Dikmen et al., 2005; Hochreiter et al., 2006; Marian et al., 2009) and Phase I/II clinical trials with imetelstat have been initiated in patients with chronic lymphocytic leukemia, refractory or relapsed solid tumors, NSCLC, multiple myeloma and breast cancer (Geron Corp., 2009).

3.3.2 Limitations and future prospects of telomerase inhibition by IND as a therapy for GBM

Although the inhibition of telomerase offers exciting therapeutic possibilities for the treatment of GBM patients, there are some potential limitations of this approach, such as the engagement of an alternative telomere-lengthening mechanism that can lead to anti-telomerase treatment (Bollmann et al., 2007). In addition, anti-telomerase therapy may be associated with a delay in efficacy because of the lag period between the initiation of anti-telomerase therapy (telomerase shortening) and the onset of therapeutically beneficial effects (cell death) (Bechter et al., 2004). The combination of IND of telomerase inhibitors with chemotherapy or radiotherapy may produce more rapid effects, and may provide an approach for minimizing the lag phase, potentially preventing or delaying tumor recurrences (Shay & Wright, 2006). The combination of imetelstat with existing chemotherapeutic agents has been demonstrated to enhance chemosensitivity in various human cancer cells (Djojosubroto et al., 2005; Godblatt et al., 2009a, 2009b). More specifically, imetelstat increased doxorubicin sensitivity of Hep3B human hepatoma cells (Djojosubroto et al., 2005), sensitized human breast cancer cells to paclitaxel and trastuzumab (Godblatt et al., 2009a, 2009b), and also enhanced hyperthermia-mediated radiosensitization in human 293 cell lines (Gomez-Millan et al., 2007). Recently, imetelstat in combination with radiation and temozolomide had a statistically significant effect on cell survival and activated the DNA damage response pathway in GBM tumor-initiating cells (Marian et al., 2010).

Further potential limitations of oligonucleotide-based therapies using IND are the low bioavailability and absorption in the nasal mucosa and tumor tissues because of low permeability and solubility (Kausch & Böhle, 2003; Dias & Stein, 2002). The poor absorption of drugs across the nasal membrane is due to low permeability of the nasal membrane, mucociliary clearance, enzymatic degradation, and efflux mechanisms, such as P-glycoprotein and ABC transporters (Dhuria et al., 2010).

3.3.3 Intranasal delivery of liposomal therapeutic agents

Liposomes can be used as biocompatible carriers to improve delivery properties across the nasal mucosa perhaps by increasing residence time of the formulation in the nasal cavity, resulting in higher concentration of encapsulated drugs in the brain. A study of IND with rivastigmine, an acetyl cholinesterase inhibitor, showed that the liposome drug formulation had a longer half-life compared to the free drug due to sustained release of rivastigmine from the liposomes (Arumugam et al., 2008). Migliore *et al* also reported that IND of the liposomal preparation resulted in a higher net delivery and longer retention of ovalbumin in the brain than the nonliposomal preparation (Migliore et al., 2010). Increased tissue retention may be a consequence of the protein's association with cationic lipids, rendering it more likely to undergo cellular binding and adsorptive endocytosis and impeding its diffusion and clearance from the brain (Kumagai et al., 1987). IND with liposomal therapeutic agents is conceptually attractive, and its appeal as a minimally invasive therapeutic strategy would facilitate its translation into clinical trials for the treatment of brain tumor patients.

4. Conclusion

IND of therapeutic agents is an innovative therapeutic strategy capable of targeting drug delivery to the brain for the treatment of brain tumors and could provide an alternative to systemic (intravascular) and/or direct (intraparechymal) drug administrations. IND is a practical and noninvasive method of bypassing the BBB, and is amenable to self-administration by patients. This technique has demonstrated promising results in the treatment of human CNS neurological disorders and rodent brain tumor without obvious toxicity. IND with GRN-163, an oligonucleotide-based telomerase inhibitor, has exhibited impressive oncolytic activity without inducing toxicity to healthy tissue (Hashizume et al., 2008). Data support further development of intranasal GRN-163 as a potential therapy for patients with brain tumors and perhaps as a means for treating multifocal brain tumors, such as metastatic brain tumors and/or pediatric brainstem tumors, which are less amenable to surgical procedures. A telomerase inhibitor, imetelstat, has reached clinical trials, and may therefore become a part of the available cancer therapeutic armamentarium in the future. IND can be further optimized by the use of liposomal drug carriers which provide stable encapsulation for various anticancer agents.

Given the promising results from current animal studies, intranasal therapeutic agents would seem to be prime candidates for clinical trials in patients with brain tumors. Initial trials of intranasal perillyl alcohol have begun in patients with recurrent malignant gliomas, and a reduction in the size of the brain tumors has been reported (Da Fonseca et al., 2006a, 2006b, 2008).

5. References

Abbott, N.J.; Patabendige, A.A.; Dolman, D.E.; Yusof, S.R. & Begley, D.J. (2009). Structure and function of the blood-brain barrier. *Neurobiology of disease*. Vol. 37, No. 1, pp. (13-25).

Aboody, K.S.; Brown, A.; Rainov, N.G.; Bower, K.A.; Liu, S.; Yang, W.; Small, J.E.; Herrlinger, U.; Ourednik, V.; Black, P.M.; Breakefield, X.O. & Snyder, E.Y. (2000). Neural stem cells display extensive tropism for pathology in adult brain: Evidence from intracranial gliomas. *Proceedings of the National Academy of Sciences of the United States of America*. Vol. 97, No. 23, pp. (12846–12851).

Akiyama, M.; Hideshima, T.; Shammas, M.A.; Hayashi, T.; Hamasaki, M.; Tai, Y.T.; Richardson, P.; Gryaznov, S.; Munshi, N.C. & Anderson, K.C. (2003). Effects of oligonucleotide N3'gP5' thio phosphoramidate (GRN163) targeting telomerase RNA in human multiple myeloma cells. *Cancer Research*. Vol. 63, No. 9, pp. (6187-6194).

Allsopp, R.C.; Vaziri, H.; Patterson, C.; Goldstein, S.; Younglai, E.V.; Futcher, A.B.; Greider, C.W. & Harley, C.B. (1992). Telomere length predicts replicative capacity of human fibroblasts. *Proceedings of the National Academy of Sciences of the United States of America*. Vol. 89, No. 21, pp. (10114-10118).

Arumugam, K.; Subramanian, G.S.; Mallayasamy, S.R.; Averineni, R.K.; Reddy, M.S. & Udupa, N. (2008). A study of rivastigmine liposomes for delivery into the brain through intranasal route. *Acta Pharmaceutica*. Vol. 58, No. 3, pp. (287-297).

Asai, A.; Oshima, Y.; Yamamoto, Y.; Uochi, T.A.; Kusaka, H.; Akinaga, S.;Yamashita, Y.; Pongracz, K.; Pruzan, R.; Wunder, E.; Piatyszek, M.; Li, S.; Chin, A.C.; Harley, C.B. & Gryaznov, S.M. (2003). A novel telomerase template antagonist (GRN163) as a potential anticancer agent. *Cancer Research*. Vol. 63, No. 14, pp. (3931-3939).

Banks, W.A.; During, M.J. & Niehoff, M.L. (2004). Brain uptake of the glucagon like peptide-1 antagonist exendin(9-39) after intranasal administration. *The Journal of pharmacology and experimental therapeutics*. Vol. 309, No. 2, pp. (469-475).

Baumgartner, T.; Heinrichs, M.; Vonlanthen, A.; Fischbacher, U. & Fehr, E. (2008). Oxytocin shapes the neural circuitry of trust and trust adaptation in humans. *Neuron*. Vol. 58, No. 4, pp. (639–650).

Bechter, O.E.; Zou, Y.; Walker, W.; Wright, W.E. & Shay, J.W. (2004). Telomeric recombination in mismatch repair deficient human colon cancer cells after telomerase inhibition. *Cancer Research*. Vol. 64, No. 10, pp. (3444-3451).

Benedict, C.; Hallschmid, M.; Hatke, A.; Schultes, B.; Fehm, H.L.; Born, J. & Kern, W. (2004). Intranasal insulin improves memory in humans. *Psychoneuroendocrinology*. Vol. 29, No. 10, pp. (1326-1334).

Bidros, D.S. & Vogelbaum, M.A. (2009). Novel drug delivery strategies in neuro-oncology. *Neurotherapeutics*. Vol. 6, No. 3, pp. (539–546).

Bollmann, F.M. (2007). Targeting ALT: The role of alternative lengthening of telomeres in pathogenesis and prevention of cancer. *Cancer Treatment Reviews*. Vol. 33, No. 8, pp. (704-709).

Boockvar, J.A.; Tsiouris, A.J.; Hofstetter, C.P.; Kovanlikaya, I.; Fralin, S.; Kesavabhotla, K.; Seedial, S.M.; Pannullo, S.C.; Schwartz, T.H.; Stieg, P.; Zimmerman, R.D.; Knopman, J.; Scheff, R.J.; Christos, P.; Vallabhajosula, S. & Riina, H.A. (2010). Safety and maximum tolerated dose of superselective intraarterial cerebral infusion of bevacizumab after osmotic blood-brain barrier disruption for recurrent malignant glioma. *Journal of Neurosurgery*. Vol. 114, No. 3, pp. (624-632).

Brightman, M.W. (1977). Morphology of blood–brain interfaces. *Experimental eye research*. Vol. 25, pp. (1–25).

CBTRUS statistical report tables: Brain Tumor Registry of The United States, Hinsdale, IL, USA, In: *CBTRUS*, (accessed April 12th 2011). *http://www.cbtrus.org/2010-NPCR-SEER/Table23.pdf*

Choi, Y.K. & Kim, K.W. (2008). Blood-neural barrier: its diversity and coordinated cell-to-cell communication. *BMB Reports*. Vol. 41, No. 5, pp. (345-352).

Coomber, B.L.; Stewart, P.A.; Hayakawa, K.; Farrell, C.L. & Del Maestro, R.F. (1985). Quantitative morphology of human glioblastoma multiforme microvessels: structural basis of blood-brain barrier defect. *Journal of Neuro-oncology*. Vol. 5, No. 4, pp. (299–307).

Corey, D.R. (2002). Telomerase inhibition, oligonucleotides, and clinical trials. *Oncogene*. Vol. 21, No. 4, pp. (631-637).

Da Fonseca, C.O.; Landeiro, J.A.; Clark, S.S.; Quirico-Santos, T.; da Costa Carvalho Mda, G. & Gattass, C.R. (2006). Recent advances in the molecular genetics of malignant gliomas disclose targets for antitumor agent perillyl alcohol. *Surgical Neurology*. Vol. 65, pp. (S1:2-S1:9).

Da Fonseca, C.O.; Masini, M.; Futuro, D.; Caetano, R.; Gattass, C.R. & Quirico-Santos, T. (2006). Anaplastic oligodendroglioma responding favorably to intranasal delivery of perillyl alcohol: a case report and literature review. *Surgical Neurology*. Vol. 66, No. 6, pp. (611-615).

Da Fonseca CO, Schwartsmann G, Fischer J, Nagel J, Futuro D, Quirico-Santos T, Gattass CR. (2008). Preliminary results from a phase I/II study of perillyl alcohol intranasal administration in adults with recurrent malignant gliomas. *Surgical Neurology*. Vol. 70, No. 3, pp. (259-267).

Danielyan, L.; Schäfer, R.; von Ameln-Mayerhofer, A.; Buadze, M.; Geisler, J.; Klopfer, T.; Burkhardt, U.; Proksch, B.; Verleysdonk, S.; Ayturan, M.; Buniatian, G.H.; Gleiter, C.H.; Frey, W.H. 2nd. (2009). Intranasal delivery of cells to the brain. *European Journal of Cell Biology*. Vol. 88, No. 6, pp. (315-324).

Dias, N. & Stein, C.A. (2002). Potential roles of antisense oligonucleotides in cancer therapy. The example of Bcl-2 antisense oligonucleotides. *European journal of pharmaceutics and biopharmaceutics*. Vol. 54, No. 3, pp. (263-269).

Deeken, J.F. & Loscher, W. (2007). The blood-brain barrier and cancer: transporters, treatment and Trojan horses. *Clinical Cancer Research*, Vol. 13, No. 6, pp. (1663-1674).

Dhuria, S.V.; Hanson, L.R. & Frey, W.H. 2nd. (2010). Intranasal delivery to the central nervous system: mechanisms and experimental considerations. *Journal of Pharmaceutical Sciences*. Vol. 99, No. 4, pp. (1654-1673).

Dhanda, D.; Frey, W.H. 2nd.; Leopold, D. & Kompella, U.B. (2006). Approaches for drug deposition in the human olfactory epithelium. *Drug Delivery Technology*. Vol. 5, No. 4, pp. (64-72).

Dikmen, Z.G.; Gellert, G.C.; Jackson, S.; Gryaznov, S.; Tressler, R.; Dogan, P.; Wright, W.E. & Shay, J.W. (2005). *In vivo* inhibition of lung cancer by GRN163L: A novel human telomerase inhibitor. *Cancer Research*. Vol. 65, No. 17, pp. (7866-7873).

Djojosubroto, M.W.; Chin, A.C.; Go, N.; Schaetzlein, S.; Manns, M.P.; Gryaznov, S.; Harley, C.B. & Rudolph, K.L. (2005). Telomerase antagonists GRN163 and GRN163L inhibit tumor growth and increase chemosensitivity of human hepatoma. *Hepatology*. Vol. 42, No. 5, pp. (1127-1136).

Domes, G.; Heinrichs, M.; Glascher, J.; Buchel, C.; Braus, D.F. & Herpertz, S.C. (2007). Oxytocin attenuates amygdala responses to emotional faces regardless of valence. *Biological Psychiatry*. Vol. 62 No. 10, pp. (1187–1190).

Domes, G.; Heinrichs, M.; Michel, A.; Berger, C. & Herpertz, S.C. (2007). Oxytocin improves "mind-reading" in humans. *Biological Psychiatry* Vol. 61, No. 6, pp. (731–733).

Ekstrand, A.J.; James, C.D.; Cavenee, W.K.; Seliger, B.; Pettersson, R.F. & Collins, V.P. (1991). *Cancer Research*. Vol. 51, No. 8, pp. (2164-2172).

ElBayoumi, T.A. & Torchilin, V.P. (2009). Tumor-targeted nanomedicines: enhanced antitumor efficacy in vivo of doxorubicin-loaded, long-circulating liposomes modified with cancer-specific monoclonal antibody. *Clinical Cancer Research*. Vol. 15, No. 6, pp. (1973-1980).

Eyal, S, Hsiao, P. & Unadkat, J.D. (2009). Drug interactions at the blood- brain barrier: fact or fantasy? *Pharmacology & Therapeutics*. Vol. 123, No. 1, pp. (80-104).

Frank, R.T.; Edmiston, M.; Kendall, S.E.; Najbauer, J.; Cheung, C.W.; Kassa, T.; Metz, M.Z.; Kim, S.U.; Glackin, C.A.; Wu, A.M.; Yazaki, P.J. & Aboody, K.S. (2009). Neural stem cells as a novel platform for tumor-specific delivery of therapeutic antibodies. *Public Library of Science one*. Vol. 4, No. 12, pp. e8314.

Feng, J.; Funk, W.D.; Wang, S.S.; Weinrich, S.L.; Avilion, A.A.; Chiu, C.P.; Adams, R.R.; Chang, E.; Allsopp, R.C. & Yu, J. (1995). The RNA component of human telomerase. *Science*. Vol. 269, No. 5228, pp. (1236-1241).

Gabizon, A.; Shmeeda, H. & Barenholz, Y. (2003). Pharmacokinetics of pegylated liposomal Doxorubicin: review of animal and human studies. *Clinical pharmacokinetics*. Vol. 42, No. 5, pp. (419-436).

Geron Corp, Menlo Park, CA, USA, (2009). Telomerase inhibitor drug - Imetelstat (GRN163L): *www.geron.com/patients/clinicaltrials/ GRN163L.aspx*

Gerstner, E.R. & Fine, R.L. (2007). Increased permeability of the blood-brain barrier to chemotherapy in metastatic brain tumors: establishing a treatment paradigm. *Journal of Clinical Oncology*. Vol. 25, No. 16, pp. (2306-2312).

Godblatt, E.M.; Erickson, P.A.; Gentry, E.R.; Gryaznov, S.M. & Herbert, B.S. (2009). Lipid-conjugated telomerase template antagonists sensitize resistant HER2-positive breast cancer cells to trastuzumab. *Breast Cancer Research and Treatment*. Vol. 118, No. 1, pp. (21-32).

Goldblatt, E.M.; Gentry, E.R.; Fox, M.J.; Gryaznov, S.M.; Shen, C. & Herbert, B.S. (2009). The telomerase template antagonist GRN163L alters MDA-MB-231 breast cancer cell morphology, inhibits growth, and augments the effects of paclitaxel. *Molecular Cancer Therpeutics*. Vol. 8, No. 7, pp. (2027-2035).

Gomez-Millan, J.; Goldblatt, E.M.; Gryaznov, S.M.; Mendonca, M.S. & Herbert, B.S. (2007). Specific telomere dysfunction induced by GRN163L increases radiation sensitivity in breast cancer cells.*International journal of radiation oncology, biology, physics*. Vol. 67, No. 3, pp. (897-905).

Guastella, A.J.; Mitchell, P.B. & Dadds, M.R. (2008). Oxytocin increases gaze to the eye region of human faces. *Biological Psychiatry*. Vol. 63, No. 1, pp. (3–5).

Graznov, S.M.; Jackson, S.; Dikmen, G.; Harley, C.; Herbert, B.S.; Wright, W.E.; Shay, J.W. (2007). Oligonucleotide conjugate GRN163L targeting human telomerase as potential anticancer and antimetastatic agent. *Nucleosides Nucleotides and Nucleic Acids*. Vol. 26, No. 10-12, pp. (1577-1579).

Greenwood, J. (1992). Experimental manipulation of the blood–brain and blood–retinal barriers. In *Physiology and Pharmacology of the Blood–Brain Barrier. Handbook of Experimental Pharmacology*, Bradbury, M.W.B. and Abbott, N.J., pp. 459–486, Springer-Verlag, Berlin, Germany

Gryaznov, S.M.; Pongracz, K.; Matray, T.; Schultz, R.; Pruzan, R.; Aimi, J.; Chin, A.; Harley, C.; Shea-Herbert, B.; Shay, J.; Oshima, Y.; Asai, A. & Yamashita, Y. (2001). Telomerase inhibitors - Oligonucleotide phosphoramidates as potential therapeutic agents. *Nucleosides Nucleotides and Nucleic Acids*. Vol. 20, No. 4-7, pp. (401-410).

Greider, C.W. & Blackburn, E.H. (1985). Identification of a specific telomere terminal transferase activity in *Tetrahymena* extracts. *Cell*. Vol. 43, No. 2, Pt 1, pp. (405-413).

Hashizume, R.; Ozawa, T.; Gryaznov, S.M.; Bollen, A.W.; Lamborn. K.R.; Frey, W.H. 2nd & Deen, D.F. (2008). New therapeutic approach for brain tumors: Intranasal delivery of telomerase inhibitor GRN163. *Neuro-Oncology*. Vol. 10, No. 2, pp. (112-1120).

Herbert, B.S.; Gellert, G.C.; Hochreiter, A.; Pongracz, K.; Wright, W.E.; Zielinska, D.; Chin, A.C.; Harley, C.B.; Shay, J.W. & Gryaznov, S.M. (2005). Lipid modification of GRN163, an N3'gP5' thio- phosphoramidate oligonucleotide, enhances the potency of telomerase inhibition. *Oncogene*. Vol. 24, No. 33, pp. (5262-5268).

Herbert, B.S.; Pongracz, K.; Shay, J.W. & Gryaznov, S.M. (2002). Oligonucleotide N3'gP5' phosphoramidates as efficient telomerase inhibitors. *Oncogene*. Vol. 21, No. 4, pp. (638-642).

Hochreiter, A.E.; Xiao, H.; Goldblatt, E.M.; Gryaznov, S.M.; Miller, K.D.; Badve, S.; Sledge, G.W. & Herbert, B.S. (2006). Telomerase template antagonist GRN163L disrupts telomere maintenance, tumor growth, and metastasis of breast cancer. *Clinical Cancer Research*. Vol. 12, No. 10, pp. (3184-3192).

Huynh, G.H.; Deen, D.F. & Szoka, F.C. Jr. (2006). Barriers to carrier mediated drug and gene delivery to brain tumors. *Journal of Control Release*. Vol. 110, No. 2, pp. (236-259).

Kausch, I. & Böhle, A. (2003). Antisense oligonucleotide therapy for urologic tumors. *Current Urology Reports*. Vol. 4, No. 1, pp. (60-69).

Kawakami, K.; Kawakami, M.; Kioi, M.; Husain, S.R. & Puri, R.K. (2004). Distribution kinetics of targeted cytotoxin in glioma by bolus or convection-enhanced delivery in a murine model.*Journal of Neurosurgery*. Vol. 101, No. 6, pp. (1004-1011).

Kim, N.W.; Piatyszek, M.A.; Prowse, K.R.; Harley, C.B.; West, M.D.; Ho, P.L.; Coviello, G.M.; Wright, W.E.; Weinrich, S.L. & Shay,J.W. (1994). Specific association of human telomerase activity with immortal cells and cancer. *Science*. Vol. 266, No. 5193, pp. (2011-2015).

Kirsch, P.; Esslinger, C.; Chen, Q.; Mier, D.; Lis, S.; Siddhanti, S.; Gruppe, H.; Mattay, V.S.; Gallhofer, B. & Meyer-Lindenberg, A. (2005). Oxytocin modulates neural circuitry for social cognition and fear in humans. *The Journal of Neuroscience*. Vol. 25, No. 49, pp. (11489–11493).

Kosfeld, M.; Heinrichs, M.; Zak, P.J.; Fischbacher, U. & Fehr, E. (2005). Oxytocin increases trust in humans. *Nature*. Vol. 435, No. 7042, pp. (673-676).

Kumagai, A.K.; Eisenberg, J.B. & Pardridge, W.M. (1987). Absorptive-mediated endocytosis of cationized albumin and a b- endorphin-cationized albumin chimeric peptide by isolated brain capillaries. Model system of blood-brain barrier transport. *The Journal of Biological Chemistry*. Vol. 262, No. 31, pp. (15214–15219).

Levy, M.Z.; Allsopp, R.C.; Futcher, A.B.; Greider, C.W. & Harley, C.B. (1992). Telomere end-replication problem and cell aging. *Journal of Molecular Biology*. Vol. 225, No. 4, pp. (951-960).

MacKay, J.A.; Deen, D.F. & Szoka, F.C. Jr. (2005). Distribution in brain of liposomes after convection enhanced delivery; modulation by particle charge, particle diameter, and presence of steric coating. *Brain Research*. Vol. 1035, No. 2, pp. (139-153).

Mamot, C.; Drummond, D.C.; Noble, C.O.; Kallab, V.; Guo, Z.; Hong, K., Kirpotin, D.B. & Park, J.W. (2005). Epidermal growth factor receptor-targeted immunoliposomes significantly enhance the efficacy of multiple anticancer drugs in vivo. *Cancer Research*. Vol. 65, No. 24, pp. (11631-11638).

Mamot, C.; Nguyen, J.B.; Pourdehnad, M.; Hadaczek, P.; Saito, R.; Bringas, J.R.; Drummond, D.C.; Hong, K.; Kirpotin, D.B.; McKnight, T.; Berger, M.S.; Park, J.W. & Bankiewicz, K.S. (2004). Extensive distribution of liposomes in rodent brains and brain tumors following convection-enhanced delivery. *Journal of Neuro- Oncology*. Vol. 68, No. 1, pp. (1-9).

Marian, C.O.& Shay, J.W. (2009). Prostate tumor-initiating cells: A new target for telomerase inhibition therapy? *Biochimica et biophysica acta*. Vol. 1792, No. 4, pp. (289-296).

Marian, C.O.; Cho, S.K.; McEllin, B.M.; Maher, E.A.; Hatanpaa, K.J.; Madden, C.J.; Mickey, B.E.; Wright, W.E.; Shay, J.W.; Bachoo, R.M. (2010). The telomerase antagonist, imetelstat, efficiently targets glioblastoma tumor-initiating cells leading to decreased proliferation and tumor growth. *Clinical Cancer Research*. Vol. 16, No. 1, pp. (154-163).

Migliore, M.M.; Vyas, T.K.; Campbell, R.B.; Amiji, M.M. & Waszczak, B.L. (2010). Brain delivery of proteins by the intranasal route of administration: a comparison of cationic liposomes versus aqueous solution formulations. *Journal of Pharmaceutical Sciences*. Vol. 99, No. 4, pp. (1745-1761).

Moreau P. (2009). Combination regimens using doxorubicin and pegylated liposomal doxorubicin prior to autologous transplantation in multiple myeloma. *Expert review of anticancer therapy*. Vol. 9, No. 7, pp. (885-890).

Murad GJ, Walbridge S, Morrison PF, Garmestani K, Degen JW, Brechbiel MW, Oldfield EH, Lonser RR. (2006). Real-time, image-guided, convection-enhanced delivery of interleukin 13 bound to pseudomonas exotoxin. *Clinical Cancer Research*. Vol. 12, No. 10, pp. (3145-3151).

Murramatsu, K.; Maitani, Y.; Takayama, K. & Nagai, T. (1999). The relationship between the rigidity of the liposomal membrane and

the absorption of insulin after nasal administration of liposomes modified with an enhancer containing insulin in rabbits. *Drug development and industrial pharmacy*. Vol. 25, No. 10, pp. (1099-1105).

Noble, C.O.; Krauze, M.T.; Drummond, D.C.; Yamashita, Y.; Saito, R.; Berger, M.S.; Kirpotin, D.B.; Bankiewicz, K.S. & Park, J.W. (2006). Novel Nanoliposomal CPT-11 Infused by Convection-Enhanced Delivery in Intracranial Tumors: Pharmacology and Efficacy. *Cancer Research*. Vol. 66, No. 5, pp. (2801-2806).

Ozawa, T.; Wang, J.; Hu, L.J.; Bollen, A.W.; Lamborn, K.R. & Deen, D.F. (2002). Growth of human glioblastomas as xenografts in the brains of athymic rats. *In Vivo*. Vol. 16, No. 1, pp. (55-60).

Ozawa, T.; Gryaznov, S.M.; Hu, L.J.; Pongracz, K.; Santos, R.A.; Bollen, A.W.; Lamborn, K.R. & Deen, D.F. (2004). Antitumor effects of specific telomerase inhibitor GRN163 in human glioblastoma xenografts. *Neuro-Oncology*. Vol. 6, No 3, pp. (218-226).

Parker, K.J.; Buckmaster, C.L.; Schatzberg, A.F. & Lyons, D.M. (2005). Intranasal oxytocin administration attenuates the ACTH stress response in monkeys. *Psychoneuroendocrinology*. Vol. 30, No. 9, pp. (924-929).

Pardridge, W.M. (1999). Non-invasive drug delivery to the human brain using endogenous blood-brain barrier transport systems. *Pharmaceutical science & technology today*. Vol. 2, No. 2, pp. (49–59).

Pardridge, W.M. (2007). Blood-brain barrier delivery. *Drug Discovery Today*. Vol. 12, No 1–2, pp. (54–61).

Phatak, P. & Burger, A.M. (2007). Telomerase and its potential for therapeutic intervention. *British Journal of Pharmacology*. Vol. 152, No. 7, pp. (1003-1011).

Rapoport, S.I. (1996). Modulation of blood–brain barrier permeability.*Journal of Drug Targeting*. Vol. 3, No. 6, pp. (417–425).

Reger, M.A.; Watson, G.S.; Green, P.S.; Wilkinson, C.W.; Baker, L.D.; Cholerton, B.; Fishel, M.A.; Plymate, S.R.; Breitner, J.C.; DeGroodt, W.; Mehta, P. & Craft, S. (2008). Intranasal insulin improves cognition and modulates beta-amyloid in early AD. *Neurology*. Vol. 70, No. 6, pp. (440-448).

Rimmele U, Hediger K, Heinrichs M, Klaver P: Oxytocin makes a face in memory familiar. *Jouranl of Neuroscience* (2009). 29 (1): 38–42.

Röth, A.; Vercauteren, S.; Sutherland, H.J. & Lansdorp, P.M. (2003). Telomerase is limiting the growth of acute myeloid leukemia cells. *Leukemia*. Vol. 17, No. 12, pp. (2410-2417).

Rousselle, C.; Clair, P.; Lefauconnier, J.M.; Kaczorek, M.; Scherrmann, J.M. & Temsamani, J. (2000). New advances in the transport of doxorubicin through the blood–brain barrier by a peptide vector- mediated strategy. *Molecular Pharmacology*. Vol. 57, No. 4, pp. (679–686).

Sakane, T.; Yamashita, S.; Yata, N. & Sezaki, H. (1999). Transnasal delivery of 5-fluorouracil to the brain in the rat. *Journal of Drug Targeting*. Vol. 7, No. 3, pp. (233-240).

Saito, R.; Bringas, J.R.; Panner, A.; Tamas, M.; Pieper, R.O.; Berger, M.S. & Bankiewicz, K.S. (2004). Convection-enhanced delivery of tumor necrosis factor-related apoptosis-inducing ligand with systemic administration of temozolomide prolongs survival in an intracranial glioblastoma xenograft model. *Cancer Research*. Vol. 64, No. 19, pp. (6858-6862).

Saito, R.; Krauze, M.T.; Noble, C.O.; Tamas, M.; Drummond, D.C.; Kirpotin, D.B.; Berger, M.S.; Park, J.W. & Bankiewicz, K.S. (2006). Tissue affinity of the infusate affects the distribution volume during convection-enhanced delivery into rodent brains: Implications for local drug delivery. *Journal of neuroscience methods*. Vol. 154, No. 1-2, pp. (225-232).

Sampson, J.H.; Akabani, G.; Archer, G.E.; Berger, M.S.; Coleman, R.E.; Friedman, A.H.; Friedman, H.S.; Greer, K.; Herndon, J.E. 2nd; Kunwar, S.; McLendon, R.E.; Paolino, A.; Petry, N.A.; Provenzale, J.M.; Reardon, D.A.; Wong, T.Z.; Zalutsky, M.R.;

Pastan, I. & Bigner, D.D. (2008). Intracerebral infusion of an EGFR-targeted toxin in recurrent malignant brain tumors. *Neuro-Oncology*. Vol. 10, No. 3, pp. (320-329).
Sandberg, D.I.; Edgar, M.A. & Souweidane, M.M. (2002). Convection-enhanced delivery into the rat brainstem. *Journal of Neurosurgery*. Vol. 96, No. 5, pp. (885-891).
Saunders, N.R.; Ek, C.J.; Habgood, M.D. & Dziegielewska, K.M. (2008). Barriers in the brain: a renaissance? *Trends in Neurosciences*. Vol. 31, No. 6, pp. (279-286).
Schlosshauer, B. (1993). The blood–brain barrier: morphology, molecules, and neurothelin. *Bioassays*. Vol. 1, pp. (341–346).
Serwer, L.; Hashizume, R.; Ozawa, T. and James, C.D. (2010). Systemic and local drug delivery for treating diseases of the central nervous system in rodent models. *Journal of visualized experiments*. Vol. 42, pii: 1992. doi: 10.3791/1992.
Shay, J.W. & Wright, W.E. (2006). Telomerase therapeutics for cancer: Challenges and new directions. *Nature Reviews Drug Discovery*. Vol. 5, No. 7, pp. (577-584).
Shingaki, T.; Sakane, T.; Yamashita, S.; Sezaki, H.; Yoshiharu, T.; Shoubu, S. (1999). Transnasal delivery of anticancer drugs to the brain tumor: A new strategy for brain tumor chemotherapy. *Drug Delivery System*. Vol. 14, No. 5, pp. (365-371).
Shingaki, T.; Inoue, D.; Furubayashi, T.; Sakane, T.; Katsumi, H.; Yamamoto, A. & Yamashita, S. (2010). Transnasal Delivery of Methotrexate to Brain Tumors in Rats: A New Strategy for Brain Tumor Chemotherapy. *Molecular Pharmaceutics*. Vol. 7, No. 5, pp. (1561–1568).
Tamai, I. & Tsuji, A. (1996). Drug delivery through the blood–brain barrier. *Advanced drug delivery reviews*. Vol. 19, pp. (401–424).
Tai, C. & Kasahara, N. (2008). Replication-competent retrovirus vectors for cancer gene therapy. *Frontiers in Bioscience*. Vol. 13, pp. (3083-3095).
Tanguay, J.S.; Ansari, J.; Buckley, L. & Fernando, I. (2009). Epithelial ovarian cancer: role of pegylated liposomal Doxorubicin in prolonging the platinum-free interval and cancer antigen 125 trends during treatment. *International journal of gynecological cancer*, Vol. 19, No. 3, pp. (361-366).
Thorne, R.G.; Pronk, G.J.; Padmanabhan, V. & Frey, W.H. 2nd. (2004). Delivery of insulin-like growth factor-I to the rat brain and spinal cord along olfactory and trigeminal pathways following intranasal administration. *Neuroscience*. Vol. 127, No. 2, pp. (481-496).
Thorne, R.G., Hanson, L.R.; Ross, T.M.; Tung, D. & Frey, W.H. 2nd. (2008). Delivery of interferon-beta to the monkey nervous system following intranasal administration. *Neuroscience*. Vol. 152, No. 3, pp. (785-797).
United States National Institutes of Health, In: *Clnicaltrial.gov*, (accessed April 12th 2011), http://clinicaltrials.gov/ct2/results?term=Convection-enhanced+delivery
Wang, D.; Gao, Y. & Yun, L. (2005). Study on brain targeting of raltitrexed following intranasal administration in rats. *Cancer Chemotherpy and Pharmacology*. Vol. 57, No. 1, pp. (1-8).
Wang, E.S.; Wu, K.; Chin, A.C.; Chen-Kiang, S.; Pongracz, K.; Gryaznov, S.; & Moore, M.A. (2004). Telomerase inhibition with an oligonucleotide telomerase template antagonist: *In vitro* and *in vivo* studies in multiple myeloma and lymphoma. *Blood*. Vol. 103, No. 1. pp. (258-266).
Yamashita, Y.; Krauze, M.T.; Kawaguchi, T.; Noble, C.O.; Drummond, D.C.; Park, J.W. & Bankiewicz, K.S. (2007). Convection-enhanced delivery of a topoisomerase I

inhibitor (nanoliposomal topotecan) and a topoisomerase II inhibitor (pegylated liposomal doxorubicin) in intracranial brain tumor xenografts. *Neuro-Oncology*. Vol. 9, No. 1, pp. (20–28).

Yong, R.L.; Shinojima, N.; Fueyo, J.; Gumin, J.; Vecil, G.G.; Marini, F.C.; Bogler, O.; Andreeff, M. & Lang, F.F. (2009). Human bone marrow-derived mesenchymal stem cells for intravascular delivery of oncolytic adenovirus Delta24-RGD to human gliomas. *Cancer Research*. Vol. 69, No. 23, pp. (8932–8940).

Zhang, Y.; Zhang, Y.F.; Bryant, J.; Charles, A.; Boado, R.J. & Pardridge, W.M. (2004). Intravenous RNA interference gene therapy targeting the human epidermal growth factor receptor prolongs survival in intracranial brain cancer. *Clinical Cancer Research*. Vol. 10, No. 11, pp. (3667–3677).

12

Transcription Factor Targets as Treatment for Medulloblastoma

Mehdi H. Shahi and Elva Díaz
Department of Pharmacology, UC Davis School of Medicine, Davis, CA U.S.A.

1. Introduction

Pediatric brain tumors are more complex disorders than other cancers due to gaps in our understanding of their cellular origins, insufficient drug therapy, and complications arising from the blood brain barrier. Nevertheless, in the last decade, there has been significant improvement in the treatment of these tumors although the survival rate is still low. Thus, new innovative approaches to treat these malignant tumors are warranted. Among pediatric brain tumors, medulloblastoma is the most common and contributes significantly to the high mortality rate among children throughout the world. Defects in Sonic Hedgehog (Shh) signal transduction are major contributors to brain tumor development, especially medulloblastoma. In this book chapter, we review recent publications that identified new Shh downstream target genes that are implicated in medulloblastoma development. The products of these genes represent novel therapeutic targets that might lead to innovative approaches to treat brain tumors.

2. Medulloblastoma biogenesis

Medulloblastoma is a member of the family of cranial primitive neuroectodermal tumors (PTEN) (Wechsler-Reya and Scott, 2001). Medulloblastoma cells are small, round, undifferentiated cells that are often located near the cerebellum. Their morphological properties and physical location are most consistent with cerebellar granule neuron precursor (GNPs), and thus, medulloblastomas are believed to originate from transformed GNPs that have failed to differentiate and continue to proliferate (Wechsler-Reya and Scott, 2001). For example, mutations in the Shh signaling pathway lead to persistent GNP proliferation and a failure to differentiate and ultimately medulloblastoma development (Wechsler-Reya and Scott, 2001). However, tumor biogenesis is a complex process that involves many genes and signaling pathways and recent studies indicate that subtypes of medulloblastoma have distinct molecular and cellular origins. For instance, mutations in the Wnt pathway lead to a discrete subtype of medulloblastoma that arise outside of the cerebellum (Gibson et al., 2010). Therefore, it is very difficult to treat tumors with one drug or pathway inhibitor. Furthermore, Shh signal transduction is important for a wide variety of cellular processes during normal development; therefore, drugs that interfere with Shh signal transduction might lead to neurodevelopmental defects. In addition, Shh downstream target genes are cross-regulated by multiple, independent pathways including Notch and

Wnt pathways. Thus, developing novel therapeutics to downstream target genes allows the ability to inhibit selectively multiple signal transduction pathways, to provide added efficacy in disease treatment, and to ameliorate possible deleterious side effects associated with inhibition of Shh signal transduction in normal development.

2.1 Sonic hedgehog signal transduction pathway

Binding of Shh to the Patched (Ptch1) receptor relieves the inhibition of another transmembrane receptor Smoothened (Smo) (Ingham and McMahon, 2001) (Figure 1). Upon Smo activation, members of the Gli family of transcription factors translocate to the nucleus and bind to the promoter of many target genes such as Ptch1, D Cyclins, and Nmyc (Browd et al., 2006; Yoon et al., 2002). In the cerebellum, Shh is produced by Purkinje neurons to promote proliferation of GNPs during the first week of postnatal development (Wechsler-Reya and Scott, 1999). Shh signalling regulates proliferation of GNPs in part via expression of Nmyc (Kenney et al., 2003; Knoepfler et al., 2002; Oliver et al., 2003). Mutations in the Shh signal transduction pathway are thought to underlie the etiology of medulloblastoma that arise from transformed GNPs that fail to cease proliferation during development (Wechsler-Reya and Scott, 2001). For example, mice with a heterozygous deletion of the Shh negative regulator Ptch1 develop tumors that resemble human medulloblastomas (Goodrich et al., 1997). The focus of this book chapter is the discovery of new Shh downstream target genes that are implicated in medulloblastoma development.

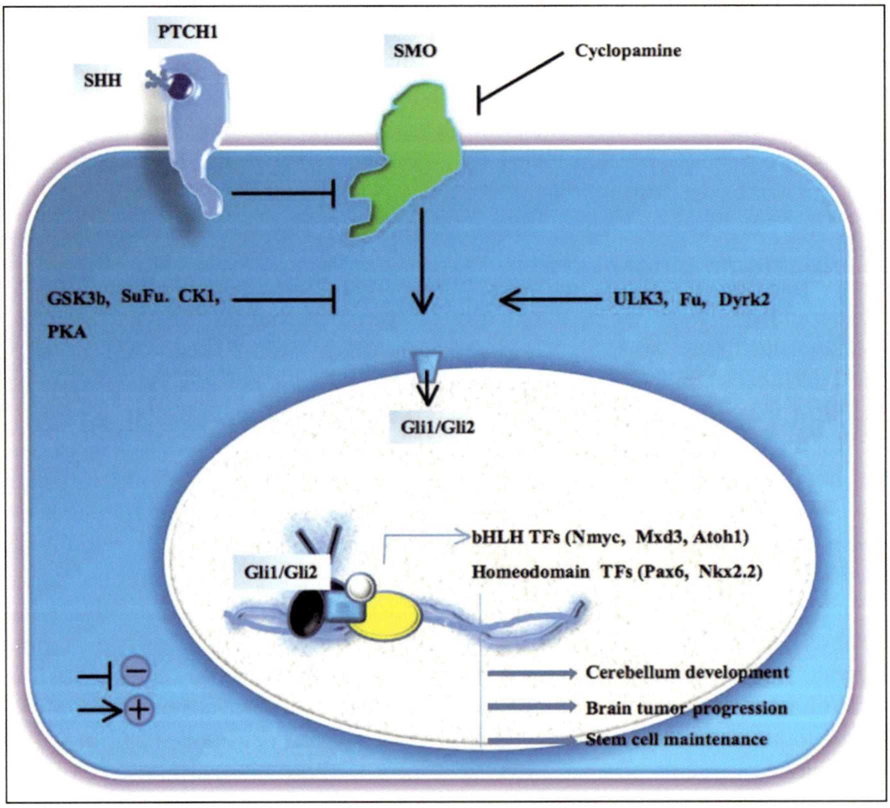

Fig. 1. The Sonic Hedgehog Signal Transduction Pathway

2.2 Cancer stem cell hypothesis

Current research suggests that a small subset of cells within the tumor mass with the capability of tumor regeneration persist even after aggressive therapies including surgery, radiation, and chemotherapy. These cells behave like stem cells and are hypothesized to be tumor stem cells (TSCs) with renewal capacity (Singh et al., 2004). Therefore, the current outlook supports the need for new approaches to target these TSCs for complete tumor eradication or at least to overcome tumor recurrence and increase the survival of the patient. A complete understanding of the biology of TSCs and the genes and pathways involved is vital towards the development of novel therapeutics to treat brain tumors. It has been reported that Oct-4, BMP (bone morphogenic protein), Janus family kinase, Notch, Shh and Wnt signaling regulate stem cell renewal (Taipale and Beachy, 2001). Among these pathways, Shh is thought to be the major contributor to brain tumor development, especially medulloblastoma, and Shh shows crosstalk with multiple stem cell renewal pathways including Wnt and Notch (Sengupta et al., 2007) (Figure 2), suggesting that mutations in the Shh pathway might lead to the development of TSCs and ultimately tumorigenesis. Indeed, a recent report has shown that a subset of medulloblastoma cells derived from Ptch1 heterozygous mice are cancer stem cells, which are capable of initiating and propagating tumors (Ward et al., 2009). However, the exact mechanism of how TSCs are regulated by Shh signaling is not well explored. This book chapter will review mechanisms of newly identified Shh downstream target genes in stem cell biology to provide insight into the role in medulloblastoma biogenesis.

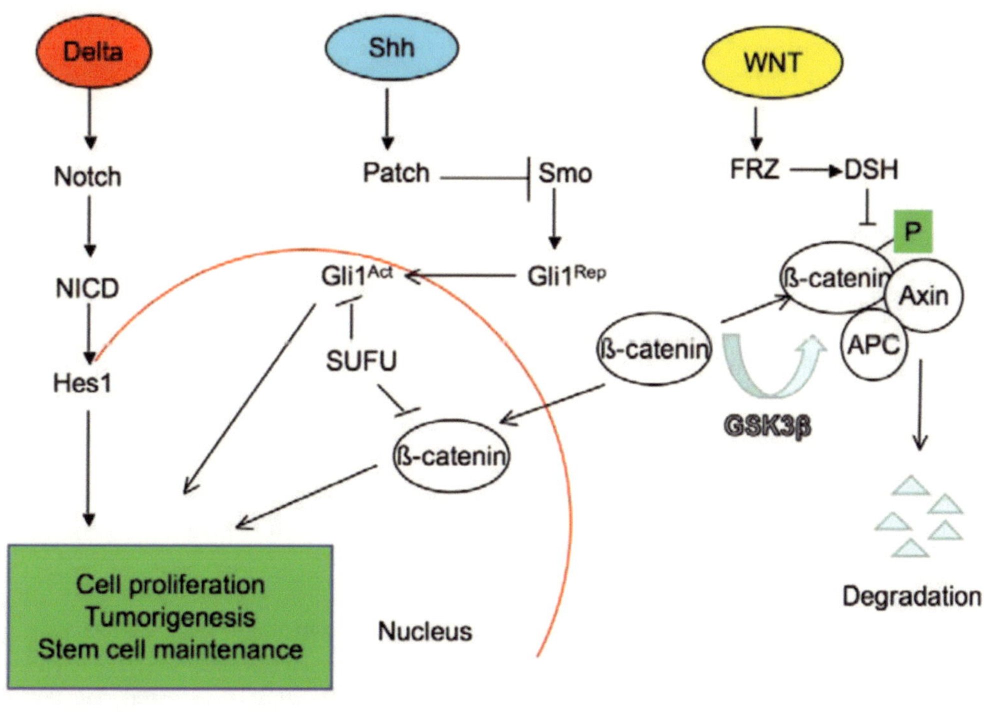

Fig. 2. Crosstalk between Sonic Hedgehog, Wnt, and Notch signal transduction pathways

3. Transcription factors implicated in Sonic Hedgehog Signal Transduction in Neural Tube

Pax6 and Nkx2.2 are homeobox transcription factors and their involvement within the Shh signaling pathway is well defined in the development of the neural tube (Briscoe et al., 2000); however, their role has only recently been explored in brain tumor development. Interestingly, both Pax6 and Nkx2.2 are targets of the major Shh downstream transcription factor Gli1 in medulloblastoma cell lines and tissues (Shahi et al., 2010). Moreover, both genes have been implicated in stem cell maintenance (Hu et al., 2009; Zhang et al., 2010); therefore, it would be fruitful to understand these genes in the context of Shh signaling in TSC-mediated medulloblastoma biogenesis.

3.1 Nkx2.2

Nkx2.2 (also known as NKX2B and NKX2-2) is a member of the homeobox transcription factor family NK-2 originally identified in Drosophila (Kim and Nirenberg, 1989). The Nk-2 homeodomain transcription factor family has four members: Nkx2.1, Nkx2.1, Nkx2.3 and Nkx2.5. These transcription factors show specific binding to the consensus sequence T(C/T)AAGTG (Chen and Schwartz, 1995; Tsao et al., 1994), a unique feature compared with other homeodomain proteins. The Nk-2 transcription factor family is defined by three domains which are conserved in all members: a) Homeodomain: 60 amino acid, helix-turn-helix motif, binds to DNA; b) Transcriptional repressor-domain (TN-domain): located at the N-terminal region of the protein; and c) Nk-2 specific domain (Nk2-SD): located at the C-terminal region of the protein (Lints et al., 1993). Nkx2.2 is a nuclear transcription factor and transport into the nucleus is mediated by nuclear localization signals (NLS) of which Nkx2.2 has two located within the homeodomain (Hessabi et al., 2000).

3.1.1 Role of Nkx2.2 in nervous system development

The role of Nkx2.2 during patterning of the ventral neural tube is well defined. Nkx2.2 is expressed in a gradient induced by Shh signaling to facilitate the subdivision of the ventral neural tube into five progenitor domains: p0, p1, p2, pMN (motor neuron) and p3 (Briscoe et al., 2000). It has been shown that the Gli transcriptional activator binds to the enhancer region of Nkx2.2 in differentiating neural progenitors (Vokes et al., 2007). Interestingly, another homeodomain transcription factor, Pax6 (discussed below), is modulated by Shh signaling to define ventral neural tube progenitor cell fate and it is repressed by Nkx2.2 at the boundary of pMN and p3 (Briscoe et al., 2000). After the establishment of ventral neural progenitor cell fate, expression of both homeodomain transcription factors Pax6 and Nkx2.2 is maintained to promote the transition of neural progenitors to specific types of postmitotic neurons: vo, v1, v2, MN and v3 (Briscoe et al., 2000). However, this stage of development is independent of the Shh target transcription factors Gli1 and Gli2, suggesting that later stages of Shh signaling act through other transcription factors (Ding et al., 1998).

3.1.2 Role of Nkx2.2 in brain cancer

Nkx2.2 transcription factor expression was surveyed in astrocytic and oligodendroglial tumors of low to high grade (Riemenschneider et al., 2004). In general, Nkx2.2 expression was high in the low grade tumors (class II and III - anaplastic astrocytoma) compared to high grade glioblastoma multiforme (class IV-GBM) (Riemenschneider et al., 2004). Nkx2.2 is also expressed in medulloblastoma cell lines and primary tumor samples and Nkx2.2

expression is dependent on Shh-Gli1 pathway (Shahi et al., 2010). Upon knockdown of Gli1 in medulloblastoma cell line with short interfering RNAs (siRNA), Nkx2.2 expression was reduced compared to control negative siRNA treated cells (Shahi et al., 2010), suggesting that Gli1 positively regulates Nkx2.2 expression. The expression pattern of Nkx2.2 in astrocytoma samples was found to be present in most of the astrocytoma cell lines while expression in tumor samples was low or absent except for some low grade (class III) astrocytoma tumor samples (Shahi et al., 2010). This high expression of Nkx2.2 in some of the low grade astrocytoma tumor samples is consistent with previous results of Riemenschneider and colleagues. In contrast, knockdown of Gli1 in the high grade astrocytoma cell line U87MG showed no change in expression pattern compared to control cells (Shahi et al., 2010), suggesting that other signaling pathways or transcription factors regulate expression of Nkx2.2 in astrocytoma. The expression of Nkx2.2 was low in the majority of neuroblastoma cell lines analyzed (72%) compared to normal control cells (Shahi et al., 2011).

3.1.3 Role of Nkx2.2 in stem cells

The origin and progression of brain tumors is a complex process that is not very well understood. However, recent advances in tumor biology research suggest that the tumor mass originates from a small number of atypical stem cells called TSCs. TSC renewal is regulated by many pathways including BMP, Notch, Shh and Wnt (Ponnusamy and Batra, 2008; Taipale and Beachy, 2001). A recent study indicated that high expression of Nkx2.2 inhibits the self-renewal characteristics of glioma TSCs that underlies the high grade tumor GBM and switches cell fate towards oligodendroglial differentiation (Muraguchi et al., 2011). This study is also supported by previous work in which human embryonic stem cells (hESCs) were induced by Shh signaling to express Nkx2.2 to form pre-oligodendrocyte precursor cells (Hu et al., 2009). These results support a negative role of Nkx2.2 in TSC proliferation and suggest that promoting the inhibitory role of Nkx2.2 is a possible therapeutic target strategy to cause TSCs to switch their fate from a proliferative nature to a differentiated state.

Interestingly, Nkx2.2 is positively regulated by the graded expression of Shh in neural tube development (Briscoe et al., 2000). However, its expression pattern in medulloblastoma, astrocytoma and neuroblastoma cell lines and primary tumor samples indicates that it may be down-regulated at least partially by Shh signaling, although other signaling pathways and transcription factors might also play a role (Shahi et al., 2010; Shahi et al., 2011). Regardless, its high expression in low grade astrocytic tumors compared to high grade tumors suggest that it would be a good marker for the prognosis of patients to define their astrocytic tumor grade (Riemenschneider et al., 2004).

3.2 Pax6

Pax6 (paired box gene 6) is a homeodomain transcription factor of which there are 9 members in this family (Pax1-9). Pax6 is highly conserved in vertebrates and is the most studied among the Pax family members for its vital role in neuronal fate determination (Mansouri et al., 1996). The vertebrate Pax6 gene encodes three isoforms: canonical Pax6, Pax6(5a) and Pax6(ΔPD). The canonical Pax6 has a paired domain (PD) at the N-terminus connected via a linker region to the paired type homeodomain (HD). The C-terminus contains a proline/serine/theronine (P/S/T) domain. Both PD and HD domains bind to

DNA whereas the P/S/T domain has transactivation activity. Isoform Pax6 (5a) is formed with the insertion of 14 residues in the PD, which affects its DNA binding activity. The linker region encodes three alternative translation start codons to generate Pax6 isoforms known as Pax6 (ΔPD) or pairless isoforms that lack a PD.

3.2.1 Role of Pax6 in nervous system development

Pax6 plays a crucial role for the establishment of ventral progenitors and specification of the ventral interneuron and motor neuron cell fates in response to graded Shh signaling in the ventral spinal cord and hindbrain. There is a low-to-high gradient of Pax6 expression from ventral to dorsal in the ventral neural tube in response to graded Shh signaling (Ericson et al., 1997). Interestingly, when Pax6 expression is suppressed during Shh signaling, expression of other transcription factors appears in the neural tube for specification of ventral neurons. After the closure of the neural tube, progenitors are destined to become forebrain, midbrain or hindbrain and the demarcation boundary is determined by the graded expression pattern of Pax6 (Mastick et al., 1997).

3.2.2 Role of Pax6 in brain cancer

Pax6 contributes significantly to neurogenesis and it is expressed throughout the ventricular zone and in the external granular layer of the developing cerebellum. High expression of Pax6 in transformed rat fibroblasts suggests that it might function as a proto-oncogene (Maulbecker and Gruss, 1993). Furthermore, Pax6 showed high expression in 78% of medulloblastoma samples (Kozmik et al., 1995). In glioma tumor samples, expression of Pax6 was high in low grade tumors (class III-anaplastic astrocytoma) and low in high grade class IV-GBM (Zhou et al., 2003). Zhou and colleagues suggest that high expression of Pax6 is favorable for patient survival compared to low expression, indicating that Pax6 would be a good prognostic marker for the transition of low grade to high grade glioma. In a recent study, Shahi and colleagues showed that Pax6 expression is regulated by Shh-Gli1 signaling in medulloblastoma and astrocytoma cell lines and primary tumor samples (Shahi et al., 2010). Knockdown of Gli1 in medulloblastoma cells led to decreased Pax6 expression compared to control negative siRNA (Shahi et al., 2010), suggesting that Gli1 upregulates Pax6 expression in medulloblastoma. Interestingly, medulloblastoma cell lines and primary tumor samples showed high expression of Pax6 compared to normal control samples (Shahi et al., 2010). Similarly, expression of Pax6 in siRNA-mediated Gli1 knockdown in astrocytoma cells led to increased Pax6 expression compared to control negative siRNA (Shahi et al., 2010), suggesting that Gli1 might also downregulate Pax6 expression in astrocytoma. Moreover, most astrocytoma and primary tumor samples showed low expression of Pax6 compared to normal controls (Shahi et al., 2010), supporting this possibility. Intriguingly, this differential regulation of Pax6 expression in medulloblastoma and astrocytoma cells suggests that Shh signaling elicits distinct outcomes for the growth of these tumors (Shahi et al., 2010). In neuroblastoma cell lines, Pax6 expression was low compared to normal control samples (Shahi et al., 2011). Moreover, another independent study revealed that Pax6 behaves like a tumor suppressor gene to inhibit the invasiveness of glioma tumors (Mayes et al., 2006). Pax6 was found to contain a hemizygous deletion in its 5′-region in subependymoma tumor (Maekawa et al., 2010), suggesting that Pax6 may switch between an oncogene and tumor suppressor and that this switching activity is variable among tumors. In favor of this hypothesis, another transcription factor, Atoh1 (discussed below), behaves as an oncogene in medulloblastoma and a tumor suppressor gene in colorectal cancer and Merkel cell carcinoma (Bossuyt et al.,

2009; Flora et al., 2009). Atoh1 is regulated by different signaling pathways in these tumors and its differential regulation is thought to underlie its onocogenic or tumor suppressive activity (Bossuyt et al., 2009; Flora et al., 2009). Therefore, Pax6 might only be a good therapeutic target in tumor types for which it behaves as an oncogene such as medulloblastoma.

3.2.2 Role of Pax6 in stem cells

Treatment of embryonic stem cells with the soluble signaling molecules BMP4 and Wnt3a induced the generation of cerebellar granule and Purkinje cell fates (Su et al., 2006). Pax6 expression was correlated with these differentiated cells (Su et al., 2006), suggesting that Pax6 functions to promote cerebellar cell fate and thus might play a role in medulloblastoma biogenesis. Pax6 also plays an indispensable role in the proliferation and expansion of the adult mammalian retinal stem cells (Xu et al., 2007). Pax6 is also important for the specification of neuroectoderm (NE) from human embryonic stem cells (hESCs) (Zhang et al., 2010). Moreover, overexpression of the isoforms Pax6 and Pax6 (5a) but not Pax6 (ΔPD) initiate differentiation of hESCs, although, Pax6 appears to be the main factor to determine the NE specification (Zhang et al., 2010). Interestingly, during the specification of NE from hESCs, Pax6 inhibits the expression of pluripotent genes; however, the mechanism of this inhibition is not known (Zhang et al., 2010). It would be intriguing to explore the role of specific Pax6 isoforms in brain tumorigenesis and the contribution of these isoforms to the stem cell origin of brain tumors.

4. Transcription factors involved in sonic hedgehog signal transduction in cerebellum

In the cerebellum, Shh is produced by Purkinje neurons to promote proliferation of GNPs during the first week of postnatal development (Wechsler-Reya and Scott, 1999). Shh signalling regulates proliferation of GNPs in part via expression of the bHLH (basic helix-loop-helix) transcription factor Nmyc (Kenney et al., 2003; Knoepfler et al., 2002; Oliver et al., 2003). Mutations in the Shh pathway are thought to underlie the etiology of medulloblastoma that arise from transformed GNPs that fail to cease proliferation during development (Wechsler-Reya and Scott, 2001). Interestingly, recent studies have implicated two additional transcription factors, Atoh1 (formerly known as Math1) and Mxd3 (formerly known as Mad3) in the Shh signalling pathway that regulate GNP proliferation and medulloblastoma biogenesis.

4.1 Atoh1

Atonal (Atoh1) was originally identified in Drosphila and is highly conserved (other known names; Hath1, Math1 and bHLHa14). Atoh1 belongs to the family of bHLH transcription factors. The protein consists of a basic domain that recognizes specific E-box sequences (5'CANNTG-3') while the two helices interact with other bHLH protein to form heterodimers (Krizhanovsky et al., 2006). Atoh1 plays a key role in specification of cerebellar cell fates (Ben-Arie et al., 1996). In the past few years, evidence has been mounting for a role of this gene in cerebellar brain tumor development.

4.1.1 Role of Atoh1 in nervous system development

The role of Atoh1 in cerebellum is well defined and its regulated expression is important for granule cell development (Ben-Arie et al., 1997). Mice lacking Atoh1 fail to form granule cells and are born with a cerebellum that is devoid of an external germinal layer (Ben-Arie et al., 1997). Overexpression of Atoh1 interferes with differentiation and causes irregularity in the maturation of granule cells (Helms et al., 2001). Interestingly, expression of Atoh1 and Neurogenin (another bHLH transcription factor) sub-divides the lower rhombic lip into discrete presumptive cell fates and this subdivision is dependent on Pax6 expression (Landsberg et al., 2005). The phenotype of Atoh1 overexpressing transgenic mice indicates that Atoh1 downregulates expression of Pax6 (Helms et al., 2001). Moreover, misexpression of Atoh1 in neural precursors is lethal for the proper development of central nervous system (Isaka et al., 1999).

4.1.2 Role of Atoh1 in brain tumors

Atoh1 plays a critical role in the coordination of proliferation and differentiation of GNPs (Ben-Arie et al., 1997). Therefore, this transcription factor might also be involved in medulloblastoma tumorigenesis. In support of this possibility, double mutant mice of poly [ADP-ribose] polymerase 1(PARP-1)$^{-/-}$/p53$^{-/-}$ mice developed medulloblastoma with high expression of Atoh1 (Tong et al., 2003), suggesting a role as an oncogene. Interestingly, the expression pattern of Atoh1 is distinct in adult and childhood medulloblastoma. In adult medulloblastoma, Atoh1 is expressed at high levels compared to childhood medulloblastoma (Salsano et al., 2004). The origin of these two categories of medulloblastomas is controversial; however, its expression provides further support for the role of Atoh1 in medulloblastoma development. Atoh1 is regulated by Shh signaling in GNPs (Kenney and Rowitch, 2000) and its expression is downregulated upon Shh signaling inhibition (Romer et al., 2004), suggesting that Atoh1 might function in medulloblastoma development. Indeed, deletion of Atoh1 disrupts Shh signaling in the developing cerebellum and prevents medulloblastoma (Flora et al., 2009), supporting an oncogenic role. Interestingly, Atoh1 appears to act directly on the Gli2 transcription factor in the Shh signaling pathway to regulate medulloblastoma biogenesis (Flora et al., 2009). It is well known that Atoh1 binds to E-box elements within target genes and accordingly Atoh1 binds to E-box sequences located in the second intron of Gli2 (Flora et al., 2009). This finding represents a new paradigm of the role of Shh signaling in cerebellum and medulloblastoma because thus far, Gli1 has been thought to be the major transcription factor of the Shh pathway. Gli2 was considered a secondary transcription factor that acts as an activator only the absence of Gli1 (Bai and Joyner, 2001). The regulation of Gli2 by Atoh1 suggests the possibility that either Atoh1 acts on Gli2 in a Gli1-independent manner or that Gli1 regulates the expression of Atoh1 and subsequently Atoh1 acts on Gli2 to promote tumorigenesis.

Ayrault and colleagues demonstrated that co-expression of Atoh1 and Gli1 in primary GNPs cells from postnatal cerebella of healthy C57BL/6 mice transformed into TSCs (Ayrault et al., 2010). Less than 200 TSCs were capable to induce medulloblastoma in the brain of transplanted naïve mice (Ayrault et al., 2010), suggesting that both Atoh1 and Gli1 cooperate to transform GNPs into TSCs. However, Ayrault and colleagues were unable to see the induction of Gli2 expression in response to Atoh1 induced expression in primary GNPs in contrast to Flora and colleagues. The authors suggest that this discrepancy is due to different genetic models for their experiments and warrants further research into the interaction of Atoh1 with Shh mediated transcription factors Gli1 and Gli2 in the development of medulloblastoma.

Although it has been suggested that Atoh1 acts as an oncogene and a possible target of Shh signaling to promote medulloblastoma development, it is important to note that other studies suggest that Atoh1 functions as a tumor suppressor gene in other cell types. For example, Atoh1 regulates proliferation and apoptosis in colorectal cancer and Markel cell carcinoma with the induction of Jun N-terminal kinase (Ntrk1) signaling pathway (Bossuyt et al., 2009).

4.1.3 Role of Atoh1 in stem cells

Many markers have been determined for the identification of TSCs including CD133, Nestin and BMI-1. Cells expressing these selective markers have the capability to generate tumors when xenotranplanted into nude mice. Among these markers, $CD133^+$ expressing cells are considered potent medulloblastoma propagating cells. However, a recent study showed that Atoh1+ and CD15+/SSEA-1 expressing cells have a higher-fold capability of generating medulloblastoma in Ptch1 mutant mice compared to $Atoh1^-/CD15^-$ cells (Read et al., 2009). Intriguingly, $CD133^+$ cells were unable to generate medulloblastoma in Ptch1 mutant mice (Read et al., 2009), suggesting that cells expressing high $Atoh1^+$ and $CD15^+$ are specified to promote proliferation and to inhibit apoptosis and differentation. Thus, it will be intriguing to understand how Atoh1 regulates TSCs that give rise to medulloblastoma.

4.2 Mxd3

Mxd3 (previously known as Mad3) is a member of the bHLH transcriptional regulators (Hurlin et al., 1995) to which Nmyc also belongs. In the classical model, Myc and Mad proteins form heterodimers with the cofactor Max and bind to E-box sequences to activate or repress, respectively, transcription (Grandori et al., 2000). Thus, it has long been thought that Mad/Max complexes function to antagonize Myc/Max complexes by competitive binding to DNA and the promotion to a Mad-dependent differentiation cell state from a Myc-dependent proliferative state. Myc is an established oncogene; thus, Mad proteins were originally hypothesized to function as tumor suppressor genes. However, recent studies for Mxd3 challenge the current model.

4.2.1 Role of Mxd3 in nervous system development

Mxd3 is transiently upregulated in GNPs during postnatal cerebellum development and it fails to be downregulated in *weaver* mice in which GNPs fail to exit the cell cycle (Diaz et al., 2002). In cultured GNPs, Mxd3 is essential for Shh-dependent GNP proliferation and Mxd3 is upregulated in response to Shh signaling (Yun et al., 2007). Mxd3 regulates GNP proliferation in part via expression of Nmyc (Yun et al., 2007). Intriguingly, Mxd3 is predicted to interact directly with Nmyc to promote GNP proliferation (Barisone et al., 2008), suggesting that Mxd3 and Nmyc function as part of a feedback loop to regulate GNP proliferation. Similar to other Mad family proteins, mice with a targeted deletion of Mxd3 are viable; however, Mxd3 null mice exhibit increased sensitivity to radiation-induced apoptosis (Queva et al., 2001). The effect of Mxd3 deletion in postnatal cerebellum development was not explored in this mouse line. Interestingly, Mxd3 expression in immature B cells has been shown to induce cell proliferation without differentiation, a phenotype of leukemia (Gore et al., 2010), suggesting that Mxd3 might also regulate proliferation of other types of cancer cells.

4.2.2 Role of Mxd3 in brain cancer

Like Nmyc, Mxd3 is upregulated in tumors and pre-tumor cells from Ptch1 heterozygous mice (Yun et al., 2007) and Mxd3 is expressed in human brain tumors including glioblastoma and medulloblastoma (Barisone et al., 2008). Together, these studies suggest that Mxd3 might also function with Nmyc to regulate tumor biogenesis. Furthermore research is required to address this intriguing possibility.

4.2.3 Role of Mxd3 in stem cells

Mxd3 has not been studied extensively and there are no published reports regarding a role for Mxd3 in regulation of stem cells. However, given the fact that Mxd3 and Nmyc function together to regulate GNP proliferation and are predicted to physically associate with each other, it is likely that Mxd3 functions with Nmyc to regulate stem cell proliferation. Additional experiments are necessary to test this interesting possibility.

Location	Function	Pathway	References
Ventral progenitors of the spinal cord	Transcription factor	Sonic hedgehog Pax6	Ericson et al., 1997; Briscoe et al., 2000
Astrocytic and oligodendroglial tumors	Tumor suppressor	Sonic hedgehog	Riemenschneider et al., 2004; Shahi et al., 2010
Medulloblastoma	Oncogene	Sonic hedgehog	Shahi et al., 2010
Neuroblastoma	Tumor suppressor	Sonic hedgehog	Shahi et al., 2010
Human embryonic stem cells	Transcription factor	Sonic hedgehog	Hu et al., 2009
Oligodendroglial cells	Transcription factor	Sonic hedgehog	Danesin et al., 2006; Muraguchi et al., 2010

Table 1. Summary of Nkx2.2 function in neural progenitor cells and tumors.

Location	Function	Pathway	References
Ventral progenitors of the spinal cord	Transcription factor	Sonic hedgehog Nkx2.2	Ericson et al., 1997
Medulloblastoma	Oncogene	Sonic hedgehog	Kozmik et al., 1995; Shahi et al., 2010
Glioma	Tumor suppressor	Sonic hedgehog	Zhou et al., 2003; Mayes et al., 2006; Shahi et al., 2010
Neuroblastoma	Tumor suppressor	Sonic hedgehog	Shahi et al., 2011
Subependymoma tumors	Tumor suppressor	PTEN, SOX	Maekawa et al., 2010
Embryonic stem cells	Transcription factor	BMP4, Wnt3a, Atoh1	Sue et al., 2006; Zhang et al., 2010
Retinal stem cells	Transcription factor	Sonic hedgehog, Sufu	Xu et al., 2007; Cwinn et al., 2011

Table 2. Summary of Pax6 function in neural progenitor cells and tumors

Location	Function	Pathway	References
Cerebellum	Transcription factor	Sonic hedgehog Pax6	Ben-Arie et al., 1997; Kenny and Rowitch 2000; Helms et al., 2006; Flora et al., 2009
Medulloblastoma	Oncogene	Sonic hedgehog Gli2	Tong et al., 2003; Salsano et al., 2004; Briggs et al., 2008; Flora et al., 2009
Tumor stem cells	Transcription factor	Sonic hedgehog	Ayrault et al., 2010; Read et al., 2009
Neural stem cells	Transcription factor	Sonic hedgehog	Isaka et al., 1999; Hu et al., 2010
Colorectral cancer and Merkel cell carcinoma	Tumor suppressor	Jun N-terminal kinase	Bossuyt et al., 2009

Table 3. Summary of Atoh1 function in neural progenitor cells and tumors

Location	Function	Pathway	References
Neural progenitor cells	Transcription factor	Unknown	Queva et al., 2001
Cerebellar granule cell precursors	Transcription factor	Sonic hedgehog	Yun et al., 2007
Medulloblastoma	Oncogene	Sonic hedgehog	Yun et al., 2007; Barisone et al., 2008
Immature B cells	Transcription factor	Id2	Gore et al., 2010

Table 4. Summary of Mxd3 function in neural progenitor cells and tumors

5. Conclusion

While many questions still remain, our understanding of the pediatric brain tumor medulloblastoma has become clearer in the past few years. Mounting evidence indicates that TSCs are the major contributor to propagate medulloblastoma and that there are many pathways that contribute to TSC maintenance. However, the precise mechanism by which these TSCs are regulated by these signaling pathways to promote tumorigenesis is not well understood. Therefore, additional studies are warranted to understand these pathways. However, the identification of new transcription factors that contribute to TSC proliferation and tumor biogenesis is a major advance in our understanding of this disease. These new transcription factors represent exciting new therapeutic targets for treatment since it is likely that a multitude of downstream molecules can be targeted with a single drug.

6. Acknowledgment

We would like to acknowledge members of the Diaz lab for discussion about the ideas discussed in this chapter. Research in the Diaz lab is funded by grants to E.D. from the National Science Foundation and the NIH Director's New Innovator Award Program.

7. References

Ayrault, O., Zhao, H., Zindy, F., Qu, C., Sherr, C.J., and Roussel, M.F. (2010). Atoh1 inhibits neuronal differentiation and collaborates with Gli1 to generate medulloblastoma-initiating cells. Cancer Res *70*, 5618-5627.

Bai, C.B., and Joyner, A.L. (2001). Gli1 can rescue the in vivo function of Gli2. Development *128*, 5161-5172.

Barisone, G.A., Yun, J.S., and Diaz, E. (2008). From cerebellar proliferation to tumorigenesis: new insights into the role of Mad3. Cell Cycle *7*, 423-427.

Ben-Arie, N., Bellen, H.J., Armstrong, D.L., McCall, A.E., Gordadze, P.R., Guo, Q., Matzuk, M.M., and Zoghbi, H.Y. (1997). Math1 is essential for genesis of cerebellar granule neurons. Nature *390*, 169-172.

Ben-Arie, N., McCall, A.E., Berkman, S., Eichele, G., Bellen, H.J., and Zoghbi, H.Y. (1996). Evolutionary conservation of sequence and expression of the bHLH protein Atonal suggests a conserved role in neurogenesis. Hum Mol Genet *5*, 1207-1216.

Bossuyt, W., Kazanjian, A., De Geest, N., Van Kelst, S., De Hertogh, G., Geboes, K., Boivin, G.P., Luciani, J., Fuks, F., Chuah, M., *et al.* (2009). Atonal homolog 1 is a tumor suppressor gene. PLoS Biol *7*, e39.

Briscoe, J., Pierani, A., Jessell, T.M., and Ericson, J. (2000). A homeodomain protein code specifies progenitor cell identity and neuronal fate in the ventral neural tube. Cell *101*, 435-445.

Browd, S.R., Kenney, A.M., Gottfried, O.N., Yoon, J.W., Walterhouse, D., Pedone, C.A., and Fults, D.W. (2006). N-myc can substitute for insulin-like growth factor signaling in a mouse model of sonic hedgehog-induced medulloblastoma. Cancer Res *66*, 2666-2672.

Chen, C.Y., and Schwartz, R.J. (1995). Identification of novel DNA binding targets and regulatory domains of a murine tinman homeodomain factor, nkx-2.5. J Biol Chem *270*, 15628-15633.

Diaz, E., Ge, Y., Yang, Y.H., Loh, K.C., Serafini, T.A., Okazaki, Y., Hayashizaki, Y., Speed, T.P., Ngai, J., and Scheiffele, P. (2002). Molecular analysis of gene expression in the developing pontocerebellar projection system. Neuron *36*, 417-434.

Ding, Q., Motoyama, J., Gasca, S., Mo, R., Sasaki, H., Rossant, J., and Hui, C.C. (1998). Diminished Sonic hedgehog signaling and lack of floor plate differentiation in Gli2 mutant mice. Development *125*, 2533-2543.

Ericson, J., Rashbass, P., Schedl, A., Brenner-Morton, S., Kawakami, A., van Heyningen, V., Jessell, T.M., and Briscoe, J. (1997). Pax6 controls progenitor cell identity and neuronal fate in response to graded Shh signaling. Cell *90*, 169-180.

Flora, A., Klisch, T.J., Schuster, G., and Zoghbi, H.Y. (2009). Deletion of Atoh1 disrupts Sonic Hedgehog signaling in the developing cerebellum and prevents medulloblastoma. Science *326*, 1424-1427.

Gibson, P., Tong, Y., Robinson, G., Thompson, M.C., Currle, D.S., Eden, C., Kranenburg, T.A., Hogg, T., Poppleton, H., Martin, J., *et al.* (2010). Subtypes of medulloblastoma have distinct developmental origins. Nature *468*, 1095-1099.

Goodrich, L.V., Milenkovic, L., Higgins, K.M., and Scott, M.P. (1997). Altered neural cell fates and medulloblastoma in mouse patched mutants. Science *277*, 1109-1113.

Gore, Y., Lantner, F., Hart, G., and Shachar, I. (2010). Mad3 negatively regulates B cell differentiation in the spleen by inducing Id2 expression. Mol Biol Cell *21*, 1864-1871.

Grandori, C., Cowley, S.M., James, L.P., and Eisenman, R.N. (2000). The Myc/Max/Mad network and the transcriptional control of cell behavior. Annu Rev Cell Dev Biol *16*, 653-699.

Helms, A.W., Gowan, K., Abney, A., Savage, T., and Johnson, J.E. (2001). Overexpression of MATH1 disrupts the coordination of neural differentiation in cerebellum development. Mol Cell Neurosci *17*, 671-682.

Hessabi, B., Schmidt, I., and Walther, R. (2000). The homeodomain of Nkx2.2 carries two cooperatively acting nuclear localization signals. Biochem Biophys Res Commun *270*, 695-700.

Hu, B.Y., Du, Z.W., Li, X.J., Ayala, M., and Zhang, S.C. (2009). Human oligodendrocytes from embryonic stem cells: conserved SHH signaling networks and divergent FGF effects. Development *136*, 1443-1452.

Hurlin, P.J., Queva, C., Koskinen, P.J., Steingrimsson, E., Ayer, D.E., Copeland, N.G., Jenkins, N.A., and Eisenman, R.N. (1995). Mad3 and Mad4: novel Max-interacting transcriptional repressors that suppress c-myc dependent transformation and are expressed during neural and epidermal differentiation. EMBO J *14*, 5646-5659.

Ingham, P.W., and McMahon, A.P. (2001). Hedgehog signaling in animal development: paradigms and principles. Genes Dev *15*, 3059-3087.

Isaka, F., Ishibashi, M., Taki, W., Hashimoto, N., Nakanishi, S., and Kageyama, R. (1999). Ectopic expression of the bHLH gene Math1 disturbs neural development. Eur J Neurosci *11*, 2582-2588.

Kenney, A.M., Cole, M.D., and Rowitch, D.H. (2003). Nmyc upregulation by sonic hedgehog signaling promotes proliferation in developing cerebellar granule neuron precursors. Development *130*, 15-28.

Kenney, A.M., and Rowitch, D.H. (2000). Sonic hedgehog promotes G(1) cyclin expression and sustained cell cycle progression in mammalian neuronal precursors. Mol Cell Biol *20*, 9055-9067.

Kim, Y., and Nirenberg, M. (1989). Drosophila NK-homeobox genes. Proc Natl Acad Sci U S A *86*, 7716-7720.

Knoepfler, P.S., Cheng, P.F., and Eisenman, R.N. (2002). N-myc is essential during neurogenesis for the rapid expansion of progenitor cell populations and the inhibition of neuronal differentiation. Genes Dev *16*, 2699-2712.

Kozmik, Z., Sure, U., Ruedi, D., Busslinger, M., and Aguzzi, A. (1995). Deregulated expression of PAX5 in medulloblastoma. Proc Natl Acad Sci U S A *92*, 5709-5713.

Krizhanovsky, V., Soreq, L., Kliminski, V., and Ben-Arie, N. (2006). Math1 target genes are enriched with evolutionarily conserved clustered E-box binding sites. J Mol Neurosci *28*, 211-229.

Landsberg, R.L., Awatramani, R.B., Hunter, N.L., Farago, A.F., DiPietrantonio, H.J., Rodriguez, C.I., and Dymecki, S.M. (2005). Hindbrain rhombic lip is comprised of discrete progenitor cell populations allocated by Pax6. Neuron *48*, 933-947.

Lints, T.J., Parsons, L.M., Hartley, L., Lyons, I., and Harvey, R.P. (1993). Nkx-2.5: a novel murine homeobox gene expressed in early heart progenitor cells and their myogenic descendants. Development *119*, 969.

Maekawa, M., Fujisawa, H., Iwayama, Y., Tamase, A., Toyota, T., Osumi, N., and Yoshikawa, T. (2010). Giant subependymoma developed in a patient with aniridia: analyses of PAX6 and tumor-relevant genes. Brain Pathol *20*, 1033-1041.

Mansouri, A., Hallonet, M., and Gruss, P. (1996). Pax genes and their roles in cell differentiation and development. Curr Opin Cell Biol *8*, 851-857.

Mastick, G.S., Davis, N.M., Andrew, G.L., and Easter, S.S., Jr. (1997). Pax-6 functions in boundary formation and axon guidance in the embryonic mouse forebrain. Development *124*, 1985-1997.

Maulbecker, C.C., and Gruss, P. (1993). The oncogenic potential of Pax genes. EMBO J *12*, 2361-2367.

Mayes, D.A., Hu, Y., Teng, Y., Siegel, E., Wu, X., Panda, K., Tan, F., Yung, W.K., and Zhou, Y.H. (2006). PAX6 suppresses the invasiveness of glioblastoma cells and the expression of the matrix metalloproteinase-2 gene. Cancer Res *66*, 9809-9817.

Muraguchi, T., Tanaka, S., Yamada, D., Tamase, A., Nakada, M., Nakamura, H., Hoshii, T., Ooshio, T., Tadokoro, Y., Naka, K., *et al.* (2011). NKX2.2 suppresses self-renewal of glioma-initiating cells. Cancer Res *71*, 1135-1145.

Oliver, T.G., Grasfeder, L.L., Carroll, A.L., Kaiser, C., Gillingham, C.L., Lin, S.M., Wickramasinghe, R., Scott, M.P., and Wechsler-Reya, R.J. (2003). Transcriptional profiling of the Sonic hedgehog response: a critical role for N-myc in proliferation of neuronal precursors. Proc Natl Acad Sci U S A *100*, 7331-7336.

Ponnusamy, M.P., and Batra, S.K. (2008). Ovarian cancer: emerging concept on cancer stem cells. J Ovarian Res *1*, 4.

Queva, C., McArthur, G.A., Iritani, B.M., and Eisenman, R.N. (2001). Targeted deletion of the S-phase-specific Myc antagonist Mad3 sensitizes neuronal and lymphoid cells to radiation-induced apoptosis. Mol Cell Biol *21*, 703-712.

Read, T.A., Fogarty, M.P., Markant, S.L., McLendon, R.E., Wei, Z., Ellison, D.W., Febbo, P.G., and Wechsler-Reya, R.J. (2009). Identification of CD15 as a marker for tumor-propagating cells in a mouse model of medulloblastoma. Cancer Cell *15*, 135-147.

Riemenschneider, M.J., Koy, T.H., and Reifenberger, G. (2004). Expression of oligodendrocyte lineage genes in oligodendroglial and astrocytic gliomas. Acta Neuropathol *107*, 277-282.

Romer, J.T., Kimura, H., Magdaleno, S., Sasai, K., Fuller, C., Baines, H., Connelly, M., Stewart, C.F., Gould, S., Rubin, L.L., *et al.* (2004). Suppression of the Shh pathway using a small molecule inhibitor eliminates medulloblastoma in Ptc1(+/-)p53(-/-) mice. Cancer Cell *6*, 229-240.

Salsano, E., Pollo, B., Eoli, M., Giordana, M.T., and Finocchiaro, G. (2004). Expression of MATH1, a marker of cerebellar granule cell progenitors, identifies different medulloblastoma sub-types. Neurosci Lett *370*, 180-185.

Sengupta, A., Banerjee, D., Chandra, S., Banerji, S.K., Ghosh, R., Roy, R., and Banerjee, S. (2007). Deregulation and cross talk among Sonic hedgehog, Wnt, Hox and Notch signaling in chronic myeloid leukemia progression. Leukemia *21*, 949-955.

Shahi, M.H., Afzal, M., Sinha, S., Eberhart, C.G., Rey, J.A., Fan, X., and Castresana, J.S. (2010). Regulation of sonic hedgehog-GLI1 downstream target genes PTCH1, Cyclin D2, Plakoglobin, PAX6 and NKX2.2 and their epigenetic status in medulloblastoma and astrocytoma. BMC Cancer *10*, 614.

Shahi, M.H., Schiapparelli, P., Afzal, M., Sinha, S., Rey, J.A., and Castresana, J.S. (2011). Expression and epigenetic modulation of sonic hedgehog-GLI1 pathway genes in neuroblastoma cell lines and tumors. Tumour Biol *32*, 113-127.

Singh, S.K., Hawkins, C., Clarke, I.D., Squire, J.A., Bayani, J., Hide, T., Henkelman, R.M., Cusimano, M.D., and Dirks, P.B. (2004). Identification of human brain tumour initiating cells. Nature *432*, 396-401.

Su, H.L., Muguruma, K., Matsuo-Takasaki, M., Kengaku, M., Watanabe, K., and Sasai, Y. (2006). Generation of cerebellar neuron precursors from embryonic stem cells. Dev Biol *290*, 287-296.

Taipale, J., and Beachy, P.A. (2001). The Hedgehog and Wnt signalling pathways in cancer. Nature *411*, 349-354.

Tong, W.M., Ohgaki, H., Huang, H., Granier, C., Kleihues, P., and Wang, Z.Q. (2003). Null mutation of DNA strand break-binding molecule poly(ADP-ribose) polymerase causes medulloblastomas in p53(-/-) mice. Am J Pathol *162*, 343-352.

Tsao, D.H., Gruschus, J.M., Wang, L.H., Nirenberg, M., and Ferretti, J.A. (1994). Elongation of helix III of the NK-2 homeodomain upon binding to DNA: a secondary structure study by NMR. Biochemistry *33*, 15053-15060.

Vokes, S.A., Ji, H., McCuine, S., Tenzen, T., Giles, S., Zhong, S., Longabaugh, W.J., Davidson, E.H., Wong, W.H., and McMahon, A.P. (2007). Genomic characterization of Gli-activator targets in sonic hedgehog-mediated neural patterning. Development *134*, 1977-1989.

Ward, R.J., Lee, L., Graham, K., Satkunendran, T., Yoshikawa, K., Ling, E., Harper, L., Austin, R., Nieuwenhuis, E., Clarke, I.D., *et al.* (2009). Multipotent CD15+ cancer stem cells in patched-1-deficient mouse medulloblastoma. Cancer Res *69*, 4682-4690.

Wechsler-Reya, R., and Scott, M.P. (2001). The developmental biology of brain tumors. Annu Rev Neurosci *24*, 385-428.

Wechsler-Reya, R.J., and Scott, M.P. (1999). Control of neuronal precursor proliferation in the cerebellum by Sonic Hedgehog. Neuron *22*, 103-114.

Xu, S., Sunderland, M.E., Coles, B.L., Kam, A., Holowacz, T., Ashery-Padan, R., Marquardt, T., McInnes, R.R., and van der Kooy, D. (2007). The proliferation and expansion of retinal stem cells require functional Pax6. Dev Biol *304*, 713-721.

Yoon, J.W., Kita, Y., Frank, D.J., Majewski, R.R., Konicek, B.A., Nobrega, M.A., Jacob, H., Walterhouse, D., and Iannaccone, P. (2002). Gene expression profiling leads to identification of GLI1-binding elements in target genes and a role for multiple downstream pathways in GLI1-induced cell transformation. J Biol Chem *277*, 5548-5555.

Yun, J.S., Rust, J.M., Ishimaru, T., and Diaz, E. (2007). A novel role of the Mad family member Mad3 in cerebellar granule neuron precursor proliferation. Mol Cell Biol *27*, 8178-8189.

Zhang, X., Huang, C.T., Chen, J., Pankratz, M.T., Xi, J., Li, J., Yang, Y., Lavaute, T.M., Li, X.J., Ayala, M., *et al.* (2010). Pax6 is a human neuroectoderm cell fate determinant. Cell Stem Cell *7*, 90-100.

Zhou, Y.H., Tan, F., Hess, K.R., and Yung, W.K. (2003). The expression of PAX6, PTEN, vascular endothelial growth factor, and epidermal growth factor receptor in gliomas: relationship to tumor grade and survival. Clin Cancer Res *9*, 3369-3375.

13

Novel Therapeutic Venues for Glioblastoma: Novel Rising Preclinical Treatment Opportunities

Siegelin Markus David and Siegelin Yasemin
Cell Biology, Columbia University, College of Physicians & Surgeons
United States of America

1. Introduction

High grade gliomas, including anaplastic glioma WHO grade III and glioblastoma WHO IV (GBM), carry a dismal prognosis. Taking all nowadays-available therapeutics options, including radiation, chemotherapy and surgery, for GBM into consideration the prognosis after initial diagnosis is about 12 month. Despite this bad prognosis, researchers gained a tremendous insight into the molecular and genetic signatures of low and high grade gliomas. Several different subtypes of GBM were demonstrated with respect to their genetic background. These genetic alterations include *p53* mutation in secondary GBMs and EGFR amplification in primary GBMs, respectively. Very recently, great excitement was raised after the discovery of *IDH1* mutation in low-grade gliomas and secondary GBMs. This discovery is of great significance since it allows further categorizing of GBMs and is helpful in distinguishing low-grade gliomas from non-neoplastic adjacent brain tissue. Despite all this progress there is an urgent need for fresh additional therapeutic strategies. In addition to the identification of novel therapeutic regimens it is of utmost importance to gain an understanding about the molecular mechanisms on how GBMs manage to evade from almost any anti-cancer treatment regimen. In experimental models of glioblastoma there are a number of novel therapeutic regimens that exhibited promising results. These novel therapeutics include, but are not limited to: Apoptosis-based therapeutics (Tumor necrosis factor alpha related apoptosis inducing ligand, TRAIL), tyrosinkinase-inhibitors, Heat-shock-protein 90 (HSP90) inhibitors, polyphenols, novel drug combinations and intracranial application based strategies. This chapter will primarily review and focus on molecular mechanisms of resistance in GBM and rising new therapeutic venues for high-grade gliomas. High-grade gliomas are a group of primary heterogenous tumors of which glioblastoma World Health Organisation, WHO IV (GBM), is the most common one. Once the diagnosis of GBM is made, the average survival time is approximately 12-15 month (Hegi, Diserens et al., 2005). Treatment usually consists of temozolomide (commonly used chemotherapeutic drug for the treatment of GBM, TMZ), radiation (either alone or in combination with chemotherapeutics) and surgery (Hegi, Diserens et al., 2005).

TMZ is a chemotherapeutic drug whose efficacy depends on the expression of the DNA repair protein MGMT (O6-methylguanine-DNA methyltransferase) in the glioblastoma tumor specimens (Krakstad&Chekenya). MGMT has been known to counteract chemotherapy-induced DNA damage by repairing the structural integrity of O^6-alkylated bases (Krakstad&Chekenya). The expression of MGMT is determined by its promoter methylation status. A hypermethylated promoter in a glioblastoma specimen indicates silenced expression of MGMT and suggests sensitivity of this patient's tumor to TMZ. Regarding the efficacy of TMZ, Stupp et al. showed that in patients suffering from GBM the combined administration of radiation and TMZ increased the median survival rate by 3 month as compared to radiotherapy alone (Hegi, Diserens et al., 2005). Furthermore, the 2 year survival rate in patients that received combined treatment (radiotherapy +TMZ) was increased from 10% to 26 % (Hegi, Diserens et al., 2005; Mercer, Tyler et al., 2009). The efficacy of combined TMZ and radiotherapy was largely dependent on the epigenetic silencing of the MGMT gene since patients with GBM harboring a methylted MGMT promoter that were treated with the therapeutic combination of radiotherapy and TMZ exhibited a median survival of approximately 22 months (Hegi, Diserens et al., 2005; Mercer, Tyler et al., 2009). Approximately 50 % of patients diagnosed with a GBM exhibit an unmethylated MGMT promoter. Unfortunately, this above mentioned patient group does not respond to TMZ treatment. Particularly for this group there is an evident need for fresh and novel treatment approaches. Overall, it can be concluded that new treatment approaches for this highly aggressive and deadly disease is warranted. In this chapter, novel-target specific and novel experimental approaches from recent preclinical developments will be illustrated.

2. Targeting novel genetic alterations in GBM

Genetically, GBM can be grouped into primary and secondary GBMs. Primary GBMs develop de novo and harbor EGFR (epidermal growth factor receptor) amplifications and alterations of PTEN (phosphatase and tensin homolog mutations), resulting in a profound activation of the PI3 - Kinase pathway that is well known to enhance apoptotic resistance, drive tumor cell proliferation and angiogenesis (Chakravarti, Zhai et al., 2004; Parsons, Jones et al., 2008). In contrast, secondary GBMs develop out of lower grade lesions and often reveal TP53 and IDH1 (isocitrate dehydrogenase 1, affected amino acid 132) mutations (von Deimling, Korshunov et al.; Parsons, Jones et al., 2008). The recent finding of IDH1 mutations in GBM and low-grade gliomas has raised great excitement in the scientific community. In 2008 the *IDH1* mutation was first identified in a comprehensive genomic analysis of 22 human GBM samples (Parsons, Jones et al., 2008). Interestingly, they found recurrent mutations in the active site of isocitrate dehydrogenase 1 (IDH1) in 12% of GBM patients (Parsons, Jones et al., 2008). They reported that these mutations were found in a large fraction of young patients and in patients with secondary GBMs (Parsons, Jones et al., 2008). Importantly, IDH1 mutations were shown to be associated with an increase in overall survival in patients (Parsons, Jones et al., 2008). The finding of IDH1 mutation in patients with GBM represents the beginning of a new molecular era. Researchers have already tried to exploit IDH1 as a therapeutic target with rather moderate effects. At this point it seems more likely that IDH1 will be a great asset for the practicing neuropathologist since recently a IDH1 mutation specific antibody was identified (Capper, Zentgraf et al., 2009) and successfully used to detect the mutatation in gliomas with both high sensitivity and specificity, respectively. This has also diagnostic implications since with the aid of this mutation specific antibody researchers were able to distinguish diffuse astrocytoma from reactive astrocytes (astrocytosis), e.g. surrounding an infarct, (Camelo-Piragua, Jansen et al.)

which is a well-known diagnostic issue for the practicing neuropathologist. An established problem in glioma research is the fact that certain genetic alteration cannot be transported into a *vitro* setting. One of the most important examples is that glioma cells with confirmed EGFR amplification lose this genetic alteration when taken into culture (Piaskowski, Bienkowski et al.). The same issue arises when reseachers were unsuccessfully trying to culture glioma cells harboring IDH1 mutations (Piaskowski, Bienkowski et al.). These results are in so far of high importance as our current culturing system of glioma cells seems not to have much in common with the relevant in vivo conditions, suggesting that based on these models it will be challenging to identify suitable treatment strategies. Nevertheless, researchers found that the IDH1 mutation at R132 might still be used as a therapeutic target. The mutated IDH1 results in a dependence on α-ketoglutarate that is produced from glutamine via the enzyme, glutaminase (Seltzer, Bennett et al.). They inhibited glutaminase both pharmacologically and genetically (siRNA approach) and found that cells harboring an IDH1 mutation grew slower than cells expressing wild-type IDH1 (Seltzer, Bennett et al.). Since there are no IDH1 mutated cell lines available, they transfected established glioma cells with a plasmid carrying IDH1 mutation and created stable IDH1-mutated clones (Seltzer, Bennett et al.). They concluded that the inhibition of glutaminase in IDH1 mutated cells might be a novel therapeutic strategy (Seltzer, Bennett et al.). In summary, the novel identification of IDH1 mutation might have both therapeutic and diagnostic implications.

3. Kinase inhibitors in GBM therapy

High grade gliomas organize a molecular network that provides them the ability to maintain massive growth and resistance towards cell death. From a mechanistic point these properties are closely linked to receptor- or intracellular kinases. With regards to receptor kinases, there are a few known receptor kinases that have gained particular importance, such as epidermal growth factor receptors (EGFR), platelet-derived growth factor receptors (PDGFR), vascular endothelial growth factor receptors (VEGFR) (Ren, Yang et al., 2007). Once their ligand has bound to the cognate receptor, an intracellular signal transduction cascade is initiated leading to the modulation of a number of important pathways, e.g. Ras/Raf/mitogen-activated protein (MAP)-kinase and phosphatidylinositol-3 kinase (PI3K)/Akt/mammalian target of rapamycin (mTOR) pathways (Ren, Yang et al., 2007) (Figure 1).

For gliomas and particularly glioblastomas, one of the most important pathway is the phosphatidylinositol-3 kinase (PI3K)/Akt pathway, because primary glioblastomas often exhibit genetic alterations in this pathway, such as PTEN and EGFR. Regarding these genes it is also worthwhile to point out that PTEN (30%) and EGFR (37%) are amongst the most frequently altered genes in glioblastoma specimens (Krakstad&Chekenya). Chakravarti et al. have recently demonstrated that an active PI3K pathway was associated with a reduction in survival in patients suffering from glioma (Chakravarti, Zhai et al., 2004). Patients with a loss of PTEN revealed a higher level of active PI3K signaling and had a significant worse prognosis with regards to survival. Considering the absolute number in this recent study, glioblastoma patients with an activated PI3K pathway revealed a median survival of only 11 month, whereas patients that had suppressed activation levels of PI3K signaling exhibited a median survival of impressive 40 month. These observations suggest that patient with an active PI3K pathway require additional targeted treatment strategies. From preclinical experiments it has been known over two decades that the PI3K pathway plays an important role in gliomas and that its inhibition is beneficial at least in preclinical settings (Ekstrand, James et al., 1991). Consequently, several PI3K were developed and nowadays are also implicated in clinicaltrials, e.g. XL765, erlotinib and geftinib (www.clinicaltrials.gov). Unfortunately, these EGFR - inhibitors targeting a key step in molecular biology of glioma reveal rather moderate efficacy in patients (Krakstad&Chekenya; Sathornsumetee, Desjardins et al.; Yung, Vredenburgh et al.). Monotherapy with EGFR inhibitors, erolotinib and geftinib, did not exhibit a dramatic increase in survival. Recently, a randomised, controlled phase II study by the European Organisation for Research and Treatment of

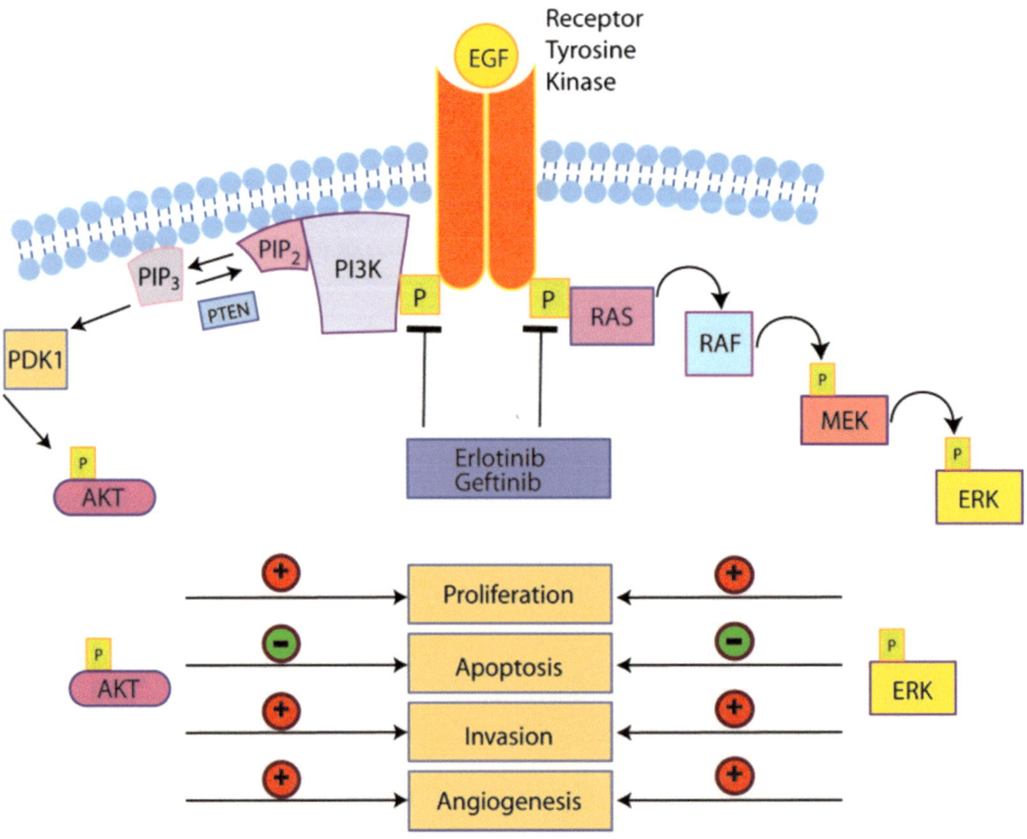

Fig. 1. Tyrosine kinase signaling. Glioblastomas often reveal genetic alterations, e.g. epidermal growth factor (EGFR). Once a ligand (EGFR) has bound to the receptor, PI3K binds to the cytosolic phosphorylated EGF-receptor. In turn, PI3K phosphorylates phosphoinositide-4,5 bisphosphate, PIP2, to phosphatidylinositol-3,4,5 triphosphate , PIP3, and PIP3 binds and phosphorylates phosphoinositide-dependent kinase 1 (PDK1). PDK1 activates proteinkinase-B, AKT, by phosphorylation (p-AKT). PTEN is a tumor suppressor that inhibits PI3K activity by dephosphorylating PIP3 to PIP2 and thereby inhibiting PI3K signaling (Krakstad&Chekenya). Similiarly to the Akt signaling, Ras binds to phosphorylated EGF-receptor and induces a phosphorylation cascade to give rise to phosphorylated ERK (p-ERK). P-ERK and P-AKT promote tumor cell proliferation, invasion and angiogenesis. They inhibit programmed cell death, apoptosis. Erlotinib and Geftinib are tyrosine kinase inhibitors and interact with the EGFR to suppress its activity.

Cancer (EORTC) was unable to demonstrate even improvement in survival and radiographic responses in erlotinib treated patients (Krakstad&Chekenya). Notably, the EORTC recently showed that neither the expression of EGFR, EGFRvIII nor PTEN in glioblastoma patients (specimens) are correlated with the responses of patients to erlotinib. Furthermore the response rate was actually worse in patients harboring the EGFRvIII genotype. This finding is in so far surprising as lung cancer patients with a EGFRvIII genotype had clinical and radiographic improvements (Krakstad&Chekenya). Overall, the effects of EGFR inhibitors seem rather moderate for GBM treatment according to the currently available literature. Nevertheless, they represent one current example of molecular-target based cancer therapy that arose out of the discovery of an alteration of a genetic pathway in glioblastoma specimens. Additional trials, experimentally modifications and novel drugs might be useful for future directions.

4. Hsp90 antagonists for preclinical glioblastoma treatment

One promising tumor druggable target is Hsp90. Hsp90 has been shown to be either over-expressed or harbors an about 100 times higher ATPase activity in tumor specimens, including malignant gliomas (Kang, Plescia et al., 2009; Siegelin, Habel et al., 2009). Hsp 90 is an abundant protein that is located in the cytosol and several organelles, including the endoplasmatic reticulum and mitochondria (Kang, Plescia et al., 2007). In addition, it is also known to be secreted, stabilizing extracellular factors. Hsp90 is closely related to proliferation, apoptosis, angiogenesis and tumor cell migration and chaperones a number of cellular proteins, Akt, survivin, BRAF, p53, JAK2, STATs, etc. , to prevent their degradation and finally drive tumor progression. Since p53 and the Akt pathway are commonly altered in high grade gliomas, it is conceivable that Hsp90 antagonist, such as Geldanamycin derivatives like 17-AAG, might target GBMs. In line with this assumption, researchers have demonstrated that 17-AAG was able to inhibit growth of human established glioblastoma and glioma-stem cell like cells *in vitro (Sauvageot, Weatherbee et al., 2009)*. Furthermore, 17-AAG was shown to synergize with radiation therapy (Sauvageot, Weatherbee et al., 2009), suggesting that 17-AAG might be an interesting candidate for a combination therapy. In addition these in vitro effects were successfully transferred into an *in vivo* model and 17-AAG administered systemically inhibited the growth of intracranial tumors and also synergized with radiation (Sauvageot, Weatherbee et al., 2009). Unfortunately, 17-AAG was not able to enhance the effects of temozolomide on glioblastoma cells *in vitro* or *in vivo*. Another recent report confirms the finding that inhibition of Hsp90 by 17-AAG does not synergize with TMZ. Nevertheless, this group found that 17-AAG at suboptimal concentrations (nanomolar range) enhanced the cytotoxicity of the DNA-crosslinking agents cisplatin and 1,3-bis(2-chloroethyl)-1-nitrosourea (Ohba, Hirose et al.). Mechanistically, this synergism was a consequence of prolonged cell cycle arrest and degradation of anti-apoptotic proteins, such as Akt and survivin (Ohba, Hirose et al.). Of note, 17 - AAG was capable to synergize with cisplatin in a nude mice based animal model (xenografted U87 cells). In addition, recent data also suggests that 17-AAG might enhance the cytotoxic effects of Tumor necrosis factor related apoptosis inducing ligand (TRAIL) which from a mechanistic point was attributed to the suppression of the anti-apoptotic molecule, survivin, an established client protein of Hsp90 (Siegelin, Habel et al., 2009). One possible obstacle in treatment of glioblastoma with Hsp90 antagonists might be that GBM cells may acquire resistance towards 17-AAG. This resistance was attributed to low activity of the mitochondrial enzyme NAD(P)H/quinone oxidoreductase 1 (NQO1) (Gaspar, Sharp et al., 2009). However, if this enzyme is the sole cause of resistance might be uncertain and remains to be determined in future analysis and there might be additional factors that contribute to the acquired resistance of 17-AAG. Another known issue with 17-AAG is the fact that it possesses unfavorable pharmacokinetics. Therefore, researchers are developing novel small-molecule compounds targeting Hsp90. One of these new molecules is the potent synthetic diarylisoxazole amide resorcinol HSP90 inhibitor, NVP-AUY922 (Gaspar, Sharp et al.). NVP-AUY922 exhibited anti-proliferative activity in a broad range of human glioblastoma cell lines. Cell death (apoptosis) was also induced by NVP-AUY922, albeit after prolonged exposure of the drug to the cells. Furthermore, in a xenograft model NVP-AUY922 (50 mg/kg i.p x 3 days) caused growth inhibition and induced apoptosis, whereas 17-AAG used at maximum tolerated dose was less effective (Gaspar, Sharp et al.). The in vivo anti-tumor activity by NVP-AUY922 was accompanied by anti-proliferative, pro-apoptotic and anti-angiogenic effects (Gaspar, Sharp et al.). Another second generation novel Hsp90 inhibitor is NXD30001 that exhibited favorable pharmacokinetics as compared to 17-AAG (Zhu, Woolfenden et al.). This compound inhibited GBM growth. Of note, this group demonstrated that NXD30001 showed anti-cancer activity in an EGFR-driven genetically engineered mouse model and concluded that the Hsp90 inhibitor NXD30001 is a therapeutically multivalent molecule, representing a compelling rationale for its use in GBM treatment (Zhu, Woolfenden et al.). Another interesting viable, rising option is targeting Hsp90 in its different subcellular compartments. Recent reports have shown that Hsp90 localizes to mitochondria, nucleus and ER. In addition, Hsp90 is also secreted by tumor cells. Strikingly, recent reports have shown that Hsp90 readily accumulates in tumor mitochondria (Kang, Plescia et al., 2007; Kang, Plescia et al., 2009). Within tumor mitochondria, Hsp90, TRAP-1 and Cyclophilin-D are part of a complex that antagonizes the cell death-promoting factor, Cyclophilin-D (Kang, Plescia et al., 2007; Kang, Plescia et al., 2009). Based on the fact that Hsp90 is over-expressed in tumor mitochondria and is involved in antagonizing tumor cell death, Kang and colleagues developed several novel Hsp90-targeted drugs that were modeled on the basis of 17-AAG (Kang, Plescia et al., 2007; Kang, Plescia et al., 2009) (Figure 2). 17-AAG was modified and linked to mitochondrial target groups, such as Triphenylphosphoniumion (TPP), giving rise to a molecule called Gamitrinib-TPP. Since these drugs are expected to target the mitochondrial matrix protein, Cyclophilin-D, and are synthesized on the 17-AAG back bone, they were called, Geldanamycin - mitochondrial - matrix - inhibitors, gamitrinibs. So far, gamitrinibs were tested successfully in a number of cell lines, including breast, prostate and colon cancer (Kang, Siegelin et al.; Kang, Plescia et al., 2009). Recent results also suggest that these molecules are capable of cell death induction in primary and established glioblastoma cell lines (Siegelin, Dohi et al.). The mechanism of action by gamitrinib on glioblastoma cells seem to be independent on the genetic background as glioma cells harboring PTEN mutation, e.g. U87 and U251, or harboring mutated p53, e.g. LN229, responded equally to gamitrinib treatment. Once glioblastoma cells were treated with Gamitrinib-TPP, a sudden loss of mitochondrial membrane potential occurred, leading to a significant loss in cellular viability.

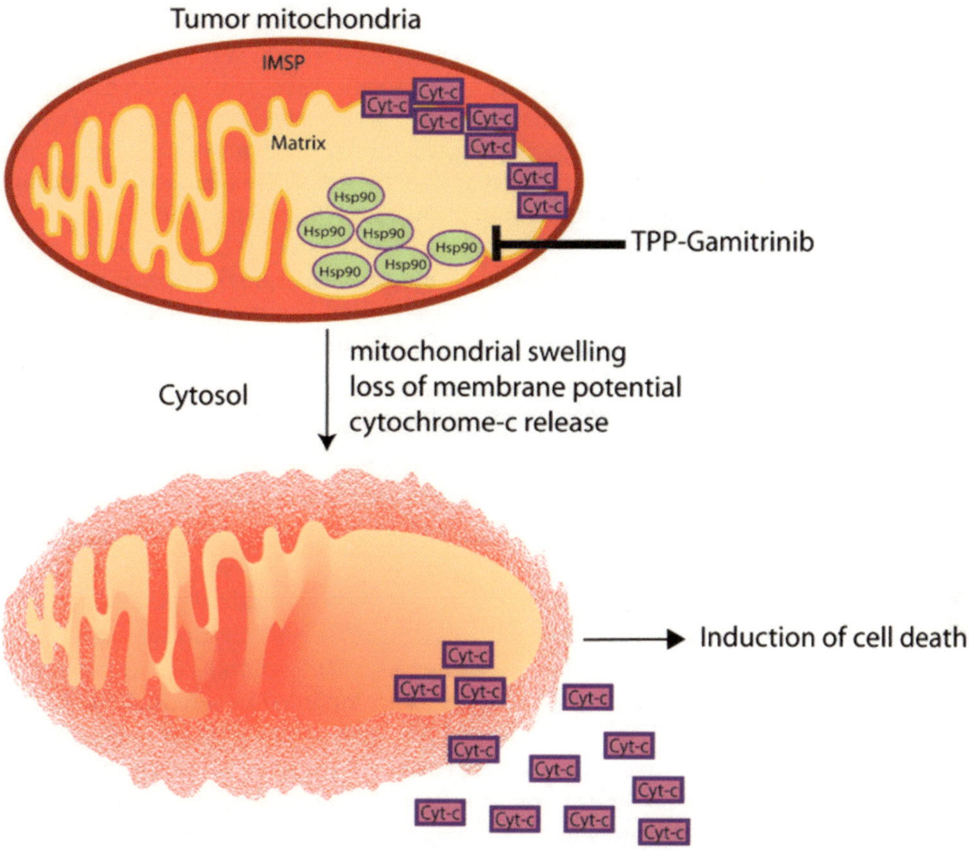

Fig. 2. Mechanism of action by TPP-Gamitrinib. TPP-Gamitrinib inhibits the mitochondrial pool of Hsp90 that is specifically over-expressed in tumor mitochondria and located in the mitochondrial matrix. Upon inhibition of Hsp90, mitochondrial swelling with loss of mitochondrial membrane potential is initiated. This leads to release of cytochrome-c from inter-membranous space (IMSP) into the cytosol. Within the cytosol, cytochrome-c induces induction of apoptosis by formation of the apoptosome and subsequently acitivation of caspases.

Mechanistically, this cell death had features of apoptosis and to some extent vacuole formation with evidence of autophagy. Inhibition of autophagy pharmacologically or genetically (siRNA mediated suppression of *atg5*) resulted in enhanced loss of cellular viability (Siegelin, Dohi et al.). Usually, mitochondrial mediated cell death is dependent on the bcl-2 family of proteins. The bcl-2 family of proteins comprises both pro-apoptotic and anti-apoptotic proteins, respectively. Finally, these proteins mediate the outer membrane permeability of the mitochondria. The bax and bak protein are known to enhance the outer membrane permeability, leading to a release of cytochrome-c from the inter-membranous mitochondrial space with the formation of the apoptosome with profound activation of caspases and induction of apoptosis (Kang, Plescia et al., 2009). Gamitrinibs do not require bax/bak protein for sufficient cell death induction (Kang, Plescia et al., 2009). In addition, gamitrinib-mediated cell death is also not inhibited by adenoviral-mediated bcl-2 overexpression (Kang, Plescia et al., 2009). Since many tumor cells, including glioblastomas, mediate therapeutic resistance by the over-expression of anti-apoptotic bcl-2 family proteins, e.g. bcl-2, Mcl-1, bcl-xL, the fact that gamitrinibs are not dependent on these molecules is a true advantage of this new class of molecules when compared for instance to established chemotherapeutic drugs. Since gamitrinibs exert anti-cancer and anti-glioma activity, additional studies are required to answer whether these reagents might synergize with either radiation and/or chemotherapy, particularly Temozolomide.

In summary, there is mounting evidence from preclinical studies that inhibition of Hsp90 by small-molecules inhibitors might represent a viable and suitable therapeutic strategy for the treatment of GBM. However, up to date no clinical trial has been launched for any Hsp90 antagonists to treat high-grade and low-grade gliomas in patients.

5. Polyphenols as a novel treatment options for gliomas

Recent research suggest a potential therapeutic value of polyphenols for cancer treatment. Polyphenols are natural compounds that can be found in a number of vegetables and fruits, green tea, roots, spices and red wine (Szliszka&Krol). According to their chemical structure, polyphenols can be subdivided by their chemical structure, consisting of flavonols, flavones, flavanols, isoflavones, flavonoligans and stilbenes (Szliszka&Krol). The main representatives of flavonols are quercetin, kaempferol and myricetin. Braghanol et al. showed that quercetin has anti-proliferative effects on U138 glioma cells (Braganhol, Zamin et al., 2006). Quercetin led to a G2 cell-cyle arrest accompanied by a reduction of mitotic rate (Braganhol, Zamin et al., 2006). In addition, this group was able to show that ischemic damage to hippocampal slice cultures was attenuated by quercetin (Braganhol, Zamin et al., 2006). These results are in so far exciting as quercetin obviously exerts anti-cancer effects on one of the most highly therapeutic resistant tumor, glioblastoma, while at the same concentrations it exhibits neuro-protection to oxygen-sensitive hippocampal neuronal cells. Other researchers have also confirmed the observation that quercetin might have anti-glioma activity. Kim et al. found that quercetin induced cell death in human glioma cells (Kim, Choi et al., 2008). Mechanistically, they found that quercetin inhibited the ERK and Akt pathway and that ectopic expression of constitutively active forms of ERK and Akt protected against quercetin mediated cell death in glioma (Kim, Choi et al., 2008). Furthermore, the inhibitor of apoptosis protein, survivin, was suppressed in a concentration dependent manner by quercetin (Kim, Choi et al., 2008). Since primary glioblastomas often exhibit loss of PTEN and/or amplification of EGFR, leading to a profound activation of the Akt pathway and possible resulting in an increased expression of survivin as survivin has been shown to be a downstream target of the Akt pathway, quercetin may be a novel welcome contribution in glioma therapy. However, additional *in vivo* studies are warranted to confirm these *in vitro* observations. In this regard, it has to be demonstrated that quercetin might inhibit the growth of xenografted human glioma cells in an orthotopic model of glioblastoma which would also indicate whether quercetin can cross the blood-brain barrier. Another interesting setting would be the combination of quercetin with established treatment modalities for glioblastoma, such as temozolomide or radiation therapy. In line with this hypothesis a recent report showed that quercetin acts in synergy with temozolomide in a astrocytoma cell line (Jakubowicz-Gil, Langner et al.) . However, so far it has not been validated whether also radiation therapy might synergize with quercetin. In summary, quercetin seems to be an interesting future drug candidate for gliomas. Kaempferol is another member of the above-mentioned group and has been shown to have activity against primary and established glioblastoma cells. In this context, it has been recently shown that kaempferol effectively sensitized glioblastoma cells to the cytotoxic effects of TRAIL (Siegelin, Reuss et al., 2008). While kaempferol and TRAIL by itself had almost no effect on cell death induction or specific induction of apoptosis, the combination of both had a dramatic effect on apoptosis induction with strong activation of the effector- and initiator caspases. This tremendous synergy effect was attributed at least in part to the suppression of the inhibitor of apoptosis protein, Survivin. Survivin inhibits the apoptotic cascasde at the core of the machinery, namely the effector caspases. Kaempferol led to a dramatic suppression of Survivin by a mechanism most likely involving the proteasome and the Akt pathway. Out of the flavanols, Epigallocatechin-3-gallate has been shown to have anti-glioma activity both as a single reagent as well as in combination with TRAIL (Siegelin, Habel et al., 2008) or even more relevant to current therapeutic approaches, temozolomide (Chen, Wang et al.). The combination of EGCG and Temozolomide was more effective than single reagents both *in vitro* and *in vivo (Chen, Wang et al.)*. Mechanistically, the anti-glioma effect of EGCG and Temozolomide was mediated through CHOP (CCAAT/enhancer binding protein homologous protein/GADD153), a stress-response transcriptional factor which was confirmed by specific siRNA mediated knock-down experiments *in vitro (Chen, Wang et al.)*. Furthermore, in an intracranial model either utilizing U251 glioblastoma cells (*p53 mutant*) or U87 glioblastoma cells (*p53 wild-type*) EGCG did not exert survival improval, whereas the combination of EGCG and Temozolomide significantly prolonged animal survival when compared to temozolomide alone (Chen, Wang et al.). Although EGCG did not increase animal survival by itself , it demonstrates efficacy in a combination regimen with temozolomide, suggesting that EGCG is capable of effectively crossing the blood-brain-barrier in orthotopic mouse glioblastoma models independent of *p53* mutational status (Chen, Wang et al.). It has also to be emphasized that EGCG and likewise temozolomide were administered orally, suggesting that even the oral route might be a suitable treatment strategy to combat glioblastoma to combat glioblastoma. Although the glioblastoma xenografts were not completely eradicated by the combined strategy, these results are nevertheless promising given the fact that the treatment was orally well tolerated and that there are only a very limit number of treatment options for GBM. In this regard, it would be interesting whether EGCG would also synergize with radiation therapy in the above-mentioned GBM xenograft models. Moreover, as U87 cells harbor a methylated MGMT promoter, one might also consider a triple therapy consisting of EGCG, temozolomide and radiation. Because glioblastomas diffusely infiltrate the adjacent brain parenchyma, it is of highest significance to inhibit tumor cell migration with regards to glioma therapy. EGCG was also capable of inhibiting migration in glioma cells by suppression of Metalloproteinase-2 (MMP-2) secretion. This finding further establishes a potential role for EGCG as an anti-glioma reagent. In summary, flavonoids might represent an interesting novel therapeutic venue for glioblastoma. Figure 3 provides a quick overview of the pathways and molecules that are inhibited by polyphneols in glioblastoma cells. Polyphenols inhibit apoptotic and proliferation pathways (c-FLIP, inhibitors of apoptosis proteins, Akt and ERK pathway). In addition they even exert anti-migratory activity by MMP-2 suppression.

Particularly exciting is the fact that these molecules are abundant in food and that there anti-glioma activity seems to be tumor specific as hippocampal neurons were even protected by polyphenol treatment after ischemic injury. Therefore, researchers often link these molecules to chemoprevention. Moreover, the fact that these molecules are able to synergize with TMZ (EGCG) and TRAIL (Quercetin) suggests even that these molecules might have a significant value in combinatorial drug treatments. Up to date, no clinical trial with polyphenol for treatment of glioblastoma has been initiated.

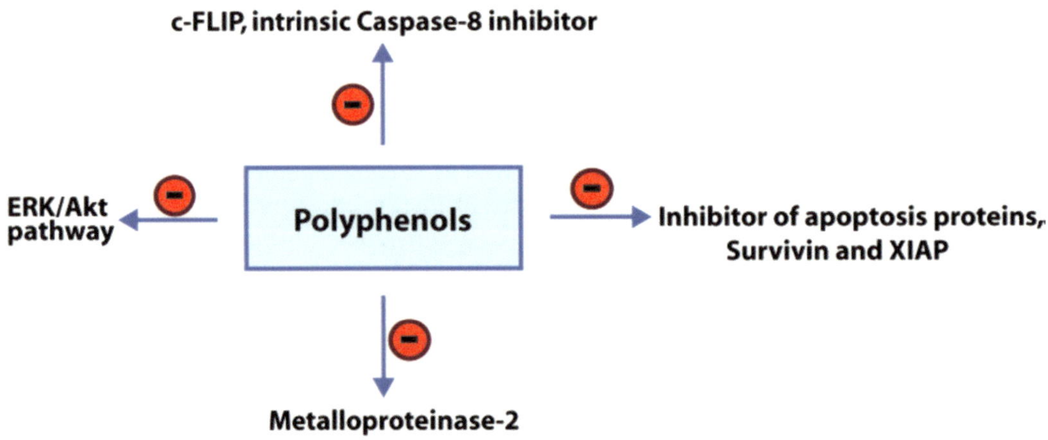

Fig. 3. Anti-glioma activity of polyphenols. Recent data suggests that polyphenols inhibit apoptotic pathways, Erk/Akt pathway, c-FLIP and the inhibitor of apoptosis proteins. They also inhibit glioma migration by suppression of Metalloproteinase-2.

6. The exploitation of the extrinsic apoptotic pathway by tumor necrosis factor alpha related apoptosis inducing ligand, TRAIL, in glioblastoma

TRAIL is a promising death receptor ligand that upon interaction with its receptors induces programmed cell death, called apoptosis. TRAIL interacts with its membrane-bound receptors (DR4/DR5), leading to the activation of caspase-8 in the tumor cells. Caspase 8 can either directly activate caspase-3 to induce apoptotic cell death (extrinsic pathway) or it can cleave the protein BID, leading to release of cytochrome –c from the mitochondria with subsequent formation of the apoptosome and activation of caspase-9 (Figure 4). In turn, caspase-9 activates caspase - 3 (intrinsic pathway). Depending on the individual cell type, there are so called type-I cells that signal straight from caspase-8 to caspase-3 for the induction of apoptosis (Figure 4). In contrast, type-II cells, which encompass the majority of glioblastoma tumor cells, require signal amplification by activation of the intrinsic pathway. This has further important implications since glioblastomas over-express a number of anti-apoptotic factors that exert their activity through inhibition of the release of cytochrome - c from the mitochondria into the cytosol.

TRAIL binds to DR4/5 (DR:death receptor), TRAIL R1/R2 (TRAIL R: TRAIL receptor), and subsequently leads to an activation process of caspase-8 (through involvement of the adaptor protein FADD). Activation of caspase-8 is inhibited by the intrinsic capase-8 inhibitor, c-FLIP. C-FLIP itself consists of several isoforms, of which the long and short isoform have gained considerable importance. Caspase-8 activates Caspase-3 to mediate apoptotic cell death (type I pathway). Caspase-8 may also cleave BID, resulting in a release of cytochrome-c from the mitochondria and formation of a complex, called apoptosome (Cytochrome-c, Apaf-1, Procaspase-9 and dATP (not shown). Within the apoptosome Caspase-9 is activated and cleaves Caspase-3 to engage apoptotic cell death (type-II pathway). The release of cytochrome-c can be inhibited by the bcl-2 familiy of proteins, e.g. Bcl-2, Bcl-Xl and Mcl-1. Effector caspase activation (Caspase-3) is intrinsically inhibited by the Inhibitor of apoptosis proteins, IAP. Examples of IAPs are XIAP and Survivin.

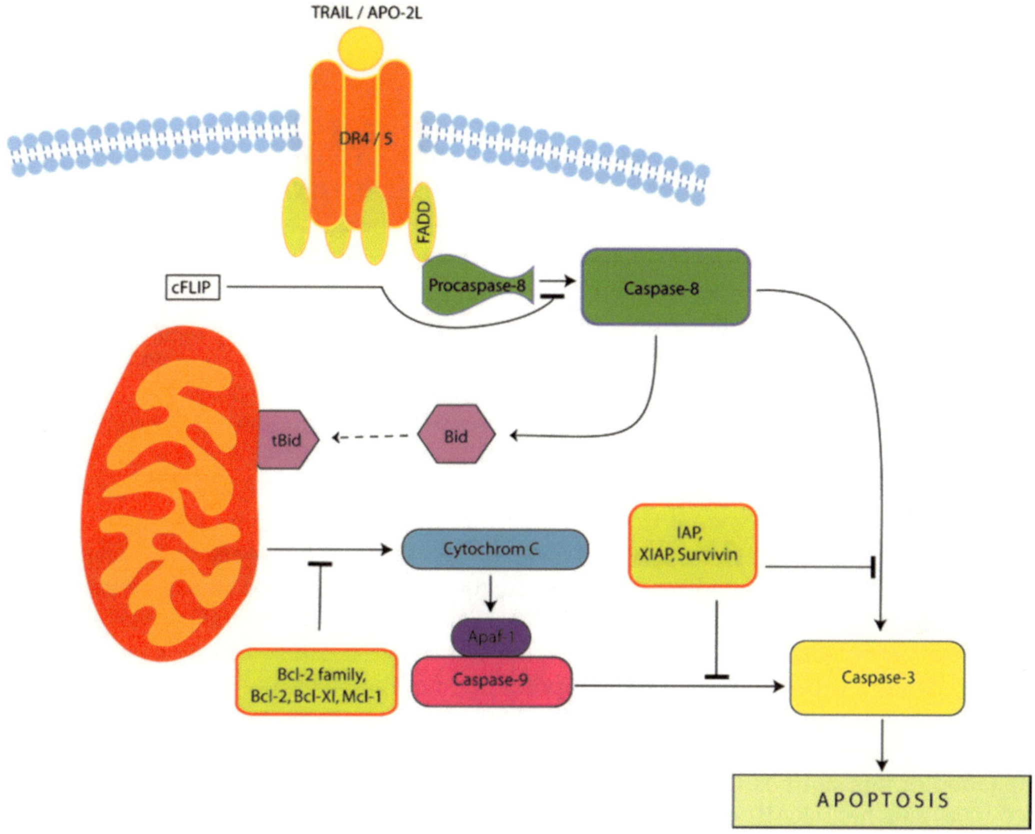

Fig. 4. Signaling pathway of TRAIL.

TRAIL was initially described and cloned based on its homology to CD95 in 1995. In 1999, two independent research groups identified TRAIL as a powerful and highly specific anti-cancer molecule. Walczak et al. created a "trimeric TRAIL" by introducing a leucine-zipper backbone into the TRAIL molecule (leucine zipper TRAIL, LZ-TRAIL) (Ashkenazi, Pai et al., 1999; Walczak, Miller et al., 1999). This led to a tremendous intrinsic activity towards cancer cells without any significant toxicity against non-neoplastic cells. In sharp contrast to CD95, which upon systemic administration to rodents led to fulminant hepatotoxicity, LZ-TRAIL was shown to be non-toxic to hepatocytes (Walczak, Miller et al., 1999). They also demonstrated that LZ-TRAIL was effective in a skin-xenograft model using human mammary adenocarcinoma cell line MDA-231 that was sensitive to LZ-TRAIL *in vitro (Walczak, Miller et al., 1999)*. Histologically, TRAIL induced an apoptotic like cell death as demonstrated by H.E. staining. In the same year, Ashkenazi and colleagues reported about another form of TRAIL that might be used for therapy (Ashkenazi, Pai et al., 1999). They presented a version of TRAIL that is devoid of tags, spans from amino acid 114 to 281 and is produced in bacteria (Ashkenazi, Pai et al., 1999). In addition, they found that TRAIL (114-281) did not kill normal cells and also injection in monkeys did not cause toxicity (Ashkenazi, Pai et al., 1999). In contrast, TRAIL had either cytotoxic or cytostatic effects on a number of tumor cell lines, including lung, breast, colon and also glioma (Ashkenazi, Pai et al., 1999). Strikingly, the in vivo administration in xenograft models was well tolerated and prolonged animal survival without detectable toxicity in non-cancerous tissues (Ashkenazi, Pai et al., 1999). The above-mentioned reports have several things in common. They clearly demonstrate that TRAIL has tumor specificity and that it effects are really dramatic in sensitive tumors. The major differences in these reports are the TRAIL formulations being employed. Walczak et al. used a version of TRAIL with a tag, whereas Ashkenazi used a tag-free version of TRAIL. Recently, the tag-free version of TRAIL (Dulanermin) has also entered several clinical trials (www.clinicaltrials.gov). One recent phase Ib, open-label, multicenter trial study in which Dulanermin was used has been completed. In this study, Dulanermin was administered in combination with rituximab in patients with low-grade lymphomas (www.clinicaltrials.gov). In addition, there are two trials involving either locally advanced or metastatic colorectal cancer, in which Dulanermin is combined with bevacizumab and the FOLFOX regimen (www.clinicaltrials.gov).

Following the discovery of TRAIL as an anti-cancer drug by Walczak et. al and Ashkenazi et al., Roth and colleagues found that TRAIL might also be effective for the treatment of Glioblastoma multiforme WHO grade IV (Roth, Isenmann et al., 1999). They nicely showed that TRAIL was also effective in the treatment for an orthotopic model of glioblastoma in nude mice. Only two repetitive doses of 2 uG of TRAIL were necessary to achieve long - term survival in these animals (>100 days) as compared to animals treated with vehicle solution (36 days) (Roth, Isenmann et al., 1999). Histologically, TRAIL induced an apoptotic like cell death as shown by TUNEL (terminal transferase-catalyzed in situ end-labeling) staining (Roth, Isenmann et al., 1999). Importantly, no obvious acute or delayed neuronal toxicity was detected upon treatment with TRAIL. Although these results are very exciting and promising particularly with regards to the dismal prognosis of GBM, the significant limitation of this study is that TRAIL was administered intracranially and therefore it was not clear whether TRAIL could cross the blood-brain barrier. Two years later in 2001, a group of scientist found that Apo2L/TRAIL given systemically was an effective treatment of orthotopic glioblastoma xenografts (mice) utilizing U87 glioma cells (Pollack, Erff et al., 2001). Specifically, they found that at a dosage of 30 mg/kg of TRAIL administered by intra-peritoneal infusion (pump system) resulted in a long-term survival (more than 120 days) of all animals (Pollack, Erff et al., 2001). These results suggested that TRAIL might be an effective drug for astrocytic brain cancers and that obviously TRAIL was able to penetrate the blood-brain barrier without any significant side effects in the animals. Of course, these results are promising but also still harbor significant caveats. The main pitfall is the requirement of constant administration of TRAIL which would be practical difficult in humans. Another important aspect is whether the dosage used in the animal studies can be translated into humans without buying serious and unwanted side effects. Nevertheless, the two reports by Pollack and Roth clearly demonstrate that TRAIL is a potential treatment strategy for malignant gliomas. Given the unfavorable pharmacokinetics of TRAIL and presence of the blood-brain barrier in the setting of malignant glioma, a new exciting strategy was recently developed to specifically transport TRAIL to the tumor side. This excellent idea entails the usage of neural stem cells. In the year 2000, a group of researchers demonstrated that neural stem cells expressing a foreign gene for the exploitation of therapy revealed a strong tropism to glioblastoma cells *in vivo* (Aboody, Brown et al., 2000; Ehtesham, Kabos et al., 2002). Importantly, neural stem cells were shown to hunt down the infiltrating glioma cells while retaining the expression of a foreign gene (Aboody, Brown et al., 2000). When injected in the contra-lateral hemisphere neural stem cells were able to migrate into the glioma and even more relevant the administration of neural stem cells outside the central nervous system resulted in effective accumulation of neural stem cells in glioma tumors (Aboody, Brown et al., 2000). To test therapeutic efficacy, this group transduced neural stem cells with cytosine deaminase and then achieved significant reduction in tumor growth in an experimental model of glioma (Aboody, Brown et al., 2000). Two years later, Aboody et al. engineered neural stem cells expressing TRAIL and assessed the efficacy of neural stem cells secreting TRAIL in an orthotopic glioma model utilizing U343MG glioma cells. It has to be pointed out that the U343MG cells are relatively sensitive to the apoptotic effects of TRAIL as compared to other glioma cells lines such as LN229 or U87 cells that would require higher TRAIL dosages or a sensitizing reagent. The established gliomas (7 days after implantation) were treated with intra-tumoral injections of neural stem cells expressing TRAIL, neural stem cells expressing a control gene or saline. While saline and neural stem cells expressing gene had the same effect, the neural stem cells secreting TRAIL reduced the size of the tumors impressively (Aboody, Brown et al., 2000). One controversial aspect is of course the fact that this group did not utilize some sort of imaging to definitely confirm the establishment of the tumors. However, according to personal and also to other research groups experience orthotopic glioma models have a nearly 100% engrafting rate.

A main obstacle of TRAIL-based therapies is that a number of glioblastoma cells are resistant to the apoptotic effects of TRAIL. This issue becomes even worse considering the lacking markers on diagnostic tissue predicting TRAIL sensitivity. As described already TRAIL signals via distinct death receptors. In glioma recent data suggests that a descent number of high-grade gliomas exhibit silenced expression of death receptor 4, which is clearly explained through an epigenetic mechanism (Elias, Siegelin et al., 2009). Remarkable is the fact that treatment with a broad demethylating reagent restores expression of death receptor 4, suggesting that this resistance mechanism is reversible and targetable. However, it has been known already for quite some time that the actual expression of TRAIL receptors is per se not an indicator for TRAIL sensitivity (Wagner, Punnoose et al., 2007). In this context, it has been revealed that the expression of peptidyl O-glycosyltransferase GALNT14 determined the susceptibility of various cancer cells to TRAIL. However, this correlation was mainly detected in pancreatic, lung and skin cancer, suggesting that GALNT14 might be a predictor with obvious limitations, indicating that further markers to predict sensitivity are still required to be identified. Given the present issues with resistance it is of utmost importance to overcome this resistance which can be achieved by antagonizing certain anti-apoptotic molecules, such as c-FLIP, anti-apoptotic proteins of the bcl-2 family and inhibitors of apoptosis proteins, such as XIAP and Survivin. To this end, Fulda and colleagues combined TRAIL with a Smac-mimetic peptide that antagonizes XIAP (Fulda, Wick et al., 2002). This combination therapy was shown to eradicate orthotopic glioblastoma xenografts, leading to a long-term survival in animals treated with this drug combination

(Fulda, Wick et al., 2002). Despite this tremendous anti-glioma activity the limitation of this study was that TRAIL was applied loco regional. Nevertheless, this demonstration of drug efficacy was quite remarkable. Since GBMs usually do not metastasize and have a tendency to recur at their initial presentation spot, locoregional treatment approaches are feasible for malignant gliomas.

Many TRAIL-based drug combinations for the treatment of GBM have been employed successfully since 1999. Since the mainstay treatment for GBM consists of radiation and/or chemotherapy with temozolomide, combining these treatment modalities with TRAIL is a main issue. So far, these combinations in the setting of an experimental glioma model include, but are not limited to, TRAIL+Temozolomide (Saito, Bringas et al., 2004), TRAIL+radiation therapy (Nagane, Cavenee et al., 2007), TRAIL+Bortezomib (Jane, Premkumar et al.; Koschny, Holland et al., 2007), TRAIL+ABT737 (Tagscherer, Fassl et al., 2008), , TRAIL+Quercetin (Siegelin, Reuss et al., 2009), TRAIL+Kaempferol (Siegelin, Reuss et al., 2008) , TRAIL+Celecoxib (Gaiser, Becker et al., 2008), TRAIL + PI-103 (a PI-3 Kinase Inhibitor) (Bagci-Onder, Wakimoto et al.), TRAIL + Troglitazone (Akasaki, Liu et al., 2006; Schultze, Bock et al., 2006), TRAIL + 17-AAG (Siegelin, Habel et al., 2009) and TRAIL + Gamitrinibs (Siegelin, Dohi et al.). Most of these combinations work by enhancing either the extrinsic or intrinsic apoptotic pathway, respectively. As an example the extrinsic apoptotic pathway is controlled by the TRAIL-receptors, Caspase-8 and the c-FLIP. C-FLIP can be present in several isoforms, e.g. a long c-FLIP (L) and a short isoform c-FLIP (S). It is well established as an inhibitor of caspase-8, thereby inhibiting either direct activation of apoptosis through caspase -3/-7 or indirect through cleavage of BID and engagement of the intrinsic apoptotic pathway through cytochrome-c release, formation of the apoptosome and activation of caspase-9. Temozolomide has been shown to modulate the expression of death receptors (Saito, Bringas et al., 2004), and the proteasomal inhibitor, Bortezombib, decreased c-FLIP protein levels in primary glioma cells (Koschny, Holland et al., 2007). The intrinsic pathway is largely controlled by the Bcl-2 family of proteins, e.g. Bcl-Xl, Mcl-1 and bcl-2. However, the intrinsic pathway is also indirectly influenced by the inhibitor of apoptosis protein family, such as XIAP and survivin. ABT-737 is an inhibitor of the bcl-2 family of proteins. ABT-737 is a molecule that requires high levels of bcl-2 and low levels of Mcl-1 in order to exert efficacy. As glioblastoma cells are known to over-express the anti-apoptotic bcl-2 proteins, ABT-737 was capable to sensitize glioblastoma cells to TRAIL-mediated apoptosis. Recently, the therapeutic efficacy of a novel PI3-kinase/mTOR inhibitor, PI-103, was evaluated in the combination with TRAIL. The importance of the mTOR and PI-3 Kinase pathway in gliomas has been well know and many GBM and tumor stem cells in gliomas rely on the activation of these two pathways giving them resistance to apoptotic stimuli by the enhancement of certain anti-apoptotic molecules regulating either the extrinisic or intrinsic apoptotic pathways, such as c-FLIP, IAPs or bcl-2 family of proteins. In an orthotopic glioblastoma animal model they showed that neural stem cell derived TRAIL in combination with PI-103 was more effective in tumor growth inhibition than either single treatments alone (Bagci-Onder, Wakimoto et al.). 17-AAG and flavonoids led to a down-regulation of survivin protein and thereby overcame TRAIL-resistance in glioma cells.

Recently, we discovered a novel mechanism to sensitize tumor cells, including glioma cells, to the cytotoxic effects of TRAIL. Tumor cells have been shown to organize a tumor-cell specific chaperone network within their mitochondria. This network consists of at least Hsp90, the mitochondrial Hsp-90 homologue, TRAP-1 and Cyclophilin-D. These proteins form a complex to antagonize the pro-apoptotic function of Cyclophilin-D (Kang, Plescia et al., 2007). Antagonizing this chaperone network might be therefore interesting for the treatment of tumors. To this end, a novel molecule that encompasses 17-AAG linked with a mitochondrial targeting sequence, called Triphenylphosphoniumion (TPP), was developed (Kang, Plescia et al., 2009). This molecule (G-TPP) was part of the family of so called Gamitrinibs, Geldanamycin-mitochondrial-matrix-inhibitors (Kang, Plescia et al., 2009). Treatment of glioma cells with G-TPP led to the induction of a mitochondrial unfolded protein response (UPR) and to the initiation of a specific transcriptional program (Siegelin, Dohi et al.). This transcritpional induction involved the up-regulation of CHOP and CEBP/beta and concomitant to a strong suppression of NF-kB activity (Siegelin, Dohi et al.). The suppression of NF-kB activity was partially responsible for the tremendous sensitization of apoptosis-resistant glioblastoma cells to TRAIL *in vitro*. Furthermore, it was demonstrated that this combination of gamitrinib and TRAIL was highly efficient in *an vivo* setting of glioblastoma. To this end, a well-known orthotopic glioblastoma model was employed. In this model, U87 glioblastoma cells (p53 wt/PTEN mutant) were transduced with a viral luciferase construct giving rise to U87-luc cells. U87-luc cells were stereotactically injected into the right striatum of nude mice. Established tumors were then treated with vehicle solution, TRAIL, Gamitrinib and the combination of TRAIL and Gamitrinibs. Remarkably, only the combination treatment exhibited significant effects on bioluminescence intensities, suggesting a significant induction of cell death and inhibition of proliferation as indicated by Ki-67 and TUNEL-staining, respectively. Given all these novel and pretty promising experimental findings on TRAIL and glioblastoma, clinical trials involving this substance either as a single reagent or in combination is warranted. Since many of the combination partners of TRAIL are already in clinical use, the threshold of approval for a combined administration of TRAIL with established therapeutics should be reasonable.

7. Conclusion

Although glioblastoma (average reported incident of 6-7/100.000 new cases (Krakstad&Chekenya)) is a relatively rare disease and might be considered as an orphan disease, viable, effective treatment strategies need to be identified. Hence, regardless of its rareness humans die from this deadly disease. Regarding to its prevalence, pharmaceutical companies might not have a reasonable financial interest to invest into novel drug discoveries for glioblastoma. That being said, non-profit organizations such as universities are in charge to identify and characterize established and novel pathways in glioblastoma. A very recent example of a significant discovery in glioma biology was the identification of IDH1 mutation in low-grade and high-grade gliomas. This finding was made independently by several non-profit organizations showing that IDH1 is mutated particularly in secondary glioblastomas. Cell lines ectopically expressing this mutation showed slower tumor growth *in vitro* and *in vivo*, and patients harboring this mutation had a longer median survival. In addition, we reviewed some of the most recent novel research on glioblastoma therapy emphasizing mostly on preclinical developments. Specifically, we focused here on EGFR inhibitors, Hsp90 antagonists, polyphenols and the activation of apoptosis by TRAIL. The EGFR inhibitors are a recent example for the practical pathway of drug discovery. First, a genetic alteration was found. Second, the role of the genetic alterations was studied regarding its importance for tumor growth in experimental, preclinical models and in patients, respectively. Third, based on these data pharmaceutical companies developed drugs (Erlotinib and Geftinib) to specifically target these genetic alterations. Unfortunately, a recent phase II trial in GBM patients with erlotinib revealed no therapeutic benefit. Therefore, additional treatment approaches targeting multiple pathways should be exploited. In this line, targeting the Hsp90 by 17-AAG might be another suitable approach for the treatment of GBM as Hsp90 binds a number of important tumor growth driving molecules in GBM and 17-AAG revealed anti-glioma effects in several preclinical models of GBM. In addition, recent evidence suggested that targeting of the mitochondrial Hsp90 pool by a drug-modified 17-AAG showed efficacy on glioblastoma cells. Finally, 17-AAG has been successfully exploited in other tumor entities in patients. Polyphenols are also a promising group of molecules for the treatment of GBM, which is at least suggested by recent experimental data. Finally, induction of apoptosis by TRAIL might be a welcome contribution to glioblastoma therapy as it preclinical activity suggests dramatic, specific anti-glioma activity, particularly when administered in combination with other reagents. Although at this point glioblastoma remains incurable, even these reported small progresses will finally lead to the identification of novel, fresh effective drug combinations in the future.

8. References

Aboody, K. S., A. Brown, N. G. Rainov, K. A. Bower, S. Liu, W. Yang, J. E. Small, U. Herrlinger, V. Ourednik, P. M. Black, X. O. Breakefield &E. Y. Snyder. (2000). Neural stem cells display extensive tropism for pathology in adult brain: evidence from intracranial gliomas. *Proc Natl Acad Sci U S A*, 97, 23, Nov 7, 12846-51

Akasaki, Y., G. Liu, H. H. Matundan, H. Ng, X. Yuan, Z. Zeng, K. L. Black &J. S. Yu. (2006). A peroxisome proliferator-activated receptor-gamma agonist, troglitazone, facilitates caspase-8 and -9 activities by increasing the enzymatic activity of protein-tyrosine phosphatase-1B on human glioma cells. *J Biol Chem*, 281, 10, Mar 10, 6165-74

Ashkenazi, A., R. C. Pai, S. Fong, S. Leung, D. A. Lawrence, S. A. Marsters, C. Blackie, L. Chang, A. E. McMurtrey, A. Hebert, L. DeForge, I. L. Koumenis, D. Lewis, L. Harris, J. Bussiere, H. Koeppen, Z. Shahrokh &R. H. Schwall. (1999). Safety and antitumor activity of recombinant soluble Apo2 ligand. *J Clin Invest*, 104, 2, Jul, 155-62

Bagci-Onder, T., H. Wakimoto, M. Anderegg, C. Cameron &K. Shah. A dual PI3K/mTOR inhibitor, PI-103, cooperates with stem cell-delivered TRAIL in experimental glioma models. *Cancer Res*, 71, 1, Jan 1, 154-63

Braganhol, E., L. L. Zamin, A. D. Canedo, F. Horn, A. S. Tamajusuku, M. R. Wink, C. Salbego &A. M. Battastini. (2006). Antiproliferative effect of quercetin in the human U138MG glioma cell line. *Anticancer Drugs*, 17, 6, Jul, 663-71

Camelo-Piragua, S., M. Jansen, A. Ganguly, J. C. Kim, D. N. Louis &C. L. Nutt. Mutant IDH1-specific immunohistochemistry distinguishes diffuse astrocytoma from astrocytosis. *Acta Neuropathol*, 119, 4, Apr, 509-11

Capper, D., H. Zentgraf, J. Balss, C. Hartmann &A. von Deimling. (2009). Monoclonal antibody specific for IDH1 R132H mutation. *Acta Neuropathol*, 118, 5, Nov, 599-601

Chakravarti, A., G. Zhai, Y. Suzuki, S. Sarkesh, P. M. Black, A. Muzikansky &J. S. Loeffler. (2004). The prognostic significance of phosphatidylinositol 3-kinase pathway activation in human gliomas. *J Clin Oncol*, 22, 10, May 15, 1926-33

Chen, T. C., W. Wang, E. B. Golden, S. Thomas, W. Sivakumar, F. M. Hofman, S. G. Louie &A. H. Schonthal. Green tea epigallocatechin gallate enhances therapeutic efficacy of temozolomide in orthotopic mouse glioblastoma models. *Cancer Lett*, 302, 2, Mar 28, 100-8

Ehtesham, M., P. Kabos, M. A. Gutierrez, N. H. Chung, T. S. Griffith, K. L. Black &J. S. Yu. (2002). Induction of glioblastoma apoptosis using neural stem cell-mediated delivery of tumor necrosis factor-related apoptosis-inducing ligand. *Cancer Res*, 62, 24, Dec 15, 7170-4

Ekstrand, A. J., C. D. James, W. K. Cavenee, B. Seliger, R. F. Pettersson &V. P. Collins. (1991). Genes for epidermal growth factor receptor, transforming growth factor alpha, and epidermal growth factor and their expression in human gliomas in vivo. *Cancer Res*, 51, 8, Apr 15, 2164-72

Elias, A., M. D. Siegelin, A. Steinmuller, A. von Deimling, U. Lass, B. Korn &W. Mueller. (2009). Epigenetic silencing of death receptor 4 mediates tumor necrosis factor-related apoptosis-inducing ligand resistance in gliomas. *Clin Cancer Res*, 15, 17, Sep 1, 5457-65

Fulda, S., W. Wick, M. Weller &K. M. Debatin. (2002). Smac agonists sensitize for Apo2L/TRAIL- or anticancer drug-induced apoptosis and induce regression of malignant glioma in vivo. *Nat Med*, 8, 8, Aug, 808-15

Gaiser, T., M. R. Becker, A. Habel, D. E. Reuss, V. Ehemann, A. Rami &M. D. Siegelin. (2008). TRAIL-mediated apoptosis in malignant glioma cells is augmented by celecoxib through proteasomal degradation of survivin. *Neurosci Lett*, 442, 2, Sep 12, 109-13

Gaspar, N., S. Y. Sharp, S. A. Eccles, S. Gowan, S. Popov, C. Jones, A. Pearson, G. Vassal &P. Workman. Mechanistic evaluation of the novel HSP90 inhibitor NVP-AUY922 in adult and pediatric glioblastoma. *Mol Cancer Ther*, 9, 5, May, 1219-33

Gaspar, N., S. Y. Sharp, S. Pacey, C. Jones, M. Walton, G. Vassal, S. Eccles, A. Pearson &P. Workman. (2009). Acquired resistance to 17-allylamino-17-demethoxygeldanamycin (17-AAG, tanespimycin) in glioblastoma cells. *Cancer Res*, 69, 5, Mar 1, 1966-75

Hegi, M. E., A. C. Diserens, T. Gorlia, M. F. Hamou, N. de Tribolet, M. Weller, J. M. Kros, J. A. Hainfellner, W. Mason, L. Mariani, J. E. Bromberg, P. Hau, R. O. Mirimanoff, J. G. Cairncross, R. C. Janzer &R. Stupp. (2005). MGMT gene silencing and benefit from temozolomide in glioblastoma. *N Engl J Med*, 352, 10, Mar 10, 997-1003

Jakubowicz-Gil, J., E. Langner, I. Wertel, T. Piersiak &W. Rzeski. Temozolomide, quercetin and cell death in the MOGGCCM astrocytoma cell line. *Chem Biol Interact*, 188, 1, Oct 6, 190-203

Jane, E. P., D. R. Premkumar &I. F. Pollack. Bortezomib sensitizes malignant human glioma cells to TRAIL, mediated by inhibition of the NF-{kappa}B signaling pathway. *Mol Cancer Ther*, 10, 1, Jan, 198-208

Kang, B. H., J. Plescia, T. Dohi, J. Rosa, S. J. Doxsey &D. C. Altieri. (2007). Regulation of tumor cell mitochondrial homeostasis by an organelle-specific Hsp90 chaperone network. *Cell*, 131, 2, Oct 19, 257-70

Kang, B. H., J. Plescia, H. Y. Song, M. Meli, G. Colombo, K. Beebe, B. Scroggins, L. Neckers &D. C. Altieri. (2009). Combinatorial drug design targeting multiple cancer signaling networks controlled by mitochondrial Hsp90. *J Clin Invest*, 119, 3, Mar, 454-64

Kang, B. H., M. D. Siegelin, J. Plescia, C. M. Raskett, D. S. Garlick, T. Dohi, J. B. Lian, G. S. Stein, L. R. Languino &D. C. Altieri. Preclinical characterization of mitochondria-targeted small molecule hsp90 inhibitors, gamitrinibs, in advanced prostate cancer. *Clin Cancer Res*, 16, 19, Oct 1, 4779-88

Kim, E. J., C. H. Choi, J. Y. Park, S. K. Kang &Y. K. Kim. (2008). Underlying mechanism of quercetin-induced cell death in human glioma cells. *Neurochem Res*, 33, 6, Jun, 971-9

Koschny, R., H. Holland, J. Sykora, T. L. Haas, M. R. Sprick, T. M. Ganten, W. Krupp, M. Bauer, P. Ahnert, J. Meixensberger &H. Walczak. (2007). Bortezomib sensitizes primary human astrocytoma cells of WHO grades I to IV for tumor necrosis factor-related apoptosis-inducing ligand-induced apoptosis. *Clin Cancer Res*, 13, 11, Jun 1, 3403-12

Krakstad, C. &M. Chekenya. Survival signalling and apoptosis resistance in glioblastomas: opportunities for targeted therapeutics. *Mol Cancer*, 9, 135

Mercer, R. W., M. A. Tyler, I. V. Ulasov &M. S. Lesniak. (2009). Targeted therapies for malignant glioma: progress and potential. *BioDrugs*, 23, 1, 25-35

Nagane, M., W. K. Cavenee &Y. Shiokawa. (2007). Synergistic cytotoxicity through the activation of multiple apoptosis pathways in human glioma cells induced by combined treatment with ionizing radiation and tumor necrosis factor-related apoptosis-inducing ligand. *J Neurosurg*, 106, 3, Mar, 407-16

Ohba, S., Y. Hirose, K. Yoshida, T. Yazaki &T. Kawase. Inhibition of 90-kD heat shock protein potentiates the cytotoxicity of chemotherapeutic agents in human glioma cells. *J Neurosurg*, 112, 1, Jan, 33-42

Parsons, D. W., S. Jones, X. Zhang, J. C. Lin, R. J. Leary, P. Angenendt, P. Mankoo, H. Carter, I. M. Siu, G. L. Gallia, A. Olivi, R. McLendon, B. A. Rasheed, S. Keir, T. Nikolskaya, Y. Nikolsky, D. A. Busam, H. Tekleab, L. A. Diaz, Jr., J. Hartigan, D. R. Smith, R. L. Strausberg, S. K. Marie, S. M. Shinjo, H. Yan, G. J. Riggins, D. D. Bigner, R. Karchin, N. Papadopoulos, G. Parmigiani, B. Vogelstein, V. E. Velculescu &K. W. Kinzler. (2008). An integrated genomic analysis of human glioblastoma multiforme. *Science*, 321, 5897, Sep 26, 1807-12

Piaskowski, S., M. Bienkowski, E. Stoczynska-Fidelus, R. Stawski, M. Sieruta, M. Szybka, W. Papierz, M. Wolanczyk, D. J. Jaskolski, P. P. Liberski &P. Rieske. Glioma cells showing IDH1 mutation cannot be propagated in standard cell culture conditions. *Br J Cancer*, Feb 15,

Pollack, I. F., M. Erff &A. Ashkenazi. (2001). Direct stimulation of apoptotic signaling by soluble Apo2l/tumor necrosis factor-related apoptosis-inducing ligand leads to selective killing of glioma cells. *Clin Cancer Res*, 7, 5, May, 1362-9

Ren, H., B. F. Yang &N. G. Rainov. (2007). Receptor tyrosine kinases as therapeutic targets in malignant glioma. *Rev Recent Clin Trials*, 2, 2, May, 87-101

Roth, W., S. Isenmann, U. Naumann, S. Kugler, M. Bahr, J. Dichgans, A. Ashkenazi &M. Weller. (1999). Locoregional Apo2L/TRAIL eradicates intracranial human malignant glioma xenografts in athymic mice in the absence of neurotoxicity. *Biochem Biophys Res Commun*, 265, 2, Nov 19, 479-83

Saito, R., J. R. Bringas, A. Panner, M. Tamas, R. O. Pieper, M. S. Berger &K. S. Bankiewicz. (2004). Convection-enhanced delivery of tumor necrosis factor-related apoptosis-inducing ligand with systemic administration of temozolomide prolongs survival in an intracranial glioblastoma xenograft model. *Cancer Res*, 64, 19, Oct 1, 6858-62

Sathornsumetee, S., A. Desjardins, J. J. Vredenburgh, R. E. McLendon, J. Marcello, J. E. Herndon, A. Mathe, M. Hamilton, J. N. Rich, J. A. Norfleet, S. Gururangan, H. S. Friedman &D. A. Reardon. Phase II trial of bevacizumab and erlotinib in patients with recurrent malignant glioma. *Neuro Oncol*, 12, 12, Dec, 1300-10

Sauvageot, C. M., J. L. Weatherbee, S. Kesari, S. E. Winters, J. Barnes, J. Dellagatta, N. R. Ramakrishna, C. D. Stiles, A. L. Kung, M. W. Kieran &P. Y. Wen. (2009). Efficacy of the HSP90 inhibitor 17-AAG in human glioma cell lines and tumorigenic glioma stem cells. *Neuro Oncol*, 11, 2, Apr, 109-21

Schultze, K., B. Bock, A. Eckert, L. Oevermann, D. Ramacher, O. Wiestler &W. Roth. (2006). Troglitazone sensitizes tumor cells to TRAIL-induced apoptosis via down-regulation of FLIP and Survivin. *Apoptosis*, 11, 9, Sep, 1503-12

Seltzer, M. J., B. D. Bennett, A. D. Joshi, P. Gao, A. G. Thomas, D. V. Ferraris, T. Tsukamoto, C. J. Rojas, B. S. Slusher, J. D. Rabinowitz, C. V. Dang &G. J. Riggins. Inhibition of glutaminase preferentially slows growth of glioma cells with mutant IDH1. *Cancer Res*, 70, 22, Nov 15, 8981-7

Siegelin, M. D., T. Dohi, C. M. Raskett, G. M. Orlowski, C. M. Powers, C. A. Gilbert, A. H. Ross, J. Plescia &D. C. Altieri. Exploiting the mitochondrial unfolded protein response for cancer therapy in mice and human cells. *J Clin Invest*, Mar 1,

Siegelin, M. D., A. Habel &T. Gaiser. (2008). Epigalocatechin-3-gallate (EGCG) downregulates PEA15 and thereby augments TRAIL-mediated apoptosis in malignant glioma. *Neurosci Lett*, 448, 1, Dec 19, 161-5

Siegelin, M. D., A. Habel &T. Gaiser. (2009). 17-AAG sensitized malignant glioma cells to death-receptor mediated apoptosis. *Neurobiol Dis*, 33, 2, Feb, 243-9

Siegelin, M. D., D. E. Reuss, A. Habel, C. Herold-Mende &A. von Deimling. (2008). The flavonoid kaempferol sensitizes human glioma cells to TRAIL-mediated apoptosis by proteasomal degradation of survivin. *Mol Cancer Ther*, 7, 11, Nov, 3566-74

Siegelin, M. D., D. E. Reuss, A. Habel, A. Rami &A. von Deimling. (2009). Quercetin promotes degradation of survivin and thereby enhances death-receptor-mediated apoptosis in glioma cells. *Neuro Oncol*, 11, 2, Apr, 122-31

Szliszka, E. &W. Krol. The role of dietary polyphenols in tumor necrosis factor-related apoptosis inducing ligand (TRAIL)-induced apoptosis for cancer chemoprevention. *Eur J Cancer Prev*, 20, 1, Jan, 63-9

Tagscherer, K. E., A. Fassl, B. Campos, M. Farhadi, A. Kraemer, B. C. Bock, S. Macher-Goeppinger, B. Radlwimmer, O. D. Wiestler, C. Herold-Mende &W. Roth. (2008). Apoptosis-based treatment of glioblastomas with ABT-737, a novel small molecule inhibitor of Bcl-2 family proteins. *Oncogene*, 27, 52, Nov 6, 6646-56

von Deimling, A., A. Korshunov &C. Hartmann. The next generation of glioma biomarkers: MGMT methylation, BRAF fusions and IDH1 mutations. *Brain Pathol*, 21, 1, Jan, 74-87

Wagner, K. W., E. A. Punnoose, T. Januario, D. A. Lawrence, R. M. Pitti, K. Lancaster, D. Lee, M. von Goetz, S. F. Yee, K. Totpal, L. Huw, V. Katta, G. Cavet, S. G. Hymowitz, L. Amler &A. Ashkenazi. (2007). Death-receptor O-glycosylation controls tumor-cell sensitivity to the proapoptotic ligand Apo2L/TRAIL. *Nat Med*, 13, 9, Sep, 1070-7

Walczak, H., R. E. Miller, K. Ariail, B. Gliniak, T. S. Griffith, M. Kubin, W. Chin, J. Jones, A. Woodward, T. Le, C. Smith, P. Smolak, R. G. Goodwin, C. T. Rauch, J. C. Schuh &D. H. Lynch. (1999). Tumoricidal activity of tumor necrosis factor-related apoptosis-inducing ligand in vivo. *Nat Med*, 5, 2, Feb, 157-63

Yung, W. K., J. J. Vredenburgh, T. F. Cloughesy, P. Nghiemphu, B. Klencke, M. R. Gilbert, D. A. Reardon &M. D. Prados. Safety and efficacy of erlotinib in first-relapse glioblastoma: a phase II open-label study. *Neuro Oncol*, 12, 10, Oct, 1061-70

Zhu, H., S. Woolfenden, R. T. Bronson, Z. M. Jaffer, S. Barluenga, N. Winssinger, A. E. Rubenstein, R. Chen &A. Charest. The novel Hsp90 inhibitor NXD30001 induces tumor regression in a genetically engineered mouse model of glioblastoma multiforme. *Mol Cancer Ther*, 9, 9, Sep, 2618-26

14

The Molecular Basis of Resistance to the Antiproliferative Effect of EGFR Inhibition in Human Glioblastoma Multiforme Cell Lines

Georg Karpel-Massler and Marc-Eric Halatsch
University of Ulm School of Medicine, Ulm
Germany

1. Introduction

Dysregulated epidermal growth factor receptor (HER1/EGFR) is found in about 50% of glioblastoma, the most common primary brain tumor (Karpel-Massler et al., 2009). Despite recent improvements of the standard of care which currently comprises gross total tumor resection, irradiation and concomitant and adjuvant chemotherapy with temozolomide, the prognosis of patients with this disease remains dismal. A variety of therapeutic strategies was developed in order to improve the clinical outcome of patients with glioblastoma. One such approach involves HER1/EGFR-targeted agents among which small-molecule tyrosine kinase (TK) inhibitors (*e.g.*, erlotinib) represent the clinically most advanced HER1/EGFR-targeted compounds (Halatsch et al., 2006). While experimental studies with erlotinib in the setting of glioblastoma showed promising results (Lal et al., 2002; Halatsch et al., 2004), clinical translation failed to prove a significant benefit (van den Bent et al., 2009). This finding might be partly explained by the fact that erlotinib was shown to exert largely variable antiproliferative effects on different human glioblastoma cell lines in vitro and in vivo (Halatsch et al., 2004). Based on the observation that there is no established correlation between HER1/EGFR baseline expression and erlotinib-induced antiproliferative effects, it seems likely that more complex genetic constellations form the molecular basis of the erlotinib-sensitive and erlotinib-resistant glioblastoma phenotypes. Identification of the molecular pattern determining the erlotinib-resistant phenotype may allow the development of a therapeutic concept to overcome resistance towards erlotinib using multi-targeting that includes those genes that confer resistance. By analyzing a set of erlotinib-sensitive, intermediately responsive and erlotinib-resistant glioblastoma cell lines in an expression analysis of 244 prospectively selected genes whose products, among others, constitute the HER1/EGFR signaling pathway, expression of two genes, *FK506-binding protein* 14 (*FKBP*14) and *Ras-related C3 botulinum toxin substrate* 1 (*RAC*1) were identified to significantly correlate with the erlotinib-resistant glioblastoma phenotype (Halatsch et al., 2008). Thus, interference with these genes may enhance the antiproliferative efficacy of erlotinib against glioblastoma.

2. HER1/EGFR-targeted therapy in glioblastoma

2.1 HER1/EGFR – a promising target

HER1/EGFR plays an important role in the regulation of diverse cellular functions such as proliferation or differentiation (Wells, 1999). It belongs to the HER family of receptors and contains an extracellular ligand-binding site, a transmembraneous portion and an intracellular tyrosine kinase (TK) domain. Activation of HER1/EGFR is triggered by binding of *e.g.* epidermal growth factor (EGF) or transforming growth factor-α (TGF-α) to the ligand-binding site. As a consequence, autophosphorylation of specific tyrosine residues within the cytoplasmic catalytic kinase domain of the receptor takes place, initiating further downward signaling *via* the ras-raf-mitogen-activated protein kinase (MAPK) or the phosphatidylinositol 3-kinase (PI3-K)/Akt pathways (Arteaga, 2003; Scagliotti et al., 2004).

Dysregulation of HER1/EGFR was shown to be associated with a variety of neoplastic disorders including glioblastoma (Earp et al., 2003). This finding can be explained by the fact that aberrant alteration of downstream signal transduction results in a shift of the cellular homeostasis towards increased proliferation, tumorigenesis, angiogenesis or invasion and/or inhibition of apoptosis, thus towards a neoplastic cellular phenotype (Halatsch et al., 2006). Gene amplification represents one of the mechanisms that lead to dysregulation of HER1/EGFR-mediated signaling and HER1/EGFR overexpression as shown for 40-50% of glioblastoma (Salomon et al., 1995). Mutational changes of the intrinsic receptor structure constitute another mechanism that may result in uncontrolled HER1/EGFR signaling. The most frequent mutant form of HER1/EGFR, termed EGFR variant III (EGFRvIII), results from an in-frame deletion of 801 base pairs in the DNA sequence encoding the extracellular ligand-binding domain of HER1/EGFR. This truncated receptor variant constitutes approximately 60% of all mutants and is characterized by continuous activation independent of ligand-binding (Frederick et al., 2000; Karpel-Massler et al., 2010).

2.2 HER1/EGFR-targeted small molecule TK inhibitors – preclinical studies

The accumulation of evidence for HER1/EGFR to play a pro-oncogenic role in glioblastoma led to the development of a multitude of HER1/EGFR-targeted therapeutic strategies such as vaccination therapy, HER1/EGFR-targeted antibodies or small-molecule TK inhibitors (Karpel-Massler et al., 2009). In glioblastoma, most clinical experience exists with small-molecule TK inhibitors such as erlotinib. The mode of action of erlotinib is based on binding to the intracellular catalytic TK domain of HER1/EGFR in competition with adenosine triphosphate, thereby inhibiting autophosphorylation of the receptor and further downstream signaling (Halatsch et al., 2006). In preclinical studies, erlotinib was shown to exert a variety of interesting antineoplastic effects in the setting of glioblastoma. Griffero et al. showed that treatment with erlotinib at a concentration of 5 μM significantly reduced cellular viability of six human glioblastoma-derived tumor-initiating cell lines (Griffero et al., 2003). This effect was shown to correlate with decreased EGF-induced phosphorylation of HER1/EGFR and subsequent inhibition of the MAPK signaling pathway. In a different study, Lal *et al.* showed that exposure of transformed D54-MG glioblastoma cells (D54-EGFRvIII) to 20 μM of erlotinib resulted in a significant downregulation of certain genes encoding pro-invasive proteins and to significantly inhibit the invasiveness of D54-EGFRvIII cells (Lal et al., 2002). In addition, Halatsch et al. showed that the extent of erlotinib-mediated inhibition of anchorage-independent growth of glioblastoma-derived cell lines correlates inversely with the cellular capability to induce HER1/EGFR mRNA, emphasizing the important role of HER1/EGFR in the pathogenesis of glioblastoma (Halatsch et al., 2004).

2.3 HER1/EGFR-targeted small molecule TK inhibitors – clinical situation

The promising findings shown by experimental studies led to the conductance of several clinical trials examining the effects of erlotinib in the setting of recurrent or newly diagnosed glioblastoma. Erlotinib was shown to fit a reasonable safety profile and was generally well tolerated as shown by phase I clinical trials (Krishnan et al., 2006; Prados et al., 2006). With regard to its clinical efficacy, varying results were derived from early phase clinical trials. In a phase II trial, the effects of erlotinib applied at a dose of 150 mg/d on 42 patients with recurrent glioblastoma and 43 patients with non-progressive glioblastoma following radiotherapy were examined (Raizer et al., 2010). Median overall survival and progression-free survival for the patients with recurrent glioblastoma were reported as 6 months and 2 months, respectively. The patients with non-progressive glioblastoma post radiotherapy reached a median overall survival of 14 months. Thus, erlotinib had minimal efficacy in patients with recurrent glioblastoma and at best slight efficacy in patients with non-progressive glioblastoma post radiotherapy compared to historical controls. Other investigators showed for 48 patients with recurrent glioblastoma who were treated with erlotinib a median overall survival and 6-month progression-free survival that exceeded historical data of patients receiving standard chemotherapy (Yung et al., 2010). However, this study had to be discontinued due to an insufficient number of responses after a planned interim analysis. In a randomized controlled phase II clinical trial, it was finally shown for patients with recurrent glioblastoma that erlotinib monotherapy was inferior to the treatment with temozolomide or BCNU in terms of clinical efficacy (van den Bent et al., 2009). Only 11.4% of the patients treated with erlotinib were free of progression after 6 months compared to 24.1% of the patients in the control group. In addition, no significant differences in median overall survival were found among the different treatment groups.

2.4 Erlotinib and standard radio-/chemotherapy

Several studies were conducted to evaluate whether treatment with erlotinib might provide a clinical benefit when combined with conventional radiochemotherapy. In a phase I/II trial, 89 patients with newly diagnosed glioblastoma were treated with erlotinib at a dose of 150 mg/d starting 1 week prior to fractionated radiotherapy (60 Gy total dose) and temozolomide at a dose of 75 mg/m^2/d (Brown et al., 2008). The treatment with erlotinib was continued during radiotherapy and accompanied by up to 6 cycles of temozolomide at a dose of 200 mg/m^2/d for 5 days every 4 weeks subsequent to the completion of radiotherapy. Median overall survival was 15.7 months which, however, was not significantly different from that of the radiotherapy plus temozolomide arm from the EORTC 26981/22981-NCIC trial (Mirimanoff et al., 2006).

In a different phase II clinical trial, 65 patients with newly diagnosed glioblastoma or gliosarcoma were treated with erlotinib and fractionated radiotherapy with concomitant and adjuvant temozolomide (Prados et al., 2009). Median progression-free survival and median overall survival were reported as 8.2 months and 19.3 months, respectively, and were thus markably prolonged when compared to a combined historical control. In contrast, rather negative results were reported in 27 patients with newly diagnosed glioblastoma that were treated with a maximum dose of 150 mg/d erlotinib and radiotherapy (60 Gy in 30 fractions) with concurrent (75 mg/m^2/d for 42 days) and adjuvant (12 four-week cycles comprising each 5 days of 150-200 mg/m^2/d) temozolomide (Peereboom et al., 2010). Due to lack of efficacy and unacceptable toxicity, this trial had to be closed preterm. Median overall survival and median progression-free survival were reported as 8.6 months and 2.8 months, respectively. Progressive disease was found in 22 patients (67%). In addition, 4 patients (15%) had an adverse event. Notably, three treatment-related deaths occurred. Based on these results, a combined treatment with erlotinib, temozolomide and radiotherapy appears antagonistic and dangerous.

2.5 Erlotinib and other agents

The fact that treatment with erlotinib alone or together with conventional adjuvant therapies does not seem to provide a substantial benefit in this disease emphasizes the necessity for a change of strategy. Combining HER1/EGFR TK inhibitors with other targeted agents represents one such new promising approach.

Inhibition of downstream key regulators such as mammalian target of rapamycin (mTOR) and PI3-K in addition to the treatment with HER1/EGFR TK inhibitors was shown to be favorable in preclinical studies. Combined treatment of phosphatase and tensin homolog deleted on chromosome 10 (PTEN)-deficient U87 and SF295 glioblastoma cells with erlotinib and rapamycin, an mTOR inhibitor, resulted in a significantly increased anti-proliferative effect when compared to cells receiving either agent alone (Wang et al., 2006). Similar results were reported by a different group (Fan et al., 2007). Moreover, in this study, an even more pronounced antiproliferative efficacy was observed when PI3-K was also inhibited by using a dual mTOR/PI3-K inhibitor (PI-103) compared to the treatment with erlotinib and either additional inhibition of mTOR or PI3-K. In the clinical setting, 22 patients with recurrent glioblastoma treated with erlotinib or gefitinib in combination with sirolimus were shown to have a 6-month progression-free survival of 25% (Doherty et al., 2006). However, a phase II clinical trial evaluating the therapeutic efficacy of a treatment with 150 mg/d (450 mg/d in patients on enzyme-inducing anti-epileptic drugs [EIAEDs]) erlotinib and 5 mg/d (10 mg/d in patients on EIAEDs) sirolimus in 32 patients with recurrent glioblastoma reported negligible anti-tumor activity (Reardon et al., 2010). Complete or partial responses were not observed, and median overall survival and median progression-free survival were 33.8 weeks and 6.9 weeks, respectively.

Recently, the clinical efficacy of a combination therapy with erlotinib and bevacizumab was examined in the setting of recurrent high-grade glioma (Sathornsumetee et al., 2010). Twenty-five patients were treated with bevacizumab at a dose of 10 mg/kg i.v. biweekly and erlotinib at a dose of 200 mg/d (500 mg/d in patients on EIAEDs). Overall survival and median progression-free survival were favorable (42 weeks and 18 weeks, respectively). In addition, in nearly half of the patients a radiographic response was observed. However, a similar progression-free survival and radiographic response were derived from historical data of patients receiving single-agent therapy with bevacizumab.

Overall, despite promising results reported by some early phase clinical trials, combining HER1/EGFR TK inhibitors with other agents has so far been not overly successful in the treatment of patients with glioblastoma. Novel targets need to be identified to overcome resistance towards HER1/EGFR TK inhibitors and to substantially enhance the latter's antineoplastic effects by compounds without overlapping toxicity profile.

3. *FKBP*14 and *RAC*1 – two candidate genes for conferring resistance towards erlotinib

The fact that alterations of HER1/EGFR and its pathway are so frequently encountered in glioblastoma while erlotinib failed in the clinical setting reflects the complex architecture of tumor-driving signaling pathway networks. This phenomenon is highlighted by findings derived from an experimental study showing that erlotinib exerts highly variable antiproliferative effects on different human glioblastoma cell lines independent of baseline HER1/EGFR expression levels (Halatsch et al., 2004). By analyzing HER1/EGFR pathway gene expression profiles of glioblastoma cell lines displaying an erlotinib-responsive, somewhat responsive and erlotinib-resistant phenotype, *FKBP*14 and *RAC*1 were identified as candidate genes conferring resistance to erlotinib (Halatsch et al., 2008). This fact may render *FKBP*14 and *RAC*1 potential therapeutic targets in the vicinity of the EGFR signaling pathway, and interference with *FKBP*14 and/or *RAC*1 may allow enhancing the efficacy of erlotinib against glioblastoma. *RAC*1 is an important contributor to cell survival in glioma and plays an established role in tumorigenesis as well as in tumor maintenance in this setting (Senger et al., 2002). With respect to *FKBP*14, less is known about its function. However, data available so far do indicate a tumor-promoting role for its gene product. FKBPs are encoded by a multigene family and exert anti-apoptotic effects. In addition, *FKBP*12, a member of this family was reported to be overexpressed in childhood astrocytomas (Khatua et al., 2003). Further studies are warranted to evaluate the potential benefit of a combinatorial therapeutic regimen including erlotinib and an inhibitor of *RAC*1 and/or *FKBP*14.

4. Conclusion

With respect to the treatment of glioblastoma, erlotinib has so far failed to shape clinical practice. A consistant therapeutic benefit could be noted neither when erlotinib was applied alone nor when it was administered in combination with standard radio-/chemotherapy. Recently, the suspicion was raised that erlotinib might even compromise patients' safety when added to temozolomide and radiotherapy (Peereboom et al., 2010). The discrepancy between the promising results erlotinib achieved in experimental studies and its clinical failure might be partly explained by insufficient penetration of the blood brain barrier and the heterogeneity of tumor cells.

In addition, another important factor underlying glioblastoma resistance towards erlotinib could be simultaneous activation of multiple receptor tyrosine kinases (RTKs) with complex converging interactions or other key factors mediating pro-neoplastic signaling. Therefore, interception of HER1/EGFR-mediated signaling by erlotinib might be compensated, leading to maintenance of the cancerous cellular phenotype. Multiple PI3-K-activating RTKs were shown to be simultaneously activated in a variety of different glioma cell lines (Stommel et al., 2007). In this study, shut-down of either the hepatocyte growth factor receptor or HER1/EGFR alone did not significantly inhibit downstream signaling, while the inhibition of both markedly decreased PI3-K activation and cell survival.

In concordance with this notion, two molecular determinants, *RAC*1 and *FKBP*14, are overexpressed in glioblastoma cell lines with erlotinib-resistant phenotype, thus representing candidate genes for conferring resistance towards erlotinib. Further studies are under way examining the potential benefit of a multitargeted therapeutic strategy including erlotinib as well as *RAC*1 and/or *FKBP*14 inhibitors.
The current clinical situation of patients with glioblastoma does not allow us to take a rest. A continuous search for novel targets and more efficient combination therapies is of ultimate urge and requires all our efforts.

5. References

Arteaga, C. (2003). HER1/EGFR: a molecular approach to cancer therapy. *Semin Oncol*, 30, pp. 3-14.

Brown, P., Krishnan, S., Sarkaria, J., Wu, W., Jaeckle, K., Uhm, J., Geoffroy, F., Arusell, R., Kitange, G., Jenkins, R., Kugler, J., Morton, R., Rowland, K., Mischel, P., Yong, W., Scheithauer, B., Schiff, D., Giannini, C. & Buckner, J. (2008). Phase I/II trial of erlotinib and temozolomide with radiation therapy in the treatment of newly diagnosed glioblastoma multiforme: north central cancer treatment group study N0177. *J Clin Oncol*, 26, pp. 5603-5609.

Doherty, L., Gigas, D., Kesari, S., Drappatz, J., Kim, R., Zimmermann, J., Ostrowsky, L. & Wen, P. (2006). Pilot study of the combination of EGFR and mTOR inhibitors in recurrent malignant gliomas. *Neurology*, 67, pp. 156-158.

Earp, H., Calvo, B. & Sartor, C. (2003). The EGF receptor family - multiple roles in proliferation, differentiation, and neoplasia with an emphasis on HER4. *Trans Am Clin Climatol Assoc*, 114, pp. 315-333.

Fan, Q.-W., Cheng, C., Nicolaides, T., Hackett, C., Knight, Z., Shokat, K. & Weiss, W. (2007). A dual phosphoinositide-3-kinase anti/mTOR inhibitor cooperates with blockade of epidermal growth factor receptor in PTEN-mutant glioma. *Cancer Res*, 67, pp. 7960-7965.

Frederick, L., Wang, X.-Y., Eley, G. & James, C. (2000). Diversity and frequency of epidermal growth factor receptor mutations in human glioblastomas. *Cancer Res*, 60, pp. 1383-1387.

Friedman, H., Prados, M., Wen, P., Mikkelsen, T., Schiff, D., Abrey, L., Yung, W., Paleologos, N., Nicholas, M., Jensen, R., Vredenburgh, J., Huang, J., Zheng, M. & Cloughesy, T. (2009). Bevacizumab alone and in combination with irinotecan in recurrent glioblastoma. *J Clin Oncol*, 27, pp. 4733-4740.

Griffero, F., Daga, A., Marubbi, D., Capra, M., Melotti, A., Pattarozzi, A., Gatti, M., Bajetto, A., Porcile, C., Barbieri, F., Favoni, R., Lo Casto, M., Zona, G., Spaziante, R., Florio, T. & Corte, G. (2003). Different response of human glioma tumor-initiating cells to epidermal growth factor receptor kinase inhibitors. *J Biol Chem*, 284, pp. 7138-7148.

Halatsch, M.-E., Gehrke, E., Vougioukas, V., Bötefür, I., Efferth, T., Gebhardt, E., Domhof, S., Schmidt, U. & Buchfelder, M. (2004). Inverse correlation of *epidermal growth factor receptor* messenger RNA induction and suppression of anchorage-independent growth by OSI-774, an epidermal growth factor receptor tyrosine kinase inhibitor, in glioblastoma multiforme cell lines. *J Neurosurg*, 100, pp. 523-533.

Halatsch, M.-E., Schmidt, U., Behnke-Mursch, J., Unterberg, A. & Wirtz, C. (2006). Epidermal growth factor receptor inhibition for the treatment of glioblastoma multiforme and other malignant brain tumours. *Cancer Treat Rev*, 32, pp. 74-89.

Halatsch, M.-E., Löw, S., Hielscher, T., Schmidt, U., Unterberg, A. & Vougioukas, V. (2008). Epidermal growth factor receptor pathway gene expressions and biological response of glioblastoma multiforme cell lines to erlotinib. *Anticancer Res*, 28, pp. 3725-3728.

Karpel-Massler, G., Schmidt, U., Unterberg, A. & Halatsch, M.-E. (2009). Therapeutic inhibition of the epidermal growth factor receptor in high-grade gliomas - where do we stand? *Mol Cancer Res*, 7, pp. 1000-1012.

Karpel-Massler, G., Wirtz, C. & Halatsch, M.-E. (2010). Ribozyme-mediated inhibition of 801-bp deletion-mutant *epidermal growth factor receptor* mRNA expression in glioblastoma multiforme *Molecules*, 15, pp. 4670-4678.

Khatua, S., Peterson, K.M., Brown, K.M., Lawlor, C., Santi, M.R., LaFleur, B., Dressman, D., Stephan, D.A. & MacDonald, T.J. (2003). Overexpression of the EGFR/FKBP12/HIF-2alpha pathway identified in childhood astrocytomas by angiogenesis gene profiling. *Cancer Res*, 63, pp. 1865-70.

Krishnan, S., Brown, P., Ballmann, K., Fiveash, J., Uhm, J., Giannini, C., Jaeckle, K., Geoffroy, F., Nabors, L. & Buckner, J. (2006). Phase I trial of erlotinib with radiation therapy in patients with glioblastoma multiforme: results of north central cancer treatment group protocol N0177. *Int J Radiat Oncol Biol Phys*, 65, pp. 1192-1199.

Lal, A., Glazer, C., Martinson, H., Friedman, H., Archer, G., Sampson, J. & Riggins, G. (2002). Mutant epidermal growth factor receptor up-regulates molecular effectors of tumor invasion. *Cancer Res*, 62, pp. 3335-3339.

Mirimanoff, R., Gorlia, T., Mason, W., van den Bent, M., Kortmann, R.-D., Fisher, B., Reni, M., Brandes, A., Curschmann, J., Villa, S., Cairncross, G., Allgeier, A., Lacombe, D. & Stupp, R. (2006). Radiotherapy and temozolomide for newly diagnosed glioblastoma: recursive partitioning analysis of the EORTC 26981/22981-NCIC CE3 phase III randomized trial. *J Clin Oncol*, 24, pp. 2563-2569.

Peereboom, D., Shepard, D., Ahluwalia, M., Brewer, C., Agarwal, N., Stevens, G., Suh, J., Toms, S., Vogelbaum, M., Weil, R., Elson, P. & Barnett, G. (2010). Phase II trial of erlotinib with temozolomide and radiation in patients with newly diagnosed glioblastoma multiforme. *J Neurooncol*, 98, pp. 93-99.

Prados, M., Chang, S., Butowski, N., DeBoer, R., Parvataneni, R., Carliner, H., Kabuubi, P., Ayers-Ringler, J., Rabbitt, J., Page, M., Fedoroff, A., Sneed, P., Berger, M., McDermott, M., Parsa, A., Vandenberg, S., James, C., Lamborn, K., Stokoe, D. & Haas-Kogan, D. (2009). Phase II study of erlotinib plus temozolomide during and after radiation therapy in patients with newly diagnosed glioblastoma multiforme or gliosarcoma. *J Clin Oncol*, 27, pp. 579-584.

Prados, M., Lamborn, K., Chang, S., Burton, E., Butowski, N., Malec, M., Kapadia, A., Rabbitt, J., Page, M., Fedoroff, A., Xie, D. & Kelley, S. (2006). Phase I study of erlotinib HCl alone and combined with temozolomide in patients with stable or recurrent malignant glioma. *Neurooncol*, 8, pp. 67-78.

Raizer, J., Abrey, L., Lassman, A., Chang, S., Lamborn, K., Kuhn, J., Yung, W., Gilbert, M., Aldape, K., Wen, P., Fine, H., Mehta, M., DeAngelis, L., Lieberman, F., Cloughesy, T., Robins, H., Dancey, J. & Prados, M. (2010). A phase II trial of erlotinib in patients with recurrent malignant gliomas and nonprogressive glioblastoma multiforme postradiation therapy. *Neurooncol*, 12, pp. 95-103.

Reardon, D., Desjardins, A., Vredenburgh, J., Gururangan, S., Friedman, A., Herndon II, J., Marcello, J., Norfleet, J., McLendon, R., Sampson, J. & Friedman, H. (2010). Phase II trial of erlotinib plus sirolimus in adults with recurrent glioblastoma. *J Neurooncol*, 96, pp. 219-230.

Salomon, D., Brandt, R., Ciardello, F. & Normanno, N. (1995). Epidermal growth factor-related peptides and their receptors in human malignancies. *Crit Rev Oncol Hematol*, 19, pp. 183-232.

Sathornsumetee, S., Desjardins, A., Vredenburgh, J., McLendon, R., Marcello, J., Herndon II, J., Mathe, A., Hamilton, M., Rich Sr, J., Norfleet, J., Gururangan, S., Friedman, H. & Reardon, D. (2010). Phase II trial of bevacizumab and erlotinib in patients with recurrent malignant glioma. *Neurooncol*, 12, pp. 1300-1310.

Scagliotti, G., Selvaggi, G., Novello, S. & Hirsch, F. (2004). The biology of epidermal growth factor receptor in lung cancer. *Clin Cancer Res*, 10, pp. 4227s-4232s.

Senger, D.L., Tudan, C., Guiot, M.C., Mazzoni, I.E., Molenkamp, G., LeBlanc, R., Antel, J., Olivier, A., Snipes, G.J. & Kaplan, D.R. (2002). Suppression of Rac activity induces apoptosis of human glioma cells but not normal human astrocytes. *Cancer Res*, 62, pp. 2131-40.

Stommel, J., Kimmelman, A., Ying, H., Nabioullin, R., Ponugoti, A., Wiedemeyer, R., Stegh, A., Bradner, J., Ligon, K., Brennan, C., Chin, L. & DePinho, R. (2007). Coactivation of receptor tyrosine kinases affects the response of tumor cells to targeted therapies. *Science*, 318, pp. 287-290.

van den Bent, M., Brandes, A., Rampling, R., Kouwenhoven, M., Kros, J., Carpentier, A., Clement, P., Frenay, M., Campone, M., Baurain, J., Armand, J., Taphoorn, M., Tosoni, A., Kletzl, H., Klughammer, B., Lacombe, D. & Gorlia, T. (2009). Randomized phase II trial of erlotinib versus temozolomide or carmustine in recurrent glioblastoma: EORTC brain tumor group study 26034. *J Clin Oncol*, 27, pp. 1268-1274.

Vredenburgh, J.J., Desjardins, A., Herndon, J.E., 2nd, Marcello, J., Reardon, D.A., Quinn, J.A., Rich, J.N., Sathornsumetee, S., Gururangan, S., Sampson, J., Wagner, M., Bailey, L., Bigner, D.D., Friedman, A.H. & Friedman, H.S. (2007). Bevacizumab plus irinotecan in recurrent glioblastoma multiforme. *J Clin Oncol*, 25, pp. 4722-9.

Wang, M., Lu, K., Zhu, S., Dia, E., Vivanco, I., Shackleford, G., Cavenee, W., Mellinghoff, I., Cloughesy, T., Sawyers, C. & Mischel, P. (2006). Mammalian target of rapamycin inhibition promotes response to epidermal growth factor receptor kinase inhibitors in PTEN-deficient and PTEN-intact glioblastoma cells. *Cancer Res*, 66, pp. 7864-7869.

Wells, A. (1999). EGF receptor. *Int J Biochem Cell Biol*, 31, pp. 637-643.

Yung, W., Vredenburgh, J., Cloughesy, T., Nghiemphu, P., Klencke, B., Gilbert, M., Reardon, D. & Prados, M. (2010). Safety and efficacy of erlotinib in first-relapse glioblastoma: a phase II open-label study. *Neurooncol*, 12, pp. 1061-1070.

15

Medical Management of Brain Metastases from Lung Cancer

Ryuya Yamanaka
Kyoto Prefectural University of Medicine
Graduate School for Health Care Science, Kamigyoku, Kyoto
Japan

1. Introduction

Brain metastases are a frequent complication in patients with lung cancer and a significant cause of morbidity and mortality. Brain metastases are found in about 10-25% of patients at the time of diagnosis, and approximately 40-50% of all patients with lung cancer develop brain metastases during the course of their disease, with greater frequency at autopsy (approximately 50%) than predicted from the presence of symptoms (1). The incidence of brain metastasis is increasing mainly due to longer patient survivals resulting from newer treatment modalities. Most patients with lung cancer metastatic to the brain have multiple lesions (2). Brain metastases are usually associated with poor outcomes and shortened survival of 3 to 6 months. Standard treatment options include symptomatic therapy with corticosteroids and whole-brain radiotherapy (WBRT) (3), and more aggressive approaches such as surgery or radiosurgery are indicated in a subset of patients (4,5). Surgical resection of accessible brain metastases combined with postoperative WBRT is the management of choice for a single metastasis (6). However, radiosurgery for brain metastases produces high rates of tumor control similar to the rates obtained by excisional surgery (7). Patients with multiple brain metastases are commonly treated with WBRT for the palliation of symptoms (8). The role of radiosurgery for multiple brain metastases is less clear, but it can be effective (9). The poor outcomes and relapses following WBRT alone indicate a need for new therapeutic options. Generally, poor prognosis occurs not from cerebral problems, but from extracranial metastases, and death is caused by systemic disease combined with the neurological condition (10). However, treatment with systemic chemotherapy is controversial because chemotherapeutic agents may not cross the blood-brain-barrier (BBB) and therefore are less effective against central nervous system (CNS) disease than against extracranial, systemic disease. However, the BBB is partially disrupted in brain metastases (11) and similar concentrations of chemotherapeutic agents are found in intracerebral and extracerebral tumors (5). Brain metastases resulting from both non-small-cell (NSCLC) and small-cell lung cancer (SCLC) are susceptible to systemic chemotherapy, and cerebral response rates up to 50% were observed even in second-line treatment of NSCLC and SCLC (1,10,11). Still, medical therapies for brain metastases are neither well-studied nor established. Here, I analyze the impact of medical treatment on survival by reviewing recent articles and provide recommendations for the management of patients with brain metastases from lung cancer.

2. Non-small cell lung cancer (NSCLC)

NSCLC accounts for approximately 75% of lung cancer cases, with the majority of patients having inoperable, locally advanced or metastatic disease at the time of diagnosis, reflected in the low 5-year survival rate for all stages (currently 13%) (12). Despite two decades of cisplatin-based chemotherapy of advanced NSCLC, the survival benefit remains modest (13). New chemotherapy combinations have minimal impact on survival compared with older regimens, with overall response rates of approximately 30%, median survival benefits of 8–9 months, and 1-year survival rates of approximately 30% (14). New therapies are required that are effective against locally advanced or metastatic NSCLC.

2.1 Front-line chemotherapy (Table 1)

Many chemotherapeutic regimens have been tested in phase II or III trials for the treatment of brain metastases arising from NSCLC. There are 8 larger reports (15-22) with more than 10 patients, published from 1994 to 2008 in English, on front-line chemotherapy of brain metastases from NSCLC. In patients with NSCLC, 17-50% of patients with previously untreated brain metastases responded to a combination of cisplatin plus fotemustine; carboplatin plus etoposide; cisplatin plus teniposide; cisplatin plus etoposide; cisplatin plus ifosfamide, CPT-11; cisplatin plus vinorelbine; carboplatin plus vinorelbine, gemcitabine; cisplatin plus paclitaxel. Systemic disease activity correlates well with activity against brain metastases, but overall survival (OS) is still 4-12 months.

Author	Regimen	No. of patients	Study design	Response rate (%)	Disease stabilization (%)	mPFS (Month)	OS (Month)
Cotto C	CDDP,Fotemustine	31	Phase II	23	51.6	5	4
Malacarne P	CBDCA,VP16	18	Phase II	17	39	n.d.	7.5
Minotti V	CDDP,Teniposide	23	Phase II	35	65	7	5
Franciosi V	CDDP,VP-16	43	Phase II	30	65	4	8
Fujita A	CDDP,IFOS,CPT-11	28	Phase I/II	50	96	4.6	12
Robinet G	CDDP,VNR	76	Phase III	27	n.d.	3.2	6
Bernardo G	CBDCA,VNR,GEM	22	Phase II	45	85	6.2	8.2
Cortes J	CDDP,Paclitaxel	26	Phase II	38	69	3.2	5.3

Table 1.CBDCA,carboplatin; CDDP, cisplatin; CPT-11, irinotecan; GEM, gemcitabine; IFOS, ifosfamide; mOS, median overall survival; mPFS, median progression free survival; n.d., not determined; VNR, vinorelbine; VP16, etoposide. Modified from: Yamanaka R. Oncol Rep 2009;22:1269-1276 with permission from Spandidos Publications

2.2 Second-line chemotherapy

2.2.1 Epidermal growth factor receptor tyrosine kinase Inhibitor

The epidermal growth factor receptor (EGFR) is expressed in a variety of tumors, including NSCLC (23), and elevated EGFR expression is associated with a poor prognosis in lung cancer patients (24). Several EGFR-targeted agents have been developed, including gefitinib (ZD1839; Iressa) and erlotinib (OSI-774; Tarceva), an orally active anilinoquinazoline compound that inhibits EGFR tyrosine kinase activity (25). In two large, well-designed phase II clinical trials, refractory patients with NSCLC experienced overall response rates of 11.8–18.4%, median survival benefits of 6.5–7.6 months, and 1-year survival rates of 29-35% (26,27), with encouraging response rates in select patients (women, non-smokers, patients with adenocarcinoma, and specific *EGFR* mutations in the kinase domain) (28-33). Although targeting EGFR-associated tyrosine kinase with gefitinib and erlotinib results in durable responses in some patients, the activity of these drugs against brain metastases has been poorly documented so far.

Gefitinib (Table 2)

Phase II studies of gefitinib on brain metastases from NSCLC indicated objective responses occur in 33% of patients (Asia) (34,35) or 9.7% of patients (Europe) (36). In comparison, WBRT with 30 to 40 Gy for brain metastases from NSCLC results in objective responses in 38% to 45% of patients (37,38). Gefitinib is well tolerated, mostly with grade 1/2 skin rashes. The severity of skin toxicity was tightly associated with tumor response and patient survival (34). Gefitinib was most effective at treating brain metastases in patients with EGFR mutations in the tyrosine kinase domain (deletion mutation in two patients and a point mutation in one patient) in one study (39). However, this analysis was performed using tissue samples from primary lung cancer and not from metastatic brain lesions. Yokouchi et al (40). reported that some patients who experienced disease progression after responding to gefitinib were sensitive to gefitinib re-administration after temporary cessation of gefitinib and other treatments. Patients may still be expected to have prolonged survival if they once responded to gefitinib and then underwent various subsequent treatments followed by re-administration of gefitinib. These findings might provide valuable information for the management of gefitinib-responders. Although the survival benefit is controversial, gefitinib may also be useful for the treatment of carcinomatous meningitis from NSCLC to improve neurological dysfunction (41,42,43). Thus, gefitinib has therapeutic potential for palliative therapy in patients with brain metastases.

Author	No. of patients	Study design	Previous WBRT/Chemo (%)	Response rate (%)	Disease stabilization (%)	mPFS (Month)	OS (Month)
Ceresoli GL	41	phase II	43.9/90.2	9.7	26.8	3	5
Chiu CH	76	phase II	n.d./84.2	33.3	63.2	5	9.9
Wu C	40	phase II	65/100	32	77	9	15

Table 2. Chemo, chemotherapy; mOS, median overall survival; mPFS, median progression free survival; n.d., not determined; WBRT, whole brain radiotherapy. Modified from: Yamanaka R. Oncol Rep 2009;22:1269-1276 with permission from Spandidos Publications.

Erlotinib

Erlotinib treatment of brain metastases from NSCLC has been reported in 20 cases (44-55). These were histologically confirmed as adenocarcinoma in the primary site. The main adverse events were Grade 1 skin rashes. Some patients had responses longer than 6 months. Erlotinib responses are higher in patients with a somatic mutation in *EGFR* or a point mutation in the activation loop of the kinase domain (56,57). Thirteen patients showed a response to erlotinib after gefitinib failure. Although gefitinib failure may result from cross-resistance to other EGFR tyrosine kinase inhibitors (EGFR-TKI), these cases suggest that re-challenging patients with EGFR-TKI may be beneficial. At the recommended dosage, erlotinib showed higher blood concentrations than gefitinib, and may also have higher in cerebral spinal fluid. In addition, two patients with intracranial lesions responded to erlotinib treatment although extra-cranial lesion progressed. In the Rupport case (51), a secondary T790M mutation associated with resistance to EGFR-TKI was found in the liver biopsy. Erlotinib was reintroduced and produced quick neurological improvement, even though the extra-cranial disease remained resistant to erlotinib. These cases also highlight the oligoclonal nature of NSCLC and its differential sensitivity to EGFR-TKIs, in that extra-cranial disease was resistant to erlotinib both initially and on re-challenge. Persistent cerebral TKI sensitivity should be considered in patients presenting with a CNS relapse after stopping EGFR-TKI, even with a T790M resistant mutation in non-cerebral metastases. In addition, erlotinib should be considered for treatment of intra-cranial disease.

2.2.2 Temozolomide (Table 3)

Temozolomide is an orally administered prodrug that is converted spontaneously to the active alkylating agent, monomethyl triazenoimidazole carboxamide, at physiologic pH, crosses the BBB, and has antitumor activity against malignant glioma, melanoma, NSCLC, and carcinoma of the ovary and colon (58). CNS concentrations reach approximately 30–40% of plasma levels, achieving therapeutic concentrations in the brain (59), and clearance of temozolomide is unaffected by co-administration with anticonvulsants, antiemetics, or dexamethasone (58,59). The dose-limiting toxicity is non-cumulative myelosuppression that rarely requires treatment delays or dose reductions. In patients with newly-diagnosed brain metastases or with progression after radiotherapy, temozolomide produces objective response rates between 5 and 10% (60-62) and is well tolerated.

Author	Regimen	No. of patients	Study design	Previous WBRT/Chemo (%)	Response rate (%)	Disease stabilization (%)	mPFS (Month)	OS (Month)
Giorgio	TMZ	30	phase II	100/100	10	20	3.6	6
Kouroussis C	TMZ	12	phase II	n.d./100	8.3	25	n.d.	n.d.
Abrey LE	TMZ	22	phase II	100/n.d.	9	45	n.d.	n.d.
Christodoulou C	TMZ	12	phase II	100/n.d.	8	n.d.	n.d.	n.d.

Table 3. TMZ,temozolomide; Chemo, chemotherapy; mOS, median overall survival; mPFS, median progression free survival; n.d., not determined; WBRT, whole brain radiotherapy. Modified from: Yamanaka R. Oncol Rep 2009;22:1269-1276 with permission from Spandidos Publications

2.2.3 Temozolomide plus other chemotherapeutic agents

Preclinical experiments and early clinical studies in other malignancies indicate that temozolomide may have additive or synergistic effects when used with other chemotherapeutic agents (64,65). In addition, its minimal toxicity allows for the combination of temozolomide with gemcitabine, gemcitabine/cisplatin, or gemcitabine/vinorelbine in NSCLC patients to produce dramatic cerebral responses (66,67). The combination of temozolomide with other chemotherapeutic agents represents a promising strategy for treating brain metastases.

2.3 Chemotherapy plus whole-brain irradiation (Table 4)

Combining chemotherapy with brain radiotherapy is attractive because chemotherapy is active against both primary tumors and brain metastases, and because chemotherapy may act as a radiosensitizer. Two studies have compared randomized chemotherapy alone with chemotherapy/WBRT. Quantin et al. (68) reported a phase II study of radiotherapy plus vinorelbine, ifosfamide, and cisplatin chemotherapy in patients with brain metastases of NSCLC. The response rate was 56% and median survival was 7.6 months. The same author also reported a phase II study with concomitant brain radiotherapy and high-dose ifosfamide in brain relapses (69). Median survival was 13 months. Myelosuppression was the main toxic effect, but remained manageable and no toxic deaths occurred. The high response rate for brain lesions and improvement in neurological symptoms deserves further exploration.

Author	Chemotherapy Regimen	No. of patients	Study design	Previous WBRT/Chemo (%)	Response rate (%)	Disease stabilization (%)	mPFS (Month)	OS (Month)
Quantin	CDDP,VNR, IFOS	23	phase II	0/0	56	65	n.d.	7.6
Quantin	high-dose IFOS	16	phase II	n.d./n.d.	25	n.d.	n.d.	13
Ma S	Gefitinib	25	phase II	0/0	81	95.2	10	13
Addeo R	TMZ	15	phase II	44/74	6.5	60	6	8.8
Cortot	CDDP,TMZ	50	phase II	6/n.d.	12	54	2.3	5
Robinet	CDDP,VNR	85	phase III	0/0	28	n.d.	2.7	5.2

Table 4. CDDP, cisplatin; Chemo, chemotherapy; IFOS, ifosfamide; mOS, median overall survival; mPFS, median progression free survival; n.d., not determined; TMZ,temozolomide; VNR,vinorelbine; WBRT, whole brain radiotherapy. Modified from: Yamanaka R. Oncol Rep 2009;22:1269-1276 with permission from Spandidos Publications

Ma et al. (70) found that treatment with concomitant gefitinib and WBRT was well tolerated, with significant improvement of neurological symptoms in a Chinese population with brain metastases from NSCLC. Addeo et al. (71) reported response rates of 6.5% using a combination of temozolomide and WBRT. Cortot et al. (72) reported response rates of 12% with temozolomide, cisplatin, and WBRT. A randomized phase II study evaluated the efficacy of concurrent temozolomide and radiotherapy versus radiotherapy alone in 58 patients with previously untreated brain metastases from different solid tumors (31 patients had NSCLC) (73). The temozolomide group showed significant improvements in cerebral response rate (96% versus 67%), and temozolomide was safe and well-tolerated. However, overall survival rates and changes in neurological function were similar in both groups. Robinet *et al.* (74) reported a phase III study comparing the timing of WBRT, either before or after chemotherapy, and found a 28% response rate in 85 patients treated with cisplatin and vinorelbine in the early WBRT arm. The median survival in this arm was 5.2 months and median time to progression (TTP) was 2.1 months. Radiotherapy timing did not change survival time. Thus, for NSCLC, WBRT should be added to initial chemotherapy if there is no treatment response.

3. Small Cell Lung Cancer

The brain is the most common metastatic site in SCLC, and is usually fatal. Approximately 18-25% of SCLC patients have brain metastases already at diagnosis, and an additional 50% will develop CNS involvement during their disease course (75-77). Although WBRT and corticosteroids are the treatment of choice, systemic chemotherapy may also have therapeutic value. Extracranial disease is almost always present in SCLC, and chemotherapy can treat both brain metastases and these other disease sites. Prophylactic cranial irradiation (PCI) for patients responsive to induction therapy markedly reduces the risk of CNS relapse and significantly improves survival (77,78). Surgical treatment for solitary lesions or systemic chemotherapy for multifocal brain metastases that are minimally symptomatic can be useful, particularly when these patients also have extracranial metastatic disease. Thus, systemic chemotherapy can complement WBRT for treatment of brain metastases in SCLC.

3.1 Front-line chemotherapy (Table 5)

There are 4 larger reports (79-82) with more than 10 patients, published from 1989 to 2008 in English, on front-line chemotherapy of brain metastases from SCLC. The chemotherapeutic regimens, including cyclophosphamide, vincristine, etoposide, doxorubicin and cisplatin, produced response rates of 27-82% Thus, chemotherapy followed by radiation therapy may be first-line treatment for patients with systemic disease and asymptomatic brain metastases.

Author	Regimen	No. of patients	Study design	Response rate (%)	Disease stabilization (%)	mPFS (Month)	OS (Month)
Lee JS	CTX,DX,VCR,VP-16	11	Phase II	82	91	6	8.5
Twelves CJ	CTX,VP-16,VCR	25	Retrospective	53	n.d.	5.5	8.5
Kristjansen PE	CDDP,VP-16,VCR	21	Phase II	52	57	4.5	3.7
Seute T	CTX,DX,VP-16	22	Phase II	27	50	n.d.	n.d.

Table 5. CTX, cyclophosphamide; DX, doxorubicin; mOS, median overall survival; mPFS, median progression free survival; n.d., not determined; VCR, vincristine; VP16, etoposide; Modified from: Yamanaka R. Oncol Rep 2009;22:1269-1276 with permission from Spandidos Publications.

3.2 Second-line chemotherapy (Table 6)

SCLC relapse may also require systemic chemotherapy, which showed efficacy in 7 small phase II studies (83-89) with chemotherapy as salvage treatment after failing systemic chemotherapy and WBRT. Response rates are generally lower and survival is decreased in patients who receive chemotherapy for brain metastases after failure following radiotherapy. Postmus et al. (83) reported a response rate of 43% in the brain after high-dose etoposide. Groen et al. (84) reported a response rate of 40% with carboplatin and Postmus et al. (85) reported a response rate of 42% with a single agent, teniposide. The response rates of the primary tumor are not given in these reports. Chen et al. (89) reported a high response rate of 65% with a combination of carboplatin and irinotecan. In an analysis by Schuette et al. (86) and Korfel et al. (88), response rates for brain metastases of 50% and 33%, respectively, were achieved with topotecan. In both, the cerebral response rate was superior to the response rate of the primary tumor, probably because the intact BBB during the first treatment round protected tumor cells of the brain metastases. However, the severe adverse events associated with these regimens would be difficult to tolerate for pretreated patients who had already received radiation and multiple regimens of myelosuppressive chemotherapy. Treatment-related mortality was observed in 7 of 13 patients treated with high-dose etoposide (83) and in 8 of 80 patients treated with teniposide (85).

Author	Regimen	No. of patients	Study design	Response rate (%)	Disease stabilization (%)	mPFS (Month)	OS (Month)
Postmus PE	HD-VP16	23	Phase II	43	52	n.d.	8
Groen H	CBDCA	20	Phase II	40	60	2	4
Postmus PE	Teniposide	80	Phase II	33	47.5	4.8	2.9
Schuette W	Topotecan	22	Phase II	50	82	n.d.	6
Postmus PE	Teniposide	60	Phase III	22	43	4.5	3.2
Korfel A	Topotecan	30	Phase II	33	60	3.1	3.6
Chen G	CBDCA, CPT-11	15	Phase II	65	86	n.d.	6

Table 6. CBDCA,carboplatin; CPT-11, irinotecan; mOS, median overall survival; mPFS, median progression free survival; n.d., not determined; HD-VP16, high dose etoposide
Modified from: Yamanaka R. Oncol Rep 2009;22:1269-1276 with permission from Spandidos Publications

Temozolomide shows low response rates when used alone. Ebert et al. (90) reported a case of a patient with SCLC with recurrent brain metastases who was treated with temozolomide and oral etoposide. This regimen was well tolerated and resulted in dramatic, durable responses. Combining temozolomide with other chemotherapeutic agents represents a promising strategy for treating patients with brain metastases from SCLC.

3.3 Chemotherapy plus whole-brain irradiation

Postmus et al. (87) reported a phase III study where 120 SCLC patients with brain metastases were randomized to receive teniposide with or without WBRT. Combined treatment produced a 57% response rate, and teniposide alone produced a 22% response rate. Combined treatment produced a longer TTP, but both regimens produced similar clinical responses outside the brain, median survival times (median survival 3.5 and 3.2 months, respectively) and symptomatic improvement. Further studies are needed to compare combinations of WBRT with chemotherapy.

4. Discussion

The impairment of physical, cognitive, and affective function that accompanies most brain metastases is highly distressing and can be seen as a "loss" of the patient even before death. Improved treatment of overt brain metastases may have palliative value and eradication of microscopic brain disease may cure patients already cured in other sites. Assumptions about BBB penetration and chemotherapy resistance have limited the use of chemotherapy for treatment of brain metastases. Small, lipid-soluble molecules can penetrate the normal BBB barrier, but large, hydrophilic molecules cannot. Furthermore, high levels of the multidrug transporter, P-gp, are expressed in the endothelial cells of brain capillaries. P-gp actively prevents drugs from passing through the BBB (91). However, macroscopic metastases, relapsed disease, and radiation therapy can disrupt the BBB (92), as shown via magnetic resonance imaging (MRI) or computed tomography (CT) of intravenous contrast inside intracerebral lesions. In addition, the concentration of chemotherapy drugs, including platinum, is similar in intracerebral and extracerebral tumors (5). Cytostatics unable to penetrate the BBB produce comparable response rates for cerebral metastases and systemic disease, and adding BBB-penetrating drugs such as procarbazine, nitrosoureas, or methotrexate to a standard combination regimen did not improve the CNS relapse frequency (93,94). The chemosensitivity of the primary tumor is the major determinant of the response to systemic treatment for brain metastases (92,95), although asymptomatic brain metastases may have lower responses than systemic tumors to systemic chemotherapy (82).

Dexamethasone and enzyme-inducing anti-epileptic drugs (EIAEDs) can induce cytochrome p450 3A isoenzymes, including CYP3A4, which metabolizes chemotherapeutic agents (96,97) including paclitaxel, irinotecan, vinorelbine, cyclophosphamide, doxorubicin, etoposide, ifosfamide, teniposide, erlotinib, and gefitinib. Therefore, co-administration of EIAEDs or dexamethasone may increase the metabolism of chemotherapeutic agents, lower plasma concentrations, and reduce efficacy.

Response and survival rates are generally lower after chemotherapy for brain metastases following radiotherapy failure (84). Combination regimens also produce side effects that would be difficult to tolerate after radiation or multiple regimens of myelosuppressive chemotherapy. Oral agents such as gefitinib, erlotinib, and temozolomide were well tolerated even in pretreated patients, confirming their favorable adverse event profile. In a molecularly selected population with brain metastases, these agents can produce high response rates.

Brain metastases resulting from both NSCLC and SCLC are susceptible to systemic chemotherapy, with cerebral response rates similar to primary tumor responses, even in second-line treatment. Clinical conditions such as a chemotherapy-sensitive primary tumor, no prior chemotherapy, or the presence of systemic metastases should indicate the use of chemotherapy. The brain is rarely the sole site of metastases in lung cancer, and patients receiving cranial irradiation alone often die of extra-cranial tumors rather than cerebral metastases. Chemotherapy can control other disease sites and is generally better tolerated than

WBRT. Chemotherapy should be initiated before WBRT because chemotherapy cannot be given for 1 month after WBRT and concomitant WBRT/chemotherapy is more toxic. Combinations of these therapeutic modalities for the management of brain metastases require further testing in randomized phase III studies. Because of the short survival times, the late effects of cranial irradiation such as dementia may be underestimated because they do not usually present until months or years after treatment. Kristensen et al. (98) showed response rates of 76% in primary brain metastases from SCLC but only 43% in relapsed metastases, similar to other SCLC metastatic sites. Chemotherapy has a clearer therapeutic impact in SCLC than NSCLC. Thus, chemotherapy should be incorporated into the management of brain metastases as part of a multimodal treatment concept.

First-line chemotherapy can be performed in patients with asymptomatic or minor neurological symptoms or other metastatic sites, as well as for relapses after radiotherapy or systemic chemotherapy. The main goal of cytostatic therapy is palliation, with clinical improvement and brief, limited duration of high-dose steroid treatments critical to this palliation. The inclusion of patients with brain metastases from lung cancer in prospective trials of new therapeutic agents or combinations should be pursued.

5. References

[1] Kristensen CA, Kristjansen PE, Hansen H: Systemic chemotherapy of brain metastases from small-cell lung cancer: a review. J Clin Oncol 10(9): 1498-1502, 1992.

[2] Wen PY, McLaren Black P, Loeffler JS: Metastatic brain cancer. In: Cancer: Principles and Practice of Oncology, 6th edition. De Vita VT Jr, Hellman S, Rosenberg SA (eds.) Lippincott Williams & Wilkins, Philadelphia, PA, pp2655–2670,1999.

[3] Lagerwaard FJ, Levendag PC, Nowak PJCM, *et al*: Identification of prognostic factors in patients with brain metastases: a review of 1292 patients. Int J Radiat Oncol Biol Phys 43: 795–803,1999.

[4] Sheenan JP, Sun MH, Kondziolka D, *et al*: Radiosurgery for non-small cell lung carcinoma metastatic to the brain: long-term outcomes and prognostic factors influencing patient survival time and local tumor control. J Neurosurg 97: 1276–1281,2002.

[5] Stewart DJ, Leavens M, Maor M, *et al*: Human central nervous system distribution of cis-diamminedichloroplatinum and use as a radiosensitizer in malignant brain tumors. Cancer Res 42(6):2474-2479,1982.

[6] Patchell RA, Tibbs PA, Walsh JW, *et al*: A randomized trial of surgery in the treatment of single metastases to the brain. N Engl J Med 322(8):494-500,1990.

[7] Kihlström L, Karlsson B, Lindquist C: Gamma Knife surgery for cerebral metastases. Implications for survival based on 16 years experience. Stereotact Funct Neurosurg 61 Suppl 1:45-50,1993.

[8] Horton J, Baxter DH, Olson KB: The management of metastases to the brain by irradiation and corticosteroids. Am J Roentgenol Radium Ther Nucl Med 111(2):334-336,1971.

[9] Fukuoka S, Seo Y, Takanashi M, *et al*: Radiosurgery of brain metastases with the Gamma Knife. Stereotact Funct Neurosurg 66 Suppl 1:193-200,1996.

[10] Siegers HP: Chemotherapy for brain metastases: recent developments and clinical considerations. Cancer Treat Rev 17(1):63-76,1990.

[11] Lesser GJ: Chemotherapy of cerebral metastases from solid tumors. Neurosurg Clin N Am 7(3):527-536,1996.

[12] Stanley K and Stjernsward J: Lung cancer—a worldwide health problem. Chest 96 Suppl 1:1S–5S, 1989.

[13] Non-small Cell Lung Cancer Collaborative Group: Chemotherapy in non-small cell lung cancer: a meta-analysis using updated data on individual patients from 52 randomised clinical trials. BMJ 311: 899–909,1995.

[14] Schiller JH, Harrington D, Belani CP, *et al*: Eastern Cooperative Oncology Group. Comparison of four chemotherapy regimens for advanced non-small-cell lung cancer. New Engl J Med 346:92–98, 2002.

[15] Cotto C, Berille J, Souquet PJ, *et al*: A phase II trial of fotemustine and cisplatin in central nervous system metastases from non-small cell lung cancer. Eur J Cancer 32A(1):69-71, 1996.

[16] Malacarne P, Santini A, Maestri A: Response of brain metastases from lung cancer to systemic chemotherapy with carboplatin and etoposide. Oncology 53(3):210-213, 1996.

[17] Minotti V, Crinò L, Meacci ML, *et al*: Chemotherapy with cisplatin and teniposide for cerebral metastases in non-small cell lung cancer. Lung Cancer 20(2):93-98,1998.

[18] Franciosi V, Cocconi G, Michiara M, *et al*: Front-line chemotherapy with cisplatin and etoposide for patients with brain metastases from breast carcinoma, nonsmall cell lung carcinoma, or malignant melanoma: a prospective study. Cancer 85(7):1599-1605, 1999.

[19] Fujita A, Ohkubo T, Hoshino H, *et al*: Phase II study of cisplatin, ifosfamide, and irinotecan with rhG-CSF support in patients with stage IIIb and IV non-small-cell lung cancer. Br J Cancer 89(6):1008-1012,2003.

[20] Robinet G, Thomas P, Breton JL, *et al*: Results of a phase III study of early versus delayed whole brain radiotherapy with concurrent cisplatin and vinorelbine combination in inoperable brain metastasis of non-small-cell lung cancer: Groupe Français de Pneumo-Cancérologie (GFPC) Protocol 95-1. Ann Oncol 12(1):59-67,2001.

[21] Bernardo G, Cuzzoni Q, Strada MR, *et al*: First-line chemotherapy with vinorelbine, gemcitabine, and carboplatin in the treatment of brain metastases from non-small-cell lung cancer: a phase II study. Cancer Invest 20(3):293-302, 2002.

[22] Cortes J, Rodriguez J, Aramendia JM, *et al*: Front-line paclitaxel/cisplatin-based chemotherapy in brain metastases from non-small-cell lung cancer. Oncology 64(1):28-35,2003.

[23] Rusch V, Baselga J, Cordon-Cardo C, *et al*: Differential expression of the epidermal growth factor receptor and its ligands in primary non-small cell lung cancers and adjacent benign lung. Cancer Res 53:2379–2385,1993.

[24] Volm M, Rittgen W, Drings P: Prognostic value of ERBB-1, VEGF, cyclin A, FOS, JUN and MYC in patients with squamous cell lung carcinomas. Br J Cancer 77:663–669,1998.

[25] Lawrence DS and Niu J: Protein kinase inhibitors: the tyrosine-specific protein kinases. Pharmacol Ther 77:81–114, 1998.

[26] Fukuoka M, Yano S, Giaccone G, *et al*: Multi-institutional randomized phase II trial of gefitinib for previously treated patients with advanced non-small-cell lung cancer. J Clin Oncol 21:2237–2246,2003.

[27] Kris MG, Natale RB, Herbst RS, *et al*: Efficacy of gefitinib, an inhibitor of the epidermal growth factor receptor tyrosine kinase, in symptomatic patients with non-small cell lung cancer. A randomized trial. JAMA 290:2149–2158, 2003.

[28] Fukuoka M, Yano S, Giaccone G, *et al*: Multi-institutional randomized phase II trial of gefitinib for previously treated patients with advanced non-small-cell lung cancer (The IDEAL 1 Trial). J Clin Oncol 21 (12):2237–2246, 2003.

[29] Kris MG, Natale RB, Herbst RS, *et al*: Efficacy of gefitinib, an inhibitor of the epidermal growth factor receptor tyrosine kinase, in symptomatic patients with non-small cell lung cancer: a randomized trial. JAMA 290 (16): 2149–2158, 2003.

[30] Tsao MS, Sakurada A, Cutz JC, *et al*: Erlotinib in lung cancer - molecular and clinical predictors of outcome. N Engl J Med 353 (2): 133–144, 2005.

[31] Cappuzzo F, Hirsch FR, Ross E, *et al*: Epidermal growth factor receptor gene and protein and gefitinib sensitivity in non-small-cell lung cancer. J Natl Cancer Inst 97 (9): 643–655,2005.

[32] Paez JG, Janne PA, Lee JC, *et al*: EGFR mutations in lung cancer: correlation with clinical response to gefitinib therapy. Science 304 (5676): 1497–1500,2004.

[33] Eberhard DA, Johnson BE, Amler LC, *et al*: Mutations in the epidermal growth factor receptor and in KRAS are predictive and prognostic indicators in patients with non-small-cell lung cancer treated with chemotherapy alone and in combination with erlotinib. J Clin Oncol 23 (25):5900–5909,2005.

[34] Chiu CH, Tsai CM, Chen YM, *et al*: Gefitinib is active in patients with brain metastases from non-small cell lung cancer and response is related to skin toxicity. Lung Cancer 47(1):129-138, 2005.

[35] Wu C, Li YL, Wang ZM, *et al*: Gefitinib as palliative therapy for lung adenocarcinoma metastatic to the brain. Lung Cancer 57(3):359-364,2007.

[36] Ceresoli GL, Cappuzzo F, Gregorc V, *et al*: Gefitinib in patients with brain metastases from non-small-cell lung cancer: A prospective trial. Ann Oncol 15:1042-1047,2004.

[37] Antoniou D, Kyprianou K, Stathopoulos GP, *et al*: Response to radiotherapy in brain metastases and survival of patients with non-small cell lung cancer. Oncol Rep 14:733-736,2005.

[38] Nieder C, Niewald M, Hagen T: Brain metastases in bronchial and breast carcinoma: Differences in metastatic behavior and prognosis (German). Radiologe 35:816-821,1995.

[39] Shimato S, Mitsudomi T, Kosaka T, *et al*: EGFR mutations in patients with brain metastases from lung cancer: association with the efficacy of gefitinib. Neuro Oncol 8(2):137-144, 2006.

[40] Yokouchi H, Yamazaki K, Kinoshita I, *et al*: Clinical benefit of readministration of gefitinib for initial gefitinib-responders with non-small cell lung cancer. BMC Cancer 7:51,2007.

[41] Sakai M, Ishikawa S, Ito H, *et al*: Carcinomatous meningitis from non-small-cell lung cancer responding to gefitinib.Int J Clin Oncol 11(3):243-245, 2006.

[42] Kim MK, Lee KH, Lee JK, *et al*: Gefitinib is also active for carcinomatous meningitis in NSCLC. Lung Cancer 50(2):265-269, 2005.

[43] So T, Inoue M, Chikaishi Y, *et al*: Gefitinib and a ventriculo-peritoneal shunt to manage carcinomatous meningitis from non-small-cell lung cancer: report of two cases. Surg Today 39(7):598-602, 2009.

[44] Lai CS, Boshoff C, Falzon M, Lee SM: Complete response to erlotinib treatment in brain metastases from recurrent NSCLC. Thorax 61(1):91,2006.

[45] Popat S, Hughes S, Papadopoulos P, *et al*: Recurrent responses to non-small cell lung cancer brain metastases with erlotinib.Lung Cancer 56(1):135-137,2007.

[46] Chang JW, Chou CL, Huang SF, *et al*: Erlotinib response of EGFR-mutant gefitinib-resistant non-small-cell lung cancer. Lung Cancer 58(3):414-417,2007.

[47] Gounant V, Wislez M, Poulot V, *et al*: Subsequent brain metastasis responses to epidermal growth factor receptor tyrosine kinase inhibitors in a patient with non-small-cell lung cancer. Lung Cancer 58(3):425-428,2007.

[48] Fekrazad MH, Ravindranathan M, Jones DV Jr: Response of intracranial metastases to erlotinib therapy. J Clin Oncol 25(31):5024-5026,2007.

[49] von Pawel J, Wagner H, Duell T, Poellinger B: Erlotinib in patients with previously irradiated, recurrent brain metastases from non-small cell lung cancer: two case reports. Onkologie31(3):123-126, 2008.

[50] Altavilla G, Arrigo C, Santarpia MC, *et al*: Erlotinib therapy in a patient with non-small-cell lung cancer and brain metastases. J Neurooncol 90(1):31-33, 2008.

[51] Ruppert AM, Beau-Faller M, Neuville A, *et al*: EGFR-TKI and lung adenocarcinoma with CNS relapse: interest of molecular follow-up. Eur Respir J 33(2):436-440,2009.

[52] Katayama T, Shimizu J, Suda K, *et al*: Efficacy of erlotinib for brain and leptomeningeal metastases in patients with lung adenocarcinoma who showed initial good response to gefitinib. J Thorac Oncol 4(11):1415-1419, 2009.

[53] Kunimasa K, Yoshioka H, Iwasaku M, *et al*: Two cases of non-small cell lung cancer which developed central nervous system metastases during gefitinib treatment, improving after changing to erlotinib treatment. Nihon Kokyuki Gakkai Zasshi 48(2):166-171, 2010.

[54] Fujikura Y, Morishima Y, Ota K, *et al*: Satisfactory outcome with erlotinib after failure with gefitinib in a patient with meningeal carcinomatosis secondary to non-small cell lung cancer. Nihon Kokyuki Gakkai Zasshi 48(5):391-396, 2010.

[55] Clarke JL, Pao W, Wu N, *et al*: High dose weekly erlotinib achieves therapeutic concentrations in CSF and is effective in leptomeningeal metastases from epidermal growth factor receptor mutant lung cancer. J Neurooncol 99(2):283-286, 2010.

[56] Pao W, Miller VA: Epidermal growth factor receptor mutations, small-molecule kinase inhibitors, and non-small-cell lung cancer: current knowledge and future directions. J Clin Oncol 23:2556–2568,2005.

[57] Tsao MS, Sakurada A, Cutz JC, *et al*: Erlotinib in lung cancer: molecular and clinical predictors of outcome. N Engl J Med 353:133–144,2005.

[58] Baker SD, Wirth M, Statkevich P, *et al*: Absorption, metabolism and excretion of 14C-temozolomide following oral administration to patients with advanced cancer. Clin Cancer Res 5:309–317,1999.

[59] Ostermann S, Csajka C, Buclin T, *et al*: Plasma and cerebrospinal fluid population pharmacokinetics of temozolomide in malignant glioma patients. Clin Cancer Res 10:3728–3736,2004.

[60] Giorgio CG, Giuffrida D, Pappalardo A, *et al*: Oral temozolomide in heavily pre-treated brain metastases from non-small cell lung cancer: phase II study. Lung Cancer 50(2):247-254, 2005.

[61] Kouroussis C, Vamvakas L, Vardakis N, *et al*: Continuous administration of daily low-dose temozolomide in pretreated patients with advanced non-small cell lung cancer: a phase II study. Oncology 76(2):112-117, 2009.

[62] Abrey LE, Olson JD, Raizer JJ, *et al*: A phase II trial of TMZ for patients with recurrent or progressive brain metastases. J Neurooncol 53:259–265,2001.

[63] Christodoulou C, Bafaloukos D, Kosmidis P, *et al*: Phase II study of temozolomide in heavily pretreated cancer patients with brain metastases. Ann Oncol 12:249–254,2001.

[64] D'Atri S, Graziani G, Lacal PM, *et al*: Attenuation of O6-methylguanine-DNA methyltransferase activity and mRNA levels by cisplatin and temozolomide in jurkat cells. J Pharmacol Exp Ther 294:664–671,2000.
[65] Piccioni D, D'Atri S, Papa G, *et al*: Cisplatin increases sensitivity of human leukemic blasts to triazene compounds. J Chemother 7:224–229, 1995.
[66] Ebert BL, Niemerko E, Shaffer K, *et al*: Use of temozolomide with other cytotoxic chemotherapy in the treatment of patients with recurrent brain metastases from lung cancer. Oncologist 8:69–75, 2003.
[67] Mangiameli A, Mineo G, Trovato G: Temozolomide (TMZ) in patients with brain metastases from NSCLC in combination with brain metastases from NSCLC in combination with gemcitabine-cisplatin (GEM+CDDP) or gemcitabine-vinorelbine (GEM+VNB). Proc Am Soc Clin Oncol 20:A2797,2001.
[68] Quantin X, Khial F, Reme-Saumon M, *et al*: Concomitant brain radiotherapy and vinorelbine–ifosfamide–cisplatin chemotherapy in brain metastases of non-small cell lung cancer. Lung Cancer 26: 25–39,1999.
[69] Quantin X, Pujol JL, Paris A, *et al*: Concomitant brain radiotherapy and high-dose ifosfamide in brain relapses of lung cancer. Ann Oncol 8(9):911-913,1997.
[70] Ma S, Xu Y, Deng Q, Yu X: Treatment of brain metastasis from non-small cell lung cancer with whole brain radiotherapy and Gefitinib in a Chinese population. Lung Cancer 65(2):198-203,2009.
[71] Addeo R, De Rosa C, Faiola V, *et al*: Phase 2 trial of temozolomide using protracted low-dose and whole-brain radiotherapy for nonsmall cell lung cancer and breast cancer patients with brain metastases. Cancer 113(9):2524-2531,2008.
[72] Cortot AB, Gerinière L, Robinet G, *et al*: Phase II trial of temozolomide and cisplatin followed by whole brain radiotherapy in non-small-cell lung cancer patients with brain metastases: a GLOT-GFPC study. Ann Oncol 17(9):1412-1417,2006.
[73] Antonodau D, Paraskevaidis M, Sarris G, *et al*: Phase II randomized trial of temozolomide and concurrent radiotherapy in patients with brain metastases. J Clin Oncol 20:3644–3650,2002.
[74] Robinet G, Thomas P, Breton JL, *et al*: Results of a phase III study of early versus delayed whole brain radiotherapy with concurrent cisplatin and vinorelbine combination in inoperable brain metastases of non-small cell lung cancer: groupe francais de pneumocancerologie (GFPC) protocol 95-1. Ann Oncol 12:59–67, 2001.
[75] van de Pol M, van Oosterhout AG, Wilmink JT, *et al*: MRI in detection of brain metastases at initial staging of small-cell lung cancer. Neuroradiology 38(3):207-210,1996.
[76] Seute T, Leffers P, ten Velde GP, Twijnstra A: Neurologic disorders in 432 consecutive patients with small cell lung carcinoma. Cancer 100(4):801-806, 2004.
[77] Komaki R, Cox JD, Whitson W: Risk of brain metastasis from small cell carcinoma of the lung related to length of survival and prophylactic irradiation. Cancer Treat Rep 65(9-10):811-814,1981.
[78] Arriagada R, Le Chevalier T, Borie F, *et al*: Prophylactic cranial irradiation for patients with small-cell lung cancer in complete remission. J Natl Cancer Inst 87(3):183-190,1995.
[79] Lee JS, Murphy WK, Glisson BS, *et al*: Primary chemotherapy of brain metastasis in small-cell lung cancer. J Clin Oncol 7(7):916-922,1989.
[80] Twelves CJ, Souhami RL, Harper PG, *et al*: The response of cerebral metastases in small cell lung cancer to systemic chemotherapy. Br J Cancer 61(1):147-150,1990.

[81] Kristjansen PE, Soelberg Sørensen P, Skov Hansen M, Hansen HH: Prospective evaluation of the effect on initial brain metastases from small cell lung cancer of platinum-etoposide based induction chemotherapy followed by an alternating multidrug regimen. Ann Oncol 4(7):579-583, 1993.

[82] Seute T, Leffers P, Wilmink JT, *et al*: Response of asymptomatic brain metastases from small-cell lung cancer to systemic first-line chemotherapy. J Clin Oncol 24(13):2079-2083,2006.

[83] Postmus PE, Haaxma-Reiche H, Sleijfer DT, *et al*: High-dose etoposide for central nervous system metastases of small cell lung cancer. Preliminary results. Eur J Respir Dis Suppl 149:65-71,1987.

[84] Groen HJ, Smit EF, Haaxma-Reiche H, Postmus PE: Carboplatin as second line treatment for recurrent or progressive brain metastases from small cell lung cancer. Eur J Cancer 29A(12):1696-1699, 1993.

[85] Postmus PE, Smit EF, Haaxma-Reiche H, *et al*: Teniposide for brain metastases of small-cell lung cancer: a phase II study. European Organization for Research and Treatment of Cancer Lung Cancer Cooperative Group. J Clin Oncol 13(3):660-665,1995.

[86] Schütte W, Manegold C, von Pawel JV, *et al*: Topotecan--a new treatment option in the therapy of brain metastases of lung cancer. Front Radiat Ther Oncol 33:354-363,1999.

[87] Postmus PE, Haaxma-Reiche H, Smit EF, *et al*: Treatment of brain metastases of small-cell lung cancer: comparing teniposide and teniposide with whole-brain radiotherapy--a phase III study of the European Organization for the Research and Treatment of Cancer Lung Cancer Cooperative Group. J Clin Onol 18(19):3400-3408,2000.

[88] Korfel A, Oehm C, von Pawel J, *et al*: Response to topotecan of symptomatic brain metastases of small-cell lung cancer also after whole-brain irradiation. a multicentre phase II study. Eur J Cancer 38(13):1724-1729,2002.

[89] Chen G, Huynh M, Chen A, *et al*: Chemotherapy for metastases in small-cell lung cancer. Clin Lung Cancer 9(1):35-38,2008.

[90] Ebert BL, Niemierko E, Shaffer K, Salgia R: Use of temozolomide with other cytotoxic chemotherapy in the treatment of patients with recurrent brain metastases from lung cancer. Oncologist 8(1):69-75, 2003.

[91] Régina A, Demeule M, Laplante A, *et al*: Multidrug resistance in brain tumors: roles of the blood brain barrier. Cancer Metastasis Rev 20: 13–25,2001.

[92] Postmus PE, Smit EF: Chemotherapy for brain metastases of lung cancer: A review. Ann Oncol 10 : 753 -759,1999.

[93] Bunn PA Jr, Nugent JL, Matthews MJ: Central nervous system metastases in small cell bronchogenic carcinoma. Semin Oncol 5(3):314-322, 1978.

[94] Neijstrom ES, Capizzi RL, Rudnick SA, *et al*: High-dose methotrexate in small cell lung cancer. Lack of efficacy in preventing CNS relapse. Cancer 51(6):1056-1061,1983.

[95] van den Bent MJ: The role of chemotherapy in brain metastases. Eur J Cancer 39(15):2114-2120,2003.

[96] McCune JS, Hawke RL, LeCluyse EL, *et al*: In vivo and in vitro induction of human cytochrome P4503A4 by dexamethasone. Clin Pharmacol Ther 68(4):356-366, 2000.

[97] Yap KY, Chui WK, Chan A: Drug interactions between chemotherapeutic regimens and antiepileptics. Clin Ther 30(8):1385-1407,2008.

[98] Kristensen CA, Kristjansen PE, Hansen HH: Systemic chemotherapy of brain metastases from small-cell lung cancer: a review. J Clin Oncol 10(9):1498-1502, 1992.

Part 3

Gene Therapy and Immunotherapy

16

Fundamentals of Gene and Viral Therapy for Malignant Gliomas

Farizan Ahmad[1,2] and Jafri Malin Abdullah[2]
[1]*Department of Biotechnology and Molecular Medicine*
A.I. Virtanen Institute for Molecular Sciences, University of Eastern Finland, Kuopio
[2]*Department of Neurosciences, School of Medical Sciences*
Universiti Sains Malaysia, Kelantan
[1]*Finland*
[2]*Malaysia*

1. Introduction

Brain tumors are one of the most devastating cancers in human with approximately 200 000 cases reported annually in United States (Khasraw M. & Lassman A.B, 2010). Among all types of brain tumors, malignant gliomas are the most frequent subtype of primary brain tumors which are categorized into low grade, anaplastic and glioblastoma multiforme depending on the histopathological appearance of the tumors. Malignant brain tumors, including high grade gliomas and brain metastases of carcinomas, are devastating forms of cancer and contribute to a high number of fatalities. According to WHO classification, malignant gliomas include grade III and IV tumors with GBM (WHO grade IV), anaplastic astrocytoma (WHO grade III), malignant oligodendroglioma (WHO grade III) and malignant ependymoma (WHO grade III).

Current treatment options for malignant brain tumors are surgical resection followed with chemotherapy and/or radiotherapy. Despite advances in therapeutic modalities, prognosis of the patients remains poor with a mean survival of 14.6 months after diagnosis and a 5-year survival rate of 9.8% (Wirth T. et al, 2009). Tumor recurrence has been reported to usually occur within 12-months after tumor resection. One of the major obstacles to fight over tumor recurrence is the highly aggressive and invasive nature of tumors which often lead to unsuccessful treatments. Therefore, advancement of therapeutic regimes for treating glioma is crucially needed.

2. Gene therapy for GBM, the history

Gene therapy is generally defined as a therapeutic approach for correcting defective genes by delivering genetic materials into cells. Application of viral vector as the main delivery mechanism is consequently called viral gene therapy. Current mostly studied gene therapies involve cancers and hereditary diseases via various approaches. The most important aspect of gene therapy not only to respond specifically in the target area but also to give favorable outcome with the least possible side effects to the patients.

Glioma is a perfect target for gene therapy for its dismal prognosis, localized growth in the restricted brain areas and absence of metastasis. Advances in gene therapy for brain tumors have started long time ago along with other malignant cancers. In 1992, the first clinical trial for brain tumors was reported by Brenner et al. They studied the delivery mechanism of IL-2 gene using retroviral vectors in neuroblastoma patients. Subsequently in the similar year, Oldfield et al, Ram et al, and Klatzmann et al have initiate another clinical trial using HSV-tk suicide gene therapy approach using Retroviral Vector Producing Cells (VPCs) with intravenous Ganciclovir (GCV). (Oldfield et al, 1993 and Ram et al, 1993)
Currently most utilized gene therapy approaches for brain tumors include suicide gene therapy, cytokine gene therapy, oncolytic virotherapy and immune gene therapy with the main use of retroviruses, herpes simplex virus and adenoviruses. Malignant gliomas are the mostly targeted group for brain tumor gene therapy. The two mainly registered clinical trials for brain tumors are cytotoxic gene therapy and suicide gene therapy methods with a total numbers of 34 and 32 respectively (Määtta et al, 2009). Along with others, a total of 91 gene therapy clinical trials have been reported until September 2009 with 62 in phase I, 17 in phase I/II, 7 in phase II, 1 in phase II/III and 4 in phase III. (www.wiley.co.uk/genetherapy/clinical).

3. Viral gene therapy/gene delivery vehicles

Viruses are obligate intra-cellular parasites which generally infecting cells, inserting its DNA into the host genome which is eventually transcribed for the purpose of viral replication. The virus genome contains the basic information of how to produce more copies of their genetic material in order to replicate increase the number of viruses in the host cells. In gene therapy approaches, this virus replication nature has been modified by removing the sequences necessary for the replication and replacing it with the therapeutic gene of interest. The modified virus is subsequently known as viral vector. This modification not only assure the production of the target therapeutic genes but also efficiently working without causing any harm to the host cells (Kanzawa et al, 2003).
Gene delivery vehicles consist of viral and non-viral vectors. Viral vectors which are most commonly used in gene therapy are described in the following table (Table 1). Non-viral vectors used for gene transfer include nucleic acid therapeutics such as antisense oligonucleotide and naked DNA plasmid (Kanzawa et al, 2003).
Delivery mechanism of genetic materials to the patients can be achieved either by direct delivery to the cells (in vivo) or by altering the genes of cells outside of the human body and transfer it back to the patients (ex vivo). Glioblastoma was the first reported cancer to use in vivo technique for gene delivery. (Engelhard H.H., 2005).

Vectors	Type	Advantages	Disadvantages
Retrovirus/ Lentivirus	RNA virus	• broad cell tropism • Stable gene expression due to viral genome integration into cell chromosomes • No toxic effect on infected cells, infect only dividing cells • Total insert capacity 8 kb	• Random insertion of viral genome, possibility of mutagenesis and oncogene activation • Possibility of replication competent virus formation • Degraded rapidly by complement • Possible recombination with

			human endogenous retroviruses
Adenovirus	DNA virus	• very high titers (10^{12} pfu/ml) • Transiently high levels of gene expression • Infect both dividing and non-dividing cells • DNA insert capacity 7-8 kb	• Inflammatory and toxic host immune responses • Host's humoral immune responses may neutralize adenoviral particles • Not suitable for long-term expression of the transgene • Complicated vector genome
Baculovirus	DNA virus	• non-human pathogenic • Infect dividing and non-dividing cells • Transient or stable transduction • High transgene capacity (>35 kb)	• Inactivated by complement factor • Immunogenicity, elevation of short term inflammatory reactions
Adeno-associated virus (AAV)	DNA virus	• Replication-defective parvovirus • High titers (10^{10} pfu/ml) • Wide range of cells can be infected, also non-dividing cells • Ability o the virus to establish latent infection • Nonpathogenic, non-toxic, small genome • Viral integration specific for human chromosome 19	• High titers of pure virus are difficult to obtain • AAV requires a helper adeno- or herpervirus • Limited capacity of foreign genes • Lack of specific integration for recombinant AAV vectors, possibly mutagenesis • Inefficient due to short-lived in patients
Herpes simplex virus (HSV)	DNA virus	• DNA virus, titers range from 10^8 to 10^{10} pfu/ml • Does not integrate into the cell genome • Long-term expression of the transgene in neuronal cells • Induce cytopathic effects in cancer cells • Transgene capacity 30 kb without affecting neither titers nor replication • Sensitive to antiherpetic agents like ganciclovir, which provides a safety mechanism by which viral replication could be abrogated	• Host immune responses, inflammatory and toxic reactions in patients • Complicated vector genome • Most people have preexisting herpes immunity, which could mpair gene delivery • Ability to infect both replicating and nonreplicating cells is undesirable for gene therapy which requires selective targeting of replicating cells

Table 1. Most commonly used viral vectors in gene therapy approaches (Kristiina T. 2006, Immonen A. et al, 2004, Kanzawa et al., 2003 and Romano et al, 2000)

4. Viral vectors for gene therapy

Viral vector is the most important vehicle in gene therapy for its efficiency and specificity to infect host cells and expressing the transgenes. In gene therapy approach for gliomas, retroviruses and adenoviruses have been heavily used in either non-replicating or replicating forms in vivo. Additionally, oncolytic viruses such as HSV-1, Measles, New Castle Disease Virus (NDV), Reovirus, Poliovirus and Vesicular Stomatitis Virus (VSV) have also been tested (Aghi and Chiocca, 2006).

4.1 Retrovirus (Rv)/lentivirus

Retrovirus belongs to the family of *Retroviridae* which is described as RNA type of virus. Rv is highly capable of infecting host cells and reverting its RNA to DNA via reverse transcriptase activity. The formed DNA is subsequently inserted into host genome before being transcribed and translated into protein. (Anson D.S., 2004)

Retroviral vectors are mostly based upon the Moloney murine leukaemia virus (Mo-MLV), an amphotrophic virus which is capable of infecting both mouse cells and human cells thus enabling vector development in mouse models and human treatment.

Rv genome is relatively small (between 8-11 kb) and easy to manipulate for the use of viral vector production. It can also be produced in high titers (10^6-10^7 pfu/ml) (Romano et al, 2000). In viral vector development, genome of Rv is modified by replacing the genes encoding for *gag*(capsid), *pol*(reverse transcriptase) and *env*(envelope glycoprotein) with specific transgene of interest (Kristiina T., 2006).

In cases of malignant glioma, Rv is known to have a vast advantages as a viral vector for its natural activity which is only infecting dividing cells not the non-dividing cells. Therefore, the postmitotic non-dividing brain tissue is left unaffected. Rv have also shown stable integration of the transgene and leads to long term expression of the target proteins. Additionally, Rv demonstrated safety with minimal risk of toxicity in the use of intracranial application (Aghi & Chiocca, 2006). However, there are also reported disadvantages including relatively low titers of the Rv packaging cells production, and small size genome limiting transgene insertion into the cassette. Due to the fact that Rv is integrating into dividing cells, there is high risk of insertional mutagenesis and oncogene activation which may eventually leading to cancer development. (Kanzawa et al, 2003 and Anson D.S., 2004).

Lentivirus (Lv) is a subclass of Rv which is considerably more complex than Rv with additional six proteins, tat, rev, vpr, vpu, nef & vif. It has been shown that lentivirus can infect both dividing and non-dividing cells in a broad range of tissues, stably integrate into the host genome and produce long term expression in brain, liver, muscles and retina (Miyoshi H. M. et al, 1998).

4.2 Adenovirus (Ad)

Adenovirus (Ad) was first isolated from adenoid tissues in 1953 with identification of more than 50 serotypes (Russell, 2009 and Volpers & Kochanek, 2004). Adenovirus infection often causes illness of respiratory system including acute respiratory infections, pharyngitis and conjunctivitis, epidemic keratoconjunctivitis, gastroentitis and pneumonia in young children.

Ad is characterized by non-enveloped type of virus, icosahedral virus with 60-90 nm in diameter and having linear double stranded DNA with genome size of 30-40 kb (Volpers & Kochanek, 2004). Structure of Ad composed of icosahedral capsid consisting of three major proteins, hexon (II), penton base (III) and knobbed fibre (IV) with some other minor proteins which give Ad molecular weight of about 150 MDa (Russell, 2009 and Volpers & Kochanek, 2004). Ad is capable of accommodating up to 10 kb size of transgene, giving it great advantages in gene therapy purposes (King et al, 2008 and Lam & Breakefield, 2001).

Ad is the most extensively used viral vector in gene therapy clinical trials. Most frequently used Ad serotypes in gene therapy are Ad2 and Ad5 (Haritha 2008 and Kristiina T. 2006) which are designed as replication defective viruses as generally used in viral vector gene therapy (Engelhard H.H., 2000). Therapeutic genes are designed to be inserted in into regions of E1A and /or E1B genes, and E2 and E4 genes replacing the original virus sequences (Lam & Breakefield, 2001). However, some drawbacks were reported from this generation of viruses including, 1) maintenance of the viral genome is rapidly lost in dividing cells, 2) viral tumorigenecity, and 3) receptor-mediated uptake of the virus through the primary Ad receptor, CAR, whose expression inversely correlates with malignancy (Aghi and Chiocca, 2006).

Ad is capable of infecting various types of quiescent and proliferating cells including lung, skeletal muscles, heart, liver, blood cells and central nervous system (Haritha 2008). In gene therapy approaches, gene expression from Ad viral vectors occurs without integration of the virus into host genome (Kanzawa et al 2003). Additional advantage of Ad viral vectors are the ability to be produced in high titers (10^{12}-10^{13} viral particles per ml) and low pathogenicity of the virus. However, Ad viral products have been reported to carry high antigenicity and have been associated with toxic and inflammatory responses in brain. Additionally, cytotoxic (CTL)-mediated immune respond often leads to clearance of vector transduced cells and to short duration of transgene expression (Volpers & Kochanek, 2004 and Lam & Breakefield, 2001).

4.3 Other viral vectors

Herpes Simplex Virus (HSV) is a DNA virus with great advantages for gene therapy application. HSV is a common human pathogen which can be found in most people and infecting both proliferating and non-proliferating cells (Lam & Breakefield, 2001). Besides the ability to replicate in neuronal cells and kill brain tumor cells, HSV has been shown to cause fatal encephalitis in humans (Biederer et al, 2002).

HSV offers great advantages including ability to be produced in high titers (10^8 to 10^{10} pfu/ml), huge size of transgene (up to 30 kb in size) can be inserted into HSV genome without affecting the titers or replication, delivery system in CNS is very effective due to neurotropism, sensitive to antiherpetic agents like ganciclovir and HSV has been shown not to integrate into host genome thus reduce the risk of insertional mutagenesis. However, due to its very large viral genome size, the manipulation of the gene becomes more complicated in vitro. Additionally, many people have been detected to have pre-existing HSV in their body thus provides immunity that could lead to gene delivery failure (Aghi & Chiocca, 2006 and Romano et al, 2000). Two types of HSV that have been used in clinical trial of glioma gene therapy are HSV-G207 and HSV-1716. These two types of viruses are conditionally replicating herpes simplex viruses with specific gene mutations and a selective ability to replicate only within dividing cancer cells, leading to oncolysis (Haritha, 2008).

Another type of virus that has shown promising results in glioma gene therapy is adeno-associated virus (AAV) a type of native human parvovirus. This virus enters the host cells by binding to heparin sulfate and able to replicate via assistance of adenovirus or herpes virus. Normally, infection of AAV does not cause any disease in human though integration of the virus genome into host genome occurs. The fact that AAV requires help from either adenovirus or herpes virus for its replication, gives a clear drawback of this virus in gene therapy approach. Additionally, possible transgene that can be inserted into AAV genome is too small (5 kbp only) and gene expression may not be so efficient (Kanzawa et al, 2003).

Other viruses that have been studied in gene therapy for gliomas include Newcastle Disease Virus (NDV), Poliovirus, Measles and Vesicular Stomatitis Virus. NDV is an enveloped negative-stranded oncolytic RNA (Aghi & Chiocca, 2006) with ability to induce necrosis in cancer. Secretion of different cytokines such as interferon and IL-1 may give anti-tumor effect in gene therapy application (Biederer et al, 2002).

Paliovirus is a RNA virus which can specifically infect and replicate in tumor cells due to tumor-specific expression of human poliovirus receptor CD 155. Paliovirus does not integrate and replicate in postmitotic cells like neurons and has been shown as nonpathogenic in primates. In one study, intracranial injection of the poliovirus resulted in 80% long-term survival at 50 days in immunodeficient mice (Aghi & Chiocca, 2006).

5. Gene therapy strategies for glioblastoma

Gene therapy undoubtedly holds a great promise for treating various types of cancer including glioblastoma. Currently, we are aware that no single therapeutic will be sufficient to eradicate tumor completely. Therefore, the combination of conventional treatments with novel gene therapy modalities seems to be the preferred choice (Germano IM., 2009). There is a remarkable potential in the rapidly growing gene therapy field for glioblastoma, however to many dismay it has not yet been proven to be a success story in terms of therapeutic options. There are numerous experimental trials on animal models that hold a great promise for malignant glioma treatment (Germano IM., 2009). Nevertheless, in clinical practice there are substantial obstacles to be considered. Currently, only several protocols were adopted in human studies with varying results. As of June 2010 there were 159 cancer gene therapy trials ongoing worldwide, out of which only 13 were targeted against glioma (http://clinicaltrials.gov/). The rate limiting steps for successful gene therapy for brain tumors lie in the efficiency, stability and safety of viral vectors. However, it is believed that the greatest shortcoming comes from the lack of efficiency that is partly caused by the treatment execution and delivery methods.

In this review, gene therapy approaches for gliomas in 4 different categories will be discussed; 1) pro-drug activation/suicide gene therapy; 2) transfer of tumor suppressor genes and cell cycle modulators; 3) genetic immune modulation; and 4) anti-angiogenic gene therapy.

5.1 Pro-drug activation/suicide gene therapy

Pro-drug activation which is also known as suicide gene therapy applies the concept of delivering a gene encodes for certain enzyme which can metabolize a non-toxic drug to become toxic (suicide gene) and subsequently kill the tumor cells.

5.1.1 Herpes simplex virus type 1/tymidine kinase-ganciclovir (HSV-tk/GCV)

HSV-tk/GCV is the most commonly used gene therapy approaches for glioma. In this two-step therapy approach, HSV-tk enzyme converts non-toxic nucleoside analogs, ganciclovir into phosphorylated compounds which kills actively dividing cells particularly tumor cells (Aghi

& Chiocca, 2006 and Wirth et al, 2009). GCV is a synthetic acyclic analogue of 2'-deoxy-guanosine, chemically designed as 9-[[2-hydroxy-1-(hydroxymethyl)ethoxy]methyl]guanine. In the pro-drug activation approach, HSV-tk presented a higher capability compared to any other mammalian enzymes to phosphorylating GCV and subsequently changes its conformation into GCV-monophosphate residue (Määtta et al, 2009 and Wirth T. et al, 2009). Further actions by intracellular kinases converts GCV-monophosphate into GCV-triphosphate (GCV-TP) which is capable to inhibit DNA polymerase or its incorporation into DNA, resulting to DNA chain termination. This mechanism of actions specifically targeting DNA replication particularly S-phase-specific, thus giving advantage that only dividing cells or in this case only tumor cells are affected (Fueyo J. et al, 1999, Aghi & Chiocca, 2006 and Wirth T. et al, 2009).

The efficiency of this approach also depends very much on the bystander effects of the enzyme activities, referring to the killing of cells that are adjacent to the cells transduced with HSV-TK/GCV. These cells do not express the enzyme but receive similar effects through cell-to-cell contact via gap junctions which allow transfer of Ganciclovir triphosphate from HSV-TK+ cells to non-transduced cells. Activation of the enzyme in the transduced and adjacent cells allow formation of the cytotoxic molecules which contribute to the increment of the treatment efficiency and cells death (Aghi and Chiocca, 2006, Kanzawa *et al.*, 2003).

Gene therapy via HSV-tk approach has undergone clinical trial (phase III) in many countries using retrovirus and most recently adenovirus (Kanzawa at al, 2003 and Asadi-Moghaddam K. and Chiocca E.A, 2009). Until September 2008, a total of 34 clinical trials were registered worldwide with malignant glioma being the biggest sub-group treated. HSV-tk has been the most widely used approach with 32 clinical trials (Maatta et al, 2010).

5.1.2 CD/5-FC combination

5-Fluoro Cytosine (5-FC) is an anti-fungal agent that is generally used to treat fungal infection (Asadi-Moghaddam K. and Chiocca E.A, 2009). In gene therapy modality, this prodrug is converted into active and toxic form of 5-fluorouracil (5-FU) by enzyme called cytosine deaminase (CD). The toxic effects of 5-FU is mediated by its intracellular metabolites, via conversion of 5-FU onto 5-fluoro-2'-deoxyuridine-5'-monophosphate, causes DNA strand breakage leading to cell death (Aghi and Chiocca, 2006).

It has been shown that tumor cells receiving CD may present CD peptides on the MHC Class I which could lead to immune response activation. CD/5-FU combination renders a strong bystander effects compared to HSV-tk due to its ability to diffuse via membrane cells and enters the nontransduced cells (Lam & Breakefield, 2003). Adenovirus has been used in the experimental studies for CD/5-FU combination. There is one registered study which is now in the stage of recruiting patients for the Phase I clinical trials (http://clinicaltrials.gov).

5.1.3 Cytochrome P450 2B1/cyclophosphamide (CPA)

Another pro-drug activating enzyme that has been well-characterized in gene therapy is rat cytochrome P450 2B1/cyclophosphamide (CPA). CPA is a pro-drug agent that can be activated by liver-specific enzyme of the cytochrome P450 family via its conversion to phosphoramide mustard (PM). PM relatively appears in a stable and diffusible form with ability to enter adjacent cells without contact-dependent bystander effects. (Aghi and Chiocca, 2006)

This approach has initially been developed for the use in brain tumor (Chen L. et al, 1997). Studies using retrovirus have shown great promise to reduce glioma formation in mice (Manome et al, 1996 and Wei et al, 1995). Additionally, manipulation of replication-conditional HSV vector has been used for carrying P450 2B1/CPA in glioma treatment (Aghi et al, 1999). Manipulated HSV-1 virus carrying P450 gene acts via 3 modes; 1) using viral oncolysis; 2) rendering the infected cells to CPA; 3) rendering the infected cells to GCV (Asadi-Moghaddam K. and Chiocca E.A, 2009).

Besides the ability to diffuse via membrane to the neighboring cells, use of cytochrome P450 also less immunogenic than other suicide gene therapy such as HSV-tk thus provides long term drug activation (Karle P. et al, 2001). However, due to the fact that cyclophosphamide's active metabolites can only be generated by liver P450 and these metabolites are poorly transported across BBB, there may be some limitation of the use in treating glioma (Aghi and Chiocca, 2006).

5.2 Transfer of p53 tumor suppressor genes

Various studies have shown that alterations of different oncogenes and tumor suppressor genes that control the cycle cycle involved in glioma progression. The alteration may cause disruption of normal functions of the genes and lead to the uncontrolled proliferation of cancer cells (Garrett, 2001). The reported mechanisms by which could abolish the normal functions of the tumor suppressor genes include loss of heterozygosity, methylation, cytogenetic aberrations, genetic mutations, gain of autoinhibitory function and polymorphism (Zingde, 2001).

One of the most widely studied is p53 tumor suppressor gene which is generally inactivated in 35-60% if human malignant gliomas (Kanzawa et al, 2003). Pre-clinical trials with adenovirus mediated p53 gene transfer demonstrated promising results with growth inhibition of transplated glioma and prolongation of the survival in the models. Lang et al in his phase I clinical trial also reported median survival of the glioma patients was 10 months and no-recurrence has been reported in 1 patient for up to 3 years. Lang et al in their studies used two-staged approach for delivering the therapeutic genes; adenovirus vector containing p53 gene was injected intratumorally via a stereotactically implanted catheter, whereafter the tumor and catheter were resected en bloc and re-injections (up to 3×10^{12} vp) were performed into the walls of the tumor cavity. (Pulkkanen & Ylä-Herttuala, 2005 and Lang et al, 2003)

There are also reports that p53 gene transfer is not effective to wild type p53 and glioma is a mixture of cells with mutated p53 and wild-type p53 resulted to partially effective p53 gene therapy. In relation to that, p53 gene therapy combinations have been introduced in order to increase the therapeutic effects. For example, p53 in combination with radiation improves the positive effects in heterogenous cells (Fueyo J. et al, 1999). Interesting study by Huang et al showed that combination therapy of p53 with HSV-tk/GCV suicide gene therapy demonstrated a synergistic effect in C6 rat glioma model (Huang et al, 2007). P53 in combination with oncolytic virotherapy has improved the survival in animal models (Geoerger et al., 2004).

Other therapeutic genes that hold great promise to glioma gene therapy include epidermal growth factor receptor gene, which is often amplified in malignant gliomas (Asadi-Moghaddam K. and Chiocca E.A, 2009).

5.3 Immuno gene therapy

The concept of immune gene modulation in cancers implies the use of various cytokines to enhance the immune response against tumor cells. Most widely studied cytokines in malignant gliomas are interleukin IL-2, IL-4, IL-12, interferon (IF)-β, IF-γ,39 and granulocyte-macrophage colony stimulating factor (GM-CSF) (Kanzawa et al, 2003 and Lam & Breakefield, 2001).

Malignant glioma is a great target for immune gene therapy because of its structure that consists of blood brain barrier (BBB) and without any drainage system. Immuno gene therapy can be achieved either via active or passive strategies. Active immunotherapy provides long-term effect immunity via up regulating the immune response. On the other hand, passive immunotherapy applies the delivery of immune effectors to achieve immediate effect but for short term immunity. Various studies are currently ongoing for both active and passive immune gene therapy for glioma (Clarke J. et al, 2010).

Inductions of cytokines production in gliomas are achieved either by direct cells transplant or genetically engineered virus which carries specific transgenes. One of the promising immune gene therapy approaches is using EGFRvIII as tumor specific antigen to induce immune system to fight against the tumor cells. This study has entered phase 2/3 clinical trial with promising results (Yamanaka, 2008).

Other cytokine that have shown efficacy in experimental animals is IFN- α. IFN- α inhibits cell cycle progression and induces apoptosis in tumor cells thereby leading to enhanced immune system reaction by increasing expression of MHC-1 (King 2005 and Yang 2004). IFN- α has shown to regress glioma in animal model when co-delivered with DCs into the tumor (Tsugawa 2004).

5.4 Anti-angiogenic gene therapy

One of the promising areas to improve the efficiency of the gene therapy is by targeting angiogenesis in the gliomas. Increasing evidences have shown that similar to any other solid tumors, malignant gliomas require sufficient blood supply to sustain growth and glioblastomas have been shown to be the most densely vascularized human tumor (Kunkel *et al.*, 2001). Since 1971, the idea of inhibition of angiogenesis has emerged and lead to extensive research towards identifying and isolating the regulators of angiogenesis, some of which represent therapeutic targets.

Angiostatin, an internal peptide fragment of plasminogen, has recently been shown to potently inhibit endothelial proliferation in vitro and tumor growth in vivo. Animal experiments carried out by Griscelli and co-workers (1998) showed decreased tumor volume, decreased tumor vascularity and increased tumor cell apoptosis in nude mouse model injected with adenovirus expressing angiostatin. Recombinant angiostatin has also been reported to inhibit growth and neovascularization of intracerebral glioma xenografts, as well as to increase tumor cell apoptosis (Rege *et al.*, 2005).

Endostatin, a 20-kDa carboxyl-terminal proteolytic cleavage fragment of collagen 18 is also a potential angiogenic inhibitor. Endostatin was originally reported to inhibit the proliferation of bovine capillary endothelial cells, but not the proliferation of cells of nonendothelial origin, and also inhibit angiogenesis in the chick chorioallantoic membrane model. However, complete tumor inhibition was not observed in either the athymic or immunocompetent animal glioma models (Rege *et al.*, 2005, Kanzawa *et al.*, 2003).

Despite some failures and ongoing research in finding anti-angiogenic therapies for gliomas, some of the researchers are interested with the potential of bevacizumab (avastin) shown in non-small-cell-lung cancer, renal cell cancer and metastatic breast cancer. Bevacizumab is anti-VEGF-A which has been approved by the US Food and Drug Administration (FDA) for the treatment of metastatic colorectal cancer in combination with 5-fluorouracil (FU)-based chemotherapy regimens. Clinical trials of bevacizumab for malignant glioma patients have been carried out by some researchers but conclusive data is not yet been published. (Vredenburgh J.J., 2007, Rose S.D and Aghi M.K, 2010)

6. Conclusion

Advances in the approach of gene therapy for gliomas via pro-drug activation/suicide gene therapy, transfer of tumor suppressor genes and cell cycle modulators, genetic immune modulation and anti-angiogenic gene therapy have shown great promises to better the current treatment regimes. Either being delivered in single or combination with other conventional treatment, gene therapy is anticipated to be able to translate the successful findings from animal experiments to clinical application. In clinical practice, the challenges are not only to fight the extreme invasive and aggressive nature enclosed in malignant gliomas, but also to overcome the difficulties of delivering modified virus vectors into the solid tumor as well as to ensure the efficiency of the genetic transfer. Currently, gene therapy for gliomas is studied in different clinical trials phases.

7. References

Aghi M., Chou T.C., Suling K., Breakefield X.O., Chiocca E.A. (1999). *Cancer Res. Multimodal cancer treatment by a replicating oncolytic virus that delivers the oxazophosphorine/rat cytochrome P4502B1 and ganciclovir/herpes simplex virus thymidine kinase gene therapies.* 59, pp. 3861-3865

Anson D. S. (2004) Genetic Vaccines and Therapy. *The use of retroviral vectors for gene therapy-what are the risks? A review of retroviral pathogenesis and its relevance to retroviral vector-mediated gene delivery.* 2, 9

Biederer C., Ries S., Brandts C.H. and Frank McCormick. (2002) J Mol Med. *Replication-selective viruses for cancer therapy.* 80, pp. 163–175

Chen L., Yu L. J. and Waxm D.J. (1997) Cancer Res. *Potentiation of Cytochrome P450/Cyclophosphamide-based Cancer Gene Therapy by Coexpression of the P450 Reductase Gene.* 57, pp 4830-4837

Clarke J, Butowski N., Chang S. (2010) Arch Neurol. *Recent Advances in Therapy for Glioblastoma.* 67, 3, pp 279-283

Engelhard H.H. (2000). Surg Neurol. *Gene Therapy for Brain Tumors: the Fundamentals.* 54, pp 3-9

Fueyo J., Gomez-Manzano C., Alfred Yung W. K., Kyritsis A.P. (1999) Arch Neurol. *Targeting in Gene Therapy for Gliomas.* 46, pp 445-448

Garrett, M. D. (2001). Current Science. *Cell cycle control and cancer.* 81, pp. 515-522

Germano IM, Binello E. (2009). J. Neurooncol. *Gene therapy as an adjuvant treatment for malignant gliomas: from bench to bedside.* 93, 1, pp. 79-87

Geoerger B., Vassal G., Opolon P., Dirven C.M., Morizet J., Laudani L., Grill J., Giaccone G., Vandertop W.P., Gerritsen W.R., van Bausechem V.W., (2004) Cancer Res. *Oncolytic activity of p53-expressing conditionally replicating adenovirus AdDelta24-p53 against human malignant glioma.* 64, pp. 5753-5759

Haritha D. Samaranayake (2008) *Combination Gene Therapy for Malignant Glioma.* Thesis for Masters Degree in Biotechnology and Molecular Medicine, Biotechnology and Molecular Medicine Department, A.I.Virtanen Institute, University of Kuopio, Finland

Huang Q., Pu P., Xia Z., You Y., (2007) J. Neurooncol. *Exogenous wt-p53 enhances the antitumor effect of HSV-TK/GCV on C6 glioma cells.* 82, pp. 239-248

Im S, Gomez-Manzano C, Fueyo J, et al. (1999) Cancer Res. *Antiangiogenesis treatment for gliomas: transfer ofantisense-vascular endothelial growth factor inhibits tumor growth in vivo.* 59, pp 895–900

Immonen A., Vapalahti, M., Tyynela, K., Hurskainen, H., Sandmair, A., Vanninen, R., Langford, G., Murray, N. & Yla-Herttuala, S. (2004) Mol Ther. *AdvHSV-tk gene therapy with intravenous ganciclovir improves survival in human malignant glioma: a randomised, controlled study.* 10, 5, pp 967-971

Kanzawa, T., Ito, H., Kondo, Y. & Kondo, S. (2003) Journal of Biomedicine and Biotechnology. *Current and Future Gene Therapy for Malignant Gliomas.* 1, pp 125-34

Karle P, Renner M, Salmons B. and Gunzburg W.H. Cancer (2001) Gene Therapy. *Necrotic, rather than apoptotic, cell death caused by cytochrome P450-activated ifosfamide.* 8, 3, pp 220-230

Kaveh Asadi-Moghaddam and E. Antonio Chiocca. (2009) Neurotherapeutics. *Gene- and Viral-Based Therapies for Brain Tumors.* 6, 3, pp 547–557

Khasraw M and Lassman A.B. (2010) Current Oncology Rep. *Advances in the Treatment of Malignant Gliomas.* 12, pp 26-33

King G.D., Curtin J.F., Candolfi M., Kroeger K., Lowenstein P.R., Castro M.G., (2005) Curr. Gene Ther. *Gene therapy and targeted toxins for glioma.* 5, pp. 535-557

King G.D., Ghulam Muhammad A.K.M, Xiong W., Kroeger K.M., Puntel M., Larocque D., Palmer D., Ng P., Pedro R. Lowenstein, and Maria G. Castro (2008) Journal of Virology. *High-Capacity Adenovirus Vector-Mediated Anti-Glioma Gene Therapy in the Presence of Systemic Antiadenovirus Immunity.* 82, 9, pp. 4680–4684

Kristiina Tyynela (2006) *Gene Therapy of Malignant Glioma.* Experimental and Clinical Studies. Doctoral Dissertation. Biotechnology and Molecular Medicine, Biotechnology and Molecular Medicine Department, A.I.Virtanen Institute, University of Kuopio, Finland

Kunkel, P., Ulbricht, U., Bohlen, P., Brockmann, M. A., Fillbrandt, R., Stavrou, D., Westphal, M. & Lamszus, K. (2001) Cancer Research. *Inhibition of glioma angiogenesis and growth in vivo by systemic treatment with a monoclonal antibody against Vascular Endothelial Growth Factor Receptor-2.* 61, pp 6624-6628

Lam, P. Y. P. & Breakefield, X. O. (2001) Human Molecular Genetics. *Potential of gene therapy for brain tumors.* 10, pp 777-787

Lang F. F., Bruner J.M, Fuller G.N, Aldape K., Prados M.D., Chang S., Berger M.S., McDermott M.W., Kunwar S.M., Junck L.R., Chandler W., Zwiebel J.A., Kaplan R.S., Alfred Yung W.K. (2003). J. Clin. Oncol. *Phase I trial of adenovirus-mediated p53 gene therapy for recurrent glioma: biological and clinical results.* 21, pp. 2508 - 2518

Määtta A., Samaranyake H., Pikkarainen J., Wirth T. and Ylä-Herttuala S. (2009) Current Gene Therapy. *Adenovirus Mediated Herpes Simplex Virus-Thymidine Kinase/Ganciclovir Gene Therapy for Resectable Malignant Glioma.* 9, 5, pp. 356-367

Manome Y, Wen P, Chen L, et al. (1996) Gene Ther. *Gene therapy for malignant gliomas using replication incompetent retroviral and adenoviral vectors encoding the cytochrome P450 2B1 gene together with cyclophosphamide. 3,* pp 513–520

Miller C, Williams C, Buchsbaum D, Gillespie G. (2002) Cancer Res. *Intratumoral 5-fluorouracil produced by cytosine deaminase/5-fluorocytosine gene therapy is effective for experimental human glioblastomas. 62,* pp 773–780

Miyoshi H., Blomer U., Takahashi M., Gage F.H. and Verma I.M. (1998) Journal of Virology. *Development of a Self-Inactivating Lentivirus Vector.* 72, 10, pp 8150–5157

Oldfield EH, Ram Z, Culver KW, Blaese RM, DeVroom HL, Anderson WF (1993) Human Gene Ther. *Gene Therapy for the treatment of brain tumors using intra-tumoral transduction with the thymidine kinase gene and intravenoud ganciclovir.* 4, 1, pp 39-69

Pulkkanen K.J and Yla-Herttuala S. (2005) Molecular Therapy. *Gene Therapy for Malignant Glioma:Current Clinical Status.* 12, 4, pp 585-598

Ram Z, Culver KW, Walbridge S, Blaese RM, Oldfield EH. (1993) Cancer Res. *In situ retroviral-mediated gene transfer for the treatment of brain tumors in rats.* 53, 1, pp 83-88

Rege, T. A., Fears, C. Y. & Gladson, C. L. (2005) Neuro-oncology. *Endogenous inhibitors of angiogenesis in malignant gliomas: Nature's antiangiogenic therapy.* 7, 2, pp 106-121

Romano G., Micheli P., Pacilio C., Giordano A. (2000). *Stem Cells Latest Developments in Gene Transfer Technology: Achievements, Perspectives, and Controversies over Therapeutic Applications.* 18, pp.19-39

Russell W. C. (2009) Journal of General Virology. *Adenoviruses: update on structure and function.* 90, pp 1–20

Samuel D. Rose and Manish K. Aghi. (2010) Clinical Neurosurgery. *Mechanisms of Evasion to Antiangiogenic Therapy in Glioblastoma.* 57, pp 123-128

Sandmair, A. M., Turunen, M., Tyynela, K., Loimas, S., Vainio, P., Vanninen, R., Vapalahti, M., Bjerkvig, R., Jane, J. & S. Yla-Herttuala. (2000) Cancer Gene Therapy. *Herpes simplex virus thymidine kinase gene therapy in experimental rat BT4C glioma model: effect of the percentage of thymidine kinase-positive glioma cells on treatment effect, survival time and tissue reactions.* 7, pp 413-421

Tjuvajev J, Gansbacher B, Desai R, et al. (1995) *Cancer Res. RG-2 glioma growth attenuation and severe brain edema caused by local production of interleukin-2 and interferon-gamma.* 55, pp 1902–1910

Tsugawa T., Kuwashima N., Sato H., Fellows-Mayle W.K., Dusak J.E., Okada K., Papworth G.D., Watkins S.C., Gambotto A., Yoshida J.,Pollack I.F., Okada H., (2004) Gene Ther. *Sequential delivery of interferon-alpha gene and DCs intracranial gliomas promotes an effective antitumor response.* 11, pp.1551-1558

Volpers C. and Kochanek S. (2004) J Gene Med. *Adenoviral vectors for gene transfer and therapy.* 6, pp. S164–S171

Vredenburgh J.J, Desjardins A., Herndon II J.E., Dowell J.M., Reardon D.A, Quinn J.A, Rich J.N, Sathornsumetee S., Gururangan S., Wagner M., Bigner D.D, Friedman A.H., and Friedman H.S. (2007) Clin Cancer Res. *Phase II Trial of Bevacizumab and Irinotecan in Recurrent Malignant Glioma.* 13, 4, pp 1253-1259

Vredenburgh J.J, Desjardins A., Herndon II J.E., Dowell J.M., Reardon D.A, Quinn J.A, Rich J.N, Sathornsumetee S., Gururangan S., Wagner M., Bigner D.D, Friedman A.H., and Friedman H.S. (2007) J Clin Oncol. *Bevacizumab plus irinotecan in recurrent glioblastoma multiforme.* 25, 30, pp 4722-4729

Wei M, Tamiya T, Rhee R, Breakefield X, Chiocca E. (1995) Clin. Cancer Res. *Diffusible cytotoxic metabolites contribute to the in vitro bystander effect associated with the cyclophosphamide/cytochrome P450 2B1 cancer gene therapy paradigm.* 1, pp 1171–1177

Wirth T., Samaranyake H., Pikkarainen J., Maatta A. & Ylä-Herttuala S. (2009) Current Opinion in Molecular. *Therapeutics Clinical trials for glioblastoma multiforme using adenoviral vectors.* 11, 5, pp 485-492

Yamanaka R. (2008) Trends Mol Med. *Cell- and peptide-based immunotherapeutic approaches for glioma.* 14, 5, pp 228-235.

Zingde, S. M. (2001) Current Science. *Cancer genes.* 81, 5, pp 508-514

Yang S.Y., Liu H., Zhang J.N., (2004) DNA Cell Biol. *Gene therapy of rat malignant gliomas using neural stem cells expressing IL-12.* 23, pp. 381-389

17

New Therapeutic Strategies in Gliomas Treatment

Gerardo Caruso, Mariella Caffo, Giuseppe Raudino, Concetta Alafaci and Francesco Tomasello

Neurosurgical Clinic, Department of Neurosciences, Psychiatry and Anaesthesiology
University of Messina
Italy

1. Introduction

Gliomas account for about 45% of all primary central nervous system (CNS) tumors and 77% of all malignant primary CNS tumors. Gliomas develop from diverse histological lineages, including oligodendrogliomas, astrocytoma and mixed oligoastrocytoma and all have the potential to become highly malignant neoplasms. Recent studies in molecular biology have better depicted the mechanisms involved in the genesis of cerebral gliomas. It is now generally understood that tumor genesis occurs either by over-expression of oncogenes or inactivation of tumor suppressor genes. Cerebral gliomas represent an interesting target for local gene therapy because of its restricted anatomical location and absence of metastases outside the CNS. This allows delivery of vectors directly to the desired site only a small risk of systemic toxicity (Immonen et al., 2004). The two main gene groups involved in brain tumor development are proto-oncogenes and tumor suppressor genes, respectively upregulated and downregulated during the tumor initiation and progression. In these processes are activated growth factors signaling pathways, marked angiogenesis, downregulation of apoptotic genes and upregulation of antiapoptotic genes. The principal proto-oncogenes involved in gliomagenesis encode for growth factors, growth factors receptors, or downstream effectors of growth factors function, including c-sis (PDGF-B chain), erb-B (EGFR), ras (second messenger for GFRs) and myc (transcription factor). Other important genes and protein functions involved in brain tumor development are bcl-2, protein kinase C-α (PKC-α), c-raf-1, protein kinase A-Type I (PKA I), telomerase, MDM2, IGF I and insulin-like growth factor I receptor (IGF-IR), HER-2 (encoded from c-erbB-2 gene), bFGF, fibroblast growth factor receptor (FGFR), TGF-α, TGF-β2, vascular endothelial growth factor (VEGF), integrins and genes and proteins involved in the cell cycle control, cell proliferation and programmed cell death, angiogenesis and invasiveness pathways. It's evident that the modulation of gene expression at more levels, such as DNA, mRNA, proteins and transduction signal pathways, may be the most effective modality to downregulate or silence specific genic functions. In addition to tumor-suppressor genes and proto-oncogenes, there are, also, the suicide genes. These last ones encodes for a non-mammalian enzyme, that is used to convert a non-toxic prodrug into its active cytotoxic metabolite within the cancerous cells.

Cancer gene therapy can be subdivided into two main strategies: immunological and molecular approaches. The first try to overcome the escape of cancer cells from immune system. Despite the initial enphasys of preclinical immune-gene therapy studies, only a few of these modalities have entered into human trials for gliomas treatment. Genetic immunotherapy can be used mainly to boost T-cell mediated immune response against cancer. This approach involves the transfer of the genes of the immune-stimulant molecules, such as cytokines. Interleukin-12 gene is one of the most studied cytokine. It has been showed complete tumor regression in murine cancer models after interleukin-12 gene transfection into hepatocellular carcinoma and adenocarcinoma cells. The production of IL-12 by tumor cells, after IL-12 gene transfection, mediates activation of cytotoxic T lymphocytes and natural killer (NK) cells (Wesseling & Adema, 2009). Direct genetic vaccination by the antigen (tumor-specific antigen)-encoding genes, like transfection of in vitro engineerized dendritic cells with specific antigens, can also induce the desired antitumoral immune reaction (El-Aneed, 2004; Passioura & Symonds, 2004).

Molecular approaches in cancer gene therapy involve the modulation of oncogenes, tumor-suppressor genes and suicide genes. One of the most investigated suicide gene/prodrug system is the herpes simplex virus thymidine kinase (HSV-tk)/ganciclovir (GCV) system. This indirect gene therapy system has been carried out through the delivery of the herpes simplex virus thymidine kinase (HSV-tk) gene to the tumor by using an adenovirus vector and by transplantating genetically in vitro engineerized cells or inoculation of a recombinant defective virus form into a target cell. Adenoviruses transfer their DNA by binding to a specific cell surface receptor to form a pore in the endosome to translocate genetic materials to the nucleus. The penetration of HSV-tk gene inside only tumoral cells allows the synthesis of thymidine kinase protein and the selective death only of these cells. This process lead to intracellular viral replication and exclusive cytolysis of targeted cancer cells; the newly released virions from a leased cell could infect the neighboring and distant cells but selectively replicate only in cancer cells (Izquierdo et al., 1996). Regarding tumor suppressor genes, because their implication in cancer initiation and progression only when they are deleted in homozygote pattern, the gene therapeutic strategy with should be directed to reach the wild type form of the specific gene function into cancer cell, differently than classic antisense therapy that lead to silence specific genic sequences, usually mutated and/or amplified oncogenes through inhibitors small RNA or DNA molecules.

The prognosis for patients affected by brain tumors is influenced by the histological features of the neoplasm, the age of the patient and the neurological condition or functional status. Despite progresses in microneurosurgical approaches, radiotherapy, radiosurgery and chemotherapy as well as in experimental immunotherapy an effective curative treatment of gliomas does not yet exist. Mortality, in particular if considered into high-grade gliomas cohort, is still close to 100% and the average survival of patients with glioblastoma multiforme (GBM) is less than 1 year when classical treatments is used (Gonzalez & Gilbert, 2005; Stupp et al., 2005). Indeed, progress in treatment of this disease has led only to a slight increase in average survival up to 15-18 months. The efficacy of current anti-cancer strategies in gliomas is limited by the lack of specific therapies against malignant cells. The blood brain barrier limits, moreover, the delivery of many chemotherapeutic agents to the central nervous system, contributing to the failure of treatment. An increased site specificity and internalization can improve the efficacy of treatment and decrease the possibility of side effects.

A potential and futurible therapeutic approach in gliomas treatment is represented by antisense therapy to block selectively glioma cells, trying to led to revert gliomagenetic molecular pathways. This aim could be reached through antisense molecules, delivered inside the brain and in particular inside tumoral cells, able to penetrate into glioma cells nucleus and to integrate with their genome to silence some specific genic functions. Among antisense molecules there are antisense oligonucleotides, ribozymes and RNA interference (iRNA). The specificity of hybridization makes antisense method an interesting strategy to selectively modulate the expression of genes involved in tumorigenesis. Glial tumors seems to be able to create a favorable environment for the invasion of glioma cells in cerebral parenchyma when they combine with the extracellular matrix (ECM) via cell surface receptors. In clinical oncology there are various interesting examples regarding the efficacy of anticancer antisense therapy. Rubenstein et al. published a very interesting findings in an in vivo murin model of human PC-3 prostate tumor. The intralesional injection of antisense oligonucleotides directed against mRNA encoding TGF-α and its target, EGFR, reached to an important hemorrhagic necrosis inside the tumor, directly correlated with cancer cell death. Moreover, although direct intratumoral injection of antisense oligonucleotides was effective, systemic administration appeared to have a better response rate (Rubenstein et al., 1996). Similar results have been obtained from Smythe et al. in malignant pleural mesothelioma lines REN (epithelial) and 1-45 (sarcomatous), using modified bcl-xl antisense oligonucleotides directed near the mRNA initiation sequence. This approach induced upregulation of apoptosis in mesothelioma cell lines (Smythe et al., 2002). In this chapter we describe the most relevant findings of antisense approach application in glioma treatment pointing out the attention on effectiveness, delivery system possibilities, targeting modalities and safety of antisense strategy.

2. Gliomagenesis

Gliomagenesis is characterized by several biological events, such as activated growth factor receptor signaling pathways, downregulation of many apoptotic mechanisms and unbalance among proangiogenic and antiangiogenic factors (El-Aneed, 2004; Idbaih et al., 2008). Several growth factor receptors, such epidermal growth factor receptor (EGFR), platelet-derived growth factor receptor (PDRGF), C-Kit, vascular endhotelial growth factor receptor (VEGFR) and others growth factors receptors, are overexpressed, amplified and/or mutaded in gliomas. Features of the glioma cells are the loss of tumor suppressor genes, which are critical for the cell growth, differentiation and function. Table 1 summarizes the main genes involved in gliomagenesis.

2.1 Genetic alterations in gliomas

Gliomagenesis can develop through two different ways, resulting in evolution of a cluster genic alteration directly from normal astrocyte to GBM or by different kinds of mutations of various genes passing gradually from normal astrocyte to low-grade glioma, to high-grade glioma, to GBM. Primary GBM shows amplification of the epidermal growth factor receptor (EGFR), deletion or mutation of homozygous cyclin-dependent kinase (CDK) inhibitor $p16^{INK4A}$/(CDKN2A), alterations in tumor suppressor PTEN on chromosome 10, and deletion in the INK4a gene with loss of p14 and p16 (Hanahan & Weinberg, 2000; Holland, 2001). Progression from low-grade to high-grade astrocytomas involve inactivating mutations of tumor-suppressor gene TP53 and elevated expression of platelet-derived growth factor (PDGF) ligands and receptors, accumulation of genetic alteration of retinoblastoma-associated cell-cycle regulatory pathways, including deletion or mutations of cyclin-dependent kinase inhibitor $p16^{INK4A}$/(CDKN2A) or the retinoblastoma susceptibility locus 1 (pRB1), as well as amplification or over-expression of cyclin-dependent kinase 4 (CDK4) and human double minute 2 (HDM2). Evolution to secondary GBM is associated with deletion of chromosome 10, which includes tumor-suppressor phosphatase and tensin homolog (PTEN). Additionally Bcl2-like 12 increased expression (BcI2L12) inhibits apoptosis (Stegh et al., 2007). The astrocyte elevated gene-1 (AEG-1) is over-expressed in the majority of malignant gliomas and stimulates cellular transformation and invasion together with the Ha-ras family of retrovirus-associated DNA sequences (RAS) (Ohgaki and Kleihues 2007). Furthermore, oncogenic Ha-ras induces AEG-1 expression by modulating the phosphatidylinositol 3-kinase (PI3K)-Akt signaling pathway and contributes to the growth of HGGs. Mitogenetic signals activate a molecular cascade known as ras-mitogen activated protein kinase (Ras/MAPK). MAPK inhibits the Rb gene, activates the transcriptional factor E2F and cells enter the S phase. The INK4a gene influences the Rb pathway by activating three cyclin kinase inhibitors: p15, p16, and p19.The final result is the blockage of cyclin-dependent kinase 2, 4 and 6, triggering cell-cycle progression by inhibiting pRb.

Genes	**Chromosome**	**Molecular alterations**	**Effects of molecular alterations**
3	Cr17p13.1	Mutation	Cell cycle control loss, proliferation
PDGF-A PDGFR-α	Cr4q11-q12	Overexpression, amplification	Proliferation, invasiveness
Unknown tumor suppressor genes	1p, 19q, 4q, 9p, 11p loss	Loss of heterozygosity	Proliferation, invasiveness
Unknown tumor suppressor genes	Cr22q	Deletion	Proliferation
Rb 1	Cr13q14.2	Mutations/deletion	Cell cycle control loss, proliferation
P16	Cr9p	CDKN2/p16 deletion	Cell cycle control loss, proliferation
PTEN	Cr10q23	LOH	Loss regulation Akt/PKB pathway proliferation, tumor growth, invasiveness, angiogenesis
BAX	Cr19q24	LOH	Pro-apoptotic action loss, proliferation
EGFR (c-erb-2)	Cr7p11-p12	Amplification, overexpression	Cell transformation, proliferation
DM2	Cr12q14.3-q15	Overexpression	Cell cycle control loss, proliferation

Table 1. Main genes involved in gliomagenesis

2.2 Angiogenesis

Malignant gliomas are characterized by extensive microvascular proliferation and a higher degree of vasculature. The formation of new blood vessels from existing microvessels is angiogenesis, an histological indicator of the degree of malignancy and prognosis of patients. The presence of marked endothelial glomeruloid-like proliferations and of a positive immunoreaction at level of basament membrane (BM) in perivascular areas demonstrates active tumor invasiveness, disruption of pre-existing anatomical structures and neoplastic cellular migration along neoangiogenic vascular channel with evidence of proliferation of new fine capillaries (Caffo et al., 2004). Neovascularization in brain tumors correlates directly with their biological aggressiveness, degree of malignancy and clinical recurrence and inversely with the post-operative survival of patients affected by gliomas. Diffuse astrocytomas tend to progress from grade II to grade III tumors with a time interval of several years, whereas, progression of grade III to grade IV is more rapid, typically 2 years. Primary and secondary GBMs are morphologically indistinguishable and show their histologic hallmarks, i.e., "glomeruloid" microvascular tufts and necrosis. Glioma vasculature is structurally and functionally abnormal and it correlates and leads to vasogenic edema, increased interstitial pressure, and eterogeneous delivery of oxygen and drugs (Jain et al., 2007). The new vessel growth is stimulated by the secretion of pro-angiogenic growth factors; these factors bind to receptors on endothelial cells thereby activating them. The vascular endothelial growth factor (VEGF) acts as a major vascular permeability factor and as a mitogen/survival promoter for endothelial cells. The variant A of VEGF (VEGF-A) is secreted by tumor cells as well as by stromal and inflammatory cells. VEGF-A can be linked in the extracellular matrix through the interaction with proteoglycans or glycosaminoglycans. The expression of the receptors VEGFR1 and VEGFR2 is regulated on the endothelial cells in gliomas. The ligands for VEGF3 (VEGF-C&D) are expressed by multiple cell types that surround the angiogenic vessels, suggesting the existence of a novel pro-angiogenic paracrine signaling pathways in these neoplasms. VEGF expression is stimulated by hypoxia and acidosis, and probably correlates with many other growth factors and their specific receptors (EGFR, HGFR, PDGFR, C-Kit, IGFR), and their downstream signaling pathways (PI3K-Akt, Ras-MAPK) upregulation and activation in gliomas. Basic fibroblast growth factor (bFGF) is expressed by vascular cells and, focally, by the tumor cells. The receptors for bFGF include FGFR1, expressed by both the tumor cells; FGFR2 expressed only by the tumor cells whereas FGFR4 is not detected in gliomas. The binding of VEGF on endothelial cells activates the phosphatidylinositol-3-hydroxyl kinase (PI3K)/protein kinase B (Akt) pathway, whereas the bFGF receptors are predominantly shown through the protein kinase Cα (PKCα) pathway. The activation of endothelial cells results in increased expression of cell adhesion receptors, such us integrins $\alpha v\beta 3$ and $\alpha 5\beta 1$, and in increased cell survival, proliferation, and migration responses. Many other proangiogenic factors are upregulated in gliomas and this aspect might explain the failure of many actual antiangiogenic therapeutic strategies in gliomas management. An important role has absolved by bFGF, IL-1beta, IL-6, IL-8, TNF-alpha and stromal-cell-derived factor (SDF)-1 alpha (Idbaih et al., 2008). The angiopoietins are endothelial growth factors nad their signal transduction pathway passes via the Tie2 receptor tyrosine kinase expressed on endothelial cells. In particular, Ang-1 and -2, have been implicated in glioma angiogenesis (Holash et al., 1999). Ang-1 mediated activation of Tie2 is required for stabilization, remodelling and maturation of blood vessels, promotes angiogenesis and tumor growth and is associated with an increased number of highly branched vessels. VEGF and Ang-1 may act in concert (proliferation and maturation), while Ang-2 has been implicated in further remodeling of the initial microvasculature (Holash et al., 1999). Binding of Ang-2 to the Tie2 receptor on endothelial cells antagonizes this receptor's phosphorylation, thereby disrupting contacts between endothelial and periendothelial support cells and disengaging pericytes from the tumor vessels during initiation of vessel sprouting or regression. Examination of the expression patterns of angiopoietins and their receptors suggest a role in GBM vasculature and malignant transformation. Ang-2 and Tie2 expression are absent in the normal brain vasculature but are induced in tumor endothelium of coopted tumor vessels prior to their regression. Treatment of glioma cell derived mouse xenografts with a dominant negative form of Tie2 results in a significant decrease in tumor growth (Zadeh et al., 2000). The discovery of hypoxia inducible factor-1 (HIF-1) and the observation that hypoxia-induced HIF-1α expression in pseudopalisading cells, into intratumoral necrotic areas, was concomitant with the expression of one of its target genes, VEGF, established a biological link between hypoxia and angiogenesis (Semenza, 2003). During embryonic development, blood vessels are newly formed from endothelial precursors and hematopoietic stem cells in a process known as vasculogenesis (Yancopoulos et al., 2000). In contrast, angiogenesis, the sprouting of new blood vessels from pre-existing ones results from an altered balance of proangiogenic factors and antiangiogenic factors. The sequence of events leading to the formation of new blood vessels is well characterized and involves an initial VEGF-mediated increase of vascular permeability leading to extravasation of plasma proteins associated with dilatation of native vessels and reduction in their pericyte coverage. Subsequently, endothelial cells migrate and proliferate. For the newly sprouting vessel is essential the deposition of proangiogenic matrix. This involves breakdown of the vascular basement membrane and extracellular matrix through the action of cathepsin B, matrix metalloproteases (MMPs) and other enzymes as well as the expression of matrix proteins such as fibronectin, laminin, tenascin-C and vitronectin (Gladson, 1999; Ljubimova et al., 2006). The angiogenic process culminates in the assembly of endothelial cells to form a vascular lumen followed by the elaboration of a new basement membrane and the recruitment of pericytes. In contrast to the accepted dogma that tumor development occurs in 2 phases (avascular and vascular), we observe that brain tumor growth follows two vascular phases. In the first vascular phase, the vessels are native cerebral vessels, which are coopted by tumor cells, while in the second phase, there is true neovascularization arising from existing vessels. During the transition period between these two phases, hypoxia driven HIF-1 expression occurs which results in VEGF secretion and the induction of neovascularization. In stage IV, angiogenesis adjacent to the necrotic area is triggered in response to increased expression of HIF-1α and VEGF, a process that rescues the remaining tumor cells. Thus, it is possible to suggest four sequential steps in glioma progression: *i)* perivascular organization, *ii)* proliferation, *iii)* vascular regression followed by necrosis, and *iv)* angiogenesis (Zagzag et al., 2000).

2.3 Invasion

Gliomas are almost invariably fatal and recur near the resection margin in almost all cases. It is unknown how invasive glioma cells survive in the setting of invasion, how they evade immune detection, how they thwart cytotoxic therapies and defer commitment to proliferation. Gliomas show a unique pattern of invasion and with rare exceptions, do not metastasize outside of the brain. The discrepancy between the tendency of gliomas to infiltrate along anatomically defined pathways with diffuse invasion of brain parenchyma and the rarity of metastases to extra-CNS domains remains enigmatic. It is probably possible to demonstrate the preference of the tumor cells to migrate along blood vessels and along myelinated fibre tracts of white matter, through the analysis of the pathways leading to the invasion of gliomas. Invading glioma cells normally migrate to distinct anatomical structures. These structures include the basement membrane of blood vessels, the subependymal space, the glial limitans externa and parallel and intersecting nerve fiber tracts in the white matter. Glioma cell invasion into perilesional tissue consists of an active translocation of glioma cells through host cellular and extracellular matrix barriers (Kohn & Liotta, 1995). Three steps are fundamental in the phenomenon of glioma invasion: a) adhesion of glioma cells to proteins of the surrounding ECM mediated by cell adhesion receptors; b) proteases secretion by glioma cells which locally degrade the ECM components; c) migration of glioma cells into the newly created space through the ECM. ECM is composed of proteoglycans, glycoproteins, glycosaminoglycans and collagens, and also contains fibronectin, laminin, type I and IV collagen, tenascin, hyaluronic acid, vitronectin. It has turned out that the function of neurons and glia can be understood only in relation to their surrounding ECM and that the ECM via specific cell surface receptors play an important role in processes such as differentiation, apoptosis, and migration both in the normal and the pathologic nervous system. In recent years the glioma invasion has also been interpreted by numerous authors in terms of interaction between neoplastic cells and ECM. Critical factors include the synthesis and deposition of ECM components by glioma and mesenchymal cells, the release of ECM-degrading activities for remodeling interstitial spaces, the presence of adhesion molecules (matrix receptors on glioma cell surfaces that specifically recognize and adhere to ECM components) and the effects of cell-matrix interactions on the behavior of glioma cells. ECM modification aids the loss of contact inhibition allowing tumor cells to freely migrate and invade the surrounding tissues. Various ECM components, such us hyaluronan, vitronectin, tenascin-C, osteopontin are regulated within the tumor stroma and at the advancing edge of the tumor within brain parenchyma. Changes in these ECM components are felt to modulate brain tumor growth, proliferation and invasion, although specific interactions and exact mechanisms are unknown. This process is realized through specific receptors expressed on their surface. The integrins, a class of adhesion molecules and the hyaluronan receptor CD44 play a major role in glioma cell-matrix adhesion. Integrins regulate many aspects of the cell behavior including survival, proliferation, migration and differentiation. Integrins of the β1 and αv classes are expressed on different cell types, including neurons, glial cells, meningeal and endothelial cells. β2 integrins are specifically expressed by leukocytes and they are found on microglia and on infiltrating leukocytes within the CNS, αvβ3 integrins is associated with elevated levels of its ligands and with vitronectin in human gliomas. The decreasing, *in vivo*, of the β1 subunit by an antisense strategy in the intracranial C6 glioma model leads to a integrin, this is highly expressed by tumor cells, at the invasive edge of the tumors and by endothelial cells associated with new blood vessels (Bello et al., 2001). Down-regulated *β1* integrin protein levels *in vivo* probably affect interactions of glioma cells with ECM components, leading to reduced migration along vascular basement membranes. These data can be interpreted as a contribute to the locally invasive behavior of astrocytic tumors, favoring the regulation of proteases activation. The proteolytic degradation of the basement membrane (BM) is mediated by proteases, such as the matrix metalloproteases (MMPs), secreted by tumor and stromal cells. MMPs are secreted as proenzymes and are activated by proteolytic cleavage of their amino-terminal domain. MMPs play an important role in human brain tumor invasion, probably due to an imbalance between the production of MMPs and tissue inhibitor of metalloproteases-1 (TIMP-1) by the tumor cells. Among these molecules, MMP-1 is the crucial enzyme able to initiate breakdown of the interstitial collagens, collagen type 1, collagen type 2 and collagen type 3; in this way it activates the other MMPs which allows the glioma cells to infiltrate normal brain tissue.

3. The antisense strategy

Over the last few years, attention has been focused on molecularly approaches. These include the development of monoclonal antibodies to specifically target cancer cells and small-molecule inhibitors of cell signalling pathways that have been linked to oncogenesis. Several approaches are available to specifically manipulate gene expression at the DNA or RNA stage of protein synthesis. In eukaryotic organisms, pre-mRNA is transcribed in the nucleus, introns are spliced out and then the mature mRNA is exported from the nucleus to cytoplasm. The small subunits of the ribosome usually starts by binding to one end of the mRNA and is joined there by other eukaryotic initiation factors, forming the initiation complex. This multi-enzymatic complex scans along the mRNA strand until it reaches a start codon, and then the large subunit of ribosome attaches to the small subunit and translation of a protein begins. This process, by which the information of a gene is converted into protein, is referred to as "gene expression". The antisense concept, regarding genic expression therapeutic modulation, is based on an understanding of nucleic acid structure and function and is dependent on Watson-Crick hybridization mechanisms. The goal of an antisense molecules-based approach is to selectively suppress the expression of a protein of interest by exploiting the genetic sequence in which it is encoded. The identification and validation of antisense inhibitors is the fastest way to identify inhibitors of gene expression. Moreover, as they are antisense inhibitors target RNA and not protein, they can be extremely specific and versatile in their action when properly used.

The antisense strategy was first proposed in 1970s. In this study the authors demonstrated the feasibility of using short antisense oligodeoxynucleotides to block the expression of targeted genes within intact cells. They already documented the use of a tridecamer oligonucleotide as a hybridization competitor to inhibit Rous sarcoma virus replication. This work provided the first evidence that oligonucleotides could be transported into cells (Stephenson & Zamecnik, 1978). The specificity of Watson–Crick hybridization is the basis for rational drug design of antisense oligonucleotides, leading to a new class of selective protein synthesis inhibitors The goal of an antisense molecules-based approach is to selectively suppress the expression of a protein by exploiting the genetic sequence in which it is encoded, acting at translational level (Jansen & Zangemeister-Wittke, 2002; Tamm, 2006; Wacheck & Zangemeister-Wittke, 2006).

Generally, systemic treatment with antisense oligonucleotides is well tolerated and side-effects are dose-dependent. Dose-limiting toxicities include thrombocytopenia, hypotension, fever, and asthenia. Furthermore, an increase in concentration of the liver enzymes aspartate aminotransferase and alanine aminotransferase, as well as complement activation and a prolonged partial thromboplastin time, have been reported. AONs are relatively small, they have short DNA or RNA fragments, 13–25 nucleotides long, with a complementary nucleotidic sequence to sense DNA or mRNA (Baker et al., 2001; Wacheck & Zangemeister-Wittke, 2006). A DNA single strand or positive sense is normally called "sequence sense", when an RNA version of the same sequence exists and is then translated or translatable into protein. Antisense molecules interact with complementary strands of nucleic acids, modifying expression of genes. For a cell to use this information, one strand of the DNA serves as a template for the synthesis of a complementary strand of RNA. The template DNA strand is called the transcribed strand with antisense sequence and the mRNA transcript is said to be sense sequence (the complement of antisense). Because the DNA is double-stranded, the strand complementary to the antisense sequence is called non-transcribed strand and has the same sense sequence as the mRNA transcript. These antisense molecules may be introduced into a cell to silence one of many genic functions through inhibiting translation of a complementary mRNA by base pairing to it and physically obstructing the translation machinery. Antisense oligonucleotides inhibit mRNA function by several mechanisms, including modulation of splicing and inhibiting protein translation by disrupting ribosome assembly. However, the most important mechanism appears to be the utilization of endogenous RNase H enzymes (Dean & Bennett, 2003; Wacheck & Zangemeister-Wittke, 2006).

The use of triple-helix forming oligonucleotides or siRNA molecules are promising alternatives to antisense oligonucleotides. Although many oligonucleotides reportedly demonstrated activity against various viral targets, no oligonucleotide drug has yet been approved for routine therapeutic use, except fomivirsen (ISIS 2922), which is an antisense oligonucleotide composed of 21 phosphorothioate-linked nucleosides (PS-ON). It is administered intraocularly and is used for treatment of cytomegalovirus (CMV) retinitis in AIDS patients. However, it needs to be mentioned that this product has only relative importance and is only used in special cases, as CMV retinitis can be better treated with small molecules like HPMPC (recently approved by FDA and previously already available through an investigational newdrug (IND) program). Nevertheless, the approval of fomivirsen in 1998 was important to antisense technology as a whole, because it demonstrated that antisense drugs can be effective in the treatment of a local disease.

RNA- and DNA-based oligonucleotides are the most prevalent and most practical antisense drugs. There is difference between RNA-based and DNA-based antisense mechanism of action. Interactions of RNA-based antisense oligonucleotides with target mRNA inhibit gene expression by interfering with protein translation without nevessarily altering mRNA stability. Differently, double-stranded DNA/RNA in mammalian cells activates RNase H-mediated degradation of the target mRNA. RNase H recognizes the mRNA-(DNA) oligonucleotide duplex and cleaves the mRNA strand leaving the antisense oligonucleotides intact (Jason et al., 2004; Passioura & Symonds, 2004). The arrest of translation by oligodeoxynucleotides which hybridize within the coding region or over the initiation codon is dependent on cleavage of the targeted mRNA by RNase H. In some cases, but not all, binding of antisense sequences to the 5' end of mRNAs was found to inhibit protein synthesis directly, presumably by interfering with the initiation of translation. Degradation of oligonucleotides in mammalian cells and in blood occurs most rapidly by exonucleases that can be blocked by end-group modifications.

Two alternative antisense-based approaches to modulate gene expression into cancer cells are RNA interference and ribozymes. RNA interference (RNAi) has emerged as an efficient and selective technique to provide stable inhibition of gene expression. This strategy, mediated by small double stranded RNA molecules, is normally an endogenous gene silencing mechanism physiologically used by eukariotes to regulate gene expression by reducing protein production and can also be exploited as a reverse genetic tool to study the function of genes associated with human diseases and as a therapeutic device to treat disease. Moreover RNA interference plays a fundamental role in diverse eukaryotic functions including viral defence, chromatin remodelling, genome rearrangement, developmental timing, brain morphogenesis, and stem cell maintenance. In mammalian cells RNAi can exist under two distinct forms of dsRNA, short interfering RNAs (siRNAs) and short hairpin RNAs (shRNAs). These last molecules then are processed into siRNAs by the multidomains enzyme DICER in an ATP dependent process. This enzyme is an endoribonuclease in the Rnase family that cleaves double-stranded RNA and pre-microRNA (miRNA) into short double-stranded RNA fragments called small interfering RNA about 20-25 nucleotides long. DICER first processes input dsRNA into small fragments called short interfering RNAs, or microRNAs, which are the hallmark of RNAi. Dicer then helps load its small RNA products into large multiprotein complexes termed RNA induced silencing complexes (RISC). RISC and RISC-like complexes use the small RNAs as guides for the sequence-specific silencing of cognate genes through mRNA degradation, translational inhibition, and heterochromatin formation (Macrae et al., 2006). These siRNAs, through a second ATP-dependent molecular step, are then unwound and associate with the complementary RNA, through the action of a multiprotein complex known as the RNAi-induced silencing complex (RISC), and the target mRNA is cleaved within the region of complementarity to the siRNA. DsRNA and siRNA activate respectively two different molecular pathways. DsRNAs activate endogenous dsRNA-dependent protein kinase (PKR), leading to phosphorylation of the translation initiation factor EIF2α and finally to a general suppression of protein synthesis and to an upregulation of apoptosis. On the other hand, in mammalian cells, siRNAs lead to the knockdown of the target gene expression. The limit in clinic and therapeutic use of siRNA to modify strongly gene expression is represented from the transient effect of siRNA. These antisense molecules in fact, because of mammalian cells lack the RNA-dependent RNA polymerase, should be require the stable transfection into target cells by plasmid vectors. A peculiar distinctive characteristic between RNA interference and the other antisense approaches (antisense oligonucleotides and ribozymes) is the extreme selectivity for substrate from siRNA. In this way these antisense molecules may inhibit selectively the expression of oncogene containing a single point mutation, without suppress the expression of the wild-type transcript. RNA interference-based therapies are available to the targeting oncogenic transcripts in which two cellular genes have become fused, leading to the generation of an oncogenic fusion protein, such as Bcr-abl in myeloid chronic leukaemia (Jason et al., 2004; Passioura & Symonds, 2004).

Ribozymes have been discovered in the early 1980s. These molecules are catalytic RNA-RNA enzymes. The first ribozyme discovered was found in the group I intervening sequence of the pre-mRNA of Tetrahymena thermophila (Cech et al., 1986) and was shown as a ribozyme with the capacity to catalyse its own excision (CIS acting ribozyme).

4. Molecular targets

In the last decade there have been various studies that have demonstrated efficacy of antisense therapy in vitro and in vivo in oncological diseases and, specifically, in brain tumor. Different target molecules at different steps and pathways, such as cell immortalization and apoptosis escape, tumor neoangiogenesis, invasion of normal tissues have been studied and chosen as a possible target of new antisense therapeutic model in glioma treatment. In table 2 are reported the mainly molecular targets.

Molecular target	Normal function	Kind of mutation	Effect of mutation
Bcl-2	Prevents the release of cytochrome C from the mitochondria.	Overexpression	Inhibition of apoptosis and increase of resistance to chemo- and radiotherapies.
PKC-α	Involved in growth-factor-mediated signal transduction pathways.	Overexpression	Upregulation of cancer cell, proliferation and tumor growth.
TGF-β2 (Glioblastoma-derived T-cell suppressor factor, G-TSF, BSC-1 cell growth inhibitor)	It suppresses the effects of interleukin dependent T-cell tumors.	Overexpression	Downregulation of apoptosis and tumor growth. Increases ECM invasion and induces escape of tumor from immunosurveillance.
Telomerase (h-TR)	Reverse transcriptase that carries its own RNA molecule, which is used as a template when it elongates telomeres.	Overexpression	Cancer cell immortalization, tumor growth.
Focal adhesion kinase (FAK) and insulin-like growth factor I receptor (IGF-IR)	FAK is a protein tyrosine kinase which is recruited at an early stage to focal adhesions, leading the cytoskeleton to interact with proteins of the ECM, and initiate events as cell migration and anchorage-dependent differentiation. Transmembrane receptor that is activated by IGF-1 and by the related growth factor IGF-2. It belongs to the large class of tyrosine kinase receptors. This receptor mediates the effects of IGF-1.	Overexpression Gene amplification	Cancer cell proliferation, downregulation of apoptosis and tumor growth.
PTEN (MMAC 1)	Tumor-suppressor gene located on human chromosome 10q23.3,	Nonsense mutation, LOH	Cancer cell proliferation, downregulation of apoptosis, tumor growth,

Molecular target	Normal function	Kind of mutation	Effect of mutation
	regulating cell growth, apoptosis, interaction with ECM and inhibiting cell migration, as well as spreading and focal adhesion.		invasion.
PI3K/AKT/PKB (pathway of bFGF, PDGF, IGF, VEGF, EGFR)	Pathway involved in cell survival. AKT has an antiapoptotic effect by inactivating the proapoptotic BAD, procaspase-9 and fork-head transcription factors (activation of Fas ligand). AKT induces NF-kB-dependent pro-survival genes expression (BCL-xL, C-Myb), modifies cell cycle progression by inhibiting p27 and p21, up-regulates transcription of cyclin D and promotes nuclear entry of mdm2.	Overexpression Gene amplification	Upregulation of cancer cell proliferation, loss of cell cycle control, increased telomerase activity, cell invasiveness and angiogenesis by stimulating secretion of MMPs and by activating endothelial nitric oxide synthase (eNOS).

Table 2. Principal molecular pathways involved in gliomagenesis and glioma angiogenesis.

4.1 BCL-2

Apoptosis is an important process involved in cell survival. In particular exist two different constitutive apoptotic pathways, the extrinsic pathway, that starting from external death signals induces the activation of the caspase pathway through initial activation of caspase-8, and the intrinsic one. This last pathway involves Bcl-2 family proteins. Inside the extrinsic apoptotic pathway, Zhou et al have demonstrated the upregulation of glioma cells apoptosis through activation of caspase 9 and 3 (Zhou et al., 2010).

Bcl-2 gene is one of the most important proto-oncogenes, proptpypical inhibitor of apoptosis, located at the breakpoints of t(14;18) chromosomal translocations in low-grade B-cell non-Hodgkin's lymphomas. BCL-2 encodes an oncogenic mitochondrial protein with transport functions and its expression level is very increased in many types of cancer, such as follicular non Hodgkin lymphoma, other lymphomas, leukemias and lung, breast, colorectal, gastric, prostate, renal cancer and neuroblastoma. BCL-2 protein prevents the release of cytochrome C from the mitochondria (GROSS 99), inhibiting in this way apoptosis. Normally, in response to DNA damage, to cellular stress and to other cellular damage signals, BCL-2 induces the release of cytochrome c from mitochondrial matrix to cytosol, where it activates caspase-9 and caspase-3 through the activation of Apaf-1 (El-

Aneed, 2004). This overexpression of BCL-2 make it a very promising target for the antisense therapy, in consideration also of the BCL-2 protein effect on chemo/radiation resistance. In fact, the BCL-2 group of proteins has been implicated not only in the pathogenesis of cancer but also in resistance to cancer treatment. Thus, the antisense modulation of BCL-2 (mRNA or protein) expression could increase the effectiveness of conventional chemotherapeutic agents. A phase II trial is underway with G3139 in combination with standard chemotherapy for patients with relapsed, chemotherapy resistant non-Hodgkin's lymphoma. Overexpression of BCL-2 is not uncommon in non-B cell malignant tumours. Human melanoma expresses BCL-2 in up to 90% of all cases. Jansen and colleagues showed that G3139 improves the chemosensitivity of human melanoma transplants in severe combined immunodeficient mice. Additionally, in a phase I/II study, Jansen's group tested the combination of G3139 and dacarbazine in patients with advanced malignant melanoma. In a within-patient dose-scalation protocol, G3139 0.6–6.5 mg/kg was given intravenously or subcutanously to 14 patients with advanced malignant melanoma along with standard dacarbazine treatment. In serial tumour biopsy samples, BCL2 concentrations were measured by immunoblot, and apoptosis of tumour cells was assayed. The combination regimen was well tolerated with no doselimiting toxicity. Haematological abnormalities were mild to moderate. Lymphopenia was common. High doses of G3139 were associated with transient fever. Four patients had liver-function abnormalities that resolved within 1 week. Steady-state plasma concentrations of G3139 were obtained within 24 h and increased with the administered dose as assessed by liquid chromatography. By day 5, daily doses of 1.7 mg/kg and higher led to a median decrease of BCL2 expression of 40% in melanoma samples compared with baseline. Reduced BCL2 expression was associated with increased apoptosis of tumour cells. Apoptosis was further enhanced after dacarbazine treatment. Six of 14 patients showed antitumour responses. The estimated median survival of all patients was more than 12 months, which compares favourably with survival of stage IV malignant melanoma patients (usually 6–9 months with and without treatment). This study is worth mentioning because it was the first antisense trial in which downregulation of the target protein in the target tissue was shown (Jansen & Zangemeister-Wittke, 2002). Based on the promising results of this study, the combination of dacarbazine and G3139 therapy in patients with malignant melanoma received fast-track approval by the FDA, and is in a phase III multicentre trial (Pirollo et al., 2003). Phase I and II studies are also being done to test G3139 in combination with docetaxel in patients with advanced breast cancer, hormone-refractory prostate cancer, and other solid tumours. Another phase I study is analysing the combination of G3139 and mitoxantrone in patients with hormone refractory prostate cancer. In 21 individuals treated so far, toxicities were transient and included neutropenia (grade 3), lymphopenia (grade 2), fatigue, arthralgias, and myalgias (all grade 1). No dose limiting toxicities were reported for the doses tested, and one patient had a greater than 50% response to prostate specific antigen with symptomatic improvement in bone pain. Another phase I study has been started to test G3139 together with salvage chemotherapy of fludarabine and cytarabine in patients with refractory or relapsed acute myelogenous leukaemia or acute lymphocytic leukaemia. Furthermore, a phase I/II trial of a combination treatment of G3139 and irinotecan has been initiated in patients with metastatic or recurrent colorectal cancer. So far, no results are available for these two trials. By using antisense oligonucleotides against the first six codons of the human bcl-2 gene transfected into malignant glioma cells (Jon52 and Roc glioblastoma cell lines), Julien et al. demonstrated a decrease in cell growth and an increase in apoptotic death (Julien et al., 2000). As to BCL2 proteins family role in apoptotic cell death regulation, Guensberg et al. showed that resistance to chemotherapy in glioblastoma is linked to the expression of antiapoptotic Bcl-2 family members, including Bcl-xL. The authors used anti-Bcl-xL antisense oligonucleotides (ISIS 16009, ISIS 16967) in M059K glioblastoma cell lines and demonstrated a strong correlation between reduction of Bcl-xL protein expression, induction of intrinsic apoptotic pathway and enhancement of cytotoxic responses to paclitaxel treatment, resulting in a chemosensitizing effect of anti-Bcl-xL therapy (Guensberg et al., 2002).

4.2 Protein Kinase C-α (PKC-α)

A key regulatorin the glioma cell differentiation and proliferation is protein kinase C-alpha (PKC-alpha). This protein, translated from the mRNA of pkc-α gene, located on chromosome 16p11.2-q12.1, is a member of family of cytoplasmic serine-threonine protein kinases, strongly involved in growth-factor-mediated signal transduction pathways, in order to reach a key role in regulating cell differentiation and proliferation. Its involvement in oncogenesis is suggested by the fact that they are the major intracellular receptors for tumour-inducing phorbol esters. Among the various PKC isoenzymes, PKC-α may show the greatest degree of overexpression in transformed cell lines as compared to normal astrocytes in brain tissue peritumoral samples. The overexpression of this transduction signal protein has been implicated in various kinds of tumors, such as breast, colon, lung, ovarian cancer, melanoma, brain tumors (Campbell & Pollack, 1997; Pirollo et al., 2003). PKC-α inhibitors such as tamoxifen and UCN-01 rich a very high amount of down-regulation of in vitro growth and in vivo tumorigenicity. Moreover, numerous in vitro and in vivo animal studies have showed the efficacy of antisense oligonucleotides against PKC-α in the cancer growth inhibition. ISIS 3521 is the most experimented in order to test the in vitro and in vivo effects of the PKC-α downregulation towards cell proliferation and tumors, such as NHL, ovarian cancer, NSCLCs, kidney clear cell carcinoma. Results of a phase I study suggested that an antisense oligonucleotide directed against PKC-alpha (ISIS 3521) might be effective in the treatment of low-grade lymphoma. In this trial ISIS 3521 was delivered over 21 days by continuous intravenous infusion followed by a 7-day rest period. In an in vitro study of A549 lung epithelia cells, McKay et al. have shown depletion of PKC-α expression by antisense oligonucleotides leading to a reduction in c-jun expression but c-fos or junB (McKay et al., 1999). This is a crucial pathway in cell growth, cell death and its proliferation. The transcription factor c-Jun is one of major targets of JNK phosphorylation. JNK activation and c-Jun phosphorylation are involved in the induction of apoptosis (Potapova et al., 2000). Inhibition of PKC-α expression, at mRNA level, by a syntetic antisense oligonucleotide has been shown to inhibit proliferation of C6 glioma cells and in vitro and in vivo growth inhibition of transformed U-87 cells transfected with a PRSV vector loading antisense anti-PKC-α oligonucleotide, and, respectively, in vivo subcutaneous tumorigenicity lost (Pollack et al., 1996). Grossman et al. studied the therapeutic efficacy and toxicity of a phosphorothioate antisense oligonucleotide (Aprinocarsen, Eli Lilly LY9000003) directed against PKC-α in patients with recurrent malignant gliomas. In this clinical phase II study no clinical benefit was seen, probably because of tumor growth or the effect of Aprinocarsen on BBB, whose mechanisms are unknown (Grossman et al., 2004).

Other potential therapeutic targets of antisense therapy are human C-raf kinase and c-Ki-RAS proteins and signal transduction kinase proteins, involved in the control of proliferation, cellular migration, differentiation and cytoskeletal rearrangements. Monia et al. demonstrated the evidence of antitumor activity of phosphorothioate antisense inhibitor C-raf Kinase (ISIS 5132 or CGP69846A) in tumor-bearing mice, demonstrating an important reduction of tumor growth (Monia et al., 1996). Chen et al study has documented a valid role of oncogenic Ha-RAS oligo (ISIS 2503) in the proliferation of T24 cells in human bladder carcinoma (Chen et al., 1996).

4.3 TGF-β2

A key role in gliomagenesis is absolved by TGF-β2 and consequently this growth factor represent an important target of antisense therapy. TGF-β2 role in brain tumor and in glioma progression in particular was investigated in 1993 by Jachimczak et al. The authors demonstrated the efficacy of specific antisense therapy in down-regulation of TGF-β2, through stimulation of antitumoral immunosurveillance. In HTZ-153, HTZ-209 and HTZ-243 glioblastoma and malignant astrocytomas cell lines, TGF-β2 specific phosphorotioate antisense oligonucleotides enhanced lymphocyte proliferation up to 2.5 fold and autologous tumor cytotoxicity up to 60%. Through an antisense therapy against TGF-β1 and-β2 in 12 glioma cell lines, another study of the same research group has showed that the effect of anti-TGF-β2 phosphorotioate antisense oligonucleotides is much stronger than anti-TGF-β1 ones (Hau et al., 2009; Jachimczak et al., 1996). This cytokine binds to TGF-β receptors (TBR) and initiates a signaling cascade via cytoplasmic signaling mediators (Smads) into the nucleus, inducing regulation of target gene expression. Besides this pathways, other intracellular TGF- β activated pathways include mitogen- activated protein kinase (MAPK), N-RAS, Ral guanine nucleotide exchange factors (Ral-GEF), PI3-K/Akt), c-Jun-NH(2)-terminal kinase (JNK), p38-P and protein phosphatase 2A (PP2A/$p70^{S6K}$). During tumorigenesis, TGF-β increases extracellular matrix invasion and induces escape of tumor from immunosurveillance. In this study antisense compound AP 12009 (antisense oligonucleotide anti TGF-β2 mRNA) enhanced the immune cell mediated cytotoxic antitumor response against tumor cells (Hau et al., 2007; Schlingensiepen, 2005, 2006). Schneider et al. have examined a "double-punched" approach to overcome the escape of glioblastoma cells to the immune surveillance, through an active specific immunization (ASI) with Newcastle-Disease-Virus infected tumor cells and blocked the TGF-β production by delivery of TGF-β antisense oligonucleotides using polybutyl cyanoacrylate NPs. This approach induced a significant decrease in plasma TGF-β2 level as well as an increase in rate of high affinity IL-2 receptor (CD25) on lymphocytes and consequently of antitumoral cytotoxicity (Schneider et al., 2008).

4.4 Human telomerase

Kondo et al. demonstrated in vitro and in vivo that anti-hTR antisense treatment suppressed tumor cell growth and survival by inducing apoptosis, by treating malignant glioma cells (U251-MG cells) in culture with 2-5A antisense oligonucleotide against telomerase RNA and by inoculating this antisense molecule directly into tumors induced in nude mice (Kondo et al., 1998). This study group showed in vitro that human telomerase antisense inhibition induced two different pathways: apoptosis and differentiation in subpopulations of malignant glioma cells that escape from apoptotic crisis. Probably, malignant glioma cells are cells in G2/M phase in contrast with the major percentage of apoptotic cells that are in S phase of the cell cycle. These results indicate that antisense hTR reduced cell cycling and caused an accumulation of cells in G2/M. Treatment of surviving nonapoptotic cells with antisense oligonucleotides against p27, but not against p21, (two important cyclin-dependent kinase inhibitors–CDKIs) induced apoptotic cell death; this suggests that p27 may have a protective role for the survival of differentiating glioma cells (Kondo et al., 1998). The efficacy in vitro and in vivo murine model combined with therapy with 2-5A anti-hTR and recombinant adenovirus p53 (Ad5CMV-p53) was showed by Komata et al. in malignant glioma cell lines with mutant p53 and in vivo GBM murine model (Komata et al., 2000). By using an antisense oligonucleotide against hTER (the RNA component of telomerase), Mukai et al. detected many telomerase-positive tumor cells in the vast majority of malignant gliomas (Mukai et al., 2000). In a recent in vitro study (U87-MG and U373-MG human malignant glioma cells cultures, cell cultures of human astrocytes expressing telomerase with or without oncogenic Ras) and in vivo (murine model) study, it was demonstrated that treatment with 2-5A-anti-hTR in the presence of N, N'-bis (2-chloroethyl)-N.nitrosourea (BCNU), cisplatin (CDDP) and temozolomide (TMZ) better enhanced the cell-killing effect if done sequentially rather than concurrently; treatment with 2-5A-anti-hTR in the presence of paclitaxel (PTX) and γ irradiation (IR) always enhanced this effect. The enhanced cell-killing resulted by up-regulation of apoptosis. 2-5A-anti-hTR did not impair the autophagy induced by treatment with TMZ or IR and a synergistic combined effect. In animal xenograft study model, TMZ enhanced the anti-tumor effect of 2-5A anti-hTR via induction of apoptosis (Iwado et al., 2007).

In an in vivo murine model, created by implantation of U-87 MG malignant glioma cells in mouse, Im et al. demonstrated the suppression of the ability of glioma cells to form tumors in mice. This result was obtained after transfection of antisense VEGF cDNA in an antisense orientation through the recombinant adenoviral vector Ad5CMV-αVEGF. Infection of U-87 MG malignant glioma cells resulted in the reduction of the level of the endogenous VEGF mRNA and drastically decreased the production of the targeted secretory form of the VEGF protein (Im et al., 1999).

Resnicoff et al. examined the role of IGF-1R in the growth of rat GBM cells and focused the attention on IGF-1R pathway, which is critical in the regulation of cell proliferation. In fact, neuroglial cell growth and CNS development are normally strongly regulated by IGF-1 and IGF-2 via IGF-1R. By introducing a plasmid expressing an antisense RNA to IGF-1R RNA, the study demonstrated the reduction of IGF-1R levels in cell growth in vitro, anchorage-independent growth and prevention of the development of tumors in rats (Resnicoff et al., 1994). Andrews et al. observed that IGF-1R AONs-treated autologous glioma cells, collected during surgical treatment, were induced toward apoptosis and that, in an in vivo murine model, they gave rise to a host response (Andrews et al., 2001).

Liu et al. showed the crucial involvement of two signal transduction pathways, respectively activated by focal adhesion kinase (FAK) and insulin-like growth factor I receptor (IGF-IR) kinase into gliomagenesis. In this in vitro and in vivo study (U87 and LN229 glioma cell lines and mice bearing intracranial glioma xenografts) the authors demonstrated that TAE226, a potent ATP-competitive inhibitor of several tyrosine kinases (such as FAK and IGF-IR kinase) down-regulated proliferation and invasion of glioma cells and inhibited cell cycle progression particularly at the G2-M checkpoint. TAE226 also gave rise to a concomitant reduction of the expression of p-cdc2 (Tyr15) and cyclin B1, increase in apoptosis and reduction in glioma invasion in an in vitro Matrigel (Liu et al., 2007). The central role of FAK has already been examined in Wu et al. study. By using anti-FAK

phosphotothioate antisense oligonucleotides packaging into liposomes in U251 MG cells, the authors showed down-regulation of expression levels of FAK and activation of apoptosis, through increase in caspase-3 activity, which is a key-mediator of apoptosis in mammalian cells. In fact, FAK activates the PI3K survival pathway with the concomitant activation of nuclear factor Kappa B (NF-kB) and induction of inhibitor of apoptosis (Wu et al., 2006).
Another possible interesting target of antisense therapy could be PTEN or MMAC 1, a tumor-suppressor gene located on human chromosome 10q23.3, regulating cell growth, apoptosis, interaction with extracellular matrix and inhibiting cell migration, as well as spreading and focal adhesion. PTEN protein has two different phosphatase activities: a lipid-phosphatase activity and a protein-phosphatase activity. Substrates of these specific phosphatase activities are phosphatidylinositol 3,4,5-triphosphate and phosphatidylinositol 3,4-biphosphate; they are both involved in the PI3K FAK pathways. In Park et al. study, it was demonstrated that PTEN has an important role in the inhibition of hyaluronic acid-induced MMP-9 secretion, in the down-regulation of basal levels of MMP-2 and in the increase in expression levels of the tissue inhibitor of metalloproteinase-1 and -2 (Park et al., 2002).

4.5 PI3K/AKT/PKB pathway

Among the different growth factors/receptors pathways involved in tumorigenesis of brain tumors, such as bFGF, PDGF, IGF, VEGF, EGFR, a crucial role plays PI3K/AKT/protein kinase B (PKB) pathway, normally involved in cell survival. AKT is a subfamily of the serine/threonine kinases that includes AKT1, AKT2 and AKT3. Growth factors and their receptors led to the activation of PI3K, which in turn phosphorilates phosphotidylinositol-3,4-biphosphate (PIP2) to phosphotidylinositol-3,4,5-triphosphate (PIP3). PIP3 binds to PH domain of AKT and gives rise to AKT activation. AKT has an antiapoptotic effect by phosphorilating and inactivating the proapoptotic BAD, procaspase-9 and fork-head transcription factors. These molecules activate Fas ligand; moreover AKT also induces NF-kB-dependent transcription of pro-survival genes including BCL-xL, C-Myb, modifies cell cycle progression by inhibiting p27 and p21, up-regulates transcription of cyclin D and promotes nuclear entry of mdm2. It also leads to degradation of p53 and to uncontrolled cell proliferation. AKT enhances telomerase activity and promotes cell invasiveness and angiogenesis by stimulating secretion of MMPs and by activating endothelial nitric oxide synthase (eNOS). In an in vitro and in vivo murine model, Pu et al. showed the down regulation of proliferation rate of C6 glioma cells transfected with antisense AKT2 cDNA construct. Parental C6 cells and C6 cells, transfected with antisense construct, were stereotactically implanted into the right caudate nucleus of rats through lipofectamine complexes. Antisense inhibition of AKT2 resulted in the reduction of growth rate and proliferation of C6 cells, as well as in the up-regulation of GFAP expression and in the induction of apoptosis (Pu et al., 2006). Inside this crucial molecular pathway, an important potential molecular target of gliomas antisense therapy is HER1/EGFR signal transduction pathway. This tyrosine kinase receptor can show various kinds of alterations such as gene amplification or overproduction of HER1/EGFR ligands. There are various mutant forms of HER1/EGFR. The most important mutated hysoform is EGFRvIII, characterized by a truncated extracellular domain, is the most studied mutant form; it lacks of a ligand-binding domain and is constitutively activated. This mutant form has been detected in several human cancers including NSCLC, breast carcinomas, ovarian carcinomas and gliomas.

Studies in human GBM cells, in human xenografts models and in GBM patients suggest that EGFRvIII promotes tumor growth and progression via constitutive activation of the PI3-K/Akt pathway; it also induces up-regulation of cell proliferation via the MAPK/ERK1/2 signal transduction pathway. New therapeutic strategies through small-molecule HER1/EGFR TK inhibitors (erlotinib and gefitinib) and monoclonal antibodies (cetuximab) may be future therapeutic perspectives in gliomas therapy. The use of antisense RNA into murine models of human glioma, through liposomes tagged with monoclonal antibodies, facilitates tumor targeting and induces reduction of HER1/EGFR expression increasing survival (Halatsch et al., 2006).

4.6 C-Met/HGF

C-Met is a tyrosine kinase receptor whose ligand is hepatocyte growth factor (HGF). This pathway is very critical in cellular proliferation, motility and invasion and it is over-expressed in gliomas. Chu et al. demonstrated in vitro and in vivo that AONs against c-Met (FAM-labeled c-Met nonsense ODNs-LIPOFECTAMINE PLUS™ GIBCO Laboratories, Grand Island, NY) markedly suppressed the expression of c-Met mRNA in human glioma cells and cell growth. Inhibition of c-Met gene expression by antisense AONs enhanced significantly the cytotoxic effect of radiation on human U251 glioma cells in culture (Chu et al., 2006). In a successive research, the same study group showed that c-Met antisense oligonucleotides, injected intratumoral in the rat, were well tolerated at therapeutic levels and did not produce any toxic effects and recently have increased sensitivity of human glioma cells to paclitaxel, leading to a potential targeted-enhanced chemotherapeutic approach tightly selective against glioma cells (Chu et al., 2010).

4.7 ECM proteins

Khazenzon et al. have demonstrated the effects of antisense inhibition of laminin-8 expression in glioma therapy through an in vitro model using human glioblastoma multiforme cell lines M059K and U-87MG co-cultured with normal human brain microvascular endothelial cells (HBMVEC). Endothelial cells contribute laminins containing α4 and α5 chains, whereas glial cells synthesize laminins containing α1 and α2 chains. In human brain capillaries, laminin-8 is the most expressed laminin. During progression of human gliomas, the expression of capillary BM laminins containing α4 chain switches from the predominant laminin-9 into lanimin-8. Laminin-8 and its receptor, integrins α3β1 and α6β1, are important for the functioning of endothelial cell BMs, which play a role in the maintenance of the BBB. Laminin-8 (α4 and β1 chains) plays an important role in glioma cell invasiveness, in combination with other proteins associated with glioma progression, such as tenascin-C, MMP-2 and MMP-9. In fact, up-regulation of laminin-8 expression in both glioma cells and glioma-adjacent capillary endothelial cells may reduce glial cell adhesion and enhance migration, which is necessary for local tumor invasiveness. The result of this study was a significant reduction of invasion of co-cultures through Matrigel and through the use of morpholino oligos against α4 and β1 chains of laminin-8 (Khazenzon et al., 2003).

4.8 uPAR

Among the possible key molecules of gliomagenesis, the urokinase-type plasminogen activator receptor (uPAR) may be particularly important in regulating plasminogen-mediated extracellular matrix proteolysis on the cell surface. Through an antisense anti-uPAR therapy, Mohanam et al. showed in vitro a markedly lower level of ECM degradation with down-regulation of MMP-2 activity and consequently a down-regulation of surrounding tissue invasion pathways (Mohanam et al., 1997).

5. Conclusions

The treatment of gliomas represents one of the most challenging areas in neurosurgery and oncology. Malignant gliomas involves multiple aberrant signaling pathways and the blood brain barrier (BBB) restricts the delivery of many chemotherapeutic agents. The efficectiveness of the actual chemotherapeutic approach, multimodal targeted therapies, differently than the other malignant extracerebral tumors, remains very modest in gliomas. Considering the multitude of molecular entities and signaling pathways regulating the proliferation and cellular survival/cell death, the inhibition of a singular target gene or transcriptional factor could not be sufficient to suppress neoplastic progression. In this intricate and complex field it seems to be very important to improve specific selective drugs delivery systems to lead to diffusion of drugs, antisense oligonucleotides, small interference RNAs, engineered monoclonal antibodies and other therapeutic molecules into CNS overcoming BBB.

Antisense therapy is an interesting field of base and translational research in cancer therapy. This approach has been applied in various kinds of tumors and showed a very high specificity and efficacy against cancer cells. Many antisense oligonucleotides have shown sharp *in vitro* reduction in target gene expression and promising activity against a variety of human malignancies. Several experimental *in vitro* and *in vivo* studies in cell lines cultures and animal models showed inhibition of genes involved in cell proliferation, apoptosis and angiogenesis. Clinical trials demonstrated a good tolerability and no increment of toxicity of antisense oligonucleotides (Caruso et al., 2010a).

However, considering the multitude of molecular entities and signalling pathways that regulate the proliferation and cellular survival/cell death, inhibition of a singular target gene or transcriptional factor could not be sufficient to suppress neoplastic progression. Glioma cell invasion is a complex and multifactorial mechanism involving a large series of molecules and cell-cell and cell-ECM interactions. These processes allow individual tumor cells to migrate and invade the surrounding brain parenchyma. ECM, proteases, cell adhesion molecules and their related signalling pathways show an important role in glioma cell migration and invasion. It is evident that the complexity and cross-talk between signal transduction pathways limits the potential efficacy of targeting a single receptor or molecule. Future possible interesting molecular target in antisense glioma therapy, tested in preclinical study, may be clusterin, eIF-4E (eukaryotic initiation factor-4E), integrins, metalloproteinases and other key molecules involved in invasion and angiogenesis.

We now are investigating about the role of HIF (Hypoxic inducing factor) isoforms and IL-8 (Interleukine-8) in glioma progression. HIF-1α appears to be a highly involved factor in the development of a characteristic tumor phenotype influencing growth rate, invasiveness and metastasis. In fact it has to be taken into account that HIF-1α does not only regulate actively downstream processes but is also itself influenced by the tumor microenviroment in many different ways. As a result, local ipoxia, due to increased proliferation or insufficient oxygen supply, inactivation of tumor suppressors, oncogenes and growth factors, along with other cell types, such as macrophages, contribute to form a tumor microenviroment capable to modulate the HIF response itself. A highly specific targeting of the organ or tissue is mandatory: HIF-1 inhibitors for cancer therapy target the HIF pathway on different levels: they decrease HIF mRNA or proteins levels, inhibit DNA binding or decrease HIF-mediated transactivation. Antisense inhibition of HIF may be a strong target for anti-angiogenic therapy. In fact, HIF is the crucial molecule and transcriptional factor produced in response to hypoxic conditions within HIF-1α/VEGF-regulation expression-dependent angiogenic pathway. In this molecular cascade HIF-1α up-regulated levels finally induce up-regulation of VEGF expression, and, at the same time, may stimulate gene expression of other genes involved in gliomagenesis. Our study group has recently showed high expression levels of PGES-1 (Prostaglandine E 1 Sinthase) and IL-8 in high grade glioma cells and microglial cells, strongly correlated with grading tumor (Caruso et al., 2010a).

During malignancy progression gliomagenesis, leukocyte infiltration and necrosis are two biological phenomena associated with the development of neovascularization. IL-8 expression is first observed in low grade astrocytoma in perivascular tumor areas expressing inflammatory cytokines. In HGGs, IL-8 further localizes in oxygen-deprived cells surrounding necrosis. Macrophages are known to produce high levels of IL-8, which has a tumorigenic activity, by inducing tumor growth and angiogenesis; IL-8 is an inflammatory chemoattractant responding to the tumor microenvironment. Tumor pseudopalisading cells secrete hypoxic inducing factor (HIF) which induces IL-8 secretion. These results support a model in which IL-8 expression, by induction of inflammatory stimuli, may be an early step in astrocytoma development. IL-8 expression later in tumor progression increases because of reduced microenvironmental oxygen pressure. It seems that augmented IL-8 directly and/or indirectly promotes angiogenesis by binding to DARC and induces leukocyte infiltration and activation by binding to CXCR1 and CXCR2. The contemporary actions of IL-8 into glioma angiogenesis and leukocyte infiltration, as well as macrophages, microglial cells and ECM components involvement, suggest IL-8 as a future interesting target in antitumoral antisense therapy. On the base of our preliminar results, we hypotize an important role of IL-8 as crucial angiogenesis mediator within HIF-1α pathway and crosstalk between hypoxia-induced high levels of HIF-1α and VEGF expression. To try to enhance an anti-angiogenic anti-tumoral effect an attractive therapeutic mechanism may be a selective antisense strategy against two molecular targets involved, at different lavels, in the same pathological pathway.

The nanoparticles-based delivery has emerged as a potential method to improve the efficacy of the existing detection and treatment options due to the non-toxicity and engineerability of nanoparticles. In gliomas treatment, the nanoparticle systems are designed to carry out other key functions, including shielding the active drug from producing systemic side effects, crossing the BBB, and targeting specific cells after his gained access to CNS (Caruso et al., 2010b).

Nanotechnology deals with structures and devices are emerging as a new field of research at the interface of science, engineering and medicine. This approach have the ability to carry antisense molecules, such as antisense oligonucleotides, short interfering RNA (siRNA) molecules and ribozymes, that, with different modalities, exert RNA interference on target gene expression after their internalization into the target tumor cells. Obviously more detailed researches about knowledge of cellular biology, and cancer biology will permit important progress in the implications of nanotechnology in cancer and naturally in malignant gliomas treatment.

Glioma gene expression and its development during gliomagenesis will may help to better understand the role of important molecules involved in tumor-safe brain parenchyma relationships. These molecules, such as ECM proteases, cell adhesion molecules and their related signaling pathways show an important role in glioma cell migration and invasion and could be selectively attack to inhibits the glioma invasive rim. It is clear that the complexity and cross-talk between signal transduction pathways limits the potential efficacy of targeting a single receptor or molecule. Antisense targeted therapy is very fashinating and probably will be one of the most important strategy to treat high-grade glioma, into a multimodal approach for brain tumor treatment. The clinical results of this molecular approach are actually very poor, because of the relatively short time of application of this kind of strategy in brain tumors, the single molecular target chosen for targeted therapy and the anatomic and physiological barriers existing in CNS. Another important aspect to valuate is represented by the similarity between the overall survival and progression free survival in glioma patients treated according the standard protocol with surgery, chemotherapy and radiotherapy versus new experimental molecular multimodal protocol. These new future possible targeted antisense-based therapy have showed very interesting results in glioma cell lines and in in vivo murine models. On the base of these preliminar results and the limits of actual standard therapeutic protocol, we think that antisense therapy may be an interesting approach to modify the biological development of gliomas, probably trying to modulate crucial pathways of gliomagenesis during precocious steps of tumor progression and possibly two or more molecular targets of the same pathway or of two different pathways.

6. References

Andrews, DW, Resnicoff, M, Flanders, AE, Kenyon, L, Curtis, M, et al. (2001). Results of a pilot study involving the use of an antisense oligodeoxynucleotide directed against the insuline-like growth factor type I receptor in malignant astrocytomas. *J Clin Oncol*, Vol.19, No.8, (April 2001), pp. 2189-2200, ISSN 0732-183X.

Baker, BF, Condon, TP, Koller, E, McKay, Ra, Siwkowski, AM. *(2001).* Discovery and analysis of antisense oligonucleotide activity in cell culture. *Methods*, Vol.23, No.2, (February 2001), pp. 191-198, ISSN 0026-1270.

Bello, L, Francolini, M, Marthyn, P, Zhang, J, Carroll, RS, et al. (2001). Alpha(v)beta3 and alpha(v)beta5 integrin expression in glioma periphery. *Neurosurgery,* Vol.49, No.2 (August 2001), pp. 380-389, ISSN 0898-4921.

Caffo, M, Germanò, A, Caruso, G, Meli, F, Galatioto, S, et al. (2004). An immunohistochemical study of extracellular matrix proteins laminin, fibronectin and type IV collagen in paediatric glioblastoma multiforme. *Acta Neurochir,* Vol.146, No.10, (October 2004), pp. 1113-1118, ISSN 0139-3006.

Campbell, W, & Pollack, IF. (1997). Growth factors in gliomas. Antisense and dominant negative mutant strategies. *J Neurooncol,* Vol.35, No.3, (December 1997), pp. 275-285, ISSN 0167-594X.

Caruso, G, Caffo, M, Raudino, G, Alafaci, C, Salpietro, FM, et al. (2010a). Antisense oligonucleotides and extracellular matrix proteins: innovative therapeutic targets in the tratment of high grade gliomas. *Recent Pat CNS Drug Discov,* Vol.5, No.1, (January 2010), pp. 53-69, ISSN 1574-8898.

Caruso, G, Raudino, G, Caffo, M, Alafaci, C, Granata, F, et al. (2010b). Nanotechnology platforms in diagnosis and treatment of primary brain tumors. *Recent Pat Nanotechnol,* Vol.4, No.2, (June 2010), pp. 119-124, ISSN 1872-2105.

Cech, TR & Bass, BL. (1986). Biological catalysis by RNA. *Ann Rev Biochem,* Vol.55, (July 1986), pp. 599-629, ISSN 0066-4154.

Chen, G, Oh, S, Monia, BP, Stacey, DW. (1996). Antisense oligonucleotides demonstrate a dominant role of c-Ki-RAS proteins in regulating the proliferation of diploid human fibroblasts. *J Biol Chem,* Vol.271, No.45, (November 1996), pp. 28259-28265, ISSN 0021-9258.

Chu, S, Ma, Y, Feng, DF, Zhang, H, Qiu, JM, et al. (2010). C-Met antisense oligodeoxynucleotides increase sensitivity of human glioma cells to paclitaxel. *Oncol Rep,* Vol.24, No.1, (July 2010), pp. 189-194, ISSN 1791-2431.

Chu, S, Zhu, Z, Yuan, X, Li, Z, Jiang, P. (2006). In vitro and in vivo potentiating the cytotoxic effect of radiation on human U251 gliomas by the c-Met antisense oligodeoxynucleotides. *J Neurooncol,* Vol.80, No.2, (November 2006), pp. 143-149, ISSN 0167-594X.

Dean, NM, & Bennett, CF. (2003). Antisense oligonucleotide-based therapeutics for cancer. *Oncogene,* Vol.22, No.56, (December 2003), pp. 9087-9096, ISSN 0950-9232.

El-Aneed, A (2004). Current strategies in cancer gene therapy. *Eur J Pharmacol,* Vol.498, No.1-3, (September 2004)pp. 1-8, ISSN 0014-2999.

Gladson, CL. (1999). The extracellular matrix of gliomas: modulation of cell function. *J Neuropathol Exp Neurol,* Vol.58, No.10, (October 1999), pp. 1029-1040, ISSN 0022-3069.

Gonzalez, J & Gilbert, MR. (2005). Treatment of astrocytomas. *Curr Opin Neurol,* Vol.18, No.6, (December 2005), pp. 632-638, ISSN 1350-7540.

Grossman, SA, Alavi, JB, Supko, JG, Carson, KA, Priet, R, et al. (2004). Efficacy and toxicity of the antisense oligonucleotide aprinocarsen directed against protein kinase C-□ delivered as a 21-day continuous intravenous infusion in patients with recurrent high-grade astrocytomas. *Neuro Oncol,* Vol.7, No.1, (January 2004), pp. 32-40, ISSN 1523-5866.

Guensberg, P, Wacheck, V, Lucas, T, Monia, B, Pehamberger, H, et al. (2002). Bcl-xL antisense oligonucleotides chemosensitize human glioblastoma cells. *Chemotherapy,* Vol.48, No.4, (September 2002), pp. 189-195, ISSN 0009-3157.

Hanahan, D, & Weinberg, RA. (2000). The hallmarks of cancer. *Cell,* Vol.100, No.1, (January 2000), pp. 57-70, ISSN 0092-8674.

Halatsch, ME, Schmidt, U, Behnke-Mursch, J, Unterberg, A, Rainer Wirtz, C. (2006). Epidermal growth factor receptor inhibition for the treatment of glioblastoma multiforme and other malignant brain tumors. *Cancer Treat Rev,* Vol.32, No.2, (April 2006), pp. 74-89, ISSN 0305-7372.

Hau, P, Jachimczak, P, Bogdahn, U. (2009). Treatment of malignant gliomas with TGF-beta2 antisense oligonucleotides. *Expert Rev Anticancer Ther,* Vol.9, No.11, (November 2009), pp. 1663-1674, ISSN 1473-7140.

Hau, P, Jachimczak, P, Schlingensiepen, R, Schulmeyer, F, Jauch, T, et al. (2007). Inhibition of TGFbeta2 with AP 12009 in recurrent malignant gliomas: From preclinical to phase I/II studies. *Oligonucleotides,* Vol.17, No.2, (Summer 2007), pp. 201-212, ISSN 1545-4576.

Holash, J, Maisonpierre, PC, Compton, D, Boland, P, Alexander, LR, et al. (1999). Vessel cooption, regression,and growth in tumors mediated by angiopoietins and VEGF. *Science,* Vol.284, No.5422, (June 1999), pp. 1994-1998, ISSN 0036-8075.

Holland, EC. (2001). Gliomagenesis: genetic alterations and mouse models. *Nat Rev Genet,* Vol.2, No.2, (February 2001), pp. 120-129, ISSN 1471-0056.

Idbaih, A, Ducray, F, Sierra del Rio, M, Hoang-Xuan, K, Delattre, JY. (2008). Therapeutic application of noncytotoxic molecular targeted therapy in gliomas: growth factor receptors and angiogenesis inhibitors. *Oncologist,* Vol.13, No.9, (September 2008), pp. 978-992, ISSN 1083-7159.

Im, SA, Gomez-Manzano, C, Fueyo, J, Liu, TJ, Ke, LD, et al. (1999). Antiangiogenesis treatment for gliomas: Transfer of antisense-vascular endothelial growth factor inhibits tumor growth in vivo. *Cancer Res,* Vol.59, No.4, (February 1999), pp. 895-900, ISSN 1538-7445.

Immonen, A, Vapalathi, M, Tyynela, K, Hurskainen, H, Sandmair, A, et al. (2004). AdvHSV-tk gene therapy with intravenous ganciclovir improves survival in human malignant glioma: a randomised, controlled study. *Mol Ther,* Vol.10, No.5, (November 2004), pp. 967-972, ISSN 1525-0016.

Iwado, E, Daido, S, Kondo, Y, Kondo, S. (2007). Combined effect of 2-5A-linked antisense against telomerase RNA and conventional therapies on human malignant glioma cells in vitro and in vivo. *Int J Oncol,* Vol.32, No.5, (November 2007), pp. 1087-1095, ISSN 1791-2423.

Izquierdo, M, Martin, V, de Felipe, P, Izquierdo, JM, Perez-Higueras, A, et al. (1996). Human malignant brain tumor response to herpes simplex thymidine kinase (HSVtk)/ganciclovir gene therapy. *Gene Ther,* Vol.3, No.6, (June 1996), pp. 491-495, ISSN 0969-7128.

Jachimczak, P, Hessdorfer, B, Fabel-Schulte, K, Wismeth, C, Brysch, W, et al. (1996). Transforming growth factor-beta mediated autocrine growth regulation of gliomas with phosphorothioate antisense oligonucleotides. *Int J Cancer,* Vol.65, No.3, (January 1996), pp. 332-337, ISSN 1097-0215.

Jain, RK, di Tomaso, E, Duda, DG, Loefflers, LB, Sorensen, AG, et al. (2007). Angiogenesis in brain tumours. *Nat Rev Neurosci,*Vol.8, No.8, (August 2007), pp. 610-622, ISSN 1471-003X.

Jansen, B, & Zangemeister-Wittke, U. (2002). Antisense therapy for cancer - the time of truth. *Lancet Oncol,* Vol.3, No.11, (November 2002), pp. 672-683, ISSN 1470-2045.

Jason, TLH, Koropatnick, J, & Berg, RW. (2004). Toxicology of antisense therapeutics. *Toxicology and Applied Pharmacology,* Vol.201, No.1, (November 2004), pp. 66-83, ISSN 0041-008X.

Julien, T, Frankel, B, Longo, S, Kyle, M, Gibson, S, et al. (2000). Antisense-mediated inhibition of the bcl-2 gene induces apoptosis in human malignant glioma. *Surg Neurol,* Vol.53, No.4, (April 2000), pp. 360-369, ISSN 0090-3157.

Khazenzon, NM, Ljubimov, AV, Lakhter, AJ, Fujita, M, Fujiwara, H, et al. (2003). Antisense inhibition of laminin-8 expression reduces invasion of human gliomas in vitro. *Mol Cancer Ther,* Vol.2, No.10, (October 2003), pp. 985-994, ISSN 1538-8514.

Kohn, EC, & Liotta, LA. (1995). Molecular insights into cancer invasion: Strategies for prevention and intervention. *Cancer Res,* Vol.55, No.2, (May 1995), pp. 1856-1862, ISSN 1538-7445.

Kondo, S, Kondo, Y, Li, G, Silverman, RH, Cowell, JK. (1998). Targeted therapy of human malignant glioma in a mouse model by 2-5A antisense directed against telomerase RNA. *Oncogene,* Vol.16, No.25, (June 1998), pp. 3323-3330, ISSN 0950-9232.

Kondo, S, Tanaka, Y, Kondo, Y, Hitomi, M, Barnett, GH, et al. (1998). Antisense telomerase treatment: induction of two distinct pathways, apoptosis and differentiation. *FASEB J,* Vol.12, No.10, (July 1998), pp. 801-811, ISSN 0892-6638.

Komata, T, Kondo, Y, Koga, S, Lo, SC, Chung, LWK, et al. (2000). Combination therapy of malignant glioma cells with 2-5A-antisense telomerase RNA and recombinant adenovirus p53. *Gene Ther,* Vol.7, No.24, (December 2000), pp. 2071-2079, ISSN 0969-7128.

Liu, TJ, La Fortune, T, Honda, T, Ohmori, O, Hatakeyama, S, et al. (2007). Inhibition of both adhesion kinase and insulin-like growth factor-I receptor kinase suppresses glioma proliferation in vitro and in vivo. *Mol Cancer Ther,* Vol. 6, No.4, (April 2007), pp. 1357-1367, ISSN 1538-8514.

Ljubimova, JY, Fujita, M, Khazenzon, NM, Ljubimov, AV, Black, KL. (2006). Changes in laminin isoforms associated with brain tumor invasion and angiogenesis. *Front Biosci,* Vol.11, (January 2006), pp. 81-88, ISSN 1093-4715.

Macrae, IJ, Zhou, K, Li, F, Repic, A, Brooks, AN, et al. (2006). Structural basis for double-stranded RNA processing by Dicer". *Science,* Vol.311, No.5758, (January 2006), pp. 195-198, ISSN 0036-8075.

McKay, RA, Miraglia, LJ, Cummins, LL, Owens, SR, Sasmor, H, et al. (1999). A Characterization of a potent and specific class of antisense oligonucleotide inhibitor of human protein kinase C-α expression. *J Biol Chem,* Vol.274, No.3, (January 1999), pp. 1715-1722, ISSN 0021-9258.

Mohanam, S, Chintala, SK, Go, Y, Bhattacharya, A, Venkaiah, B. (1997). In vitro inhibition of human glioblastoma cell line invasiveness by antisense uPA receptor. *Oncogene,* Vol.14, No.11, (March 1997), pp. 1351-1359, ISSN 0950-9232.

Monia, BP, Sasmor, H, Johnston, J, Freier, SM, Lesnik, EA, et al. (1996). Sequence-specific antitumor activity of a phosphorothioate oligodeoxyribonucleotide targeted to human C-raf kinase supports an antisense mechanism of action in vivo. *Proc Natl Acad Sci USA,* Vol.93, No26, (December 1996), pp. 15481-15484, ISSN 1091-6490.

Mukai, S, Kondo, Y, Koga, S, Komata, T, Barna, BP, et al. (2000). 2-5A antisense telomerase RNA therapy for intracranial malignant gliomas. *Cancer Res,* Vol.60, No.16, (August 2000), pp. 4461-4467, ISSN 1538-7445.

Ohgaki, H, & Kleihues, P. (2007). Genetic pathways to primary and secondary glioblastoma. *Am J Pathol,* Vol.170, No.5, (May 2007), pp. 1445-1453, ISSN 0887-8005.

Park, MJ, Kim, MS, Park, IC, Kang, KS, Yoo, H, et al. (2002). PTEN suppresses hyaluronic acid-induced matrix metalloproteinases-9 expression in U87MG glioblastoma cells through focal adhesion kinase dephosphrylation. *Canc Res,* Vol.62, No.21, (November 2002), pp. 6318-6322, ISSN 1538-7445.

Passioura, T, & Symonds, G. (2004). Cancer gene suppression strategies: issues and potential. *Curr Issues Mol Biol,* Vol.6, No.2, (July 2004), pp. 89-102, ISSN 1467-3037.

Paterson, BM, Roberts, BE, & Kuff, EL. (1977). Structural gene identification and mapping by DNA-mRNA hybrid arrested cell-free translation. *Proc Nat Acad Sci,* Vol.74, No.10, (October 1977), pp. 4370-4374, ISSN 1091-6490.

Pirollo, KF, Rait, A, Sleers, LS, Chang, EH. (2003). Antisense therapeutics: from theory to clinical practice. *Pharmacol Ther*, Vol.99, No.1, (July 2003), pp. 55-77, ISSN 0327-6309.

Pollack, IF, Kawecki, S, & Lazo, JS. Blocking of glioma proliferation in vitro and in vivo and potentiating the effects of BCNU and cisplatin: UCN-01, a selective protein kinase C inhibitor. *J Neurosurg*, Vol.84, No.6, (June 1996), pp. 1024-1032, ISSN 0022-3085.

Potapova, O, Gorospe, M, Dougherty, RH, Dean, NM, Gaarde, WA, et al. (2000). Inhibition of c-Jun N-terminal kinase 2 expression suppresses growth and induces apoptosis of human tumor cells in a p53-dependent manner. *Mol Cell Biol*, Vol.20, No.5, (March 2000), pp. 1713-1722, ISSN 1098-5549.

Pu, P, Kang, C, Li, J, Jiang, H, Cheng, J. (2006). The effects of antisense AKT2 RNA on the inhibition of malignant glioma cell growth in vitro and in vivo. *J Neurooncol*, Vol.76, No.1, (June 2006), pp. 1-11, ISSN 0167-594X.

Resnicoff, M, Sell, C, Rubini, M, Coppola, D, Sell, C, et al. (1994). Rat glioblastoma cells expressing an antisense RNA to the insuline-like growth factor-1 (IGF-1) receptor are nontumorigenic and induce regression of wild-type tumors. *Cancer Res*, Vol.54, No.8, (April 1994), pp. 2218-2222, ISSN 1538-7445.

Rubenstein, M, Mirochnik, Y, Chou, P, Guinan, P. (1996). Antisense oligonucleotides intralesional therapy for human PC-3 prostate tumors carried in athymic nude mice. *J Surg Oncol*, Vol.62, No.3, (July 1996), pp. 194-200, ISSN 1096-9098.

Schlingensiepen, R, Goldbrunner, M, Szyrach, MN, Stauder, G, Jachimczak, P, et al. (2005). Intracerebral and intrathecal infusion of the TGF-□2-specific antisense phosphorotioate oligonucleotide AP 12009 in rabbits and primates: toxicology and safety. *Oligonucleotides*, Vol.15, No.2 (Summer 2005), pp. 94-104, ISSN 1545-4576.

Schlingensiepen, KH, Schlingensiepen, R, Steinbrecher, A, Hau, P, Bogdhan, U, et al. (2006). Targeted tumor therapy with the TGF-β2 antisense compound AP 12009. *Cytokine Growth Factor Rev*, Vol.17, No.1-2, (February-April 2006), pp. 129-139, ISSN 1359-6101.

Schneider, T, Becker, A, Ringe, K, Reinhold, A, Firscing, R, et al. (2008). Brain tumor therapy by combined vaccination and antisense oligonucleotide delivery with nanoparticles. *J Neuroimmunol*, Vol.195, No.1-2, (March 2008), pp. 21-27, ISSN 0165-5728.

Semenza, GL. (2003). Targeting HIF-1 for cancer therapy. *Nat Rev Cancer*, Vol.3, No.10, (October 2003), pp. 721-732, ISSN 1474-175X.

Smythe, WR, Mohuiddin, I, Ozveran, M, Cao, XX. (2002). Antisense therapy for malignant mesothelioma with oligonucleotides targeting the bcl-xl gene product. *J Thorac Cardiovasc Surg*, Vol.123, No.6, (June 2002), pp. 1191-1198, ISSN 0022-5223.

Stegh, AH, Kim, H, Bachoo, RM, Forloney, KL, Zhang, J, et al. (2007). Bcl2L12 inhibits post-mitochondrial apoptosis signaling in glioblastoma. *Genes Dev*, Vol.21, No.1, (January 2007), pp. 98-111, ISSN 0890-9369.

Stephenson, ML, & Zamecnik, PC. (1978). Inhibition of Rous sarcoma virus replication and cell transformation by a specific oligodeoxynucleotide. *Proc Nati Acad Sci*, Vol.75, No.1, (January 1978), pp. 280-284, ISSN 1091-6490.

Stupp, R, Mason, WP, van den Bent, MJ, Weller, M, Taphoorn, MJ, et al. (2005). Radiotherapy plus concomitant and adjuvant temozolamide for glioblastoma. *N Engl J Med*, Vol.352, No.10, (March 2005), pp. 987-996, ISSN 0028-4793.

Tamm, I. (2006). Antisense therapy in malignant disease: status quo and quo vadis? *Clin Sci*, Vol.110, No.4, (April 2006), pp. 427-442, ISSN 0143-5221.

Wacheck, V, & Zangemeister-Wittke, U. (2006). Anisense molecules for targeted cancer therapy. *Oncol Hematol*, Vol.59, No.1, (July 2006), pp. 65-73, ISSN 1536-3678.

Wesseling, P, & Adema, GJ. (2009). Immunotherapy of diffuse gliomas: helping the brain fight back!. *Brain Pathology*, Vol.19, No.4, (October 2009), pp. 674-693, ISSN 1750-3639.

Whitesell, L, Rosolen, A, & Neckers, LM. (1991). In vivo *m*odulation of Nmyc expression by continuous perfusion with an antisense oligonucleotide. *Antisense Res Dev*, Vol.1, No.4, (Winter 1991), pp. 343-350, ISSN 1050-5261.

Wu, ZM, Yuan, XH, Jiang, PC, Li, ZQ, Wu, T. (2006). Antisense oligonucleodes targeting the focal adhesion kinase inhibit proliferation, induce apoptosis and cooperate with cytotoxic drugs in human glioma cells. *J Neurooncol*, Vol.77, No,2, (April 2006), pp. 117-123, ISSN 0167-594X.

Yancopoulos, GD, Davis, S, Gale, NW, Rudge, JS, Wiegand, SJ, et al. (2000). Vascular-specific growth factors and blood vessel formation. *Nature*, Vol.407, No.6801, (September 2000), pp. 242-248, ISSN 0028-0836.

Zadeh, G, Qian, B, Okhowat, A, Sabha, N, Kontos, CD, et al. (2004). Targeting the Tie2/Tek receptor in astrocytomas. *Am J Pathol*, Vol.164, No.2, (February 2004), pp. 467-476, ISSN 0887-8005.

Zagzag, D, Amirnovin, R, greco, MA, Yee, H, Holash, J, et al. (2000). Vascular apoptosis and involution in gliomas precede neovascularization: a novel concept for glioma growth and angiogenesis. *Lab Invest*, Vol.80, No.6, (June 2000), pp. 837-849, ISSN 0023-6837.

Zhou, X, Zhang, J, Jia, Q, Ren, Y, Wang, Y, et al. (2010). Reduction of miR-21 induces glioma cell apoptosis via activating caspase 9 and 3. *Oncol Rep*, Vol. 24, No.1, (July 2010), pp. 195-201, ISSN 1791-2431.

18

Cellular Immunotherapy for Malignant Brain Tumors

Catherine Flores and Duane A. Mitchell
Duke Brain Tumor Immunotherapy Program
Duke University
USA

1. Introduction

Glioblastoma multiforme (GBM) is the most common and most aggressive adult brain tumor with a patient median survival of 15 months from the time of diagnosis, and less than 20 weeks for patients with recurrent tumors. Current standard of care consists of multi-modality therapy including image-guided tumor resection, fractionated radiotherapy, and chemotherapy. This aggressive therapy is non-specific and highly toxic, leaving collateral damage to surrounding normal brain and systemic tissue, and is often debilitating to patients. Thus, there is a dire need for a more effective therapy that more specifically targets tumor cells while minimizing damage to surrounding eloquent cerebral cortex. Immunotherapy is based on the premise that the inherent sensitivity and specificity of immunologic reactivity could deliver tumor cell-specific therapy. Cellular immunotherapy aims to utilize the patient's own immune cells that are harvested, expanded *ex vivo*, primed against tumor antigens, and returned to the host, in order to direct an anti-tumor immune response with specificity and efficiency.

During early efforts in immunotherapy, tumor specific antigens were unknown and it was unclear whether tumor antigens could be recognized and targeted by the immune system. The identification of tumor antigens began with those expressed in malignant melanoma, and soon there was an explosion in the development of antigen specific immunologic treatments against solid tumors. In the past several years, pre-clinical models of cancer have reliably demonstrated that the immune system is capable of targeting tumor antigens and eradicating malignancies. It has also been demonstrated clinically that the human immune system is capable of recognizing antigens within malignant tumor cells with precision, and current immunotherapy research aims to induce potent antitumor immune responses to prolong patient survival. It was initially unclear if a potent immune response was inducible against brain tumors because of the immunoprivileged nature of the nervous system, but studies have demonstrated that immune effector cells can infiltrate the central nervous system (CNS) and induce efficient immune responses against intracranial tumors.

Current research in cellular immunotherapy against cancer is directed at eliciting a specific immune response against tumor antigens using active immunization with cellular vaccines or adoptive transfer of *ex vivo* activated lymphocytes. Clinical studies testing the safety and efficacy of cellular vaccines in patients with grade III or grade IV gliomas include the administration of dendritic cell (DC) vaccines, autologous tumor cell vaccines, and tumor cell-antigen presenting cell fusions. Clinical studies using adoptive cell transfer employ a variety of techniques to expand tumor-specific lymphocytes *in vitro* prior to adoptive transfer to recipients with invasive brain tumors. This chapter will discuss both pre-clinical and clinical research in cellular immunotherapy targeting malignant gliomas.

2. Immune privilege

Cellular immune responses must afford protection without causing collateral damage to normal tissue. This is particularly important in the brain where passive and active mechanisms maintain a state of immunological privilege that limits the magnitude of the immune response. It has been demonstrated that immune responses in the CNS can be induced, the magnitude of this response is strictly regulated by the presence of the blood-brain barrier. Cerebral interstitial fluid (CIF) is secreted at the blood-brain barrier and flows within the spaces of the brain parenchyma. Cerebrospinal fluid (CSF) is formed by the choroid plexus within the ventricles and subarachnoid membrane, then flows through the ventricles to the basal cisterns, then through the subarachnoid space [1-3]. Antigens within the CNS enter the lymph nodes via the CSF which drains into the Virchow-Robbin spaces to the deep cervical lymphatic's via perivascular sheaths and through the subnasal mucosa [2, 4, 5]. The flow of CSF exits the subarachnoid space through the arachnoid granulations and through drainage along the olfactory nerve across the cribriform plate into blood circulation and cervical lymph nodes [4, 6, 7]. Antigens draining to cervical lymph nodes encounter cognate B cells and can also be processed and presented to T cells [4, 6, 7].

Immune activation occurs with a distinct hierarchy in terms of the types of responses induced [6]. Antigens that drain into the periphery via the cervical lymph nodes induce a response characteristic of a strong antibody response and the priming of cytotoxic T cell responses, but an absence of delayed-type hypersensitivity (DTH) responses with a skewing towards a Th2 phenotype [1, 2, 6, 8]. Strong humoral responses are induced in response to antigenic challenge. T cells are not endogenously found in the brain, but T cells and antibodies [9] have access to antigens in the brain, indicating that the blood-brain barrier does not entirely prohibit immune responses. Activated T cells "patrol" the CNS and return to systemic circulation, exiting through the cribriform plate, through the nasal mucosa, and then the cervical lymph nodes [1, 10]. Some studies suggest that T cells that encounter their cognate antigen are retained within the CNS [11], but do not proliferate and undergo apoptosis [12]. Alternatively, other studies have demonstrated that T cells encountering cognate antigen proliferate and differentiate into tumor-specific T cells, with enhanced effector function [1].

Professional antigen presenting cells (APC) such as DCs have not been described in the CNS. Microglia are the resident antigen presenting cells in the CNS, but DCs are present in the choroid plexus and meninges [10, 11, 13, 14]. Immunologic responses in the CNS require complex interactions between resident immune cells such as microglia and astrocytes, and peripheral macrophages, lymphocytes, and DCs [14-18]. Microglia constitutively express MHC class II antigens and T cell co-stimulatory molecules. Microglia are bone marrow derived cells that are capable of presenting antigen to T helper cells *in vivo* [19].

3. Glioma Immunology

In the past decade, tumor-associated antigens that are recognizable by cytotoxic T lymphocytes (CTL) have been identified and have the been the basis of cancer immunotherapy. In cancer patients, tumor-specific endogenous immunity can be elicited when tumor antigens are overexpressed, however the immune response is incapable of preventing tumor growth. The immunosuppressive tumor microenvironment, the low avidity of the T cells for tumors, and the low grade immune response are all contributing factors to the inhibition of the endogenous antitumor response. Glioma cells secrete immunosuppressive cytokines including transforming growth factor beta (TGF-β) and vascular endothelial growth factor (VEGF) [20-22] that contribute to tumor immune evasion. In addition, the increased frequency of T regulatory cells in tumor bearing patients plays a critical role in tumor tolerance [23-25].

Cancer vaccines are designed to augment patient immunity by boosting low-level immunity and stimulating the proliferation of higher-avidity T cells. Clinical studies have reported that immunotherapy by systemic administration of antigen-specific DCs and peptide antigens is capable of inducing an antitumor response against malignancies, including CNS malignancies [26-30].

In 1991, van der Bruggen *et al.* [31] identified a gene encoding a tumor-associated antigen recognizable by cytotoxic T lymphocytes in melanoma. Tumor associated genes and peptides were subsequently identified with potential use for cancer vaccines [32]. Peptide based vaccines consist of amino acids capable of binding to a major histocompatibility complex (MHC) class I antigen with the ability to activate tumor reactive T lymphocytes [20]. The immune response targets specific antigenic proteins generally classified as tumor specific antigens (TSA) or tumor associated antigens (TAA). TSAs are antigenic proteins uniquely expressed by tumor tissue while TAAs have a relatively much higher degree of antigen expression relative to normal tissue. Tumor antigens expressed by malignant neoplasms are broadly classified as (i) differentiation antigens, (ii) the products of viral, mutated, differentially spliced, or over-expressed genes, or (iii) metabolic pathway antigens[20]. There have been a few glioma associated antigens identified that are over-expressed in GBM, a few examples include interleukin 13 receptor alpha 2 (IL13Rα2) [33]which is a member of a group of antigens called cancer-testes antigens, and is thought to activate downstream transforming growth factor beta-1 (TGFβ-1) [34]. EphA2 is a tyrosine kinase receptor thought to play a role in mediating developmental processes, and is an antigen also over-expressed on the plasma membrane of GBM tumor cells and tumor-associated vasculature [35]. Survivin expression, which is documented in both gliomas and medulloblatomas [36, 37], inhibits caspase activation, leading to the negative regulation of apoptosis in tumor cells [38]. Telomerase is a ribonucleoprotein that maintains the length of telomeres and thus controls cell proliferation [39], and high telomerase activity has been documented in brain tumor cells [40, 41], particularly brain tumor stem cells [42]. The expression of cytomegalovirus (CMV) antigens IE1 and pp65 have been identified in glioma tissue, and in very low to undetectable levels in non-tumor tissue in the brain [43]. EGFRvIII is an exquisitely tumor-specific antigen and has the most potential for specific immunotherapy.

4. Immunosuppression in GBM

Patients with brain malignancies have impaired B and T cell immune function in part due to tumor secreted factors, but greatly due to depressed cellular immunity and increased levels of T regulatory cells [25, 44]. T regulatory cell frequency is increased CD4+ T cell subset in lymphopenic patients bearing malignant gliomas [25, 45]. Peripheral blood lymphocytes from glioma patients proliferate poorly in response to T cell mitogens, anti CD3, and T and B cell dependent mitogens [46-48]. The total T cell compartment has limited capabilities to respond to mitogen stimulation [46, 47, 49, 50].

4.1 Immunosuppressive cytokines

Two immunosuppressive cytokines secreted by gliomas are TGF-β and VEGF. TGF-β has been isolated from malignant glioma cell supernatants, and the gene encoding for TGF-β2 was cloned from a glioma cell line [51]. TGF-β suppresses the generation of cytotoxic T lymphocytes from PBLs and tumor-infiltrating lymphocytes by inhibiting IL-2 receptor expression on T cells, reducing IL-1 and IL-2, and depressing natural killer cell activation. TGF-β also inhibits the differentiation of cytotoxic T lymphocytes, reduces IFNγ production, and downregulates MHC class II-dependent antigen expression [52, 53]. In an *in vivo* experiment using a highly immunogenic fibrosarcoma cell line, tumor cells were transfected with TGF-β cDNA and stable clones were used *in vitro* and *in vivo* to determine the effects of TGF-β on the induction of immune responses [54]. Tumor cells producing TGF-β failed to stimulate cytotoxic T lymphocyte responses, and TGF-β expressing tumors grew progressively *in vivo*, promoting a means for a immune escape [54], subsequently negatively impacting any potential antitumor efficacy of immunotherapies.

VEGF is produced by most solid tumor cells and plays an important role in tumor immunosuppression by inhibiting the maturation of bone marrow derived DCs [55, 56] by inhibiting NF-KB signaling in hematopoietic progenitor cells. In the context of DC vaccination in tumor bearing mice, inhibition of VEGF production with a blocking anti-VEGF monoclonal antibody enhanced antitumor efficacy [57], demonstrating that attenuating VEGF-mediated immunosuppression is vital to proper function of immunotherapy. VEGF and TGF-β production by tumors contribute to tumor vascularization and immune evasion, contributing to the systemic immunosuppression found in glioma patients. Monoclonal antibodies against VEGF are used therapeutically (bevacizumab) and have been shown to be efficacious against malignant gliomas [58-60]. Preclinical studies conducted in xenogeneic systems with human brain tumor bearing immunodeficient mice have demonstrated that inhibition of VEGF is efficient in prohibiting angiogenesis, leading to subsequent growth suppression of tumors [61].

4.2 T regs

The $CD4^{+}FOXP3^{+}CD25^{+}$ T regulatory cell subset normally comprises of 5-10% of the total $CD4^{+}$ compartment [62-64]. T regulatory cells inhibit T cell cytokine secretion while inhibiting endogenous or induced immune responses [65, 66]. T regulatory cells play a significant role in hindering immunity to normal and tumor antigens [67, 68], and represent an increased frequency of CD4+ cells in the peripheral blood of GBM patients [44]. Targeting T regulatory cell activity to counter their immunosuppressive effects enhances antitumor immunity in murine and human hosts. Fecci *et al.* [44] demonstrated that in a murine model of a spontaneously arising GBM, administration of anti-CD25 antibody eliminated T regulatory cell immunosuppressive function. Though T regulatory cell numbers were only partially reduced, anti-CD25 administration inhibited their function, and anti-CD25 monoclonal antibodies enabled T lymphocyte proliferation and IFNγ responses and increased tumor-specific lysis *in vitro*. In tumor challenged mice, administration of anti-CD25 in combination with DC vaccination provided 100% tumor protection without inducing autoimmunity. Further developing strategies to deplete and inhibit T regulatory cells using monoclonal antibodies, CD25-binding immunotoxins, or pharmacologic inhibition of T regulatory cell activity is important in augmenting immunosuppression in brain tumor patients [25, 67, 68].

5. Immunotherapy

5.1 Antibody-based immunotherapy

Therapeutic use of antibodies aims to alter patient immunity by delivering monoclonal antibodies (mAb) that are targeted against TSAs or TAAs. Antitumor antibodies have been used as either naked antibodies or as vehicles to deliver radioisotopes or toxins to tumors. It is imperative that the mAb can recognize and bind to tumor tissue with high specificity and affinity, without accumulation in normal tissue. Antibody based immunotherapy has been successful for lymphomas (rituximab) and breast cancer (trastuzumab). Bevacizumab, a monoclonal antibody against the angiogenic regulator, vascular endothelial growth factor (VEGF), was approved by the FDA for the treatment of recurrent glioblastoma in 2009 [69]. Blocking VEGF is effective in normalizing abnormal tumor vasculature and increasing tumor response to radiation and chemotherapy [70].

EGFRvIII is currently the only TSA found on malignant glioma cells, but is absent from normal brain tissue. EGFRvIII consists of an in-frame deletion of exons 2-7 from the extracellular domain of the EGFR that splits a codon and produces a novel glycine at the fusion junction [71, 72]. The new glycine inserted at the fusion junction of normally distant parts of the extracellular domain results in a tumor-specific epitope not found in any normal tissue. This tumor-specific mutation encodes a constitutively active tyrosine kinase that enhances tumorigenicity [73-75] and migration of tumor cells that confers radiation and chemotherapy resistance [76-78]. The EGFRvIII mutation is expressed on the plasma membrane of up to 100% of glioma cells and is frequently found in GBM patients [79, 80]. Through the use of reverse transcriptase-polymerase chain reaction (RT-PCR) and fluorescent in situ hybridization (FISH) studies have detected the EGFRvIII mutation on 6-21% of grade III/IV gliomas that have amplified EGFR [80-82]. In addition, analysis using FACS found EGFRvIII expression in 50% of GBM samples [83]. The expression of this mutation confers a negative prognosis for GBM patients. The tumor-specific clonal expression of EGFRvIII on GBMs and its absence from normal tissues make EGFRvIII an ideal target for anti-tumor immunotherapy.

In pre-clinical systems, EGFRvIII expressing cell lines or PEPvIII, an EGFRvIII-specific 14-amino acid peptide, has been used for the generation of EGFRvIII-specific antibodies [79, 84-86], induction of cellular immune responses, or derivation of targeted toxins [87, 88]. Both murine and human chimeric EGFRvIII antibodies have been cloned for use in diagnostic immunohistochemistry and FACS [79]. Monoclonal antibodies binding EGFRvIII are rapidly internalized and have been successfully used *in vivo* in models for therapeutic radioimmunotherapy [86, 89-91]. Unarmed antibodies against EGFRvIII have demonstrated significant antitumor efficacy *in vitro* and *in vivo* in murine models. With a single intratumoral injection of Y10, an unarmed IgG_{2a} anti-EGFRvIII antibody, median survival significantly increased in mice bearing an EGFRvIII expressing intracranial tumor by an average of 286% [85] and produced 26% long-term survivors (n=117). *In vitro* experiments demonstrated that Y10 inhibits DNA synthesis and cell proliferation in tumor cells expressing EGFRvIII by inducing complement mediated, and antibody dependent cell-mediated cytotoxicity [85, 92]. The mechanism identified for Y10 antitumor activity was shown to be Fc receptor dependent. A human chimeric antibody based on Y10 has been developed for clinical use and has been shown to induce lysis of human EGFRvIII positive malignant glioma cell lines. These data on the specificity of anti-EGFRvIII antibody mediated responses support the logic for further investigation into using tumor-specific antibodies as biologic response modifiers.

It has long been established that EGFR and its downstream signaling pathway plays a role in oncogenesis and tumor progression in malignant brain tumors. Thus arose efforts to block the EGFR pathway with the aim of inhibiting tumor cell proliferation with anti-EGFR monoclonal antibodies developed for clinical use. Faillot *et al.* [92], demonstrated the ability of anti-EGFR antibody EMD55900 to bind specifically to malignant gliomas in human patients when administered in a single dose [92]. A phase I/II clinical trial involving multiple intravenous administration of EMD55900 in 16 patients, however, did not observe measurable tumor regression [93], despite evidence of antibody accumulation at the tumor site. Imaging studies have demonstrated that systemically administered anti-EGFR antibodies are capable of reaching intracranial tumors.

EGFRvIII has also been shown to be immunogenic in humans [94]. While anti-EGFRvIII antibodies have not been identified in normal volunteers, patients with malignant gliomas develop EGFRvIII specific antibodies. Weak CTL epitopes restricted by MHC class I and class II have been identified and are sufficient to induce EGFRvIII-specific lymphocyte proliferation and cytokine production. Phase I/II clinical trials targeting this mutation demonstrated that vaccines targeting EGFRvIII are capable of inducing antitumor immunity. In a phase II multicenter trial between Duke University Medical Center and M.D. Anderson Cancer Center (FDA BB-IND-9944), 18 patients with EGFRvIII expressing primary GBMs were treated with an EGFRvIII peptide vaccine called PEPvIII, which is a 13- amino-acid peptide with an additional terminal cysteine that spans the entire *EGFRvIII* mutation [95]. The progression free survival from time of histologic diagnosis was 14.2 months. Six months after histologic diagnosis, 94% of patients were alive without evidence of progression. Six months after PEPvIII vaccination, 67% of patients were alive and progression free. Six patients developed EGFRvIII-specific antibody responses, and their median overall survival from histologic diagnosis was 47.7 months. However, those who did not develop antibody responses had an overall survival time of 22.8 months [95]. In another multicenter phase II trial at Duke University and M.D. Anderson Cancer Center, PEPvIII vaccinations were administered in 22 patients undergoing either standard-doses of temozolomide (TMZ) (200mg/m^2 per 5 days) or dose-intensified (DI) TMZ (100mg/m^2 per 21 days) [96]. This study assessed the immunogenicity of the EGFRvIII peptide vaccine under different degrees of lymphopenia in patients. At 6 months after vaccination, 75% of patients who received standard TMZ were alive and lacked evidence of radiographic progression, while 90% of patients who received DI TMZ were alive and lacked evidence of progression. According to Curran's recursive partitioning analysis, 17 of 22 vaccinated patients had better outcomes than expected when compared to historical controls (p=0.008) [96]. Anti EGFRvIII vaccines have demonstrated the capacity to induce antitumor immunity in the clinical setting, thus warrants investigation in a phase III trial.

5.2 Radiolabeled antibodies

Unlabelled antibodies can be used as delivery vehicles to administer effector molecules such as toxins or radiation directly to tumors. The specificity of tumor associated antigens guide molecules to targets using the specificity of antibodies. The most common effectors conjugated to antibodies are radionucleotides. Despite the expression of EGFRvIII, tenascin has been the most widely evaluated antigenic target. Tenascin is an extracellular matrix protein that is highly expressed in gliomas [97] and its expression increases with tumor progression and is a logical target of trials using radioimmunotherapy. Conjugating antibodies with radioisotopes has been a focus in clinical studies.

The antibody 81C6 is a radiolabeled antibody used in a number of clinical studies [98-102]. 81C6 reacts with an alternatively spliced segment of tenascin at the fibronectin type III domain. Its tumor reactivity and specificity to gliomas is superior to other anti-glioma mAbs and has been proven to be clinically safe. In a safety study at Duke University, antitenascin 81C6 labeled with 131-I was administered into the surgical resection cavity of 21 newly diagnosed GBM patients to achieve a 44-Gy boost specifically to the 2-cm margin of the resection cavity [103]. In 17 patients, 131-I was administered prior to external beam radiotherapy (XRT), and 3 patients 131-I was administered after XRT. Conventional XRT and chemotherapy was then administered. One patient opted not to receive XRT or chemotherapy. Twenty out of twenty-one total patients enrolled received the targeted 44-Gy boost and at a median follow-up of 151 weeks, medial overall survival times for all patients was 96.6 weeks [103]. This study demonstrated that this radioimmunotherapy was well tolerated with encouraging survival in patients with malignant gliomas. Other studies have demonstrated that 81C6 increased survival in patients with leptomeningeal neoplasm as well as recurrent and newly diagnosed gliomas [98, 99, 101, 102]. In a study conducted conducted at Duke University [102], 33 patients with previously untreated malignant glioma (GBM, n=27; anaplastic astrocytoma, n=4; anaplastic oligodendroglioma, n=2) were given 81C6 into the surgical resection cavity followed by conventional XRT and chemotherapy. The observed median survival for all patients was 86.7 weeks, and 79.4 weeks for GBM patients. The median survival of patients treated with 131-I in this study exceeded that of historical controls treated with conventional therapy.

211At is an alpha-emitting radionucleotide, and also emits K X-ray of sufficient energy to allow both γ-counting of tissue samples and external imaging [104]. This α-emiting nucleotide is more advantageous to gliomas than other isotopes. For example, since damage to normal tissue in the brain is most detrimental to the patient's cognitive function, specificity of isotope delivery is essential. The range of 211At particles is only up to 2 mm, thus toxicity is confined to the peritumoral area, minimizing collateral damage to normal tissue. 211At α-particles have a linear energy transfer that is ideal for maximizing biologic efficacy. The distance between ionizing events is approximately the distance between DNA strands, thus increasing the likelihood of inducing irreparable DNA breaks, thereby increasing cytotoxicity [104]. In a phase I safety study, 18 patients with histologic diagnosis of recurrent supratentorial primary malignant brain tumors were treated with 211At-labeled anti-tenascin mAb administered into the surgical resection cavity and treated with salvage chemotherapy [105]. No toxicities of grade 3 or higher were observed. The median survival in patients with recurrent GBM was 54 weeks, patients with anaplastic astrocytoma or oligodendroglioma had a median survival of 52 and 116 weeks respectively. Local administration of 211At-81C6 is safe, feasible, and may potentially provide a survival benefit in recurrent malignant brain tumor patients.

5.3 Dendritic cells and tumor immunotherapy

DCs induce, regulate, and maintain T cell immunity and are essential for the foundation of immunotherapy [106, 107]. DCs take-up and process antigens, thus playing a critical role in T cell priming and regulation of the immune response. DCs are equipped with antigen-processing machinery (APM) essential for uptake and processing of tumor-derived antigens so that tumor-derived epitopes can be cross-presented to T cells [20]. Immature (non-activated) DCs present self-antigens to T cells, inducing a tolerizing immune response by activating T regulatory cells [108]. Immature DCs do not have the ability to stimulate naïve or antigen-specific T memory cells [109, 110]. Immature DCs can take-up antigens via receptor- or nonreceptor-mediated mechanisms. Upon internalization, tumor antigens are processed and split into peptides in the cytosol or endocytic vesicles, then expressed on the cell surface in association with MHC molecules [20, 111].

Activated mature antigen-loaded DCs are responsible for antigen-specific immune responses that lead to T cell activation and proliferation into T helper and effector cells [111]. The two major DC subsets are the classical DCs (myeloid DCs) and plasmacytiod DCs. Plasmacytoid DCs are responsible for the antiviral immune response, producing high amounts of type I IFNα/β in response to viruses [112]. Classical DCs are further categorized in subsets displaying different phenotypes and functions. The skin contains Langerhans cell (LC) found in human epidermis, and the dermal layer contains two subsets, $CD1a^+$ DCs and $CD14^+$ DCs [113, 114]. $CD14^+$ DCs are geared toward mounting humoral immunity. LCs prime high avidity antigen-specific $CD8^+$ T lymphocytes [115].

Ex vivo generation of DCs has been used as a therapeutic vaccine in patients with metastatic disease for over a decade [107, 116]. DCs have the ability to activate and expand T cells that are specific for self-proteins overexpressed in tumors. To generate *ex vivo* derived DC-based vaccines from patient leukapheresed peripheral blood, the combination of cytokines used to differentiate monocytes into DCs may play a role in determining the quality of the elicited T cell response [111, 116]. DCs generated with GM-CSF and IFNα are highly potent in priming T cells [117]. DCs generated in GM-CSF and IL-15 are phenotypically Langerhans cells and are more efficient in priming melanoma antigen-specific $CD8^+$ T cells *in vitro* than DCs generated in GM-CSF and IL-4 [118]. Not all DC maturation signals are equal, thus the selection of methods for activating DCs *in vitro* also represents a critical factor in designing DC vaccines [111]. The capacity to generate large numbers of DCs *in vitro* has led to the emergence of *ex vivo* loading of DCs with tumor antigens, thus cellular DC vaccination for the induction of antitumor immunity.

A number of phase I safety and feasibility clinical studies have evaluated the use of antigen-loaded DC vaccination for the treatment of malignant glioma [26, 27, 119-121]. Yu *et al.* [122] was the first study to demonstrate that tumor-specific cytotoxicity was developed in four out of seven patients who received autologous glioma peptide-pulsed DCs. Two of the four that underwent a second surgical resection demonstrated a robust CD8+ and CD45RO+ memory T cell infiltration into the tumor [122].

EGFRvIII is an evident target for tumor-targeted immunotherapy since it is the only tumor-specific antigen in gliomas. Duke University Medical Center conducted a phase I clinical trial whereby 16 glioma patients received intradermal immunizations with autologous DCs pulsed with PEPvIII, a keyhole limpet hemocyanin (KLH) conjugate of a peptide spanning the mutated region of EGFRvIII. The logic follows that DCs injected intradermally will migrate to lymph nodes, subsequently presenting antigen to T lymphocytes [123, 124]. The patients in this study were adults with malignant gliomas who underwent resection and radiotherapy. Patients underwent leukapheresis to collect autologous peripheral blood mononuclear cells from which to generate DCs *in vitro* using GM-CSF and IL-4. DCs were then pulsed with PEPvIII and matured in a combination of TNF-α, IL-1β, and IL-6 before administered to the patient in three bi-weekly intradermal injections [125]. No adverse events occurred upon completion of the vaccinations. Prior to vaccination, none of the patients had positive DTH reaction to neither KLH nor PEPvIII; however, after vaccination 13 of 13 evaluable patients reacted to KLH, and 5 of 13 responded to PEPvIII. *In vitro* culture of patients' cells demonstrated *in vitro* proliferation of lymphocytes in response to PEPvIII in 10 of 13 patients, and to KLH in 12 of 13 patients. Two patients in the study had a nearly complete response and remained stable for 66.7 and 56.9 months. Of the 14 patients without radiographically evident disease, the median time to progression was 13.2 months. For the patients with GBM in this study the median survival time was 110.8 weeks, significantly prolonged over the 60 week median survival of patients who undergo the standard of care. This study suggests that autologous tumor specific PEPvIII-pulsed DCs are safe and might potentially induce a potent antitumor response in glioma patients.

In a phase I trial, 12 GBM patients were given DCs pulsed with peptides eluted from the surface of resected autologous tumor in three bi-weekly intradermal injections [119]. In addition to demonstrating no adverse events occurring after DC vaccinations, the study demonstrated increased systemic and intracranial immunologic responses against autologous tumor in 50% of treated patients with a median survival of 23.4 months[119].

De Vleeschouwer *et al.* [126] reported the results of 56 patients with recurrent GBM given at least three vaccinations with autologous tumor lysate-pusled autologous mature DCs. Only one serious adverse event occurred of vaccine-related edema in a patient with gross residual disease. The total population median progression free survival was 3 months, while overall survival was 9.6 months. Fourteen percent of patients had an overall survival of 2 years. Patients were divided into three cohorts, each with shorter vaccination intervals per cohort. The authors observed an improved progression free survival in patients with the shorter vaccination intervals of four vaccinations a week apart, plus a boost with an intradermal injection of tumor lysate [126]. Although there was a limited clinical response, an observed two-year overall survival in some patients is encouraging.

Wheeler *et al.* [127] demonstrated a correlation between vaccination and immune response in GBM patients. Patients who received tumor lysate-pulsed DCs demonstrated a statistically significant correlation between vaccine-induced immunity and time to tumor progression and time to survival. Patients who received tumor lysate-pulsed DCs had a greater than a 1.5 fold increase of IFNγ production relative to pre-vaccination levels. Time to survival was significantly longer ($p=0.041$) in responders, 642 ± 61 days, than in non-responders, 430 ± 50 days when both recurrent and newly diagnosed GBM patients were analyzed.

Prins *et al.* [128] conducted a safety and feasibility trial using autologous tumor lysate-pulsed DC vaccination coupled with toll-like receptor (TLR) agonists in GBM patients. Patients received either imiquimod, a TLR-7 agonist, or poly-ICLC, a TLR-3 agonist. Previous preclinical studies by this group demonstrated that TLR agonists are capable of enhancing DC activation and migration, and T cell antitumor immunity in glioma models [128, 129]. In this clinical study, 23 GBM patients were enrolled and received three biweekly injections of glioma lysate-pulsed DCs followed by either imiquimod or poly-ICLC adjuvant until tumor progression. The median overall survival was 31 months with a 47% three year survival rate.

5.4 RNA-pulsed DCs

Vaccine treatments dependent on large amounts of autologous tumor tissue can be limited in patients with brain tumors because of small amounts of material available after resection. Small amounts of tumor tissue is also a limitation to tumor-lysate based DC therapy because It has been argued that continuous boosting is required to maintain antitumor protection [130, 131]. The use of tumor antigen RNA-pulsed DCs demonstrably stimulates potent antitumor immunity in both murine and human cells [132, 133]. Both murine and human tumor-derived RNA can be isolated and amplified without loss of function, thus an RNA based platform will not be limited by the availability of tumor tissue [132]. RNA transfection has also been demonstrated to be a superior method for antigen-loading of DCs [134-136], in addition, RNA-loaded DCs have been found to be better stimulators of antigen-specific T cells than other methods of loading DCs [135]. In an *in vitro* comparison, electroporation is a superior method of loading RNA into DCs than lipofection and passive pulsing of RNA [134].

In early studies with prostate cancer, DCs transfected with prostate-specific antigen RNA and were capable of inducing cytotoxic T lymphocyte responses specifically against prostate-specific antigens, but not kallikrein antigens, a protein that shares homology with prostate-specific antigens. This demonstrates the specificity of the elicited immune response [133]. RNA-pulsed DC responses are not restricted to single MHC haplotype, nor a specific T cell subtype, enabling activation of both cytotoxic T lymphocytes and T helper cells [137-139].

In a phase I clinical study by Caruso *et al.* [140], tumor-RNA-loaded DCs were used to vaccinate 7 children with recurrent brain malignancies: anaplastic astrocytoma (n=1), GBM (n=2), ependymoma (n=2), pleomorphic xanthoastrocytoma (n=1), ependymoma (n=1) [141]. Two patients mounted tumor-specific immunity, and clinical responses were observed by magnetic resonance (MR) imaging in three patients (2 with stable disease, and 1 partial response). Because of the low number of patients in the study, the authors cannot demonstrate a clinical benefit, but have demonstrated the potential of this platform to elicit antitumor immunity.

Preclinical murine models of tumor challenge have demonstrated that DCs pulsed with unselected tumor-derived antigens induce potent protective immune responses without toxicity due to autoimmunity [142-145]; however in studies modeling large solid tumors, much stronger immune responses were required for protection [146, 147]. When such responses were generated against tumor-associated antigens not exclusive to tumors, severe autoimmunity was observed in some but not all mice [147]. This platform is capable of engendering a range of immune responses, and further studies are essential to find the balance between antitumor efficacy and prevention of toxicity.

Given the immense potential for the clinical use of DC-based tumor-specific immunotherapy, studies to examine strategies of maximizing DC potential are necessary. In the past decade, the ability of DC-based strategies to induce effective T-cell responses against malignant astrocytomas has been demonstrated using human DCs. DCs generated from tumor-bearing patients were fused with autologous tumor cells or pulsed with total tumor RNA or tumor lysate. Their respective abilities to generate a tumor-specific T cell proliferation and cytotoxic response *in vitro* were examined and no significant differences were found between the various DC treatments in their capacities to stimulate T cell proliferation and induce cytotoxicity. The preclinical development of DC-based immunotherapy for gliomas warrants further investigation in the clinical setting.

5.5 Adoptive cell transfer

Adoptive transfer involves the transfusion of cells that were manipulated *ex vivo* into the patient. In the past decade, different cell types have been studied to best induce antitumor immunity in tumor bearing hosts. Different cell types that have been used include (i) peripheral blood mononuclear cells (PBMCs) or peripheral blood lymphocytes (PBL)[148, 149], (ii) lymphokine-activated killer cells (LAKS)[150-152], (iii) mitogen-activated killer cells (MAKs)[153, 154], (iv) tumor infiltrating lymphocytes (TILs)[155], and (v) antigen specific cytotoxic lymphocytes [156, 157].

In 1992, Riddell *et al.* [158] reported that the adoptive transfer of T cell clones restored viral immunity in patients undergoing hematopoietic stem cell transplant. Adoptive transfer of T cells was a way of preventing cytomegalovirus (CMV) reactivation post-transplant. Allogeneic donor peripheral blood lymphocytes (PBL) were cultured *in vitro* with CMV infected autologous fibroblasts, subsequently expanding clonogenic CMV specific CD8+ T cells, and were then transferred back into the patients. Additionally, transplants can cause reactivation of latent Epstein-Barr virus (EBV) infections that can subsequently lead to post-transplant lymphoproliferative disease (PTLD), and occurs in up to 20% of solid organ transplants. In 1994, Papadopoulos *et al.* [159] demonstrated that adoptive transfer of *ex vivo* expanded allogeneic cytotoxic T lymphocytes is capable of effectively treating EBV-associated PTLD. This was the basis of adoptive cell transfer and approaches have been expanded to target viral-associated malignancies. The development of adoptive transfer for the treatment of non-viral malignancies primarily occurred in the context of allogeneic hematopoietic stem cell transplants for treatment of hematologic malignancies and melanoma. Adoptive cell transfer was first studied in hematopoietic stem cell transplant in a non-myeloablative setting used for the treatment of chronic myeloid leukemia [160] and was further developed for solid tumors.

In 1984, Steinbok *et al.* [148] was the first to demonstrate the safety and feasibility if adoptive immunotherapy for brain malignancies, but saw no measurable benefit to patient outcome. This landmark study was based on previous observations that GBM patients had observed lymphocytic infiltrates at tumor sites [148], suggesting that there was an attempt to mount an immune response by endogenous immune cells [161, 162]. The logic follows that perhaps other systemic factors were preventing these lymphocyte infiltrates from properly reaching the tumor site, or preventing lymphocyte activation. To circumvent this and the known immune deficits of glioma patients, Steinbok and colleagues[148] collected PBMCs from patients and re-infused the cells into their post-surgical cavities. Though no beneficial clinical outcomes were observed, this study established the feasibility and beginnings of adoptive immunotherapy in CNS malignancies.

5.6 LAK cells

Lymphokine-activated killer cells (LAK) are *in vitro* activated PBMCs cultured in IL-2 that have cytotoxic capabilities. These cells demonstrably lyse autologous and allogeneic tumors, but not healthy tissue, as demonstrated in human melanoma [163]. Early human trials to treat solid tumors with LAK cells are limited however, because of dose-dependent toxicity observed from the infusion of IL-2 into patients in attempts to expand LAK cells *in vivo*. To avoid the systemic toxicity by IL-2, Jacobs *et al.* [164] infused LAKS cells that were *ex vivo* expanded with IL-2 directly into the brain. Although this trial demonstrated a minimal benefit to patients, it did not show overall safety [165-167]. Hayes *et al.* [150] was able to demonstrate that autologous LAK cells delivered into the surgical resection cavity plus IL-2 therapy increased median survival in patients with recurrent GBM from 26 weeks in historical control patients receiving standard therapy, to 53 weeks in patients who received LAK cell therapy.

In another clinical trial, 40 GBM patients received $2.0 \pm 1.0 \times 10^9$ autologous LAK cells into their post-surgical cavity. The median interval from time of diagnosis to receiving LAK cell treatment was 10.9 months.The median survival from initial diagnosis for 31 GBM patients was 17.5 months [168]. Although this trial did not have clear survival benefits, it demonstrated the safety and feasibility of adoptive transfer of *ex vivo* manipulated cells into the CNS. The mechanisms of tumor recognition and cytotoxicity by LAK cells are unknown. Although the cells seem promising, there was limited specificity of LAK cells to tumors *in vivo*.

5.7 TILS and tumor-draining-lymph node T cells

In attempts to increase T cell specificity of adoptively transferred cells, Kitahara *et al.* [157] generated CTLs by isolating PBLs from cancer patients and cultured them *in vitro* with autologous tumor cells and IL-2. These *ex vivo* expanded cells were then re-administered back into the patient intracranially. Although this strategy generated activated tumor-specific cells, it was technically more cumbersome since it required the isolation of limited numbers of human tumor cells.

Another means of isolating tumor-specific lymphocytes is to isolate lymphocytes directly from the tumor. Autologous tumor infiltrating lymphocytes (TILS) were first demonstrated to mediate tumor regression in melanoma in 1988 [163]. In this early study, the response rate was 33%. Further studies in host preconditioning substantially increased the antitumor efficacy of TILS in melanoma [169], with clinical responses in up to 50% of patients.

The recovered TILS are found in the tumor by the time surgical resection occurs. These cells are already 'primed' against the tumor and thus have tumor-specific activation. In clinical studies, TILS were recovered from tumors and re-administered into the tumor post-surgical cavity in addition to IL-2 to enhance T cell proliferation. This was most studied in melanoma patients, but in a study by Quattrocchi *et al.* [155], six recurrent malignant glioma patients received TILS in a safety trial. Autologous TILs were isolated, *ex vivo* expanded in the presence of IL-2, then administered on treatment days 1 and 14 concurrently with IL-2. Patients also received standard chemotherapy. The study demonstrated that TILs had a dose-dependent cytotoxicity against autologous tumor, allogeneic tumor, and tumor cell lines. No significant therapy associated complications occurred above Grade 2 (by the NCI Common Toxicity Scale criteria). At the three and six month follow-up, three patients had a partial response, two had stable disease, and one patient progressed. At a 45 month follow-up, one patient had a complete response, 2 had partial responses at 48 and 47 month follow-up, and three patients expired (at 12, 12, and 18 months post-TIL administration). This pilot study demonstrated that immunotherapy with TIL intracranial administration is both safe and feasible without toxicity, but due to the small patient number of this trial, the authors cannot deduce a definitive clinical benefit [155].

In another trial, Kruse *et al.* [170]hypothesized that alloreactive cytoloxic T lymphocytes (CTL) that were sensitized to the MHC protein of the patients would provide tumor-selective targeted killing of glioma cells that express MHC. The authors collected CTLs from normal donors and cultured them with irradiated patient lymphocytes, sensitizing the normal CTLs to the patients' MHC over a 2 to 3 week period. *In vitro* assays demonstrated that the CTLs lysed targets expressing the patient MHC. CTLS were initially implanted into the tumor cavity, then patients received one to five treatment cycles every other month. Authors observed a transient toxicity at Grade 1-3. One patient showed no evidence of progression for 30 months from the start of adoptive immunotherapy. Two patients with oligodendroglioma had no evidence of disease after 80 months.

The adoptive transfer of *ex vivo* manipulated T cells that are targeted against tumor-specific antigens is an ideal platform for cellular immunotherapy. The fact that there are no known tumor-specific antigens that have been identified specifically in all glioma cells proves to be a limiting factor. Studies have successfully targeted EGFRvIII with precision using vaccination strategies, but no records of using T-cell mediated adoptive immunotherapy to target EGFRvIII have been demonstrated. Other potential glioma target antigens include IL-13R2a, survivin [171], and telomerase [172]. Interestingly, several groups have found viral antigens from human cytomegalovirus (CMV) to be expressed in nearly all GBMs, but not in surrounding healthy tissue [173]. CMV antigens could thus be an ideal target for immunotherapy. All these mentioned antigens lend themselves to generating highly tumor-specific T cell populations for the use in adoptive cell transfer.

Incredible advances in adoptive immunotherapy have been made in metastatic melanoma to maximize the clinical benefits of adoptive transfer methods by optimizing host conditioning, genetic manipulation of T cells, and optimizing *in vitro* T cell expansion conditions. Adoptive cell therapy in the context of lymphodepletion is the currently the most effective treatment for advanced refractory melanoma with objective responses greater than 50% [174].

6. Host conditioning and homeostatic proliferation

Lymphodepletion is well known to significantly enhance the antitumor efficacy of adoptive cell transfer and DC vaccination strategies in tumor bearing hosts. Lymphodepletion removes inhibitory T regulatory cells, decreases competition for homeostatic cytokines between host and transferred cells, and induces homeostatic proliferation of the few remaining host T lymphocytes. Homeostatic proliferation is a rapid expansion of T cells with the purpose of recovering normal lymphocyte counts [175]. An increase in serum levels of IL-7 and IL-15 help induce rapid proliferation of T cells with a lower activation threshold [175, 176] and differentiate into effector memory T cells that respond to antigen [45]. Lymphocytes must encounter cognate antigens and compete for these cytokines. Following this logic, B and T cells that are antigen-specific such as those provided as vaccines or as adoptively transferred antigen-specific T lymphocytes, have a competitive advantage over depleted host lymphocytes [177, 178]. Antigen-specific lymphocytes disproportionately expand to become over-represented in the host circulation both in murine models and human patients [177-179], therefore enhancing antitumor immunity [177, 178, 180].

In preclinical and clinical studies of adoptive immunotherapy in metastatic melanoma, lymphodepletion enhanced the expansion of adoptively transferred tumor-specific T cells and resulted in increased clinical responses with a greater than 50% objective clinical response [174, 181-185]. Adoptively transferred cells undergo dramatic expansion and can constitute up to 90% of host T cell repertoire and persist for months [174]. These studies by Dudley and Rosenberg demonstrate a correlation between clinical regression of systemic disease, the frequency of tumor-specific T cells in peripheral blood, and the persistence of transferred cells *in vivo* [186]. In further studies, increased lymphodepletion to myeloablative levels that required bone marrow stem cell rescue further enhanced antigen-specific T cell proliferation as well as an increased antitumor efficacy [187]. Clinical trials conducted at the National Cancer Institute using tumor-reactive TILS and IL-2 infusion demonstrated that increasing intensity of lymphodepletion enhanced clinical responses. With maximum doses of lymphodepletion, 72% of patients demonstrated an objective response and 32% of patients had complete tumor regression [188]. Only 1 of 16 patients who achieved complete response recurred after 84 months.

7. Conclusion

Cellular immunotherapy is a highly specific therapy that is directed at eliciting an immune response against tumor antigens using passive or active immunization with cellular vaccines or adoptive transfer of ex vivo activated lymphocytes. Preclinical studies have demonstrated the clear antitumor efficacy of these therapeutic modalities. The breadth of clinical studies conducted demonstrates a lack of adverse toxicity related to immunotherapies. The curative potential of cellular immunotherapy has been successful in other solid and hematological malignancies and is currently in the early stages of use in CNS malignancies.

8. References

[1] Heimberger, A.B. and J.H. Sampson, *Immunotherapy coming of age: what will it take to make it standard of care for glioblastoma?* Neuro Oncol, 2011. 13(1): p. 3-13.

[2] Harling-Berg, C., *et al.*, *Role of cervical lymph nodes in the systemic humoral immune response to human serum albumin microinfused into rat cerebrospinal fluid.* J Neuroimmunol, 1989. 25(2-3): p. 185-93.

[3] Cserr, H.F., et al., *Afferent and efferent arms of the humoral immune response to CSF-administered albumins in a rat model with normal blood-brain barrier permeability.* J Neuroimmunol, 1992. 41(2): p. 195-202.

[4] Cserr, H.F., C.J. Harling-Berg, and P.M. Knopf, *Drainage of brain extracellular fluid into blood and deep cervical lymph and its immunological significance.* Brain Pathol, 1992. 2(4): p. 269-76.

[5] Weller, R.O., B. Engelhardt, and M.J. Phillips, *Lymphocyte targeting of the central nervous system: a review of afferent and efferent CNS-immune pathways.* Brain Pathol, 1996. 6(3): p. 275-88.

[6] Harling-Berg, C.J., et al., *Hierarchy of immune responses to antigen in the normal brain.* Curr Top Microbiol Immunol, 2002. 265: p. 1-22.

[7] Fabry, Z., C.S. Raine, and M.N. Hart, *Nervous tissue as an immune compartment: the dialect of the immune response in the CNS.* Immunol Today, 1994. 15(5): p. 218-24.

[8] Mosmann, T.R. and R.L. Coffman, *TH1 and TH2 cells: different patterns of lymphokine secretion lead to different functional properties.* Annu Rev Immunol, 1989. 7: p. 145-73.

[9] Bullard, D.E. and D.D. Bigner, *Applications of monoclonal antibodies in the diagnosis and treatment of primary brain tumors.* J Neurosurg, 1985. 63(1): p. 2-16.
[10] Goldmann, J., et al., *T cells traffic from brain to cervical lymph nodes via the cribroid plate and the nasal mucosa.* J Leukoc Biol, 2006. 80(4): p. 797-801.
[11] Masson, F., et al., *Brain microenvironment promotes the final functional maturation of tumor-specific effector CD8+ T cells.* J Immunol, 2007. 179(2): p. 845-53.
[12] Aloisi, F., F. Ria, and L. Adorini, *Regulation of T-cell responses by CNS antigen-presenting cells: different roles for microglia and astrocytes.* Immunol Today, 2000. 21(3): p. 141-7.
[13] Serot, J.M., et al., *Ultrastructural and immunohistological evidence for dendritic-like cells within human choroid plexus epithelium.* Neuroreport, 1997. 8(8): p. 1995-8.
[14] Gehrmann, J., Y. Matsumoto, and G.W. Kreutzberg, *Microglia: intrinsic immuneffector cell of the brain.* Brain Res Brain Res Rev, 1995. 20(3): p. 269-87.
[15] Ford, A.L., et al., *Microglia induce CD4 T lymphocyte final effector function and death.* J Exp Med, 1996. 184(5): p. 1737-45.
[16] Sedgwick, J.D., et al., *Central nervous system microglial cell activation and proliferation follows direct interaction with tissue-infiltrating T cell blasts.* J Immunol, 1998. 160(11): p. 5320-30.
[17] Hatalski, C.G., W.F. Hickey, and W.I. Lipkin, *Evolution of the immune response in the central nervous system following infection with Borna disease virus.* J Neuroimmunol, 1998. 90(2): p. 137-42.
[18] Hatalski, C.G., W.F. Hickey, and W.I. Lipkin, *Humoral immunity in the central nervous system of Lewis rats infected with Borna disease virus.* J Neuroimmunol, 1998. 90(2): p. 128-36.
[19] Hickey, W.F. and H. Kimura, *Perivascular microglial cells of the CNS are bone marrow-derived and present antigen in vivo.* Science, 1988. 239(4837): p. 290-2.
[20] Yamanaka, R., *Dendritic-cell- and peptide-based vaccination strategies for glioma.* Neurosurg Rev, 2009. 32(3): p. 265-73; discussion 273.
[21] Naumov, G.N., et al., *A model of human tumor dormancy: an angiogenic switch from the nonangiogenic phenotype.* J Natl Cancer Inst, 2006. 98(5): p. 316-25.
[22] [Schneider, T., et al., *Increased concentrations of transforming growth factor beta1 and beta2 in the plasma of patients with glioblastoma.* J Neurooncol, 2006. 79(1): p. 61-5.
[23] Sakaguchi, S., *Naturally arising Foxp3-expressing CD25+CD4+ regulatory T cells in immunological tolerance to self and non-self.* Nat Immunol, 2005. 6(4): p. 345-52.
[24] Grauer, O.M., et al., *CD4+FoxP3+ regulatory T cells gradually accumulate in gliomas during tumor growth and efficiently suppress antiglioma immune responses in vivo.* Int J Cancer, 2007. 121(1): p. 95-105.
[25] Fecci, P.E., et al., *Increased regulatory T-cell fraction amidst a diminished CD4 compartment explains cellular immune defects in patients with malignant glioma.* Cancer Res, 2006. 66(6): p. 3294-302.
[26] [Yamanaka, R., et al., *Vaccination of recurrent glioma patients with tumour lysate-pulsed dendritic cells elicits immune responses: results of a clinical phase I/II trial.* Br J Cancer, 2003. 89(7): p. 1172-9.
[27] Kikuchi, T., et al., *Vaccination of glioma patients with fusions of dendritic and glioma cells and recombinant human interleukin 12.* J Immunother, 2004. 27(6): p. 452-9.

[28] Kikuchi, T., et al., *Results of a phase I clinical trial of vaccination of glioma patients with fusions of dendritic and glioma cells.* Cancer Immunol Immunother, 2001. 50(7): p. 337-44.

[29] Rutkowski, S., et al., *Surgery and adjuvant dendritic cell-based tumour vaccination for patients with relapsed malignant glioma, a feasibility study.* Br J Cancer, 2004. 91(9): p. 1656-62.

[30] Yajima, N., et al., *Immunologic evaluation of personalized peptide vaccination for patients with advanced malignant glioma.* Clin Cancer Res, 2005. 11(16): p. 5900-11.

[31] van der Bruggen, P., et al., *A gene encoding an antigen recognized by cytolytic T lymphocytes on a human melanoma.* Science, 1991. 254(5038): p. 1643-7.

[32] Chen, Y.T., et al., *A testicular antigen aberrantly expressed in human cancers detected by autologous antibody screening.* Proc Natl Acad Sci U S A, 1997. 94(5): p. 1914-8.

[33] Debinski, W., et al., *Receptor for interleukin 13 is abundantly and specifically over-expressed in patients with glioblastoma multiforme.* Int J Oncol, 1999. 15(3): p. 481-6.

[34] Fichtner-Feigl, S., et al., *IL-13 signaling through the IL-13alpha2 receptor is involved in induction of TGF-beta1 production and fibrosis.* Nat Med, 2006. 12(1): p. 99-106.

[35] Wykosky, J., et al., *Interleukin-13 receptor alpha 2, EphA2, and Fos-related antigen 1 as molecular denominators of high-grade astrocytomas and specific targets for combinatorial therapy.* Clin Cancer Res, 2008. 14(1): p. 199-208.

[36] Das, A., et al., *Expression of survivin in primary glioblastomas.* J Cancer Res Clin Oncol, 2002. 128(6): p. 302-6.

[37] Chakravarti, A., et al., *Quantitatively determined survivin expression levels are of prognostic value in human gliomas.* J Clin Oncol, 2002. 20(4): p. 1063-8.

[38] Shankar, S.L., et al., *Survivin inhibition induces human neural tumor cell death through caspase-independent and -dependent pathways.* J Neurochem, 2001. 79(2): p. 426-36.

[39] Jeon, B.G., et al., *Characterization and comparison of telomere length, telomerase and reverse transcriptase activity and gene expression in human mesenchymal stem cells and cancer cells of various origins.* Cell Tissue Res, 2011.

[40] Sallinen, P., et al., *Increased expression of telomerase RNA component is associated with increased cell proliferation in human astrocytomas.* Am J Pathol, 1997. 150(4): p. 1159-64.

[41] DeMasters, B.K., et al., *Differential telomerase expression in human primary intracranial tumors.* Am J Clin Pathol, 1997. 107(5): p. 548-54.

[42] Beck, S., et al., *Telomerase activity-independent function of TERT allows glioma cells to attain cancer stem cell characteristics by inducing EGFR expression.* Mol Cells, 2011. 31(1): p. 9-15.

[43] Scheurer, M.E., et al., *Detection of human cytomegalovirus in different histological types of gliomas.* Acta Neuropathol, 2008. 116(1): p. 79-86.

[44] Fecci, P.E., et al., *Systemic anti-CD25 monoclonal antibody administration safely enhances immunity in murine glioma without eliminating regulatory T cells.* Clin Cancer Res, 2006. 12(14 Pt 1): p. 4294-305.

[45] Liyanage, U.K., et al., *Prevalence of regulatory T cells is increased in peripheral blood and tumor microenvironment of patients with pancreas or breast adenocarcinoma.* J Immunol, 2002. 169(5): p. 2756-61.

[46] Elliott, L.H., W.H. Brooks, and T.L. Roszman, *Cytokinetic basis for the impaired activation of lymphocytes from patients with primary intracranial tumors.* J Immunol, 1984. 132(3): p. 1208-15.

[47] Elliott, L.H., W.H. Brooks, and T.L. Roszman, *Activation of immunoregulatory lymphocytes obtained from patients with malignant gliomas.* J Neurosurg, 1987. 67(2): p. 231-6.
[48] McVicar, D.W., D.F. Davis, and R.E. Merchant, *In vitro analysis of the proliferative potential of T cells from patients with brain tumor: glioma-associated immunosuppression unrelated to intrinsic cellular defect.* J Neurosurg, 1992. 76(2): p. 251-60.
[49] Roszman, T.L. and W.H. Brooks, *Immunobiology of primary intracranial tumours. III. Demonstration of a qualitative lymphocyte abnormality in patients with primary brain tumours.* Clin Exp Immunol, 1980. 39(2): p. 395-402.
[50] Morford, L.A., et al., *T cell receptor-mediated signaling is defective in T cells obtained from patients with primary intracranial tumors.* J Immunol, 1997. 159(9): p. 4415-25.
[51] de Martin, R., et al., *Complementary DNA for human glioblastoma-derived T cell suppressor factor, a novel member of the transforming growth factor-beta gene family.* EMBO J, 1987. 6(12): p. 3673-7.
[52] Kehrl, J.H., et al., *Production of transforming growth factor beta by human T lymphocytes and its potential role in the regulation of T cell growth.* J Exp Med, 1986. 163(5): p. 1037-50.
[53] Zuber, P., M.C. Kuppner, and N. De Tribolet, *Transforming growth factor-beta 2 down-regulates HLA-DR antigen expression on human malignant glioma cells.* Eur J Immunol, 1988. 18(10): p. 1623-6.
[54] Torre-Amione, G., et al., *A highly immunogenic tumor transfected with a murine transforming growth factor type beta 1 cDNA escapes immune surveillance.* Proc Natl Acad Sci U S A, 1990. 87(4): p. 1486-90.
[55] Ohm, J.E. and D.P. Carbone, *VEGF as a mediator of tumor-associated immunodeficiency.* Immunol Res, 2001. 23(2-3): p. 263-72.
[56] Aoki, M., et al., *Effects of vascular endothelial growth factor and E-selectin on angiogenesis in the murine metastatic RCT sarcoma.* Tumour Biol, 2001. 22(4): p. 239-46.
[57] Gabrilovich, D.I., et al., *Antibodies to vascular endothelial growth factor enhance the efficacy of cancer immunotherapy by improving endogenous dendritic cell function.* Clin Cancer Res, 1999. 5(10): p. 2963-70.
[58] Lien, S. and H.B. Lowman, *Therapeutic anti-VEGF antibodies.* Handb Exp Pharmacol, 2008(181): p. 131-50.
[59] Vredenburgh, J.J., et al., *Bevacizumab plus irinotecan in recurrent glioblastoma multiforme.* J Clin Oncol, 2007. 25(30): p. 4722-9.
[60] Vredenburgh, J.J., et al., *Phase II trial of bevacizumab and irinotecan in recurrent malignant glioma.* Clin Cancer Res, 2007. 13(4): p. 1253-9.
[61] Bao, S., et al., *Stem cell-like glioma cells promote tumor angiogenesis through vascular endothelial growth factor.* Cancer Res, 2006. 66(16): p. 7843-8.
[62] Seddon, B. and D. Mason, *Regulatory T cells in the control of autoimmunity: the essential role of transforming growth factor beta and interleukin 4 in the prevention of autoimmune thyroiditis in rats by peripheral CD4(+)CD45RC- cells and CD4(+)CD8(-) thymocytes.* J Exp Med, 1999. 189(2): p. 279-88.
[63] Bagavant, H., et al., *Differential effect of neonatal thymectomy on systemic and organ-specific autoimmune disease.* Int Immunol, 2002. 14(12): p. 1397-406.
[64] Hori, S., et al., *Specificity requirements for selection and effector functions of CD25+4+ regulatory T cells in anti-myelin basic protein T cell receptor transgenic mice.* Proc Natl Acad Sci U S A, 2002. 99(12): p. 8213-8.

[65] Ng, W.F., et al., *Human CD4(+)CD25(+) cells: a naturally occurring population of regulatory T cells.* Blood, 2001. 98(9): p. 2736-44.
[66] Ermann, J., et al., *CD4(+)CD25(+) T cells facilitate the induction of T cell anergy.* J Immunol, 2001. 167(8): p. 4271-5.
[67] Somasundaram, R., et al., *Inhibition of cytolytic T lymphocyte proliferation by autologous CD4+/CD25+ regulatory T cells in a colorectal carcinoma patient is mediated by transforming growth factor-beta.* Cancer Res, 2002. 62(18): p. 5267-72.
[68] Curiel, T.J., et al., *Specific recruitment of regulatory T cells in ovarian carcinoma fosters immune privilege and predicts reduced survival.* Nat Med, 2004. 10(9): p. 942-9.
[69] Reardon, D.A., et al., *A Review of VEGF/VEGFR-Targeted Therapeutics for Recurrent Glioblastoma.* J Natl Compr Canc Netw, 2011. 9(4): p. 414-27.
[70] Lucio-Eterovic, A.K., Y. Piao, and J.F. de Groot, *Mediators of glioblastoma resistance and invasion during antivascular endothelial growth factor therapy.* Clin Cancer Res, 2009. 15(14): p. 4589-99.
[71] Libermann, T.A., et al., *Amplification, enhanced expression and possible rearrangement of EGF receptor gene in primary human brain tumours of glial origin.* Nature, 1985. 313(5998): p. 144-7.
[72] Bigner, S.H., et al., *Characterization of the epidermal growth factor receptor in human glioma cell lines and xenografts.* Cancer Res, 1990. 50(24): p. 8017-22.
[73] Batra, S.K., et al., *Epidermal growth factor ligand-independent, unregulated, cell-transforming potential of a naturally occurring human mutant EGFRvIII gene.* Cell Growth Differ, 1995. 6(10): p. 1251-9.
[74] Nishikawa, R., et al., *A mutant epidermal growth factor receptor common in human glioma confers enhanced tumorigenicity.* Proc Natl Acad Sci U S A, 1994. 91(16): p. 7727-31.
[75] Huang, H.S., et al., *The enhanced tumorigenic activity of a mutant epidermal growth factor receptor common in human cancers is mediated by threshold levels of constitutive tyrosine phosphorylation and unattenuated signaling.* J Biol Chem, 1997. 272(5): p. 2927-35.
[76] Lammering, G., et al., *Inhibition of the type III epidermal growth factor receptor variant mutant receptor by dominant-negative EGFR-CD533 enhances malignant glioma cell radiosensitivity.* Clin Cancer Res, 2004. 10(19): p. 6732-43.
[77] Nagane, M., et al., *A common mutant epidermal growth factor receptor confers enhanced tumorigenicity on human glioblastoma cells by increasing proliferation and reducing apoptosis.* Cancer Res, 1996. 56(21): p. 5079-86.
[78] [Montgomery, R.B., et al., *Expression of oncogenic epidermal growth factor receptor family kinases induces paclitaxel resistance and alters beta-tubulin isotype expression.* J Biol Chem, 2000. 275(23): p. 17358-63.
[79] Wikstrand, C.J., et al., *Monoclonal antibodies against EGFRvIII are tumor specific and react with breast and lung carcinomas and malignant gliomas.* Cancer Res, 1995. 55(14): p. 3140-8.
[80] Frederick, L., et al., *Diversity and frequency of epidermal growth factor receptor mutations in human glioblastomas.* Cancer Res, 2000. 60(5): p. 1383-7.
[81] [81] Schlegel, J., et al., *Amplification of the epidermal-growth-factor-receptor gene correlates with different growth behaviour in human glioblastoma.* Int J Cancer, 1994. 56(1): p. 72-7.
[82] Sugawa, N., et al., *Identical splicing of aberrant epidermal growth factor receptor transcripts from amplified rearranged genes in human glioblastomas.* Proc Natl Acad Sci U S A, 1990. 87(21): p. 8602-6.

[83] Wikstrand, C.J., et al., *Cell surface localization and density of the tumor-associated variant of the epidermal growth factor receptor, EGFRvIII.* Cancer Res, 1997. 57(18): p. 4130-40.
[84] Humphrey, P.A., et al., *Anti-synthetic peptide antibody reacting at the fusion junction of deletion-mutant epidermal growth factor receptors in human glioblastoma.* Proc Natl Acad Sci U S A, 1990. 87(11): p. 4207-11.
[85] Sampson, J.H., et al., *Unarmed, tumor-specific monoclonal antibody effectively treats brain tumors.* Proc Natl Acad Sci U S A, 2000. 97(13): p. 7503-8.
[86] Reist, C.J., et al., *Tumor-specific anti-epidermal growth factor receptor variant III monoclonal antibodies: use of the tyramine-cellobiose radioiodination method enhances cellular retention and uptake in tumor xenografts.* Cancer Res, 1995. 55(19): p. 4375-82.
[87] Lorimer, I.A., et al., *Immunotoxins that target an oncogenic mutant epidermal growth factor receptor expressed in human tumors.* Clin Cancer Res, 1995. 1(8): p. 859-64.
[88] Archer, G.E., et al., *Regional treatment of epidermal growth factor receptor vIII-expressing neoplastic meningitis with a single-chain immunotoxin, MR-1.* Clin Cancer Res, 1999. 5(9): p. 2646-52.
[89] Reist, C.J., et al., *In vitro and in vivo behavior of radiolabeled chimeric anti-EGFRvIII monoclonal antibody: comparison with its murine parent.* Nucl Med Biol, 1997. 24(7): p. 639-47.
[90] Reist, C.J., et al., *Improved targeting of an anti-epidermal growth factor receptor variant III monoclonal antibody in tumor xenografts after labeling using N-succinimidyl 5-iodo-3-pyridinecarboxylate.* Cancer Res, 1997. 57(8): p. 1510-5.
[91] Reist, C.J., et al., *Astatine-211 labeling of internalizing anti-EGFRvIII monoclonal antibody using N-succinimidyl 5-[211At]astato-3-pyridinecarboxylate.* Nucl Med Biol, 1999. 26(4): p. 405-11.
[92] Faillot, T., et al., *A phase I study of an anti-epidermal growth factor receptor monoclonal antibody for the treatment of malignant gliomas.* Neurosurgery, 1996. 39(3): p. 478-83.
[93] Stragliotto, G., et al., *Multiple infusions of anti-epidermal growth factor receptor (EGFR) monoclonal antibody (EMD 55,900) in patients with recurrent malignant gliomas.* Eur J Cancer, 1996. 32A(4): p. 636-40.
[94] Purev, E., et al., *Immune responses of breast cancer patients to mutated epidermal growth factor receptor (EGF-RvIII, Delta EGF-R, and de2-7 EGF-R).* J Immunol, 2004. 173(10): p. 6472-80.
[95] Sampson, J.H., et al., *Immunologic escape after prolonged progression-free survival with epidermal growth factor receptor variant III peptide vaccination in patients with newly diagnosed glioblastoma.* J Clin Oncol, 2010. 28(31): p. 4722-9.
[96] Sampson, J.H., et al., *Greater chemotherapy-induced lymphopenia enhances tumor-specific immune responses that eliminate EGFRvIII-expressing tumor cells in patients with glioblastoma.* Neuro Oncol, 2011. 13(3): p. 324-33.
[97] Kurpad, S.N., et al., *Tumor antigens in astrocytic gliomas.* Glia, 1995. 15(3): p. 244-56.
[98] Bigner, D.D., et al., *Iodine-131-labeled antitenascin monoclonal antibody 81C6 treatment of patients with recurrent malignant gliomas: phase I trial results.* J Clin Oncol, 1998. 16(6): p. 2202-12.
[99] Brown, M.T., et al., *Intrathecal 131I-labeled antitenascin monoclonal antibody 81C6 treatment of patients with leptomeningeal neoplasms or primary brain tumor resection cavities with subarachnoid communication: phase I trial results.* Clin Cancer Res, 1996. 2(6): p. 963-72.
[100] Bigner, D.D., et al., *Phase I studies of treatment of malignant gliomas and neoplastic meningitis with 131I-radiolabeled monoclonal antibodies anti-tenascin 81C6 and anti-*

chondroitin proteoglycan sulfate Me1-14 F (ab')2--a preliminary report. J Neurooncol, 1995. 24(1): p. 109-22.

[101] Reardon, D.A., et al., *Salvage radioimmunotherapy with murine iodine-131-labeled antitenascin monoclonal antibody 81C6 for patients with recurrent primary and metastatic malignant brain tumors: phase II study results.* J Clin Oncol, 2006. 24(1): p. 115-22.

[102] Reardon, D.A., et al., *Phase II trial of murine (131)I-labeled antitenascin monoclonal antibody 81C6 administered into surgically created resection cavities of patients with newly diagnosed malignant gliomas.* J Clin Oncol, 2002. 20(5): p. 1389-97.

[103] Reardon, D.A., et al., *A pilot study: 131I-antitenascin monoclonal antibody 81c6 to deliver a 44-Gy resection cavity boost.* Neuro Oncol, 2008. 10(2): p. 182-9.

[104] Turkington, T.G., et al., *Measuring astatine-211 distributions with SPECT.* Phys Med Biol, 1993. 38(8): p. 1121-30.

[105] Zalutsky, M.R., et al., *Clinical experience with alpha-particle emitting 211At: treatment of recurrent brain tumor patients with 211At-labeled chimeric antitenascin monoclonal antibody 81C6.* J Nucl Med, 2008. 49(1): p. 30-8.

[106] Steinman, R.M. and J. Banchereau, *Taking dendritic cells into medicine.* Nature, 2007. 449(7161): p. 419-26.

[107] Melief, C.J., *Cancer immunotherapy by dendritic cells.* Immunity, 2008. 29(3): p. 372-83.

[108] Steinman, R.M., D. Hawiger, and M.C. Nussenzweig, *Tolerogenic dendritic cells.* Annu Rev Immunol, 2003. 21: p. 685-711.

[109] Dhodapkar, M.V. and R.M. Steinman, *Antigen-bearing immature dendritic cells induce peptide-specific CD8(+) regulatory T cells in vivo in humans.* Blood, 2002. 100(1): p. 174-7.

[110] Wakkach, A., et al., *Characterization of dendritic cells that induce tolerance and T regulatory 1 cell differentiation in vivo.* Immunity, 2003. 18(5): p. 605-17.

[111] Palucka, K., H. Ueno, and J. Banchereau, *Recent developments in cancer vaccines.* J Immunol, 2011. 186(3): p. 1325-31.

[112] Sampson, J.H., et al., *Intracerebral infusion of an EGFR-targeted toxin in recurrent malignant brain tumors.* Neuro Oncol, 2008. 10(3): p. 320-9.

[113] Zaba, L.C., et al., *Normal human dermis contains distinct populations of CD11c+BDCA-1+ dendritic cells and CD163+FXIIIA+ macrophages.* J Clin Invest, 2007. 117(9): p. 2517-25.

[114] Klechevsky, E., et al., *Functional specializations of human epidermal Langerhans cells and CD14+ dermal dendritic cells.* Immunity, 2008. 29(3): p. 497-510.

[115] Celluzzi, C.M. and L.D. Falo, Jr., *Epidermal dendritic cells induce potent antigen-specific CTL-mediated immunity.* J Invest Dermatol, 1997. 108(5): p. 716-20.

[116] Palucka, K., et al., *Dendritic cells and immunity against cancer.* J Intern Med, 2011. 269(1): p. 64-73.

[117] Lapenta, C., et al., *Potent immune response against HIV-1 and protection from virus challenge in hu-PBL-SCID mice immunized with inactivated virus-pulsed dendritic cells generated in the presence of IFN-alpha.* J Exp Med, 2003. 198(2): p. 361-7.

[118] Dubsky, P., et al., *IL-15-induced human DC efficiently prime melanoma-specific naive CD8+ T cells to differentiate into CTL.* Eur J Immunol, 2007. 37(6): p. 1678-90.

[119] Liau, L.M., et al., *Dendritic cell vaccination in glioblastoma patients induces systemic and intracranial T-cell responses modulated by the local central nervous system tumor microenvironment.* Clin Cancer Res, 2005. 11(15): p. 5515-25.

[120] Yamanaka, R., et al., *Clinical evaluation of dendritic cell vaccination for patients with recurrent glioma: results of a clinical phase I/II trial.* Clin Cancer Res, 2005. 11(11): p. 4160-7.

[121] Yu, J.S., et al., *Vaccination with tumor lysate-pulsed dendritic cells elicits antigen-specific, cytotoxic T-cells in patients with malignant glioma.* Cancer Res, 2004. 64(14): p. 4973-9.

[122] Yu, J.S., et al., *Vaccination of malignant glioma patients with peptide-pulsed dendritic cells elicits systemic cytotoxicity and intracranial T-cell infiltration.* Cancer Res, 2001. 61(3): p. 842-7.

[123] Morse, M.A., et al., *Migration of human dendritic cells after injection in patients with metastatic malignancies.* Cancer Res, 1999. 59(1): p. 56-8.

[124] Barratt-Boyes, S.M., et al., *Maturation and trafficking of monocyte-derived dendritic cells in monkeys: implications for dendritic cell-based vaccines.* J Immunol, 2000. 164(5): p. 2487-95.

[125] Mitchell, D.A., P.E. Fecci, and J.H. Sampson, *Immunotherapy of malignant brain tumors.* Immunol Rev, 2008. 222: p. 70-100.

[126] De Vleeschouwer, S., et al., *Postoperative adjuvant dendritic cell-based immunotherapy in patients with relapsed glioblastoma multiforme.* Clin Cancer Res, 2008. 14(10): p. 3098-104.

[127] Wheeler, C.J., et al., *Vaccination elicits correlated immune and clinical responses in glioblastoma multiforme patients.* Cancer Res, 2008. 68(14): p. 5955-64.

[128] Prins, R.M., et al., *Gene expression profile correlates with T-cell infiltration and relative survival in glioblastoma patients vaccinated with dendritic cell immunotherapy.* Clin Cancer Res, 2011. 17(6): p. 1603-15.

[129] Prins, R.M., et al., *The TLR-7 agonist, imiquimod, enhances dendritic cell survival and promotes tumor antigen-specific T cell priming: relation to central nervous system antitumor immunity.* J Immunol, 2006. 176(1): p. 157-64.

[130] Kundig, T.M., et al., *On the role of antigen in maintaining cytotoxic T-cell memory.* Proc Natl Acad Sci U S A, 1996. 93(18): p. 9716-23.

[131] Matzinger, P., *An innate sense of danger.* Semin Immunol, 1998. 10(5): p. 399-415.

[132] Boczkowski, D., et al., *Induction of tumor immunity and cytotoxic T lymphocyte responses using dendritic cells transfected with messenger RNA amplified from tumor cells.* Cancer Res, 2000. 60(4): p. 1028-34.

[133] Heiser, A., et al., *Human dendritic cells transfected with RNA encoding prostate-specific antigen stimulate prostate-specific CTL responses in vitro.* J Immunol, 2000. 164(10): p. 5508-14.

[134] Wintterle, S., et al., *Expression of the B7-related molecule B7-H1 by glioma cells: a potential mechanism of immune paralysis.* Cancer Res, 2003. 63(21): p. 7462-7.

[135] Dong, H., et al., *Tumor-associated B7-H1 promotes T-cell apoptosis: a potential mechanism of immune evasion.* Nat Med, 2002. 8(8): p. 793-800.

[136] Parsa, A.T., et al., *Loss of tumor suppressor PTEN function increases B7-H1 expression and immunoresistance in glioma.* Nat Med, 2007. 13(1): p. 84-8.

[137] Kugler, A., et al., *Regression of human metastatic renal cell carcinoma after vaccination with tumor cell-dendritic cell hybrids.* Nat Med, 2000. 6(3): p. 332-6.

[138] Blank, C. and A. Mackensen, *Contribution of the PD-L1/PD-1 pathway to T-cell exhaustion: an update on implications for chronic infections and tumor evasion.* Cancer Immunol Immunother, 2007. 56(5): p. 739-45.

[139] Yao, S. and L. Chen, *Reviving exhausted T lymphocytes during chronic virus infection by B7-H1 blockade.* Trends Mol Med, 2006. 12(6): p. 244-6.

[140] Caruso, D.A., et al., *Results of a phase 1 study utilizing monocyte-derived dendritic cells pulsed with tumor RNA in children and young adults with brain cancer.* Neuro Oncol, 2004. 6(3): p. 236-46.

[141] Thompson, R.H., et al., *B7-H1 glycoprotein blockade: a novel strategy to enhance immunotherapy in patients with renal cell carcinoma.* Urology, 2005. 66(5 Suppl): p. 10-4.

[142] Kirsch, M., H. Fischer, and G. Schackert, *Activated monocytes kill malignant brain tumor cells in vitro.* J Neurooncol, 1994. 20(1): p. 35-45.

[143] Wahl, S.M., et al., *Transforming growth factor-beta is a potent immunosuppressive agent that inhibits IL-1-dependent lymphocyte proliferation.* J Immunol, 1988. 140(9): p. 3026-32.

[144] Rook, A.H., et al., *Effects of transforming growth factor beta on the functions of natural killer cells: depressed cytolytic activity and blunting of interferon responsiveness.* J Immunol, 1986. 136(10): p. 3916-20.

[145] Strome, S.E., et al., *B7-H1 blockade augments adoptive T-cell immunotherapy for squamous cell carcinoma.* Cancer Res, 2003. 63(19): p. 6501-5.

[146] Curiel, T.J., et al., *Blockade of B7-H1 improves myeloid dendritic cell-mediated antitumor immunity.* Nat Med, 2003. 9(5): p. 562-7.

[147] Suda, T., et al., *Molecular cloning and expression of the Fas ligand, a novel member of the tumor necrosis factor family.* Cell, 1993. 75(6): p. 1169-78.

[148] Steinbok, P., et al., *Intratumoral autologous mononuclear cells in the treatment of recurrent glioblastoma multiforme. A phase 1 (toxicity) study.* J Neurooncol, 1984. 2(2): p. 147-51.

[149] Young, H., A. Kaplan, and W. Regelson, *Immunotherapy with autologous white cell infusions ("lymphocytes") in the treatment of recurrrent glioblastoma multiforme: a preliminary report.* Cancer, 1977. 40(3): p. 1037-44.

[150] Hayes, R.L., et al., *Improved long term survival after intracavitary interleukin-2 and lymphokine-activated killer cells for adults with recurrent malignant glioma.* Cancer, 1995. 76(5): p. 840-52.

[151] Blancher, A., et al., *Local immunotherapy of recurrent glioblastoma multiforme by intracerebral perfusion of interleukin-2 and LAK cells.* Eur Cytokine Netw, 1993. 4(5): p. 331-41.

[152] Jacobs, S.K., et al., *Interleukin-2 or autologous lymphokine-activated killer cell treatment of malignant glioma: phase I trial.* Cancer Res, 1986. 46(4 Pt 2): p. 2101-4.

[153] Jeffes, E.W., 3rd, et al., *Therapy of recurrent high grade gliomas with surgery, and autologous mitogen activated IL-2 stimulated killer (MAK) lymphocytes: I. Enhancement of MAK lytic activity and cytokine production by PHA and clinical use of PHA.* J Neurooncol, 1993. 15(2): p. 141-55.

[154] Ingram, M., et al., *Immunotherapy for recurrent malignant glioma: an interim report on survival.* Neurol Res, 1990. 12(4): p. 265-73.

[155] Quattrocchi, K.B., et al., *Pilot study of local autologous tumor infiltrating lymphocytes for the treatment of recurrent malignant gliomas.* J Neurooncol, 1999. 45(2): p. 141-57.

[156] Tsurushima, H., et al., *Reduction of end-stage malignant glioma by injection with autologous cytotoxic T lymphocytes.* Jpn J Cancer Res, 1999. 90(5): p. 536-45.

[157] Kitahara, T., et al., *Establishment of interleukin 2 dependent cytotoxic T lymphocyte cell line specific for autologous brain tumor and its intracranial administration for therapy of the tumor.* J Neurooncol, 1987. 4(4): p. 329-36.
[158] Riddell, S.R., et al., *Phase I study of cellular adoptive immunotherapy using genetically modified CD8+ HIV-specific T cells for HIV seropositive patients undergoing allogeneic bone marrow transplant. The Fred Hutchinson Cancer Research Center and the University of Washington School of Medicine, Department of Medicine, Division of Oncology.* Hum Gene Ther, 1992. 3(3): p. 319-38.
[159] Papadopoulos, E.B., et al., *Infusions of donor leukocytes to treat Epstein-Barr virus-associated lymphoproliferative disorders after allogeneic bone marrow transplantation.* N Engl J Med, 1994. 330(17): p. 1185-91.
[160] Kolb, H.J., et al., *Donor leukocyte transfusions for treatment of recurrent chronic myelogenous leukemia in marrow transplant patients.* Blood, 1990. 76(12): p. 2462-5.
[161] Brooks, W.H., et al., *Relationship of lymphocyte invasion and survival of brain tumor patients.* Ann Neurol, 1978. 4(3): p. 219-24.
[162] Palma, L., N. Di Lorenzo, and B. Guidetti, *Lymphocytic infiltrates in primary glioblastomas and recidivous gliomas. Incidence, fate, and relevance to prognosis in 228 operated cases.* J Neurosurg, 1978. 49(6): p. 854-61.
[163] Rosenberg, S.A., *The development of new immunotherapies for the treatment of cancer using interleukin-2. A review.* Ann Surg, 1988. 208(2): p. 121-35.
[164] Jacobs, S.K., et al., *Interleukin-2 and autologous lymphokine-activated killer cells in the treatment of malignant glioma. Preliminary report.* J Neurosurg, 1986. 64(5): p. 743-9.
[165] Merchant, R.E., et al., *Intralesional infusion of lymphokine-activated killer (LAK) cells and recombinant interleukin-2 (rIL-2) for the treatment of patients with malignant brain tumor.* Neurosurgery, 1988. 23(6): p. 725-32.
[166] Blacklock, J.B. and E.A. Grimm, *Lymphokine-activated killer lymphocytes: LAK and interleukin-2 in the treatment of malignancies of the central nervous system.* Immunol Ser, 1989. 48: p. 93-9.
[167] Lillehei, K.O., et al., *Long-term follow-up of patients with recurrent malignant gliomas treated with adjuvant adoptive immunotherapy.* Neurosurgery, 1991. 28(1): p. 16-23.
[168] Dillman, R.O., et al., *Intracavitary placement of autologous lymphokine-activated killer (LAK) cells after resection of recurrent glioblastoma.* J Immunother, 2004. 27(5): p. 398-404.
[169] Dudley, M.E., et al., *Cancer regression and autoimmunity in patients after clonal repopulation with antitumor lymphocytes.* Science, 2002. 298(5594): p. 850-4.
[170] Kruse, C.A., et al., *Treatment of recurrent glioma with intracavitary alloreactive cytotoxic T lymphocytes and interleukin-2.* Cancer Immunol Immunother, 1997. 45(2): p. 77-87.
[171] Kawada, M., et al., *Vaccination of fusion cells of rat dendritic and carcinoma cells prevents tumor growth in vivo.* Int J Cancer, 2003. 105(4): p. 520-6.
[172] Komata, T., et al., *Telomerase as a therapeutic target for malignant gliomas.* Oncogene, 2002. 21(4): p. 656-63.
[173] Sampson, J.H. and D.A. Mitchell, *Is Cytomegalovirus a Therapeutic Target in Glioblastoma?* Clin Cancer Res, 2011.
[174] Itoh, M., et al., *Thymus and autoimmunity: production of CD25+CD4+ naturally anergic and suppressive T cells as a key function of the thymus in maintaining immunologic self-tolerance.* J Immunol, 1999. 162(9): p. 5317-26.

[175] Bruder, C.E., et al., *High resolution deletion analysis of constitutional DNA from neurofibromatosis type 2 (NF2) patients using microarray-CGH.* Hum Mol Genet, 2001. 10(3): p. 271-82.

[176] Pacholczyk, R., P. Kraj, and L. Ignatowicz, *Peptide specificity of thymic selection of CD4+CD25+ T cells.* J Immunol, 2002. 168(2): p. 613-20.

[177] Wolf, A.M., et al., *Increase of regulatory T cells in the peripheral blood of cancer patients.* Clin Cancer Res, 2003. 9(2): p. 606-12.

[178] Ichihara, F., et al., *Increased populations of regulatory T cells in peripheral blood and tumor-infiltrating lymphocytes in patients with gastric and esophageal cancers.* Clin Cancer Res, 2003. 9(12): p. 4404-8.

[179] Sasada, T., et al., *CD4+CD25+ regulatory T cells in patients with gastrointestinal malignancies: possible involvement of regulatory T cells in disease progression.* Cancer, 2003. 98(5): p. 1089-99.

[180] Woo, E.Y., et al., *Regulatory CD4(+)CD25(+) T cells in tumors from patients with early-stage non-small cell lung cancer and late-stage ovarian cancer.* Cancer Res, 2001. 61(12): p. 4766-72.

[181] Kappler, J.W., N. Roehm, and P. Marrack, *T cell tolerance by clonal elimination in the thymus.* Cell, 1987. 49(2): p. 273-80.

[182] Kisielow, P., et al., *Tolerance in T-cell-receptor transgenic mice involves deletion of nonmature CD4+8+ thymocytes.* Nature, 1988. 333(6175): p. 742-6.

[183] Schmitz, M., et al., *Identification of a naturally processed T cell epitope derived from the glioma-associated protein SOX11.* Cancer Lett, 2007. 245(1-2): p. 331-6.

[184] Wekerle, H., et al., *The shaping of the brain-specific T lymphocyte repertoire in the thymus.* Immunol Rev, 1996. 149: p. 231-43.

[185] Asano, M., et al., *Autoimmune disease as a consequence of developmental abnormality of a T cell subpopulation.* J Exp Med, 1996. 184(2): p. 387-96.

[186] Rosenberg, S.A., et al., *Adoptive cell transfer: a clinical path to effective cancer immunotherapy.* Nat Rev Cancer, 2008. 8(4): p. 299-308.

[187] Wrzesinski, C., et al., *Hematopoietic stem cells promote the expansion and function of adoptively transferred antitumor CD8 T cells.* J Clin Invest, 2007. 117(2): p. 492-501.

[188] Morgan, R.A., M.E. Dudley, and S.A. Rosenberg, *Adoptive cell therapy: genetic modification to redirect effector cell specificity.* Cancer J, 2010. 16(4): p. 336-41.

19

Immunotherapeutic Strategies for Brain Tumors

Mitsugu Fujita[1] and Hideho Okada[2]
[1]*Division of Immunology and Neurosurgery, Aichi Cancer Center Research Institute*
[2]*Brain Tumor Program, University of Pittsburgh Cancer Institute*
[1]*Japan*
[2]*United States of America*

1. Introduction

Cancer immunotherapy is the use of the immune system to reject cancers. The main premise is to harness the patient's immune system to attack the malignant tumor cells. This area of research has made tremendous progresses, and the United States Food and Drug Administration recently approved a vaccine for prostate cancers as the first approval for vaccines against non-viral cancers (Kantoff et al., 2010). However, when it comes to central nervous system (CNS) tumors, while early phase immunotherapy trials showed encouraging outcomes, the immunological microenvironment of the CNS and tumors arising in the CNS is still believed to be suboptimal for sufficient antitumor immune responses to mediate clinically-meaningful changes *in situ* (Okada, H. et al., 2009; Walker, P. R. et al., 2003). In this chapter, we first discuss recent advances in the CNS and CNS tumor immunology. We address factors that may promote immune escape of gliomas. We also review advances in passive and active immunotherapy strategies for glioma, with an emphasis on lessons learned from recent early phase clinical trials. We also discuss novel immunotherapy strategies that have been recently tested in non-CNS tumors with great potential for application to CNS tumors. We will finally discuss how each of these promising strategies can be combined to achieve clinical benefit for patients with CNS tumors.

2. Immunology of gliomas

2.1 Immunology of CNS

For many decades, the brain has been considered an immune-privileged site due to the presence of a blood brain barrier (BBB) and the lack of lymphatics (Ransohoff et al., 2003). More recent studies have revealed crucial components involved in the process of leukocyte migration towards the CNS and the mechanisms of neuroinflammatory reactions in the CNS (Ransohoff et al., 2003). This section will focus on three key issues of CNS immunology: 1) factors limiting inflammation in the CNS, 2) antigen-specific immune response in the CNS, and 3) immune cell trafficking towards the CNS. In-depth understanding of these aspects will allow us to gain a framework to improve current treatment strategies harnessing the immune system to treat brain tumors.

2.1.1 Factors limiting inflammation in the CNS

Cells composing the CNS are extremely sensitive to the toxic effects of exogenous substances. Therefore, the CNS and the neurovasculature system therein have evolved specialized mechanisms to control both molecular and cellular migration into and out of the CNS parenchyma and cerebral spinal fluid (CSF). Capillary endothelial cells in the CNS are termed the BBB due to their ability to restrict passive diffusion and maintain low pinocytotic activity, and neuroimmunologists synonymously use the term BBB to describe both the capillary and post capillary vessels, the latter of which is the site of T-cell migration into the brain (Ransohoff et al., 2003). This "barrier" results from the selectivity of the tight junctions (TJs) between endothelial cells in the CNS vessels that restrict the passage of large hydrophilic molecules (i.e. peptides and proteins) and cells (Abbott et al., 2006).

Many extracellular proteins have been studied as TJ proteins: primarily the occludin, claudin, and junctional adhesion molecule (JAM) families. Experimental characterization of each has shown that mice carrying a null mutation in the occludin gene develop normal TJs whereas claudins have been shown to be independently sufficient for TJ formation (Engelhardt, 2008), suggesting the importance of claudins in TJ formation and regulation. Additionally, intravenous injection of monoclonal antibodies blocking JAM into mice inhibits leukocyte accumulation in CSF and brain parenchyma presumably through blocking leukocyte transmigration at the BBB (Engelhardt, 2008).

2.1.2 Induction of Immune responses to CNS antigens

The classic paradigm of specific immune activation is achieved through antigen uptake by antigen-presenting cells (APCs), which migrate to the lymph nodes via draining lymphatics where APCs subsequently activate T-cells. In the systemic immune system, dendritic cells (DCs) are considered to be the most potent APCs. In the CNS, a variety of cell populations have been postulated as primary CNS APCs, including vascular endothelial cells, smooth muscle cells, astrocytes, perivascular macrophages, choroid plexus epithelial cells, neurons, and DCs (Dunn et al., 2007). Among them, microglia has been proposed to be the primary resident APCs in the CNS (Aloisi, 2001).

Presentation of CNS antigens can occur through multiple mechanisms (Walker, P. R. et al., 2003): 1) APC uptake antigen within the CNS and migrate to lymph nodes to present antigens; 2) antigen drains to lymph nodes where APCs take them up to present, and 3) cells that express the antigen directly drain to lymph nodes and present their own antigen (direct presentation as opposed to cross presentation by DCs). Indeed, DCs injected in brain tumors have been shown to migrate to the cervical lymph nodes (CLNs) (Dunn et al., 2007). In addition, autoantigens from brain lesions have been shown to drain to CLNs in both primate models of experimental allergic encephalomyelitis and human multiple sclerosis (de Vos et al., 2002). Concurrently, it has been shown that tumor-specific T-cells can be primed in CLNs in murine glioma models (Fujita et al., 2009; Kuwashima et al., 2005; Okada, N. et al., 2005).

2.1.3 Migration of immune cells towards the CNS

Lymphocytes traffic to the CNS through the following 4 steps: 1) tethering/rolling, 2) activation, 3) adhesion, and 4) transmigration (Engelhardt, 2008). Interactions between carbohydrates on leukocytes and adhesion molecules (usually selectins) on endothelial cells slow down the leukocytes. Chemokines (e.g. CXCL10) are released from a site of inflammation and form a concentration gradient in endothelial membrane and attract responsible leukocytes such as activated T-cells (Fujita et al., 2009; Nishimura et al., 2006). At a reduced velocity, the leukocytes sense chemokines on the endothelial cells, become activated through G-protein signaling, and up-regulate integrins such as very late antigen 4 (VLA-4) (Sasaki et al., 2007; Sasaki et al., 2008a; Sasaki et al., 2008b; Sasaki et al., 2009). Lymphocyte function-associated molecules (LFAs) on lymphocytes allow for a stable interaction to their ligands vascular cell adhesion proteins (VCAMs) and inter-cellular adhesion molecules (ICAMs) on endothelial cells. Finally, with this tight interaction in place, the cells transmigrate into the parenchyma.

2.2 Immunosuppression by gliomas

Previously characterized immunological impairments in glioma patients have included low peripheral lymphocyte counts, reduced delayed-type hypersensitivity reactions to recall antigens, and impaired proliferating responses by peripheral blood mononuclear cells (PBMCs). Gliomas are known to achieve these by producing imunosuppressive molecules and inducing immunosuppressive leukocytes.

2.2.1 Immunosuppressive factors

Transforming growth factor β (TGF-β)

TGF-β is the most potent immunosuppressive cytokine; its biological effects are multiple and complex (Gorelik et al., 2002). They include the inhibition of 1) APC maturation 2) antigen presentation of APCs, 3) T-cell activation, and 4) their differentiation towards effector cells. Recent studies have shown that TGF-β is up-regulated in glioma cell clones that are resistant to the cytotoxic effects of allogeneic cytotoxic T-cells (CTLs), suggesting the significance of TGF-β in glioma immune escape mechanisms (Gomez et al., 2007; Ueda et al., 2009).

Interleukin 10 (IL-10)

IL-10 is also known to be a strong immunosuppressive cytokine (Moore et al., 2001). Like TGF-β, this cytokine has pleiotropic effects in immunoregulation and inflammation. It down-regulates the expression of Th1 cytokines, MHC class II antigens, and costimulatory molecules on APCs. The expression levels of IL-10 in glioma tissue correlate with glioma grade as well as a degree of brain invasiveness (Huettner et al., 1997; Nitta et al., 1994).

Prostaglandin E_2 (PGE_2)

PGE_2 is a product of arachadonic acid metabolism. It is produced at sites of inflammation or tissue damage where it exerts many effects including the enhancement of vascular permeability. As PGE_2 has profound modulatory effects on T-cell activation and gliomas synthesize PGE_2, it is associated with the suppressed T-cell function observed in patients with gliomas (Castelli et al., 1989). In addition, we recently demonstrated that PGE_2 production from murine gliomas induces accumulation of tumor-associated myeloid cells that promote growth of gliomas (Fujita et al., 2011).

CCL2; macrophage chemoattractive protein 1 (MCP-1)

CCL2, also known as MCP-1, is a chemokine secreted by a variety of glioma cell lines and expressed in glioblastoma multiforme (GBM) (Desbaillets et al., 1994; Takeshima et al., 1994). In addition to its angiogenetic effects (Salcedo et al., 2000), it is associated with recruitment of immunosuppressive leukocytes, such as tumor-associated macrophages and regulatory T cells (Fujita et al., 2010; Fujita et al., 2011; Huang et al., 2007; Jordan et al., 2008).

Fas receptor/ligand

The Fas receptor is a death receptor on the surface of cells that leads to apoptosis. Malignant gliomas express Fas ligand, which induces apoptotic cell death of adjacent immune cells infiltrating into tumors sites (Walker, P. R. et al., 1997). In addition, Fas receptor expressed on glioma cells induces proinflammatory and angiogenic mediators, which in turn protect and support tumors growth (Shinohara et al., 2000).

B7-homologue 1 (B7-H1); programmed death ligand-1 (PD-L1)

The B7 family consists of co-stimulatory molecules that positively and negatively regulate immune responses. Among them, B7-H1, also known as PD-L1, exerts immunosuppressive functions when interacting with its receptor PD-1 (Chen, 2004). Glioma cells express B7-H1, which subsequently inhibits T-cell functions by decreasing cytokine production levels (IFN-γ, IL-2, and IL-10) and expression levels of the T-cell activation marker CD69 (Wintterle et al., 2003). Glioma cells often exhibit mutations in a tumor-suppressor gene phosphatase and tensin homolog (PTEN), and loss of functions in PTEN also leads to up-regulation of B7-H1 (Parsa et al., 2007).

2.2.2 Immunosuppressive leukocytes

A large number of observations suggest that certain types of immune cells in the tumor micrienvironment (TME) are not innocent bystanders at brain tumor sites, but they actively promote tumor development and progression. Inflammatory cells, primarily macrophage/microglia and regulatory T-cells, may affect these processes via their ability to express a large variety of factors, including immunoregulatory cytokines. These cytokines may be secreted not only by inflammatory cells, but also by the tumor cells and stroma cells, together establishing a network of factors that significantly affects brain tumor.

Macrophages/microglia

In the CNS, macrophage/microglial cells constitute the first line of cellular defense against a variety of stressors, participating in the regulation of innate and adaptive immune responses (Graeber et al., 2002). Resident microglias are $CD11b^+/CD45^{dim}$ whereas macrophages are $CD11b^+/CD45^{high}$. Intratumoral macrophage/microglia density is higher than in normal brain and abundance of microglia correlates with the grade of malignancy (Badie et al., 2000).

In contrast, the defense functions of macrophage/microglia against glioma are compromised in the TME. Although these cells express Toll-like receptors (TLRs), critical components for APCs to mediate innate immune responses and activate adaptive immune responses, those in the TME are unable to activate T-cells properly (Hussain et al., 2006). Consistently, macrophages/microglia release many factors, including extracellular matrix proteases (MMPs) and cytokines, which may directly or indirectly influence tumor migration/invasiveness and proliferation (Watters et al., 2005). In addition, glioma cell migration is stimulated by the presence of macrophage/microglia (Bettinger et al., 2002). Taken together, macrophages/microglias in gliomas promote the invasive phenotype of these tumors.

Regulatory T-cells (Treg)

The suppressive activity of Tregs has been implicated as an important factor limiting immune-mediated destruction of tumor cells. The presence of $CD4^+FoxP3^+$ Tregs correlates with impairment of T-cell proliferation in peripheral blood specimens in GBM patients (Fecci et al., 2006). Moreover, tumor infiltration by Tregs correlates with tumor grade and prognosis (Heimberger et al., 2008).

$CD4^+FoxP3^+$ Tregs in gliomas have been shown to express CD25, CTLA-4, GITR, and CXCR4 at high levels (Grauer et al., 2007). Intratumoral accumulation and activation of $CD4^+FoxP3^+$ Treg act as a dominant immune escape mechanism of gliomas and underline the importance of controlling tumor-infiltrating Treg in glioma immunotherapy.

3. Immunotherapy for gliomas

In this section, we will first discuss molecular targets for gliomas. Then, we will discuss two modalities: adoptive T-cell therapy (passive immunotherapy) and glioma vaccine (active immunotherapy).

3.1 Target molecules for gliomas

It is essential to know about potent target molecules for glioma immunotherapy. The following section will discuss selected human glioma-associated antigen (GAA)-derived epitopes that appear to be promising based on relatively restricted expression (compared with the normal brain) as well as well-characterized immunogenicity.

IL-13Rα2

IL-13Rα2 is a membrane glycoprotein that is overexpressed by >80% of malignant gliomas but is not expressed in normal brain tissues or other normal organs except for testes (Debinski et al., 1999). Therefore, IL-13Rα2 has attracted significant attention as a target for glioma therapy (Kahlon et al., 2004). We recently found that an analogue peptide of natural IL-13Rα2$_{345-353}$, in which the first and ninth amino-acid residues tryptophan and isoleucine have been replaced by valine and alanine, respectively, can elicit a greater CTL response against HLA-A2$^+$ IL-13Rα2$^+$ glioma cells compared with the natural peptide (IL-13Rα2$_{345-353:1A9V}$) (Eguchi et al., 2006).

EphA2

EphA2 is a tyrosine kinase receptor that plays a role in carcinogenesis (Dodelet et al., 2000). We have reported that EphA2$_{883-891}$ is expressed on gliomas and able to elicit an HLA-A2-restricted CTL response against glioma cell lines (Hatano et al., 2005). Furthermore, EphA2 mRNA overexpression was found to correlate inversely with survival in a panel of 21 GBMs (Liu et al., 2006). These findings support the idea that targeting of EphA2 by immunotherapy may provide a major impact in controlling tumor growth and prolonging patients' survival.

Survivin

Survivin is an apoptosis inhibitor protein overexpressed in most human cancers including gliomas (Blanc-Brude et al., 2002; Uematsu et al., 2005). Therefore, induction of immune response against Survivin appears to be an attractive strategy. Of interest, high level expression of Survivin was correlated with poor prognosis in patients with grade II or III astrocytomas (Uematsu et al., 2005).

Wilm's tumor 1 (WT1)

WT1 is a transcription factor oncogene that is overexpressed in various types of leukemia and solid tumor cells (Oka et al., 2002). Inhibition of WT1 in leukemic cell lines led to decrease in proliferation and increase in apoptosis of tumor cells (Glienke et al., 2007). Human gliomas also express WT1 at high levels (Izumoto et al., 2008; Rushing et al., 2010; Schittenhelm et al., 2008). These finding imply that elimination of tumor cells that overexpress WT1 may allow efficient control against glioma growth.

Sry-related high mobility group box (SOX)

SOX is a family of transcriptional cofactors implicated in the control of diverse developmental processes and exhibit highly dynamic expression patterns during development of diverse tissues and cell types, especially during embryogenesis (Wegner, 1999). Indeed, SOX2 (Gangemi et al., 2009), SOX5 (Ueda et al., 2007), SOX6 (Ueda et al., 2004), and SOX11 (Schmitz et al., 2007) are highly expressed in glioma cell lines and a majority of glioma tissues. Their preferential expression in glioma and immunogenicity indicate that SOX proteins are attractive targets for immunotherapy.

Type III variant of the EGFR mutation (EGFRvIII)

EGFRvIII is present in 30-50% of patients with GBM. Despite the limited frequency in gliomas, EGFRvIII and IL-13Rα2 are expressed most restrictedly in primary glioma tissues compared with normal tissues (Saikali et al., 2007). Therefore, this antigen also appears to be an attractive target for glioma immunotherapy.

Cytomegalovirus (CMV)

Recent reports have demonstrated the presence of the cytomegalovirus (CMV) proteins as well as CMV mRNA in a majority of human GBMs (Barami, 2010; Cobbs et al., 2002; Lucas et al., 2010; Mitchell et al., 2008; Scheurer et al., 2008). Therefore, CMV in gliomas could serve as an immunotherapeutic target for glioma. In addition, the facilitation of an immune response against viral antigens contrasts with the difficulty of immunization against self antigens. It will be intriguing to introduce the CMV-derived epitope to multiepitope-based vaccine for glioma.

3.2 Adoptive T-cell therapy (ACT) for gliomas

ACT involves passive infusion or transfer of autologous CTLs specific for tumor antigens to the host. Although ACT are currently evaluated as experimental therapy for limited types of cancers (Gattinoni et al., 2006; Morgan et al., 2006), this strategy may hold promise as an attractive future immunotherapeutic intervention against gliomas. In particular, based on strong findings that CTLs have the capacity to migrate into brain parenchyma (Ransohoff et al., 2003), the approach has been vastly improved by the use of recent advances in several areas of human T-cell biology including *in vitro* human T-cell culture and *ex vivo* genetic manipulation. This section will focus on recent technological advances in ACT as well as a current and future ACT for glioma with an emphasis on recent perspectives from human studies.

3.2.1 Source of glioma-reactive CTLs

Peripheral Bloods

PBMCs from glioma patients can be expanded *in vitro* through multiple cycles of antigenic stimulation. Subsequently, cells with a monoclonal specificity to the particular GAA will be generated. Although few numbers of GAA-reactive CTLs might be obtained this method may be feasible as, this strategy has demonstrated favorable anti-tumor responses in cancer patients (Gattinoni et al., 2006).

Glioma tissues

Another important source of the GAA-specific CTLs is a glioma tissue itself. A tumor nodule contains tumor-reactive CTLs that can be first polyclonally expanded *ex vivo* in the presence of IL-2 and later selected for antigen specificity (Rosenberg, 2008). These CTLs derived from tumor nodules have been used for ACT in melanoma patients (Dreno et al., 2002; Dudley et al., 2005).

3.2.2 Manipulation of glioma-reactive CTLs *ex vivo*

Choice of T-cell subtypes

In general, an effector T-cell subset (T_E) is predominantly enriched during *ex vivo* expansion for ACT. T_E are generally considered to be terminally differentiated CTLs that have the highest cytotoxic capacity but lack appreciable proliferating capacity (Wherry et al., 2003). These cells would not be able to establish a long-term persisting population of tumor-specific CTLs. There is a significant association between clinically favorable responses and the persistence of *ex vivo* expanded melanoma-specific CTL clones after infusion (Robbins et al., 2004). Therefore, efforts have been made to generate long-term persisting CTLs. In contrast to the T_E subset, memory cells have enhanced proliferative potential and survival, and the potential to provide more robust and enduring protectin aganist tumors (Perret et al., 2008). In particular, recent studies have highlighted the potential of central memory T-cells (T_{CM}) as a source of T_E for ACT (Wang et al., 2011; Yang et al., 2011). Yang *et al.* have shown that a large parcentage of *in vitro* generated antitumor CTLs mimick a T_{CM}-like phenotype and function (Yang et al., 2011). In addition, Wang *et al.* have demonstrated that T_{CM} are less prone to apoptosis and able to establish a persistent reservoir of functional T-cells in mice (Wang et al., 2011). Furthermore, recent studies with human T-cell subsets have revealed that naïve $CD8^+$ cells were not only the most abundant subset but also the population most capable of *in vitro* expansion and T-cell receptor (TCR) transgene expression. Despite increased expansion, naïve-derived cells displayed minimal effector differentiation, a quality associated with greater efficacy after cell infusion (Hinrichs et al., 2011).

Cloning of high-avidity T-cell receptors (TCRs)

Since the majority of GAAs are poorly immunogenic to raise CTLs that possess TCRs with low avidity, a number of modification have been made for ACT. One of attempts is to systematically search tumor-specific $CD8^+$ T-cells for clone(s) with higher TCR avidity, clone TCRα and β genes, and exogenously induce the high-avidity TCR exogenously in bulk $CD8^+$ T-cells. Li *et al.* used phage display to search for a high-avidity TCR against an HLA-A0201-restricted epitope in a NY-ESO-1 antigen (Li et al., 2005). Moreover, ACT using high-avidity TCR transgenic T-cells have been shown to sustain in blood circulation at high levels engineered cells were observed at 1 year after infusion in 2 of 15 patients who both demonstrated objective regression of metastatic melanoma lesions (Morgan et al., 2006). These data suggest the therapeutic potential of genetically engineered high-avidity TCR clones for glioma immunotherapy.

Establishment of chimeric antigen receptors (CARs)

An interesting alternative to expression of high-avidity TCRs on T-cells is to express a chimeric molecule that has antigen-binding domains of a monoclonal antibody fused with a signal transduction domain of CD3 (Gross et al., 1989), namely chimeric antigen receptors

(CAR). A significant advantage of CARs over TCRs is that the antigen recognition is not restricted by expression of certain MHC class I molecules. Recently, CARs have been used to treat a number of cancers (Cartellieri et al., 2010). CAR-based approaches are currently being developed for gliomas as well (Kahlon et al., 2004; Ohno et al., 2010).

3.2.3 Current attempts of ACT for gliomas

There have been a number of clinical trials for malignant gliomas using ACT (Table1) (Vauleon et al., 2010). Among them, three Phase I trials (Holladay et al., 1996; Plautz et al., 1998; Wood et al., 2000) and two pilot studies (Plautz et al., 2000; Sloan et al., 2000) used CTLs obtained from lymph nodes or PBMCs after intradermal vaccination. Holladay *et al.* first conducted an ACT-based Phase I clinical trial and reported disease-free survival ≥ 8 months in 7 of 15 patients (Holladay et al., 1996). Later, Wood *et al.* demonstrated a correlation between clinical response and the predominance of $CD8^{+}$ T-cells to $CD4^{+}$ cells in the injected cells (Wood et al., 2000). In addition, DTH response to autologous tumors was shown to correlate with clinical response (Sloan et al., 2000; Wood et al., 2000). However, CTLs used in these studies were not specific for GAAs. Therefore, it is necessary to generate a library of human CTL clones against GAAs using advanced techniques described above. With such refinement of *ex vivo* T-cell manipulation, ACT may become a mainstream therapeutic intervention for malignant gliomas.

Study	Type of trials	Patients	Immune responses	Clinical responses
Holladay et al., 1996	Phase I	N = 15 recurrent HGG 12 GBM, 3 AA	DTH (15/15)	No PR or SD Median FPS: ≥8 mo
Plautz et al., 1998)	Phase I	N = 10 recurrent HGG 9 GBM, 1 AA		3 PR Median FPS: > 12 mo
Plautz et al., 2000	Pilot study	N =9 recurrent HGG 6 GBM, 3 Gr3	DTH (9/9)	3 PR
Wood et al., 2000	Phase I	N =12 newly diagnosed glioma 6 GBM, 2 Gr2, 4 Gr3	DTH (12/12)	4 PR, 2 SD *Correlation between clinical response and CD4/CD8 composition of infused cells*
Sloan et al., 2000	Pilot study	N =19 recurrent HGG 16 GBM, 2 AA, 1 gliosarcoma	DTH (17/19)	1 CR, 7 PR, 9 SD Median OS : 12 mo *Correlation between survival and DTH response*

*Abbreviations used in this table. AA: anaplastic astrocytoma; CR: complete response; DTH: delayed-type hypersensitivity; GBM: gliobrastoma; Gr2: WHO grade II glioma; Gr3: WHO grade III glioma; HGG: high-grade glioma; mo: month(s); OS: overall survival; PFS: progression-free survival; PR: partial response; SD: stable disease.

Table 1. ACT-based clinical trials for glioma

3.3 Glioma vaccines

In addition to the ACT strategy described above, we will discuss glioma vaccine strategies in this section. They include 1) whole glioma cell vaccines, 2) peptide-based vaccines targeting glioma-associated antigens, and 3) DC vaccines.

3.3.1 Whole glioma cell vaccines

Initial vaccination strategies for gliomas consisted of subcutaneous inoculations of irradiated, autologous (Wikstrand et al., 1980) or allogeneic (Zhang et al., 2007) glioma cells. This type of vaccine has the advantage of providing a panel of multiple potential GAAs that are naturally expressed by glioma cells. Especially, autologous glioma cells should allow immunizations against the most relevant GAAs expressed in the patient's tumor (i.e. tailored medicine). Potential downsides of this approach, however, include: 1) cumbersome procedures and quality control (QC)/quality assurance (QA) issues associated with large scale cultures of autologous glioma cells and 2) theoretical risks of autoimmune encephalomyelitis (Wikstrand et al., 1980). Nevertheless, this type of vaccine strategy has been carefully examined (Table 2). Schneider *et al.* (Schneider et al., 2001) and Steiner *et al.*(Steiner et al., 2004) reported pilot clinical trials using autologous glioma cells modified

Study	Type of trials	Patients	Tumor cell modification	Immune responses	Clinical responses
Schneider et al., 2001	Pilot study	N =11 newly diagnosed GBM	infected with NDV, inactivated with cisplatinum	DTH (11/11) T cell infiltrate (4/4)	No survival benefit
Andrews et al., 2001	Pilot study	N =12 8 GBM, 4 AA	IGF-RA/AS ODN	T cell infiltrate (4/9)	2 CR, 4 PR, 2 SD
Steiner et al., 2004	Pilot study	N =23 GBM	infected with NDV	DTH (15/15) ELISPOT (3/3) T cell infiltrate (6/7)	1 CR Median OS: 100 wks
Parney et al., 2006	Pilot study	N =6 3 recurrent GBM 3 melanoma	transduced with B7-2 and GM-CSF	No CTL activity	Longer PFS (3/6 GBM)
Ishikawa et al., 2007	Pilot study	N =12 8 newly diagnosed GBM, 4 recurrent GBM	formalin-fixed	DTH (9/12)	1 CR, 1 PR, 2 MR Median OS: 10.7 mo
Clavreul et al., 2010	Phase I	N =5 recurrent HGG 4 GBM, 1 AOA	irradiated	DTH (2/5)	3 SD

*Abbreviations used in this table. AOA: anaplastic oligoastrocytoma; CTL: cytotoxic T-cells; ELISPOT: enzyme-linked immunosorbent spot; IGF-RA/AS ODN: insulin-like growth factoro type I receptor antisence oligodeoxynucleotide; MR: minor response; NDV: Newcastle-Disease-Virus; wk: week(s).

Table 2. Autologous whole glioma cell vaccine trials.

with Newcastle-Disease-Virus (NDV), which is known to serve as an vaccine adjuvant and therefore to improve the efficacy of glioma vaccines. Recently, Ishikawa *et al.* reported a Phase I clinical trial using formalin-fixed glioma tissues as a source of antigens (Ishikawa et al., 2007). The advantage of this strategy is that formalin fixation preserves the specific antigenicity of glioma cells. These studies reported no major adverse events.

3.3.2 Peptide-based vaccines targeting glioma-associated antigens

In vaccines using synthetic peptides for shared GAA-epitopes, advantages and disadvantages are distinct from those in whole glioma cell approaches. While synthetic GAA peptide-based vaccines may not adequately target antigens in each patient's tumor, these vaccines have less concern for autoimmunity and provide "off the shelf" feasibility. Indeed, a wide range of peptide-based vaccines have been clinically evaluated (Table 3). Yajima *et al.* reported a phase I study of peptide-based vaccinations in patients with recurrent malignant gliomas (Yajima et al., 2005). In this study, prior to the first vaccine, each patient's PBMCs were evaluated *in vitro* for cellular and humoral responses against a panel of antigens, and peptides that induced positive response were used for vaccinations. The regimen was well tolerated and resulted in an 89-week median survival of treated patients. However, there is little evidence that the antigens used in this study are expressed in gliomas at high levels. More recently, as the extension of the approach, Terasaki *et al.* reported a Phase I trial using 14 HLA-A24-binding peptides (Terasaki et al., 2011). They evaluated immune responses with dose escalation of peptides and defined 3 mg/peptide as the Phase II-recommended dose. Izumoto *et al.* reported a Phase II clinical trial using a single WT1 peptide (Izumoto et al., 2008). In this study, they reported a median progression-free survival (PFS) of 20 weeks and a possible association between the WT1 expression levels and clinical responses. When single or oligo antigens are selected and targeted by vaccines, it also seems necessary to harness the concepts of epitope spreading to address the problems of tumor immune escape, while avoiding the augmentation of deleterious CNS autoimmune responses (Vanderlugt et al., 2002). Sampson *et al.* recently reported a Phase II study targeting the EGFRvIII epitope in newly diagnosed GBM patients who received gross total resection (Sampson et al., 2010). They reported a median PFS of 14.2 months and a median overall survival (OS) of 26.0 months. In addition, they identified that the development of specific antibody or delayed-type hypersensitivity responses to EGFRvIII significantly correlated with the OS.

Study	Type of trials	Patients	Peptide(s)	Immune responses	Clinical responses
Yajima et al., 2005	Phase I	N = 25 17 GBM, 8 Gr3	multiple	DTH (11/21) CTL activity (14/21)	5 PR, 8 SD Median OS: 89 wks
Izumoto et al., 2008	Phase II	N = 21 recurrent GBM	WT1	DTH (21/21)	2 PR, 10 SD Median PFS: 20 wks
Sampson et al., 2010	Phase II	N = 18 newly diagnosed GBM	EGFRvIII	DTH (5/9) CTL activity (10/12)	Median PFS: 14.2 months Median OS: 26.0 mo
Terasaki et al., 2011	Phase I	N = 12, recurrent GBM	multiple	CTL activity (8/12)	1 PR, 7 SD Median PFS: 2.3 mo Median OS: 18.9 mo

Table 3. Peptide-based vaccine trials for glioma.

3.3.3 DC vaccines

DCs are the most potent antigen-presenting cells, driving the activation of T-cells in response to invading microorganisms (Banchereau et al., 2000). The availability to culture DCs from human peripheral blood monocytes has generated significant interest in using DCs in novel cancer vaccination strategies (Banchereau et al., 2000).

To induce tumor-specific immune reaction via DCs, antigen elusion from tumor cells has been performed (Table 4). Yu *et al.* reported a Phase I trial of vaccinations using DCs pulsed with peptides eluted from autologous glioma cells (Yu et al., 2001). Later, Liau *et al.* also reported a Phase I trial in patients with newly diagnosed GBM using DCs pulsed with acid-eluted glioma peptides (Liau et al., 2005). In this study, the authors reported the median OS of 23.4 months and that the benefit of the vaccine treatment was more evident in the subgroup of patients with slowly-progressing tumors and in those with tumors expressing low levels of TGF-β2.

Study	Type of trials	Patients	Immune responses	Clinical responses
Yu et al., 2001	Phase I	N = 9 newly diagnosed HGG 7 GBM, 2 AA	CTL activity (4/7) T cell infiltrate (2/4)	Median OS: 455 d
Wheeler et al., 2004	Phase I/II	N = 25 newly diagnosed GBM	CTL activity (8/24)	3 PR
Liau et al., 2005	Phase I	N = 12 GBM 5 recurrent 7 newly diagnosed	CTL activity (6/12) T cell infiltrate (4/8)	1 PR Median OS: 23.4 mo

Table 4. DC-based vaccine trials using acid-eluted peptides.

However, pulsing DCs with eluted peptides requires a large culture of autologous glioma cells and time-consuming procedures, for which QC/QA is not always feasible. To overcome this issue, glioma cell lysate has been used to pulse DCs in a number of trials (Table 5). Yamanaka *et al.* reported a Phase I/II study using DC pulsed with glioma lysate. Patients received either DCs matured with OK-432 or DCs without OK-432-mediated maturation (Yamanaka et al., 2003; Yamanaka et al., 2005). GBM patients receiving mature DCs had longer survival than those receiving DCs without OK-432-mediated maturation. Furthermore, patients receiving both intratumoral and intradermal DC administrations demonstrated longer overall survival than those with intradermal administrations alone (Yamanaka et al., 2005). Wheeler *et al.* reported another Phase II clinical trial with lysate-pulsed DCs (Wheeler et al., 2008). IFN-γ production levels from post-vaccine PBMC correlated significantly with patients' survival and time to progression. Prins *et al.* recently reported a Phase I clinical trial in glioma patients using lysate-pulsed DCs (Prins et al., 2011). Interestingly, their gene expression profiling in the participants' GBM tissues demonstrated that the mesenchymal gene expression profile may represent a population of patients with favorable responses to their vaccines.

Study	Type of trials	Patients	Immune responses	Clinical responses
Yamanaka et al., 2003	Phase I/II	N = 10 7 GBM, 3 recurrent Gr3	DTH (3/6) ELISPOT (2/5) T cell infiltrate (2/2)	2 MR, 4 SD Median OS: > 200 wks
Yu et al., 2004	Phase I	N = 14 1 GBM, 1 AA, 9 recurrent GBM, 3 recurrent AA	CTL activity (4/9) T cell infiltrate (3/6)	Median OS: 133 wks
Rutkowski et al., 2004	Phase I	N = 12 recurrent HGG 11 GBM, 1 others	DTH (7/8)	2 CR, 1 PR, 1 SD Median OS: 10.5 mo
Yamanaka et al., 2005	Phase I/II	N = 24 recurrent HGG 18 GBM, 6 Gr3	DTH (8/17) ELISPOT (7/16)	1PR, 3MR, 10 SD Median OS: 480 d *Longer survival if DC maturation or IC injection*
Okada, H. et al., 2007	Phase I	N = 5 newly diagnosed GBM	No response	No response
Wheeler et al., 2008	Phase II	N = 34 GBM 23 recurrent 11 newly diagnosed	ELISPOT (17/34)	3 CR, 1 PR Median OS: 642 d *Correlation between survival and IFN-γ production*
De Vleeschouwer et al., 2004	Phase I/II	N = 56 recurrent GBM	DTH (11/ 23)	Median OS: 9.6 mo
Walker, D. G. et al., 2008	Phase I	N = 13 9 GBM, 4 AA	T cell infiltrate (3/3)	2 CR, 3 PR
Ardon et al., 2010	Phase I/II	N = 8 newly diagnosed GBM	DTH (2/5) ELISPOT (5/8)	Median OS: 24 mo
Prins et al., 2011	Phase I	N = 23 GBM 8 recurrent 15 newly diagnosed	increase in systemic TNF-α and IL-6	Median OS: 31.4 mo *Better imune response if mesenchymal gene expression presents*

Table 5. DC-based vaccine trials using autologous tumor cell lysates.

While these studies demonstrate early success of DC-based vaccines in glioma patients, based on our preclinical data demonstrating that type-1 CTLs are capable of mediating effective anti-CNS tumor immunity (Fujita et al., 2008; Nishimura et al., 2006), we recently completed a Phase I/II study of vaccines evaluating safety and immunological activities of vaccines using α-type-1-polarized DCs (αDC1) that are able to produce high levels of IL-12 and induce long-lived type-1 T-cell responses (Okada, H. et al., 2011). In this study, patients with recurrent malignant glioma received intra-lymphnodal injection of αDC1 loaded with synthetic peptides for GAA epitopes and administration of polyinosinic-polycytidylic acid [poly(I:C)] stabilized by lysine and carboxymethylcellulose (poly-ICLC) in HLA-A2+ patients with recurrent malignant gliomas. GAAs for these peptides are EphA2, IL-13R-α2, YKL-40, and gp100. The regimen was well-tolerated and induced positive immune responses against at least one of the vaccination-targeted GAAs in peripheral blood mononuclear cells in 58% of patients. Peripheral blood samples demonstrated significant up-regulation of type 1 cytokines and chemokines, including interferon-α and CXCL10. For at least 12 months, nine patients achieved progression-free status. One patient with recurrent GBM demonstrated a sustained complete response. IL-12 production levels by αDC1 positively correlated with time to progression. These data support safety, immunogenicity, and preliminary clinical activity of poly-ICLC-boosted αDC1-based vaccines and warrant further development of this approach. Although these Phase I/II studies demonstrate preliminary clinical efficacy, the ultimate judgment for clinical activity has to be made by rigorous evaluation in randomized studies.

Study	Type of trials	Patients	Antigen Source	Immune responses	Clinical responses
Kikuchi et al., 2001	Phase I	N =8 5 GBM, 2 AA, 1 AO	Fused tumor cells	ELISPOT (6/6)	1 MR, 6 SD
Caruso et al., 2004	Phase I	N =7 recurrent tumors 2 GBM, 1 AA, 4 others	tumor RNA	No PBMC respnse	1 PR, 4 SD
Kikuchi et al., 2004	Phase I	N =15 recurrent HGG 6 GBM, 7 AA, 2 OAA	Fused tumor cells	DTH (15/15) CTL activity (2/8)	4 PR, 2 SD, 1 MR
Sampson et al., 2009	Phase I	N =12 newly diagnosed GBM	EGFRvIII	DTH (5/9) CTL activity (10/12)	Median OS: 22.8 mo
Okada, H. et al., 2011	Phase I/II	N = 22 13 GBM, 5 AA, 3 AO, 1 AOA	EphA2, IL-13R-α2, YKL-40, gp100	ELISPOT (10/22) increase in systemic Th1 cytokines	Median PFS: 4 mo (GBM) 13 mo (AG) *Correlation between survival and DC-derived IL-12 levels*

Table 6. Other DC-based vaccine trials for glioma.

4. Conclusion

We reviewed recent progress in the field of brain and brain tumor immunology. We also reported recent progress and current challenges in immunotherapeutic strategies for brain tumors. It is clear that the CNS and gliomas are equipped with numerous and layered immunosuppressive and immune escape mechanisms, perhaps including ones that we have not yet identified. These discoveries, however, allow us to develop strategies to overcome each of these mechanisms.

Remaining unique challenges against gliomas include relative difficulties in obtaining tumor tissues following immunotherapeutic treatments. Unlike other cancers, intracranial glioma tissues are not readily accessible following vaccine treatment. Designing neo-adjuvant settings with vaccines is not always feasible because recurrent malignant gliomas, for which surgical resection is clinically indicated, typically do not allow us to wait for weeks before surgery and often require treatment with high dose corticosteroids.
As reviewed in this article, the concept of immunotherapy has a diverse scope of strategies and target molecules. Extensive review of each field in this article has led us to identify the challenge for each strategy. Such challenges, however, may be overcome by appropriate combinations with other strategies. For example, ACT strategies may need to be combined with appropriate adjuvants and/or vaccinations to promote long lasting memory responses and anti-tumor immunosurveillance. However, when each of these agents is owned by separate industries with intellectual properties, such creative combinatorial strategies may not be implemented as efficiently as we would wish. Although several early phase clinical trials demonstrated promising therapeutic outcomes to date, clinical trials of immunotherapy for gliomas have not yet demonstrated objective proof of clinical efficacy in randomized studies. The eventual success of immunotherapies for brain tumors will be dependent upon not only an in-depth understanding of immunology behind the brain and brain tumors, but also the implementation of molecularly targeted trials that address multiple layers of challenges in brain tumors.

5. Acknowledgement

Financial Support: the National Institute of Health 2R01NS055140, 2P01NS40923, 1P01CA132714, P3CA047904.

6. References

Abbott, N. J.; Ronnback, L. & Hansson, E. (2006). Astrocyte-endothelial interactions at the blood-brain barrier, *Nature Review Neuroscience*, Vol. 7, No. 1, (January 2006), pp. 41-53, ISSN 1471-003X

Aloisi, F. (2001). Immune function of microglia, *Glia*, Vol. 36, No. 2, (November 2001), pp. 165-179, ISSN 0894-1491

Andrews, D. W.; Resnicoff, M.; Flanders, A. E.; Kenyon, L.; Curtis, M.; Merli, G.; Baserga, R.; Iliakis, G. & Aiken, R. D. (2001). Results of a pilot study involving the use of an antisense oligodeoxynucleotide directed against the insulin-like growth factor type I receptor in malignant astrocytomas, *Journal of Clinical Oncology*, Vol. 19, No. 8, (April 2001), pp. 2189-2200, ISSN 0732-183X

Ardon, H.; Van Gool, S.; Lopes, I. S.; Maes, W.; Sciot, R.; Wilms, G.; Demaerel, P.; Bijttebier, P.; Claes, L.; Goffin, J.; Van Calenbergh, F. & De Vleeschouwer, S. (2010). Integration of autologous dendritic cell-based immunotherapy in the primary treatment for patients with newly diagnosed glioblastoma multiforme: a pilot study, *Journal of Neuro-Oncology*, Vol. 99, No. 2, (September 2010), pp. 261-272, ISSN 0167-594X

Badie, B. & Schartner, J. M. (2000). Flow cytometric characterization of tumor-associated macrophages in experimental gliomas, *Neurosurgery*, Vol. 46, No. 4, (April 2000), pp. 957-961; discussion 961-952, ISSN 0148-396X

Banchereau, J.; Briere, F.; Caux, C.; Davoust, J.; Lebecque, S.; Liu, Y. J.; Pulendran, B. & Palucka, K. (2000). Immunobiology of dendritic cells, *Annual Review of Immunology*, Vol. 18, (June 2000), pp. 767-811, ISSN 0732-0582

Barami, K. (2010). Oncomodulatory mechanisms of human cytomegalovirus in gliomas, *Journal of Clinical Neuroscience*, Vol. 17, No. 7, (July 2010), pp. 819-823, ISSN 0967-5868

Bettinger, I.; Thanos, S. & Paulus, W. (2002). Microglia promote glioma migration, *Acta Neuropathologica*, Vol. 103, No. 4, (April 2002), pp. 351-355, ISSN 0001-6322

Blanc-Brude, O. P.; Yu, J.; Simosa, H.; Conte, M. S.; Sessa, W. C. & Altieri, D. C. (2002). Inhibitor of apoptosis protein survivin regulates vascular injury, *Nature Medicine*, Vol. 8, No. 9, (September 2002), pp. 987-994, ISSN 1078-8956

Cartellieri, M.; Bachmann, M.; Feldmann, A.; Bippes, C.; Stamova, S.; Wehner, R.; Temme, A. & Schmitz, M. (2010). Chimeric antigen receptor-engineered T cells for immunotherapy of cancer, *Journal of Biomedicine & Biotechnology*, Vol. 2010, (May 2010), pp. 956304, ISSN 1110-7243

Caruso, D. A.; Orme, L. M.; Neale, A. M.; Radcliff, F. J.; Amor, G. M.; Maixner, W.; Downie, P.; Hassall, T. E.; Tang, M. L. & Ashley, D. M. (2004). Results of a phase 1 study utilizing monocyte-derived dendritic cells pulsed with tumor RNA in children and young adults with brain cancer, *Neuro-Oncology*, Vol. 6, No. 3, (July 2004), pp. 236-246, ISSN 1522-8517

Castelli, M. G.; Chiabrando, C.; Fanelli, R.; Martelli, L.; Butti, G.; Gaetani, P. & Paoletti, P. (1989). Prostaglandin and thromboxane synthesis by human intracranial tumors, *Cancer Research*, Vol. 49, No. 6, (March 1989), pp. 1505-1508, ISSN 0008-5472

Chen, L. (2004). Co-inhibitory molecules of the B7-CD28 family in the control of T-cell immunity, *Nature Reviews Immunology*, Vol. 4, No. 5, (May 2004), pp. 336-347, ISSN 1474-1733

Clavreul, A.; Piard, N.; Tanguy, J. Y.; Gamelin, E.; Rousselet, M. C.; Leynia, P. & Menei, P. (2010). Autologous tumor cell vaccination plus infusion of GM-CSF by a programmable pump in the treatment of recurrent malignant gliomas, *Journal of Clinical Neuroscience*, Vol. 17, No. 7, (July 2010), pp. 842-848, ISSN 0967-5868

Cobbs, C. S.; Harkins, L.; Samanta, M.; Gillespie, G. Y.; Bharara, S.; King, P. H.; Nabors, L. B.; Cobbs, C. G. & Britt, W. J. (2002). Human cytomegalovirus infection and expression in human malignant glioma, *Cancer Research*, Vol. 62, No. 12, (June 2002), pp. 3347-3350, ISSN 0008-5472

De Vleeschouwer, S.; Van Calenbergh, F.; Demaerel, P.; Flamen, P.; Rutkowski, S.; Kaempgen, E.; Wolff, J. E.; Plets, C.; Sciot, R. & Van Gool, S. W. (2004). Transient local response and persistent tumor control in a child with recurrent malignant glioma: treatment with combination therapy including dendritic cell therapy. Case report, *Journal of Neurosurgery*, Vol. 100, No. 5, (May 2004), pp. 492-497, ISSN 0022-3085

de Vos, A. F.; van Meurs, M.; Brok, H. P.; Boven, L. A.; Hintzen, R. Q.; van der Valk, P.; Ravid, R.; Rensing, S.; Boon, L.; t Hart, B. A. & Laman, J. D. (2002). Transfer of central nervous system autoantigens and presentation in secondary lymphoid organs, *Journal of Clinical Oncology*, Vol. 169, No. 10, (November 2002), pp. 5415-5423, ISSN 0022-1767

Debinski, W.; Gibo, D. M.; Hulet, S. W.; Connor, J. R. & Gillespie, G. Y. (1999). Receptor for interleukin 13 is a marker and therapeutic target for human high-grade gliomas, *Clinical Cancer Research*, Vol. 5, No. 5, (May 1999), pp. 985-990, ISSN 1078-0432

Desbaillets, I.; Tada, M.; de Tribolet, N.; Diserens, A. C.; Hamou, M. F. & Van Meir, E. G. (1994). Human astrocytomas and glioblastomas express monocyte chemoattractant protein-1 (MCP-1) in vivo and in vitro, *International Journal of Cancer*, Vol. 58, No. 2, (July 1994), pp. 240-247, ISSN 0020-7136

Dodelet, V. C. & Pasquale, E. B. (2000). Eph receptors and ephrin ligands: embryogenesis to tumorigenesis, *Oncogene*, Vol. 19, No. 49, (November 2000), pp. 5614-5619, ISSN 0950-9232

Dreno, B.; Nguyen, J. M.; Khammari, A.; Pandolfino, M. C.; Tessier, M. H.; Bercegeay, S.; Cassidanius, A.; Lemarre, P.; Billaudel, S.; Labarriere, N. & Jotereau, F. (2002). Randomized trial of adoptive transfer of melanoma tumor-infiltrating lymphocytes as adjuvant therapy for stage III melanoma, *Cancer Immunology Immunotherapy*, Vol. 51, No. 10, (November 2002), pp. 539-546, ISSN 0340-7004

Dudley, M. E.; Wunderlich, J. R.; Yang, J. C.; Sherry, R. M.; Topalian, S. L.; Restifo, N. P.; Royal, R. E.; Kammula, U.; White, D. E.; Mavroukakis, S. A.; Rogers, L. J.; Gracia, G. J.; Jones, S. A.; Mangiameli, D. P.; Pelletier, M. M.; Gea-Banacloche, J.; Robinson, M. R.; Berman, D. M.; Filie, A. C.; Abati, A. & Rosenberg, S. A. (2005). Adoptive cell transfer therapy following non-myeloablative but lymphodepleting chemotherapy for the treatment of patients with refractory metastatic melanoma, *Journal of Clinical Oncology*, Vol. 23, No. 10, (April 2005), pp. 2346-2357, ISSN 0732-183X

Dunn, G. P.; Dunn, I. F. & Curry, W. T. (2007). Focus on TILs: Prognostic significance of tumor infiltrating lymphocytes in human glioma, *Cancer Immunity*, Vol. 7, (August 2007), pp. 12, ISSN 1424-9634

Eguchi, J.; Hatano, M.; Nishimura, F.; Zhu, X.; Dusak, J. E.; Sato, H.; Pollack, I. F.; Storkus, W. J. & Okada, H. (2006). Identification of interleukin-13 receptor $\alpha 2$ peptide analogues capable of inducing improved antiglioma CTL responses, *Cancer Research*, Vol. 66, No. 11, (June 2006), pp. 5883-5891, ISSN 0008-5472

Engelhardt, B. (2008). The blood-central nervous system barriers actively control immune cell entry into the central nervous system, *Current Pharmaceutical Design*, Vol. 14, No. 16, (August 2008), pp. 1555-1565, ISSN 1381-6128

Fecci, P. E.; Mitchell, D. A.; Whitesides, J. F.; Xie, W.; Friedman, A. H.; Archer, G. E.; Herndon, J. E., 2nd; Bigner, D. D.; Dranoff, G. & Sampson, J. H. (2006). Increased regulatory T-cell fraction amidst a diminished CD4 compartment explains cellular immune defects in patients with malignant glioma, *Cancer Research*, Vol. 66, No. 6, (March 2006), pp. 3294-3302, ISSN 0008-5472

Fujita, M.; Zhu, X.; Sasaki, K.; Ueda, R.; Low, K. L.; Pollack, I. F. & Okada, H. (2008). Inhibition of STAT3 promotes the efficacy of adoptive transfer therapy using type-1 CTLs by modulation of the immunological microenvironment in a murine intracranial glioma, *Journal of Immunology*, Vol. 180, No. 4, (February 2008), pp. 2089-2098, ISSN 0022-1767

Fujita, M.; Zhu, X.; Ueda, R.; Sasaki, K.; Kohanbash, G.; Kastenhuber, E. R.; McDonald, H. A.; Gibson, G. A.; Watkins, S. C.; Muthuswamy, R.; Kalinski, P. & Okada, H. (2009). Effective immunotherapy against murine gliomas using type 1 polarizing dendritic cells-significant roles of CXCL10, *Cancer Research*, Vol. 69, No. 4, (February 2009), pp. 1587-1595, ISSN 0008-5472

Fujita, M.; Scheurer, M. E.; Decker, S. A.; McDonald, H. A.; Kohanbash, G.; Kastenhuber, E. R.; Kato, H.; Bondy, M. L.; Ohlfest, J. R. & Okada, H. (2010). Role of type 1 IFNs in antiglioma immunosurveillance-using mouse studies to guide examination of novel prognostic markers in humans, *Clinical Cancer Research*, Vol. 16, No. 13, (July 2010), pp. 3409-3419, ISSN 1078-0432

Fujita, M.; Kohanbash, G.; Fellows-Mayle, W.; Hamilton, R. L.; Komohara, Y.; Decker, S. A.; Ohlfest, J. R. & Okada, H. (2011). COX-2 blockade suppresses gliomagenesis by inhibiting myeloid-derived suppressor cells, *Cancer Research*, Vol. 71, No. 7, (April 2011), pp. 2664-2667, ISSN 0008-5472

Gangemi, R. M.; Griffero, F.; Marubbi, D.; Perera, M.; Capra, M. C.; Malatesta, P.; Ravetti, G. L.; Zona, G. L.; Daga, A. & Corte, G. (2009). SOX2 silencing in glioblastoma tumor-initiating cells causes stop of proliferation and loss of tumorigenicity, *Stem Cells*, Vol. 27, No. 1, (January 2009), pp. 40-48, ISSN 1066-5099

Gattinoni, L.; Powell, D. J., Jr.; Rosenberg, S. A. & Restifo, N. P. (2006). Adoptive immunotherapy for cancer: building on success, *Nature Reviews Immunology*, Vol. 6, No. 5, (May 2006), pp. 383-393, ISSN 1474-1733

Glienke, W.; Maute, L.; Koehl, U.; Esser, R.; Milz, E. & Bergmann, L. (2007). Effective treatment of leukemic cell lines with wt1 siRNA, *Leukemia*, Vol. 21, No. 10, (October 2007), pp. 2164-2170, ISSN 0887-6924

Gomez, G. G. & Kruse, C. A. (2007). Cellular and functional characterization of immunoresistant human glioma cell clones selected with alloreactive cytotoxic T lymphocytes reveals their up-regulated synthesis of biologically active TGF-β, *Journal of Immunotherapy*, Vol. 30, No. 3, (April 2007), pp. 261-273, ISSN 1524-9557

Gorelik, L. & Flavell, R. A. (2002). Transforming growth factor-beta in T-cell biology, *Nature Reviews Immunology*, Vol. 2, No. 1, (January 2002), pp. 46-53, ISSN 1474-1733

Graeber, M. B.; Scheithauer, B. W. & Kreutzberg, G. W. (2002). Microglia in brain tumors, *Glia*, Vol. 40, No. 2, (November 2002), pp. 252-259, ISSN 0894-1491

Grauer, O. M.; Nierkens, S.; Bennink, E.; Toonen, L. W.; Boon, L.; Wesseling, P.; Sutmuller, R. P. & Adema, G. J. (2007). CD4+FoxP3+ regulatory T cells gradually accumulate in gliomas during tumor growth and efficiently suppress antiglioma immune responses in vivo, *International Journal of Cancer*, Vol. 121, No. 1, (July 2007), pp. 95-105, ISSN 0020-7136

Gross, G.; Waks, T. & Eshhar, Z. (1989). Expression of immunoglobulin-T-cell receptor chimeric molecules as functional receptors with antibody-type specificity, *Proceedings of the National Academy of Sciences of the United States of America*, Vol. 86, No. 24, (December 1989), pp. 10024-10028, ISSN 0027-8424

Hatano, M.; Eguchi, J.; Tatsumi, T.; Kuwashima, N.; Dusak, J. E.; Kinch, M. S.; Pollack, I. F.; Hamilton, R. L.; Storkus, W. J. & Okada, H. (2005). EphA2 as a glioma-associated antigen: a novel target for glioma vaccines, *Neoplasia*, Vol. 7, No. 8, (August 2005), pp. 717-722, ISSN 1522-8002

Heimberger, A. B.; Abou-Ghazal, M.; Reina-Ortiz, C.; Yang, D. S.; Sun, W.; Qiao, W.; Hiraoka, N. & Fuller, G. N. (2008). Incidence and prognostic impact of FoxP3+ regulatory T cells in human gliomas, *Clinical Cancer Research*, Vol. 14, No. 16, (August 2008), pp. 5166-5172, ISSN 1078-0432

Holladay, F. P.; Heitz-Turner, T.; Bayer, W. L. & Wood, G. W. (1996). Autologous tumor cell vaccination combined with adoptive cellular immunotherapy in patients with grade III/IV astrocytoma, *Journal of Neuro-Oncology*, Vol. 27, No. 2, (February 1996), pp. 179-189, ISSN 0167-594X

Huang, B.; Lei, Z.; Zhao, J.; Gong, W.; Liu, J.; Chen, Z.; Liu, Y.; Li, D.; Yuan, Y.; Zhang, G. M. & Feng, Z. H. (2007). CCL2/CCR2 pathway mediates recruitment of myeloid suppressor cells to cancers, *Cancer Letters*, Vol. 252, No. 1, (July 2007), pp. 86-92, ISSN 0304-3835

Huettner, C.; Czub, S.; Kerkau, S.; Roggendorf, W. & Tonn, J. C. (1997). Interleukin 10 is expressed in human gliomas in vivo and increases glioma cell proliferation and motility in vitro, *Anticancer Research*, Vol. 17, No. 5A, (September 1997), pp. 3217-3224, ISSN 0250-7005

Hussain, S. F.; Yang, D.; Suki, D.; Aldape, K.; Grimm, E. & Heimberger, A. B. (2006). The role of human glioma-infiltrating microglia/macrophages in mediating antitumor immune responses, *Neuro-Oncology*, Vol. 8, No. 3, (July 2006), pp. 261-279, ISSN 1522-8517

Ishikawa, E.; Tsuboi, K.; Yamamoto, T.; Muroi, A.; Takano, S.; Enomoto, T.; Matsumura, A. & Ohno, T. (2007). Clinical trial of autologous formalin-fixed tumor vaccine for glioblastoma multiforme patients, *Cancer Science*, Vol. 98, No. 8, (August 2007), pp. 1226-1233, ISSN 1347-9032

Izumoto, S.; Tsuboi, A.; Oka, Y.; Suzuki, T.; Hashiba, T.; Kagawa, N.; Hashimoto, N.; Maruno, M.; Elisseeva, O. A.; Shirakata, T.; Kawakami, M.; Oji, Y.; Nishida, S.; Ohno, S.; Kawase, I.; Hatazawa, J.; Nakatsuka, S.; Aozasa, K.; Morita, S.; Sakamoto, J.; Sugiyama, H. & Yoshimine, T. (2008). Phase II clinical trial of Wilms tumor 1 peptide vaccination for patients with recurrent glioblastoma multiforme, *Journal of Neurosurgery*, Vol. 108, No. 5, (May 2008), pp. 963-971, ISSN 0022-3085

Jordan, J. T.; Sun, W.; Hussain, S. F.; DeAngulo, G.; Prabhu, S. S. & Heimberger, A. B. (2008). Preferential migration of regulatory T cells mediated by glioma-secreted chemokines can be blocked with chemotherapy, *Cancer Immunology Immunotherapy*, Vol. 57, No. 1, (January 2008), pp. 123-131, ISSN 0340-7004

Kahlon, K. S.; Brown, C.; Cooper, L. J.; Raubitschek, A.; Forman, S. J. & Jensen, M. C. (2004). Specific recognition and killing of glioblastoma multiforme by interleukin 13-zetakine redirected cytolytic T cells, *Cancer Research*, Vol. 64, No. 24, (December 2004), pp. 9160-9166, ISSN 0008-5472

Kantoff, P. W.; Higano, C. S.; Shore, N. D.; Berger, E. R.; Small, E. J.; Penson, D. F.; Redfern, C. H.; Ferrari, A. C.; Dreicer, R.; Sims, R. B.; Xu, Y.; Frohlich, M. W. & Schellhammer, P. F. (2010). Sipuleucel-T immunotherapy for castration-resistant prostate cancer, *New England Journal of Medicine*, Vol. 363, No. 5, (July 2010), pp. 411-422, ISSN 1533-4406

Kikuchi, T.; Akasaki, Y.; Irie, M.; Homma, S.; Abe, T. & Ohno, T. (2001). Results of a phase I clinical trial of vaccination of glioma patients with fusions of dendritic and glioma cells, *Cancer Immunology Immunotherapy*, Vol. 50, No. 7, (September 2001), pp. 337-344, ISSN 0340-7004

Kikuchi, T.; Akasaki, Y.; Abe, T.; Fukuda, T.; Saotome, H.; Ryan, J. L.; Kufe, D. W. & Ohno, T. (2004). Vaccination of glioma patients with fusions of dendritic and glioma cells and recombinant human interleukin 12, *Journal of Immunotherapy*, Vol. 27, No. 6, (November 2004), pp. 452-459, ISSN 1524-9557

Kuwashima, N.; Nishimura, F.; Eguchi, J.; Sato, H.; Hatano, M.; Tsugawa, T.; Sakaida, T.; Dusak, J. E.; Fellows-Mayle, W. K.; Papworth, G. D.; Watkins, S. C.; Gambotto, A.; Pollack, I. F.; Storkus, W. J. & Okada, H. (2005). Delivery of dendritic cells engineered to secrete IFN-α into central nervous system tumors enhances the efficacy of peripheral tumor cell vaccines: dependence on apoptotic pathways, *Journal of Immunology*, Vol. 175, No. 4, (August 2005), pp. 2730-2740, ISSN 0022-1767

Li, Y.; Moysey, R.; Molloy, P. E.; Vuidepot, A. L.; Mahon, T.; Baston, E.; Dunn, S.; Liddy, N.; Jacob, J.; Jakobsen, B. K. & Boulter, J. M. (2005). Directed evolution of human T-cell receptors with picomolar affinities by phage display, *Nature Biotechnology*, Vol. 23, No. 3, (March 2005), pp. 349-354, ISSN 1087-0156

Liau, L. M.; Prins, R. M.; Kiertscher, S. M.; Odesa, S. K.; Kremen, T. J.; Giovannone, A. J.; Lin, J. W.; Chute, D. J.; Mischel, P. S.; Cloughesy, T. F. & Roth, M. D. (2005). Dendritic cell vaccination in glioblastoma patients induces systemic and intracranial T-cell responses modulated by the local central nervous system tumor microenvironment, *Clinical Cancer Research*, Vol. 11, No. 15, (August 2005), pp. 5515-5525, ISSN 1078-0432

Liu, F.; Park, P. J.; Lai, W.; Maher, E.; Chakravarti, A.; Durso, L.; Jiang, X.; Yu, Y.; Brosius, A.; Thomas, M.; Chin, L.; Brennan, C.; DePinho, R. A.; Kohane, I.; Carroll, R. S.; Black, P. M. & Johnson, M. D. (2006). A genome-wide screen reveals functional gene clusters in the cancer genome and identifies EphA2 as a mitogen in glioblastoma, *Cancer Research*, Vol. 66, No. 22, (November 2006), pp. 10815-10823, ISSN 0008-5472

Lucas, K. G.; Bao, L.; Bruggeman, R.; Dunham, K. & Specht, C. (2010). The detection of CMV pp65 and IE1 in glioblastoma multiforme, *Journal of Neuro-Oncology*, Vol. 103, No. 2, (September 2010), pp. 231-238, ISSN 0167-594X

Mitchell, D. A.; Xie, W.; Schmittling, R.; Learn, C.; Friedman, A.; McLendon, R. E. & Sampson, J. H. (2008). Sensitive detection of human cytomegalovirus in tumors and peripheral blood of patients diagnosed with glioblastoma, *Neuro-Oncology*, Vol. 10, No. 1, (February 2008), pp. 10-18, ISSN 1522-8517

Moore, K. W.; de Waal Malefyt, R.; Coffman, R. L. & O'Garra, A. (2001). Interleukin-10 and the interleukin-10 receptor, *Annual Review of Immunology*, Vol. 19, (March 2001), pp. 683-765, ISSN 0732-0582

Morgan, R. A.; Dudley, M. E.; Wunderlich, J. R.; Hughes, M. S.; Yang, J. C.; Sherry, R. M.; Royal, R. E.; Topalian, S. L.; Kammula, U. S.; Restifo, N. P.; Zheng, Z.; Nahvi, A.; de Vries, C. R.; Rogers-Freezer, L. J.; Mavroukakis, S. A. & Rosenberg, S. A. (2006). Cancer regression in patients after transfer of genetically engineered lymphocytes, *Science*, Vol. 314, No. 5796, (October 2006), pp. 126-129, ISSN 0036-8075

Nishimura, F.; Dusak, J. E.; Eguchi, J.; Zhu, X.; Gambotto, A.; Storkus, W. J. & Okada, H. (2006). Adoptive transfer of type 1 CTL mediates effective anti-central nervous system tumor response: critical roles of IFN-inducible protein-10, *Cancer Research*, Vol. 66, No. 8, (April 2006), pp. 4478-4487, ISSN 0008-5472

Nitta, T.; Hishii, M.; Sato, K. & Okumura, K. (1994). Selective expression of interleukin-10 gene within glioblastoma multiforme, *Brain Research*, Vol. 649, No. 1-2, (June 1994), pp. 122-128, ISSN 0006-8993

Ohno, M.; Natsume, A.; Ichiro Iwami, K.; Iwamizu, H.; Noritake, K.; Ito, D.; Toi, Y.; Ito, M.; Motomura, K.; Yoshida, J.; Yoshikawa, K. & Wakabayashi, T. (2010). Retrovirally engineered T-cell-based immunotherapy targeting type III variant epidermal growth factor receptor, a glioma-associated antigen, *Cancer Science*, Vol. 101, No. 12, (December 2010), pp. 2518-2524, ISSN 1347-9032

Oka, Y.; Tsuboi, A.; Elisseeva, O. A.; Udaka, K. & Sugiyama, H. (2002). WT1 as a novel target antigen for cancer immunotherapy, *Current Cancer Drug Targets*, Vol. 2, No. 1, (March 2002), pp. 45-54, ISSN 1568-0096

Okada, H.; Lieberman, F. S.; Walter, K. A.; Lunsford, L. D.; Kondziolka, D. S.; Bejjani, G. K.; Hamilton, R. L.; Torres-Trejo, A.; Kalinski, P.; Cai, Q.; Mabold, J. L.; Edington, H. D.; Butterfield, L. H.; Whiteside, T. L.; Potter, D. M.; Schold, S. C., Jr. & Pollack, I. F. (2007). Autologous glioma cell vaccine admixed with interleukin-4 gene transfected fibroblasts in the treatment of patients with malignant gliomas, *Journal of Translational Medicien*, Vol. 5, (December 2007), pp. 67, ISSN 1479-5876

Okada, H.; Kohanbash, G.; Zhu, X.; Kastenhuber, E. R.; Hoji, A.; Ueda, R. & Fujita, M. (2009). Immunotherapeutic approaches for glioma, *Critical Reviews in Immunology*, Vol. 29, No. 1, (April 2009), pp. 1-42, ISSN 1040-8401

Okada, H.; Kalinski, P.; Ueda, R.; Hoji, A.; Kohanbash, G.; Donegan, T. E.; Mintz, A. H.; Engh, J. A.; Bartlett, D. L.; Brown, C. K.; Zeh, H.; Holtzman, M. P.; Reinhart, T. A.; Whiteside, T. L.; Butterfield, L. H.; Hamilton, R. L.; Potter, D. M.; Pollack, I. F.; Salazar, A. M. & Lieberman, F. S. (2011). Induction of CD8+ T-cell responses against novel glioma-associated antigen peptides and clinical activity by vaccinations with α-type 1 polarized dendritic cells and polyinosinic-polycytidylic acid stabilized by lysine and carboxymethylcellulose in patients with recurrent malignant glioma, *Journal of Clinical Oncology*, Vol. 29, No. 3, (January 2011), pp. 330-336, ISSN 0732-183X

Okada, N.; Mori, N.; Koretomo, R.; Okada, Y.; Nakayama, T.; Yoshie, O.; Mizuguchi, H.; Hayakawa, T.; Nakagawa, S.; Mayumi, T.; Fujita, T. & Yamamoto, A. (2005). Augmentation of the migratory ability of DC-based vaccine into regional lymph nodes by efficient CCR7 gene transduction, *Gene Therapy*, Vol. 12, No. 2, (January 2005), pp. 129-139, ISSN 0969-7128

Parney, I. F.; Chang, L. J.; Farr-Jones, M. A.; Hao, C.; Smylie, M. & Petruk, K. C. (2006). Technical hurdles in a pilot clinical trial of combined B7-2 and GM-CSF immunogene therapy for glioblastomas and melanomas, *Journal of Neuro-Oncology*, Vol. 78, No. 1, (May 2006), pp. 71-80, ISSN 0167-594X

Parsa, A. T.; Waldron, J. S.; Panner, A.; Crane, C. A.; Parney, I. F.; Barry, J. J.; Cachola, K. E.; Murray, J. C.; Tihan, T.; Jensen, M. C.; Mischel, P. S.; Stokoe, D. & Pieper, R. O. (2007). Loss of tumor suppressor PTEN function increases B7-H1 expression and immunoresistance in glioma, *Nature Medicine*, Vol. 13, No. 1, (January 2007), pp. 84-88, ISSN 1078-8956

Perret, R. & Ronchese, F. (2008). Memory T cells in cancer immunotherapy: which CD8 T-cell population provides the best protection against tumours?, *Tissue Antigens*, Vol. 72, No. 3, (September 2008), pp. 187-194, ISSN 0001-2815

Plautz, G. E.; Barnett, G. H.; Miller, D. W.; Cohen, B. H.; Prayson, R. A.; Krauss, J. C.; Luciano, M.; Kangisser, D. B. & Shu, S. (1998). Systemic T cell adoptive immunotherapy of malignant gliomas, *Journal of Neurosurgery*, Vol. 89, No. 1, (July 1998), pp. 42-51, ISSN 0022-3085

Plautz, G. E.; Miller, D. W.; Barnett, G. H.; Stevens, G. H.; Maffett, S.; Kim, J.; Cohen, P. A. & Shu, S. (2000). T cell adoptive immunotherapy of newly diagnosed gliomas, *Clinical Cancer Research*, Vol. 6, No. 6, (June 2000), pp. 2209-2218, ISSN 1078-0432

Prins, R. M.; Soto, H.; Konkankit, V.; Odesa, S. K.; Eskin, A.; Yong, W. H.; Nelson, S. F. & Liau, L. M. (2011). Gene expression profile correlates with T-cell infiltration and relative survival in glioblastoma patients vaccinated with dendritic cell immunotherapy, *Clinical Cancer Research*, Vol. 17, No. 6, (March 2011), pp. 1603-1615, ISSN 1078-0432

Ransohoff, R. M.; Kivisakk, P. & Kidd, G. (2003). Three or more routes for leukocyte migration into the central nervous system, *Nature Reviews Immunology*, Vol. 3, No. 7, (July 2003), pp. 569-581, ISSN 1474-1733

Robbins, P. F.; Dudley, M. E.; Wunderlich, J.; El-Gamil, M.; Li, Y. F.; Zhou, J.; Huang, J.; Powell, D. J., Jr. & Rosenberg, S. A. (2004). Cutting edge: persistence of transferred lymphocyte clonotypes correlates with cancer regression in patients receiving cell transfer therapy, *Journal of Immunology*, Vol. 173, No. 12, (December 2004), pp. 7125-7130, ISSN 0022-1767

Rosenberg, S. A. (2008). Overcoming obstacles to the effective immunotherapy of human cancer, *Proceedings of the National Academy of Sciences of the United States of America*, Vol. 105, No. 35, (September 2008), pp. 12643-12644, ISSN 0027-8424

Rushing, E. J.; Sandberg, G. D. & Horkayne-Szakaly, I. (2010). High-grade astrocytomas show increased Nestin and Wilms's tumor gene (WT1) protein expression, *International Journal of Surgical Pathology*, Vol. 18, No. 4, (August 2010), pp. 255-259, ISSN 1066-8969

Rutkowski, S.; De Vleeschouwer, S.; Kaempgen, E.; Wolff, J. E.; Kuhl, J.; Demaerel, P.; Warmuth-Metz, M.; Flamen, P.; Van Calenbergh, F.; Plets, C.; Sorensen, N.; Opitz, A. & Van Gool, S. W. (2004). Surgery and adjuvant dendritic cell-based tumour vaccination for patients with relapsed malignant glioma, a feasibility study, *British Journal of Cancer*, Vol. 91, No. 9, (November 2004), pp. 1656-1662, ISSN 0007-0920

Saikali, S.; Avril, T.; Collet, B.; Hamlat, A.; Bansard, J. Y.; Drenou, B.; Guegan, Y. & Quillien, V. (2007). Expression of nine tumour antigens in a series of human glioblastoma multiforme: interest of EGFRvIII, IL-13Rα2, gp100 and TRP-2 for immunotherapy, *Journal of Neuro-Oncology*, Vol. 81, No. 2, (January 2007), pp. 139-148, ISSN 0167-594X

Salcedo, R.; Ponce, M. L.; Young, H. A.; Wasserman, K.; Ward, J. M.; Kleinman, H. K.; Oppenheim, J. J. & Murphy, W. J. (2000). Human endothelial cells express CCR2 and respond to MCP-1: direct role of MCP-1 in angiogenesis and tumor progression, *Blood*, Vol. 96, No. 1, (July 2000), pp. 34-40, ISSN 0006-4971

Sampson, J. H.; Archer, G. E.; Mitchell, D. A.; Heimberger, A. B.; Herndon, J. E., 2nd; Lally-Goss, D.; McGehee-Norman, S.; Paolino, A.; Reardon, D. A.; Friedman, A. H.; Friedman, H. S. & Bigner, D. D. (2009). An epidermal growth factor receptor variant III-targeted vaccine is safe and immunogenic in patients with glioblastoma multiforme, *Molecular Cancer Therapy*, Vol. 8, No. 10, (October 2009), pp. 2773-2779, ISSN 1535-7163

Sampson, J. H.; Heimberger, A. B.; Archer, G. E.; Aldape, K. D.; Friedman, A. H.; Friedman, H. S.; Gilbert, M. R.; Herndon, J. E., 2nd; McLendon, R. E.; Mitchell, D. A.; Reardon, D. A.; Sawaya, R.; Schmittling, R. J.; Shi, W.; Vredenburgh, J. J. & Bigner, D. D. (2010). Immunologic escape after prolonged progression-free survival with epidermal growth factor receptor variant III peptide vaccination in patients with newly diagnosed glioblastoma, *Journal of Clinical Oncology*, Vol. 28, No. 31, (November 2010), pp. 4722-4729, ISSN 0732-183X

Sasaki, K.; Zhu, X.; Vasquez, C.; Nishimura, F.; Dusak, J. E.; Huang, J.; Fujita, M.; Wesa, A.; Potter, D. M.; Walker, P. R.; Storkus, W. J. & Okada, H. (2007). Preferential expression of very late antigen-4 on type 1 CTL cells plays a critical role in trafficking into central nervous system tumors, *Cancer Research*, Vol. 67, No. 13, (July 2007), pp. 6451-6458, ISSN 0008-5472

Sasaki, K.; Pardee, A. D.; Okada, H. & Storkus, W. J. (2008a). IL-4 inhibits VLA-4 expression on Tc1 cells resulting in poor tumor infiltration and reduced therapy benefit, *European Journal of Immunology*, Vol. 38, No. 10, (October 2008), pp. 2865-2873, ISSN 0014-2980

Sasaki, K.; Zhao, X.; Pardee, A. D.; Ueda, R.; Fujita, M.; Sehra, S.; Kaplan, M. H.; Kane, L. P.; Okada, H. & Storkus, W. J. (2008b). Stat6 signaling suppresses VLA-4 expression by CD8+ T cells and limits their ability to infiltrate tumor lesions in vivo, *Journal of Immunology*, Vol. 181, No. 1, (July 2008), pp. 104-108, ISSN 0022-1767

Sasaki, K.; Pardee, A. D.; Qu, Y.; Zhao, X.; Ueda, R.; Kohanbash, G.; Bailey, L. M.; Okada, H.; Muthuswamy, R.; Kalinski, P.; Basse, P. H.; Falo, L. D. & Storkus, W. J. (2009). IL-4 suppresses very late antigen-4 expression which is required for therapeutic Th1 T-cell trafficking into tumors, *Journal of Immunotherapy*, Vol. 32, No. 8, (October 2009), pp. 793-802, ISSN 1524-9557

Scheurer, M. E.; Bondy, M. L.; Aldape, K. D.; Albrecht, T. & El-Zein, R. (2008). Detection of human cytomegalovirus in different histological types of gliomas, *Acta Neuropathologica*, Vol. 116, No. 1, (July 2008), pp. 79-86, ISSN 0001-6322

Schittenhelm, J.; Mittelbronn, M.; Nguyen, T. D.; Meyermann, R. & Beschorner, R. (2008). WT1 expression distinguishes astrocytic tumor cells from normal and reactive astrocytes, *Brain Pathology*, Vol. 18, No. 3, (July 2008), pp. 344-353, ISSN 1015-6305

Schmitz, M.; Wehner, R.; Stevanovic, S.; Kiessling, A.; Rieger, M. A.; Temme, A.; Bachmann, M.; Rieber, E. P. & Weigle, B. (2007). Identification of a naturally processed T cell epitope derived from the glioma-associated protein SOX11, *Cancer Letters*, Vol. 245, No. 1-2, (January 2007), pp. 331-336, ISSN 0304-3835

Schneider, T.; Gerhards, R.; Kirches, E. & Firsching, R. (2001). Preliminary results of active specific immunization with modified tumor cell vaccine in glioblastoma multiforme, *Journal of Neuro-Oncology*, Vol. 53, No. 1, (May 2001), pp. 39-46, ISSN 0167-594X

Shinohara, H.; Yagita, H.; Ikawa, Y. & Oyaizu, N. (2000). Fas drives cell cycle progression in glioma cells via extracellular signal-regulated kinase activation, *Cancer Research*, Vol. 60, No. 6, (March 2000), pp. 1766-1772, ISSN 0008-5472

Sloan, A. E.; Dansey, R.; Zamorano, L.; Barger, G.; Hamm, C.; Diaz, F.; Baynes, R. & Wood, G. (2000). Adoptive immunotherapy in patients with recurrent malignant glioma: preliminary results of using autologous whole-tumor vaccine plus granulocyte-macrophage colony-stimulating factor and adoptive transfer of anti-CD3-activated lymphocytes, *Neurosurgical Focus*, Vol. 9, No. 6, (July 2000), pp. e9, ISSN 1092-0684

Steiner, H. H.; Bonsanto, M. M.; Beckhove, P.; Brysch, M.; Geletneky, K.; Ahmadi, R.; Schuele-Freyer, R.; Kremer, P.; Ranaie, G.; Matejic, D.; Bauer, H.; Kiessling, M.; Kunze, S.; Schirrmacher, V. & Herold-Mende, C. (2004). Antitumor vaccination of patients with glioblastoma multiforme: a pilot study to assess feasibility, safety, and clinical benefit, *Journal of Clinical Oncology*, Vol. 22, No. 21, (November 2004), pp. 4272-4281, ISSN 0732-183X

Takeshima, H.; Kuratsu, J.; Takeya, M.; Yoshimura, T. & Ushio, Y. (1994). Expression and localization of messenger RNA and protein for monocyte chemoattractant protein-1 in human malignant glioma, *Journal of Neurosurgery*, Vol. 80, No. 6, (June 1994), pp. 1056-1062, ISSN 0022-3085

Terasaki, M.; Shibui, S.; Narita, Y.; Fujimaki, T.; Aoki, T.; Kajiwara, K.; Sawamura, Y.; Kurisu, K.; Mineta, T.; Yamada, A. & Itoh, K. (2011). Phase I trial of a personalized peptide vaccine for patients positive for human leukocyte antigen -A24 with recurrent or progressive glioblastoma multiforme, *Journal of Clinical Oncology*, Vol. 29, No. 3, (January 2011), pp. 337-344, ISSN 0732-183X

Ueda, R.; Iizuka, Y.; Yoshida, K.; Kawase, T.; Kawakami, Y. & Toda, M. (2004). Identification of a human glioma antigen, SOX6, recognized by patients' sera, *Oncogene*, Vol. 23, No. 7, (February 2004), pp. 1420-1427, ISSN 0950-9232

Ueda, R.; Yoshida, K.; Kawase, T.; Kawakami, Y. & Toda, M. (2007). Preferential expression and frequent IgG responses of a tumor antigen, SOX5, in glioma patients, *International Journal of Cancer*, Vol. 120, No. 8, (April 2007), pp. 1704-1711, ISSN 0020-7136

Ueda, R.; Fujita, M.; Zhu, X.; Sasaki, K.; Kastenhuber, E. R.; Kohanbash, G.; McDonald, H. A.; Harper, J.; Lonning, S. & Okada, H. (2009). Systemic inhibition of transforming growth factor-β in glioma-bearing mice improves the therapeutic efficacy of glioma-associated antigen peptide vaccines, *Clinical Cancer Research*, Vol. 15, No. 21, (November 2009), pp. 6551-6559, ISSN 1078-0432

Uematsu, M.; Ohsawa, I.; Aokage, T.; Nishimaki, K.; Matsumoto, K.; Takahashi, H.; Asoh, S.; Teramoto, A. & Ohta, S. (2005). Prognostic significance of the immunohistochemical index of survivin in glioma: a comparative study with the MIB-1 index, *Journal of Neuro-Oncology*, Vol. 72, No. 3, (May 2005), pp. 231-238, ISSN 0167-594X

Vanderlugt, C. L. & Miller, S. D. (2002). Epitope spreading in immune-mediated diseases: implications for immunotherapy, *Nature Reviews Immunology*, Vol. 2, No. 2, (February 2002), pp. 85-95, ISSN 1474-1733

Vauleon, E.; Avril, T.; Collet, B.; Mosser, J. & Quillien, V. (2010). Overview of cellular immunotherapy for patients with glioblastoma, *Clinical & Developmental Immunology*, Vol. 2010, (October 2010), pp. 689171, ISSN 1740-2522

Walker, D. G.; Laherty, R.; Tomlinson, F. H.; Chuah, T. & Schmidt, C. (2008). Results of a phase I dendritic cell vaccine trial for malignant astrocytoma: potential interaction with adjuvant chemotherapy, *Journal of Clinical Neuroscience*, Vol. 15, No. 2, (February 2008), pp. 114-121, ISSN 0967-5868

Walker, P. R.; Saas, P. & Dietrich, P. Y. (1997). Role of Fas ligand (CD95L) in immune escape: the tumor cell strikes back, *Journal of Immunology*, Vol. 158, No. 10, (May 1997), pp. 4521-4524, ISSN 0022-1767

Walker, P. R.; Calzascia, T.; de Tribolet, N. & Dietrich, P. Y. (2003). T-cell immune responses in the brain and their relevance for cerebral malignancies, *Brain Research. Brain Research Reviews,*Vol. 42, No. 2, (May 2003), pp. 97-122

Wang, X.; Berger, C.; Wong, C. W.; Forman, S. J.; Riddell, S. R. & Jensen, M. C. (2011). Engraftment of human central memory-derived effector CD8+ T cells in immunodeficient mice, *Blood*, Vol. 117, No. 6, (February 2011), pp. 1888-1898, ISSN 0006-4971

Watters, J. J.; Schartner, J. M. & Badie, B. (2005). Microglia function in brain tumors, *Journal of Neuroscience Research*, Vol. 81, No. 3, (August 2005), pp. 447-455, ISSN 0360-4012

Wegner, M. (1999). From head to toes: the multiple facets of Sox proteins, *Nucleic Acids Research*, Vol. 27, No. 6, (March 1999), pp. 1409-1420, ISSN 0305-1048

Wheeler, C. J.; Das, A.; Liu, G.; Yu, J. S. & Black, K. L. (2004). Clinical responsiveness of glioblastoma multiforme to chemotherapy after vaccination, *Clinical Cancer Research*, Vol. 10, No. 16, (August 2004), pp. 5316-5326, ISSN 1078-0432

Wheeler, C. J.; Black, K. L.; Liu, G.; Mazer, M.; Zhang, X. X.; Pepkowitz, S.; Goldfinger, D.; Ng, H.; Irvin, D. & Yu, J. S. (2008). Vaccination elicits correlated immune and clinical responses in glioblastoma multiforme patients, *Cancer Research*, Vol. 68, No. 14, (July 2008), pp. 5955-5964, ISSN 0008-5472

Wherry, E. J.; Teichgraber, V.; Becker, T. C.; Masopust, D.; Kaech, S. M.; Antia, R.; von Andrian, U. H. & Ahmed, R. (2003). Lineage relationship and protective immunity of memory CD8 T cell subsets, *Nature Immunology*, Vol. 4, No. 3, (March 2003), pp. 225-234, ISSN 1529-2908

Wikstrand, C. J. & Bigner, D. D. (1980). Immunobiologic aspects of the brain and human gliomas. A review, *American Journal of Pathology*, Vol. 98, No. 2, (February 1980), pp. 517-568, ISSN 0002-9440

Wintterle, S.; Schreiner, B.; Mitsdoerffer, M.; Schneider, D.; Chen, L.; Meyermann, R.; Weller, M. & Wiendl, H. (2003). Expression of the B7-related molecule B7-H1 by glioma cells: a potential mechanism of immune paralysis, *Cancer Research*, Vol. 63, No. 21, (November 2003), pp. 7462-7467, ISSN 0008-5472

Wood, G. W.; Holladay, F. P.; Turner, T.; Wang, Y. Y. & Chiga, M. (2000). A pilot study of autologous cancer cell vaccination and cellular immunotherapy using anti-CD3 stimulated lymphocytes in patients with recurrent grade III/IV astrocytoma, *Journal of Neuro-Oncology*, Vol. 48, No. 2, (June 2000), pp. 113-120, ISSN 0167-594X

Yajima, N.; Yamanaka, R.; Mine, T.; Tsuchiya, N.; Homma, J.; Sano, M.; Kuramoto, T.; Obata, Y.; Komatsu, N.; Arima, Y.; Yamada, A.; Shigemori, M.; Itoh, K. & Tanaka, R. (2005). Immunologic evaluation of personalized peptide vaccination for patients with advanced malignant glioma, *Clinical Cancer Research*, Vol. 11, No. 16, (August 2005), pp. 5900-5911, ISSN 1078-0432

Yamanaka, R.; Abe, T.; Yajima, N.; Tsuchiya, N.; Homma, J.; Kobayashi, T.; Narita, M.; Takahashi, M. & Tanaka, R. (2003). Vaccination of recurrent glioma patients with tumour lysate-pulsed dendritic cells elicits immune responses: results of a clinical phase I/II trial, *British Journal of Cancer*, Vol. 89, No. 7, (October 2003), pp. 1172-1179, ISSN 0007-0920

Yamanaka, R.; Homma, J.; Yajima, N.; Tsuchiya, N.; Sano, M.; Kobayashi, T.; Yoshida, S.; Abe, T.; Narita, M.; Takahashi, M. & Tanaka, R. (2005). Clinical evaluation of dendritic cell vaccination for patients with recurrent glioma: results of a clinical phase I/II trial, *Clinical Cancer Research*, Vol. 11, No. 11, (June 2005), pp. 4160-4167, ISSN 1078-0432

Yang, S.; Luca, G.; Liu, F.; Ji, Y.; Yu, Z.; Restifo, N. P.; Rosenberg, S. A. & Morgan, R. A. (2011). In vitro generated anti-tumor T lymphocytes exhibit distinct subsets mimicking in vivo antigen-experienced cells, *Cancer Immunology Immunotherapy*, Vol. 60, No. 5,(February 2011), pp. pp. 739-749 ISSN 0340-7004

Yu, J. S.; Wheeler, C. J.; Zeltzer, P. M.; Ying, H.; Finger, D. N.; Lee, P. K.; Yong, W. H.; Incardona, F.; Thompson, R. C.; Riedinger, M. S.; Zhang, W.; Prins, R. M. & Black, K. L. (2001). Vaccination of malignant glioma patients with peptide-pulsed dendritic cells elicits systemic cytotoxicity and intracranial T-cell infiltration, *Cancer Research*, Vol. 61, No. 3, (February 2001), pp. 842-847, ISSN 0008-5472

Yu, J. S.; Liu, G.; Ying, H.; Yong, W. H.; Black, K. L. & Wheeler, C. J. (2004). Vaccination with tumor lysate-pulsed dendritic cells elicits antigen-specific, cytotoxic T-cells in patients with malignant glioma, *Cancer Research*, Vol. 64, No. 14, (July 2004), pp. 4973-4979, ISSN 0008-5472

Zhang, J. G.; Eguchi, J.; Kruse, C. A.; Gomez, G. G.; Fakhrai, H.; Schroter, S.; Ma, W.; Hoa, N.; Minev, B.; Delgado, C.; Wepsic, H. T.; Okada, H. & Jadus, M. R. (2007). Antigenic profiling of glioma cells to generate allogeneic vaccines or dendritic cell-based therapeutics, *Clinical Cancer Research*, Vol. 13, No. 2, (January 2007), pp. 566-575, ISSN 1078-0432

20

Immunotherapy with Dendritic Cells and Newcastle Disease Virus in Glioblastoma Multiforme

Thomas Neßelhut[1], Dagmar Marx[1], Jan Neßelhut[1] and Fred Fändrich[2]
[1]*Institute for Tumortherapy, Duderstadt*
[2]*Clinic for Applied Cellular Medicine, University of Kiel*
Germany

1. Introduction

Malignant gliomas are the most prevalent type of primary brain tumors in adults. The most aggressive form, glioblastoma multiforme (GBM, WHO grade IV glioma), is characterized as incurable with average survivals less than 18 months (Buckner, 2003; Curran et al., 1993; De Angelis, 2001). Standard therapy consists of surgical resection to the extent that is safely feasible, followed by radiotherapy and adjuvant chemotherapy. A meta-analysis based on 12 randomized trials has supported the use of adjuvant chemotherapy treatment as compared to radiotherapy alone. A five percent increase in survival at two years, from 15 percent to 20 percent was reported (Stewart, 2002). In this context, an oral alkylating agent, temozolomide, has demonstrated antitumor activity as a single agent in the treatment of glioblastoma patients (Newlands et al., 1997; Stupp et al., 2001, 2005; Yung et al., 2000). At a median follow-up of 28 months, temozolomide treatment prolonged the median survival from 12.1 months with radiotherapy alone to 14.6 months when administered with concomitant radiotherapy (Stupp et al., 2005). Adjuvant administration of carmustine, a nitrosourea drug, has not resulted in beneficial prolongation of survival, although some long-term survivors in the chemotherapy groups have been documented in some of the non-randomized phase III trials (Chang et al., 1983; Green et al., 1983). Despite these advances in combined radio- chemotherapy treatment strategies along with surgical resection, the prognosis of patients with malignant glioma is poor and ≥ 80% of the patients survive less than 2 years. Salvage treatments upon recurrence are palliative at best and rarely provide a significant survival benefit. The minor clinical benefit of radio-chemotherapy is supposed to be mainly based on tumour stem cells, which in analogy to normal stem cells are resistant to radio- and chemotherapy (Liu et al., 2006; Singh et al., 2003). Therefore, the development of new treatment modalities is extremely important.

It is known that defects in the immune system play a crucial role in the development of cancer as well as in the host defense against cancer. Thus, specific immune therapeutic therapy approaches have been tested for a long time. Tumor-associated antigens recognized by tumor-reactive cytotoxic T lymphocytes (CTL) have been identified during the last two decades (Janeway et al., 2004). Also in patients with GBM such tumor antigen specific CD8+ T cells have been identified in the circulating blood (Tang et al., 2005). A specific cancer immunotherapy can be based on the use of antibodies directed against specific antigens, which are expressed in tumors. However, the more recently described immunological therapy strategy for GBM with an antibody (Bevacizumab), which blocks angiogenesis by binding to the vascular endothelial growth factor also shows insufficient results (Lai et al., 2010). The more promising strategy seems to be the use of tumor specific vaccines, which induce a specific cellular immune reaction by induction of tumor specific CTL.

2. Dendritic cells in cancer therapy

A specific cellular immune response against tumors is based on the uptake and presentation of tumor antigens on MHC molecules by professional antigen presenting cells leading to the induction of antigen specific CTL, which can then attack the tumor. Dendritic cells (DC) are the most potent antigen presenting cells and have been shown to be able to induce an efficient and specific immune response (Banchereau & Steinman, 1998; Steinman, 1991; Whiteside & Odoux, 2004). In comparison to other antigen presenting cells, like B cells, which induce and activate only memory T cells, dendritic cells can stimulate naive T cells (Banchereau & Steinman, 1998; Steinman, 1991; Whiteside & Odoux, 2004). Thus, today one of the most promising immunological therapy approaches in treatment of various types of human cancer is a specific immunotherapy with autologous dendritic cells (Engleman, 2003; Gilboa, 2007; Nestle, 2000).

According to their phenotype and functional properties dendritic cells can be classified as immature and mature type (Banchereau & Steinman, 1998). Immature dendritic cells are able to capture and internalize particles and soluble antigens from the environment (Banchereau & Steinman, 1998). Upon being internalized, antigens are processed and split into peptides, which are then presented on the cell surface in association with MHC molecules (Banchereau & Steinman, 1998). In response to micro-environmental signals immature DC switch to a mature phenotype with T cell stimulatory capacity (Vieira et al., 2000; Whiteside & Odoux, 2004). Mature dendritic cells express higher levels of major histocompatibility complex class I and class II molecules as well as co-stimulatory molecules like CD80 and CD86 (Dietz et al., 2000; Whiteside & Odoux, 2004). During the maturation process DC lose their ability to take up and process antigens (Dietz et al., 2000; Whiteside & Odoux, 2004). Mature dendritic cells are characterised by a distinct cytokine expression profile and their increased ability to produce Interleukin 12 (IL-12) in response to environmental signals, a cytokine known to be necessary for induction of TH1-T cell response leading to production and proliferation of CTL (Whiteside & Odoux, 2004, Rouard et al., 2002).

Until now several methods have been published to generate dendritic cells in vitro from monocytes isolated from the peripheral blood of volunteers or cancer patients, called monocytes-derived dendritic cells (MoDC) in the presence of GM-CSF and IL-4 (Morse et al., 2002; Peters et al., 1996; Romani et al., 1996, Sallusto & Lanzavecchia 1994, Zhou & Tedder, 1996). Immature MoDC can be loaded either with tumor-cell-lysate, known tumor specific peptides or with specific RNA or DNA. Upon exposure to various maturation stimuli the antigen loaded immature MoDC can be matured and are able to induce a clinical antitumor response in patients with various types of tumors through induction of tumor specific CTL, which can then attack the tumor (Engleman, 2003; Gilboa, 2007; Morse et al., 2002; Nestle, 2000; Romani et al., 1996, Zhou & Tedder, 1996).

2.1 Dendritic cell based immunotherapy in patients with GBM

Although the tumor is hidden behind the blood brain barrier immune cells can be recruited into the central nervous system (Tambuyzer et al., 2009; Vauleon et al., 2010; Wilson, et al., 2010). Macrophages and dendritic cells are found in perivacscular zones, the choid plexus and the meninges (Vauleon et al., 2010). In gliomas infiltration of CD8+ as well as CD4+ T cells have been reported (Barcia et al., 2009; Mittelbronn et al, 2007). Thus, several types of immune reactions take place in primary brain tumors. In this context Ueda and coworkers have found T cells directed against two glioma antigens (IL13Ra2 and EphA2) within the peripheral blood mononuclear cells from a long surviving patient with an anaplastic astrocytoma (Ueda et al., 2007), showing that an efficient immune reaction in brain tumors is generally possible. Hoverer, the tumor itself shows variety of so-called "tumor escape mechanisms" which are able to dampen tumor antigen-specific immune responses. These include an immunosuppressive environment by secretion of immunosuppressive cytokines and factors such as transforming growth factor beta (TGFβ) (Schneider et al., 2006) and vascular endothelial growth factor (Naumov et al., 2006), which increase the number of tumor infiltrating regulatory T cells and lower the number of cytotoxic killer cells and others. Moreover, the high expression of HLA-4 on gliomas, upon binding to NKG2A7B has a negative effect on T and NK cell activity (Wischhusen et al., 2005). Thus, in GBM the immune reactions are mostly not effective as shown by the unfavorable course of the disease and the high level of recurrences. A specific immunotherapy based on ex vivo generated antigen loaded monocyte-derived dendritic cells may overcome this inhibition leading to a re-induction of an efficient immune reaction against GBM. Such immune responses require antigen recognition. Several groups demonstrated an over-expression of several antigens including a mutated form of the Epidermal Growth Factor Receptor (EGFRvIII), GP 100 and MAGE 1 (Okada et al., 2009; Saikali et al., 2007), which could be used as targets for induction of an antigen specific immune response by priming the MoDC with peptides from these antigens. However, using the whole tumor cell lysate as well as tumor RNA as antigen source may probably reduce the risk of an immune evasion due to clonal expansion of antigen-loss tumor cell variants (Jäger et al, 1996, Vauleon et al., 2010).

Several reports have demonstrated that specific cellular immunotherapy using dendritic cells is capable of inducing a clinical antitumor response within the immunologically privileged brain, confirming that the central nervous system (CNS) is accessible to this kind of immunotherapy. Table I gives an overview on clinical studies with dendritic cell vaccines performed for glioma patients. The published data are based on phase I and II trials as well as on case reports including in total over 200 patients with GBM and over 100 patients with anaplastic astrocytomas or other malignant brain tumors (table 1). Two studies and one case report include children or young adults (Ardon et al., 2010a; Caruso et al., 2004; De Vleeschouwer et al., 2004). The dendritic cells used in these studies were ex-vivo generated from patients blood monocytes using the described standard procedure and primed with peptides, autologous tumor cell lysates or tumor-derived RNA. In two trials dendritic cells were fused with autologous tumor cells (Kikuchi et al., 2001, 2004). Dendritic cells were further matured by exposure to various maturation stimuli (Ardon et al., 2010a, 2010b; De Vleeschouwer et al.; 2008; Kikuchi et al., 2004; Okada et al., 2007; Rutkowski et al., 2004; Yamanaka et al., 2005) or were used without further maturation signals (Caruso et al., 2004; De Vleeschouwer et al., 2004; Kikuchi et al., 2001; Liau et al., 2000, 2005; Yamanaka et al., 2003; Yu et al., 2001, 2004).

Antigen source	type of trial	responses	author
tumor cell lysate + TLR-7 ligand (children)	Phase I	median OS: 12.2 months	Ardon et al., 2010a
tumor cell lysate	Phase I/II	median OS: 24 months	Ardon et al., 2010b
tumor RNA (children, young adults)	Phase I (relapsed brain tumors)	1 PR, 4 SD	Caruso et al., 2004
tumor cell lysate (4-year old child)	case report (recurrent GBM)	CR over 2 years	De Vleeschouver et al. 2004
tumorc ell lysate	Phase I/II (recurrent GBM)	median OS: 9.6 months	De Vleeschouver et al. 2008
tumor cell lysate	case report (recurrent GBM)	median OS: 11 months	Khan & Yaquin, 2006
fusion with tumor cells	Phase I	1 MR, 4 SD, 2 SD	Kikuchi et al., 2001
fusion with tumor cells	Phase I (recurrent GBM)	1 SD in GBM	Kikuchi et al., 2004
peptides	case report (recurrent GBM)	no survival benefit	Liau et al., 2000
tumor cell lysate	Phase I de novo vs. recurrent GBM	median OS: 23.4 months vs. 18.3 months	Liau et al., 2005
tumor cell lysate or irradiated tumor cells	Phase I	2 PR irradiated tumor cells	Okada et al., 2007
tumor cell lysate	Phase I (recurrent GBM)	median OS : 10,5 months	Rutkowski et al., 2004
EGFRvIII antigen	Phase I	median OS: 22.8 months	Sampson et al., 2009
inactivated tumor cells	Phase I	12-/18-months survival: 46%/23%	Walker et al., 2008
tumor cell lysate	Phase I/II vaccine + chemo vs. vaccine alone	2-year-survival 42% vs. 8%	Wheeler et al., 2004
tumor cell lysate	Phase II (de novo vs. recurrent GBM)	median OS: 642 vs. 430 days	Wheeler et al., 2008
tumor cell lysate	Phase I/II	OS: > 200 weeks	Yamanaka et al., 2003
tumor cell lysate + TLR-4 ligand	Phase I/II (recurrent GBM)	median OS: 480 (+ TLR-4 ligand) vs. 400 days	Yamanaka et al., 2005
antigens	Phase I	median OS: 455 days	Yu et al., 2001

Abbreviations: OS: Overall Survival; PR: Partial Remission; CR: Complete Remission; SD: Stable Disease

Table 1. Clinical Studies for GBM treated with autologous DC

For all used methods of MoDC generation a clinical response was described. With the exception of one trial (Yamanaka et al., 2003), where some patients receive an intracerebral injection of dendritic cells, the vaccines were administered intradermally or subcutaneously. The reported side effects were in general low besides one case with grade IV neurotoxicity (Yamanaka et al., 2005). Such reactions are probably based on an excessive inflammatory process within the brain leading to the development of severe edema. Based on our experiences, in those cases, an immune suppressive treatment with corticosteroids has to be accompanied to modulate the highly inflammatory process, which can of course counteract the efficacy of the immune response. The reported major side effects are short term flu like symptoms like fever, headaches and chill. Thus, this treatment is well tolerable without having a negative impact on the quality of life.

Clinical responses based on radiological findings, which were performed for a part of the treated patients (n=108 patients with GBM) consisted of complete remissions (3.7 %), partial remissions (4.6 %), stable diseases (12.9 %) and mixed responses (5.5 %). In some trials a prolongation of the overall survival compared with historical data or non randomized control groups are described (Ardon et al., 2010b; De Vleeschouwer et al., 2008; Liau et al., 2005; Sampson et al., 2009; Rutkowski et al., 2004; Wheeler et al., 2008; Yamanaka et al., 2003, 2005; Yu et al., 2001, 2004). In a pilot trial published by Ardon and coworkers 8 patients with de novo diagnosed GBM received an immunotherapy with tumor cell lysate pulsed dendritic cells after surgery and radio-chemotherapy. The median overall survival was 24 months ranging from 13 to 44 months (Ardon et al., 2010b). Comparable results with a median survival of 22.8 months are reported from Sampson and coworkers using dendritic cells pulsed with the mutated EGFRvIII antigen coupled to KLH (Sampson et al., 2009). Even in patients with relapsed GBM a dendritic cell therapy is reported to be successful. De Vleeschouwer and coworkers reported a case of a 4 year old child, who received a dendritic cell therapy after surgery of recurrence. 2 years after onset of the immune therapy the child still remains in a complete remission (De Vleeschouwer et al., 2004). In a phase I/II trial performed by the same group (De Vleeschouwer et al., 2008) 56 patients were treated with dendritic cells pulsed with tumor cell lysate after surgery of recurrences. The median overall survival was 9.6 months with a 2-year survival rate of 14.8 % after onset of the therapy.

Besides these very promising results the objective clinical responses are low and a lot of patients fail to respond to the therapy. One main reason for low clinical efficacy of MoDC-based anticancer therapies could be due to low IL-12 and high IL-10 production by the MoDC favoring a TH2 rather than a TH1 immune response. In fact, a lot of clinically approved maturation protocols mature MoDC insufficiently in a TH1-polarizing direction (Hildenbrandt et al., 2007, 2008; Mailliard et al., 2004; Zobywalski et al., 2007). Hildenbrandt and coworkers found that the used cytokine cocktail with TNF-a, IL-1ß, IL-6 and PGE2 according to Jonuleit et al. (Jonuleit et al., 1997) induce the phenotypic characteristics of fully matured MoDC expressing high levels of CD83, MHC, costimulatory molecules and CCR7, but secrete high levels of IL-10 and only low levels of IL-12p70 suggesting a preference for a TH2-polarisation (Hildenbrandt et al., 2008). For this reason, improved maturation protocols are required. In this context the activation of Toll-like receptors (TLR) by adding TLR-ligands to the MoDC cultures becomes an interesting alternative to mature monocytes-derived dendritic cells.

2.1.1 Toll-like receptor agonists in maturation protocols for dendritic cells

The expression of certain Toll-like receptors (TLR), a family yet 11 identified transmembrane receptors, expressed on dendritic cells plays a crucial role in the recognition of microbial or viral infections (Medzhitov, 2001). TLR mediated activation of dendritic cells is supposed to be vital for the generation of a TH1 effector response (Schnare et al., 2001). Thus, TLR ligands, which are molecular signatures of microbial or viral infections, may signal the presence of an infection (danger signal), which leads to maturation of DC with a TH1 polarization profile (Akira et al., 2001; Medzhitov, 2001). Interestingly, the TLR 3, a cell surface receptor for double-stranded RNA as well as for the synthetic analogue poly I:C, is predominantly expressed on dendritic cells (Alexopoulou et al., 2001; Muzio et al., 2000). Bone marrow derived immature dendritic cells activated by poly I:C produce large amounts of IL-12 and up-regulate MHC as well as co-stimulatory molecules on their surface (Alexopoulou et al., 2001).

Several TLR are also expressed on monocytes and immature monocytes-derived dendritic cells (Visintin et al., 2001). Moreover, it has been shown that immature MoDC have an increase in TLR 3 expression as compared to monocytes, indicating that in MoDC this TLR may play an important role (Visintin et al., 2001). At the ASCO meeting 2007 our group have show that immature MoDC from patients with GBM when activated by adding the TLR 3 ligand poly I:C switch to a mature phenotype with up-regulation of the maturation marker CD83 and of co-stimulatory molecules. After short time exposure to IFN-γ these matured MoDC were able to produce IL-12p70 at a higher level than IL-10 which clearly favours a TH1 response (Nesselhut et al., 2007). Moreover the IL-12/IL-10 ratio seems to be correlated to clinical response. The use of poly I:C is currently tested in a phase I/II trial and recent published data show that poly I:C boosted DC are safe and have clinical anti tumor activity (Okada et al., 2010). Furthermore, the authors found a correlation between the IL-12 production level and the time to progression (Okada et al, 2010). Comparable data was seen by Yamanaka and coworkers using DC matured with a ligand to TLR 4. Patients who received TLR matured DC had longer survival than those vaccinated with immature DC (Yamanaka et al., 2005). Van Gool et al. reported an improvement of the progression free survival of glioma patients, when the skin at the injection site of the mature DC was pretreated with the TLR-7 agonist Imiquimod (van Gool et al., 2009). Concordant with findings from our group Hildebrandt et al. found that the addition of INF-γ to TLR-agonists can improve the maturation status as well as the TH1 polarization of MoDC (Hildenbrandt et al., 2008). However, most TLR-agonists are not clinically approved and therefore are not allowed to be used in clinical trials, yet. In this context it is interesting, that Hildenbrandt et al. could show that IFN-γ when added to the clinical-grade cytokine cocktail (Jonuleit et al., 1997) induces the production of lower levels of IL-10 and higher levels of IL-12p70, demonstrating the TH1-prolarizing capacity of this cytokine (Hildenbrandt et al., 2008).

2.1.2 Impact of cancer induced immune suppression on the efficacy of denditic cell therapy

During the last years several investigations show an increasing evidence of a strong association between chronic infection, inflammation and cancer development as well as tumor progression (Balkwill & Mantovani, 2001; Coussens & Werb, 2002). Inflammation is a physiological process occurring after tissue damage, infections caused by microbial or viral pathogen, chemical irritation or wounding (Philipp et al., 2004.) In fact, many of the same inflammatory mediators that are secreted by wounds are found in the tumor microenvironment. Immune cells infiltrate into the developing tumor site and establish an inflammatory tumor microenvironment (Balkwill & Mantovani, 2001; Whiteside, 2008). As wound healing is self limited cancer can be described as "wounds that do not heal" (Dvorak,

1986). Meanwhile it is well established that the tumor per se can change the immunological balance into an inflammatory microenvironment by release of certain cytokines and chemokines leading not only to the promotion of tumor growth but also to the inhibition of an efficient immune response. This may be one of the reasons for an unsuccessful immunotherapy for GBM patients based on dendritic cells (Couldwell et al., 1991, Nitta et al., 1994, Hishii et al, 1995, Weller & Fontana, 1995). An example is the intratumoral expression of TGF-ß, which can suppress an adaptive antigen specific immune response. Moreover, TGF- ß expression was shown to be a predictive factor for the clinical outcome in vaccinated patients (Liau et al., 2005).

Taken together, an efficient induction of a clinical antitumor response requires both a polarization of MoDC in a TH1 direction as well as a change of the immune suppressive tumor associated microenvironment. Beside several cytokines which promote an immune suppressive microenvironment, regulatory T cells (T-reg), which are required for maintaining immunological self tolerance (Sakaguchi, 2005), play an important role in the regulation of an immune response and thus may limit an antigen specific immune response in cancer (Borsellino et al. 2007; Deaglio et al. 2007; Mandapathil et a., 2009; Nizar et al, 2009).

Several subpopulations of T-reg have been described (Sakaguchi, 2005; Seddiki et al., 2006). Most commonly used is the CD4+, CD25 $+^{high}$, CD127-/dim phenotype with intracellular expression of the transcription factor FoxP3 (Seddiki et al., 2006). More recently, a sub-population of CD39+ T-reg was described (Borsellino et al. 2007; Deaglio et al., 2007). CD39 belongs to the family of ecto-nucleoside triphosphate-diphosphatehydrolase-1 and hydrolyses extracellular ATP. This leads to a pericellular accumulation of the nucleoside adenosine, which is known to play an important role in inhibiting effector functions of activated T cells (Borsellino et al. 2007, Huang et al., 1997). The authors propose that the immune suppressive activity of T-reg is partly due to this enzymatic activity of CD39 and thus may play a crucial role in inhibition of antigen specific T cell response. Woo et al. were the first who reported an increased percentage of T-reg cells in tumor infiltrating lymphocytes in non-small-cell-lung cancer and ovarian cancer (Woo et al., 2001). Meanwhile accumulating T-reg cells are detected in the tumor microenvironment, ascites as well as in the peripheral blood of cancer patients and have been associated with poor prognosis (Beyer & Schultze 2010; Nizar et al. 2009, Wolf et al., 2003).

Our group have shown that subpopulations of T-reg characterized by a CD4+, CD25 $+^{high}$ as well as CD127-/dim or CD39+ expression profile can be detected in the peripheral blood of healthy donors, tumor free patients as well as patient with tumor load (Neßelhut et al., 2009). The percentage of T-reg was significantly higher in cancer patients, including patients with GBM, as compared to healthy donors. Moreover, patients with advanced tumors show higher levels of T-reg cells as compared to patients with no evidence of disease. Several other groups reported an increase of T-reg cells in GBM patients in peripheral blood as well as within the tumor microenvironment (Fecci et al., 2006a; Grauer et al., 2007; Hussain et al., 2006, El Andaloussi et al., 2006). Measurement of T-reg cells along with an immune therapy may be useful to discriminate between non- responding and responding patients. In fact, first analysis of our group show that rising T-reg numbers are partly associated with lack of clinical response to a dendritic cell therapy in patients with GBM. Thus, the elimination of excessive T-reg cell numbers seems to be a promising approach to improve the efficacy of a dendritic cell based immune therapy.

Several chemotherapeutical agents have immune stimulatory and T-reg modulating effects when used at lower dosages with reduced toxic effects (Nizar et al., 2009). Beside this option there are some reagents which target T-reg directly through recognition of CD25 (Morse et al., 2008, Fecci 2006 b) or through CTLA-4 blockade (Ribas et al., 2009). Some of these approaches are tested in association with DC therapy in cancer (Chiringelli et al, 2004, Ribas et al. 2009, Morse et al., 2008) including GBM (Fecci ate al. 2006 b, Maes et al., 2009). Interestingly, in a rat glioma model low dose temozolamide could also decrease the number of T-reg cells. (Banissi et al, 2009). In this context it is noteworthy that Wheeler et al. show that GBM patients, who responded to DC therapy, also exhibited a better response to a following chemotherapy (Wheeler et al., 2004). In the study published by Ardon et al. immunotherapy based on dendritic cells started after radio-chemotherapy (Ardon et al., 2010b). One can suppose that the chemotherapy with temozolamide has lead to a decrease of T-reg cells and thus enhanced the immunological response causing the high 24 months median survival for the treated patients. The combination of dendritic cell therapy and adjuvant chemotherapy was also tested in malignant astrocytomas (Walker et al., 2008). The 12- and 18-months survival rates were 46% and 23%, respectively. Depletion or inhibition of T-reg may thus improve the efficacy of dendritic cell based therapy.

2.1.3 Newcastle disease virus in treatment of GBM; a tool for improving DC therapy

Besides dendritic cell therapy another promising approach for the treatment of malignant brain tumors is the treatment with replication-selective viruses, also called oncolytic viruses. This is based on the fact that most tumor cells are more or less unable of an effective virus defense. This approach is also known as virotherapy. The application of viruses for cancer treatment is based on reports since the beginning of the 20th century on temporary improvement of cancer following natural viral infections or vaccinations against viral diseases. (DePace 1912). Meanwhile several replication competent viruses (mainly herpes and adenoviruses) were tested in vitro, in animal models as well as in phase I/II clinical trials for treatment of malignant brain tumors (Shah et al., 2003; Rainov & Ren, 2003; Wollmann et al., 2005). However, the viruses have to be genetically modified in a way that makes sure that they selectively infect and replicate in tumor cells. Within the viruses tested for human anticancer treatment the Newcastle Disease Virus (NDV), an enveloped poultry virus with single strained RNA as genetic material, seems to be one of the most promising candidates. NDV is not a pathogen for humans, and is absolutely harmless causing only mild flu-like symptoms or conjunctivitis in the worst of cases (Lorence et al., 2001; Reichard et al., 1992). NDV shows a natural distinct tropism for cancer cells. Cancer cells infected with NDV can be killed directly by the virus within a short time after infection, whereas normal infected cells are not lysed by NDV.

As described earlier tumor cell lysate may be the better antigen source for priming of dendritc cells because it contains the whole antigen repertoire of the tumor. However, it has to be taken in mind that most of the antigens expressed in tumors are poor inducers of immune response and are often recognized by the immune system as self antigens (Vergati et al., 2010). Opposed to this adjuvant active specific immunization based on tumor cells modified with a low pathogenic strain of the NDV has been reported to achieve sustained immune responses in patients with advanced colonic cancer and liver metastasis (Lehner et al., 1990 Schulze et al., 2009). NDV can have lytic activity on tumor cells directly as well as

immune stimulating properties that affect both innate and adaptive immune responses. Infection of tumor cells with live NDV results in a potent up-regulation of cell adhesion molecules on the tumor cells surface (Lehner et al. 190; Wasburn et al., 2002). Moreover, NDV infection of tumor cells leads to an improved tumor cell / T cell interaction and an increased T cell co-stimulatory activity (Ertel et al., 1993; Termeer et al., 2000). Expression of viral proteins on the tumor cell surface and presence of virus derived pathogen-associated molecular patterns (e.g. double-stranded RNA) result in breaking of host tolerance towards the tumor in vitro (Bai et al., 2002). The T cell stimulatory action of dendritic cells pulsed with lysates of NDV infected tumor cells as well as the antitumor cytotoxicity of macrophages and monocytes is increased (Schirrmacher et al., 2000; Washburn et al., 2003; Zeng et al., 2002). Finally, NDV induces an increased production of various cytokines, e.g. Interferon-α as well as chemokines, influencing the migration, the activation status and cytotoxic activity of various immune cells (Lokuta et al., 1996; Schirrmacher 2005, Schlag et al., 1992). Clinical phase I and II studies in various tumor entities have proven the safety of active specific immunization with NDV-modified tumor cells. A detailed description of the mechanisms of action of NDV modified tumor cell vaccines and results from other studies in cancer patients were reviewed by Schirrmacher (Schirrmacher, 2005).
In malignant brain tumors case reports as well as clinical phase I/II studies have shown that treatment with intravenously applied NDV as well as with vaccines utilizing NDV modified tumor cells can induce a clinical anti-tumor response in malignant brain tumors with objective clinical responses as well as with a trend towards improvement of overall survival (Csatary & Bakacs, 1999, Csatary et al., 2004; Freeman et al., 2005; Schneider et al., 2001; Wagner et al., 2006). Recent results from our group show that a therapy with dendritic cells in combination with the NDV virotherapy may improve the clinical anti-tumor response in patients with GBM (Neßelhut et al., 2007, 2011). Patients were pre-treated with intravenously administration of NDV. Dendritic cells were primed with NDV modified tumor cells or with NDV alone in patient with tumor recurrence. When tested in vitro, NDV primed MoDC of such treated patients induce the activation of autologous CD8+ T cells with release of IFN-γ. This leads to the hypothesis that, if viral antigens are expressed on the tumor cell surface, a NDV specific dendritic cell based therapy may lead to the induction of NDV specific CD8+ T cells and thus to the induction of a specific immune response against the virus infected cancer cell (Neßelhut et al., 2011).

3. Conclusion

Taken together a dendritic cell therapy as well as the NDV virotherapy have shown clinical efficacy and have been proven to be safe with only minimal side-effects. Especially patients with primary resistance against temozolamide caused by the MGMT status could benefit from such alternative therapy strategies. Furthermore, new insights in the nature and biology of glioma tumor stem cells may improve an immunological concept by using tumor stem cell specific antigens as targets in dendritic cell therapy as it was recently shown (Pellegatta et al., 2006, Stupp & Hegi, , Xu et al., 2009). An immunotherapy with dendritic cells can either be used in adjuvant, curative settings to avoid or delay tumor recurrence or in palliative settings to keep the disease stable offering the patients a chance for prolonged overall survival. Based on current results it has to be supposed that patients with minor tumor burden or no evidence of disease are the best candidates for an immunotherapy.

The main reasons for a deficient anti-tumor immune response are most likely the immune suppressive tumor microenvironment and the up-regulation of immune suppressive cells. Thus, a combination with therapies, which can modulate the tumor microenvironment as well as lower the percentage of the immune suppressive T-reg cells should be considered as treatment prior to or in combination with dendritic cell based immune therapy. Additionally, glioma cells are considered to be poor antigen-presenting cells. In order to promote antigen-specific recognition and avidity of potential anti-tumor effector cells, the biology of antigens expressed by malignant glioma cells must be taken into consideration while designing protocols for programming autologous dendritic cells and defining the appropriate patient. For example, Prins and coworkers could recently shown that the gene expression profile of the individual glioma can identify a subgroup of patients, that may be more responsive to dendritic cell based immunotherapy (Prins et al., 2011). In this context the combination with NDV seems to be a promising tool to modify tumor cells in vitro as well as in vivo to a more immunogenic phenotype resulting in better immune recognition as well as in better immune response.
The encouraging results of phase I/II trials have to be confirmed in phase III studies with special emphasis on the maturation protocols for improvement of TH1-polarisation of dendritic cells, which so far are still a matter of controversial discussion. Moreover, the optimal antigen source, cell number of injected dendritic cells, frequency of vaccinations as well as the right time point for vaccination are still not fully defined. Future studies should also involve an immune monitoring of vaccinated patients. Immune monitoring methods can include quantification of CD8+ and CD4+ T cells generated in response to the antigen or measurement of the functional status of T cells analyzed by cytokine production. However, it has to be taken into account that in vitro measurement of T cell responses do not always correlate with clinical outcome (Carpentier & Meng, 2006). Thus, the best immunological monitoring strategy is still intensively debated.
Finally, clinical trials for the evaluation of immune therapeutical approaches have to be designed in a different way as for chemotherapeutical drugs. In this context the overall survival rather than the reduction of tumor burden is probably the best primary endpoint. Based on such a study design Provenge™, an immunological treatment based on antigen presenting cells, received the FDA approval for treatment of hormone refractory prostate cancer in spring 2010.

4. References

Akira, S., Takeda, K. & Kaisho, T. (2001). Toll-like receptors: critical proteins linking innate and acquired immunity. *Nature Immunology*, Vol. 2, No. 8, (Aug 2001), pp. 675-680

Alexopoulou, L, Czopik-Holt, A, Medzhitov, R & Flavell, R (2001). Recognition of double stranded RNA and activation of NF-kb by Toll-like receptor 3. *Nature*, Vol. 413, No. 6857, (Oct 2001), pp. 732-738

Ardon, H., De Vleeschouwer, S., Van Calenbergh, F, Claes, L., Kramm, CM. et al. (2010a). Adjuvant dendritic cell-based tumour vaccination for children with malignant brain tumours. *Pediatric Blood and Cancer*, Vol. 54, No. 4, (April 2010), pp. 519–525

Ardon, H., Van Gool, S., Lopes IS. Maes, W., Sciot, R. et al. (2010b). Integration of autologous dendritic cell-based immunotherapy in the primary treatment for patients with newly diagnosed glioblastoma multiforme: a pilot study. *Journal of Neurooncology*, Vol. 99, No. 2, (Sep 2010), pp. 261–272

Bai, L., Koopmann, J., Fiola, C., Fournier, P. & Schirrmacher, V. (2002). Dendritic cells pulsed with viral oncolysates potently stimulate autologous T cells from cancer patients. *International Journal of Oncology*, Vol. 21, No. 4, (Oct 2002), pp. 685-694

Balkwill, F. & Mantovani, A. (2001). Inflammation and cancer: back to Virchow? *Lancet*, Vol. 357, No. 9255, (Feb 2001), pp. 539-545

Banchereau, J. & Steinman, RM. (1998). Dendritic cells and the control of immunity. *Nature*, Vol. 392, No. 6673, (Mar 1998), pp. 245-252

Banissi C., Chiringhelli F., Chen, L. & Carpentier, AF. (2009). Treg depletion with a low-dose metronomic temozolomide regimen in a rat glioma model. *Cancer Immunology Immunotherapy*, Vol. 58, No. 10, (Oct 2009), pp. 1627–1634

Barcia, C., Gomez, A., Gallego-Sanchez, JM., Perez-Vallés, A., Castro, MG. et al. (2009). Infiltrating CTLs in human glioblastoma establish immunological synapses with tumorigenic cells. *American Journal of Pathology*, Vol. 175, No. 2, (Aug 2009), pp. 786-789

Beyer, M. & Schultze, JL. (2006). Regulatory T cells in cancer. *Blood*, Vol. 108, No. 3, (Aug 2006), pp. 804-811

Borsellino, G., Kleinewietfeld, M., Di Mitri, D., Sternjak, A,, Diamantini, A. et al. (2007). Expression of ectonucleotidase CD39 by Foxp3+ Treg cells: hydrolysis of extracellular ATP and immune suppression. *Blood*, Vol. 110, N0. 4, (Aug 2007), pp. 1225-1232

Buckner, JC. (2003). Factors influencing survival in high-grade gliomas. *Seminars in Oncology*, Vol. 30, Suppl. 19, pp. 10-14

Carpentier, AF. & Meng, Y. (2006). Recent advances in immunotherapy for human glioma. *Current Opinion Oncology*, Vol. 18, No. 6, (Nov 2006), pp. 631-636

Caruso, DA., Orme, LM., Neale, AM., Radcliff, FJ., Amor, GM. et al. (2004). Results of a phase 1 study utilizing monocyte-derived dendritic cells pulsed with tumor RNA in children and young adults with brain cancer. *Journal of Neurooncology*, Vol. 6, No. 3, (Jul 2004), pp. 236–246

Chang, CH., Horton, J, Schoenfeld, D., Salazer, O., Perez-Tamayo, R. et al. (1983). Comparison of postoperative radiotherapy and combined postoperative radiotherapy and chemotherapy in the multidisciplinary management of malignant gliomas: a joint Radiaton Therapy Oncology Group and Eastern Cooperative Oncology Group study. *Cancer*, Vol. 52, pp. 997-1007

Couldwell, WT., Dore-Duffy, P., Apuzzo, MLJ. & Antel, JP. (1991). Malignant glioma modulation of immune function: relative contribution of different soluble factors. *Journal of Neuroimmunology*, Vol. 33, No. 2, (Aug 1991), pp. 89–96

Coussens, LM. & Werb, Z. (2002). Inflammation and cancer. *Nature*, Vol. 420, No. 6917), (Dec 2002), pp. 860-867

Csatary, LK. & Bakacs, T. (1999). Newcastle disease virus vaccine (MTH-68/H) in a patient with high-grade glioblastoma. *Jama*, Vol. 281, No. 17, (May 1999), pp. 1588-1589

Csatary, LK., Gosztonyi, G., Szeberenyi, J., Fabian, Z., Liszka, V. et al. (2004). MTH-68/H oncolytic viral treatment in human high-grade gliomas. *Journal of Neurooncology*, Vol. 67, No. 1-2, (Mar-Apr), pp. 83-93

Curran, WJ. Jr., Scott, CB., Horton, J., Nelson, JS., Weinstein, AS. et al. (1993). Recursive portioning analysis of prognostic factors in three Radiation Therapy Oncology

Group malignant glioma trials. *Journal of National Cancer Institute*, Vol. 85, No. 9, (May 1993), pp. 704-710

Deaglio, S., Dwyer, KM., Gao,. W, Friedman, D., Usheva, A., et al. (2007). Adenosine generation catalyzed by CD39 and CD73 expressed on regulatory T cells mediates immune suppression. *Journal of Experimental Medicine*, Vol. 204, No. 6, (Jun 2007), pp. 1257-65

De Angelis, LM. (2001). Brain tumors. *New England Journal of Medicine*, Vol., 344, No. 2, (Jan 2001), pp. 114-123

De Pace, NG. (1912). Sulla scomparsa di un enorme cancro vegetante del callo dell`utero senza cura chirurgica. *Ginecologia*, Vol. 9, (1912), pp. 82-88

De Vleeschouwer, S., Van Calenbergh, F., Demaerel, P., Flamen, P., Rutkowski, S. et al. (2004). Transient local response and persistent tumor control in a child with recurrent malignant glioma: treatment with combination therapy including dendritic cell therapy: case report. *Journal of Neurosurgery*, Vol. 100, No. 5, (May 2004), pp. 492–497

De Vleeschouwer, S., Fieuws, S, Rutkowski, S. Van Calenbergh, F., Van Loon, J. et al. (2008). Postoperative adjuvant dendritic cell-based immunotherapy in patients with relapsed glioblastoma multiforme. *Clinical Cancer Research*, Vol. 14, No. 10, (May 2008), pp. 3098–3104

Dvorak, HF. (1986). Tumors: wounds that do not heal. Similarities between tumor stroma generation and wound healing. *New England Journal of Medicine*, Vol. 315, No. 26, (Dec 1986), pp. 1650-1659

Dietz, AB., Bulur, PA., Knutson, GJ., Matasic, R. & Vuk-Pavlovic, S. (2000). Maturation of human monocyte-derived dendritic cells studied by microarray hybridization. *Biochem Biophys Res Commun*, Vol. 275, No. 3, (Sep 2000), pp. 731-738

El Andaloussi, A & Lesniak, MS. (2006). An increase in CD4+ CD25+FOXP3+ regulatory T cells in tumor-infiltrating lymphocytes of human glioblastoma multiforme. *Neurooncology*, Vol. 8, No. 3, (Jul 2006), pp. 234–243

Engleman, EG. (2003). Dendritic cell-based cancer immunotherapy. *Seminars in Oncology*, Vol. 30, No. 3, (Jun 2003), pp. 23-29

Ertel, C., Millar, NS., Emmerson, PT., Schirrmacher, V. & von Hoegen, P. (1993). Viral hemaglutinin augments peptide-specific cytotoxic T cell responses. *European Journal of Immunology*, Vol. 23, No. 10, (Oct 1993), pp. 2592-2596

Fecci, PE., Mitchell, DA., Whitesides JF., Xie, W., Friedmann, AH. et al. (2006). Increased regulatory T-cell fraction amidst a diminished CD4 compartment explains cellular immune defects in patients with malignant glioma. *Cancer Research*, Vol. 66, No. 6, (Mar 2006), pp. 3294–3302

Fecci, PE., Sweeney, AE., Grossi, PM., Nair, SK., Learn, CA. et al. (2006). Systemic anti-CD25 monoclonal antibody administration safely enhances immunity in murine glioma without eliminating regulatory T cells. *Clinical Cancer Research*, Vol. 12, No. 14, (Jul 2006), pp. 4294-4305

Freeman, AI., Zackay-Rones, Z., Gomori, JM., Linetsky, E., Rasooly, L. et al. (2005). Phase I/II trial of intravenous NDV-HUJ oncolytic virus in recurrent glioblastoma multiforme. *Molecular Therapy*, Vol. 13, No. 1, (Jan 2005), pp. 221-228

Ghiringhelli, F., Larmonier, N., Schmitt, E., Parcellier, A., Cathelin, D. et al. (2004). CD4+CD25+ regulatory T cells suppress tumor immunity but are sensitive to cyclophosphamide which allows immunotherapy of established tumors to be curative. *European Journal of Immunology*, Vol. 34, No. 2, (Feb 2004), pp. 336–344

Gilboa, E. (2007). DC-based cancer vaccines. *Journal of Clinical Investigation*, Vol. 117, No. 5, (May 2007), pp. 1195-1203

Grauer, OM., Nierkens, S., Bennink, E., Toonen, LW., Boon, L. et al. (2007). CD4+FoxP3+ regulatory T cells gradually accumulate in gliomas during tumor growth and efficiently suppress antiglioma immune responses in vivo. *International Journal of Cancer*, Vol. 121, No. 1, (Jul 2007), pp. 95-105

Green, SB., Byar, DP., Walker, MD., Pistenmaa, DA., Alexander, E.Jr. et al. (1983). Comparisons of carmustine, procarbazine, and high-dose methylprednisolone as additions to surgery and radiotherapy for the treatment of malignant glioma. *Cancer Treat Rep*, Vol. 67, No.2, (Feb 1983), pp. 121-132

Hildenbrand, B., Sauer, B., Kalis, O., Stoll, C., Freudenberg, MA. et al. (2007). Immunotherapy of patients with hormone-refractory prostate carcinoma pre-treated with interferon-gamma and vaccinated with autologous PSA-peptide loaded dendritic cells - A pilot study. *Prostate*, Vol. 67, No. 2, (Apr 2007), pp. 500-508

Hildenbrand, B., Lorenzen, D., Sauer, B., Hertkorn, C., Freudenberg MA. et al. (2008). IFN-g enhances TH1 polarization of monocyte-derived dendritic cells matured with clinical-grade cytokines using serum-free conditions. *Anticancer Research*, Vol. 28, No. 3A, (May-Jun 2008), pp. 1467-1476

Hishii, M., Nitta, T., Ishida, H., Ebato, M., Kurosu,. A. et al. (1995). Human glioma derived interleukin-10 inhibits antitumor immune responses in vitro. *Neurosurgery*, Vol. 37, No. 6, (Dec 1995), pp. 1160–1166

Huang, S., Apasov, S., Koshuba, M. & Sitkowski, M. (1997). Role of A2a extracellular adenosine receptor-mediated signaling in adenosine-mediated inhibition of T-cell activation and expansion. *Blood*, Vol. 90, No. 4, (Aug 1997), pp. 1600-1610

Hussain, SF., Yang, D., Suki, D., Grimm, E. & Heimberger, AB. (2006). Innate immune functions of microglia isolated from human glioma patients. *Journal of Translational Medicine*, Vol. 4, Article ID, (Jul 2006), pp 15

Jäger, E., Ringhoffer, M., Karbach, J., Arand, M., Oesch, F. & Knuth, A. (1996). Inverse relationship of melanocyte differentiation antigen expression in melanoma tissues and CD8+ cytotoxic-T-cell responses: evidence of immune selection of antigen-loss variants in vivo. *International Journal of Cancer*, Vol. 66, No. 4, (May 1996), pp. 470-476

Janeway, CA., Shlomchik, MJ., Travers, P. & Walport, M. (2004). Using the immune response to attack tumors, In: *Immunobiology 6th edn.*, Janeway CA, Shlomchik MJ, Travers P, Walport J (eds), pp 630-642, Garland Science, New York,

Jonuleit, H., Kuhn U, Muller G, Steinbrink, K., Paragnik L. et al. (1997). Pro-inflammatory cytokines and prostaglandins induce maturation of potent immunostimulatory dendritic cells under fetal calf serum- free conditions. *European Journal of Immunology*, Vol. 27, No. 12, (Dec 1997), pp. 3135–3142

Kikuchi, T., Akasaki, Y., Irie, M., Homma, S., Abe, T. & Ohno,T. (2001). Results of a phase I clinical trial of vaccination of glioma patients with fusions of dendritic and glioma cells. *Cancer Immunology Immunotherapy*, Vol. 50, No. 7, (Sep 2001), pp. 337–344

Kikuchi, T., Akasaki, Y., Abe, T., Fukuda, T., Saotome, H. et al. (2004). Vaccination of glioma patients with fusions of dendritic and glioma cells and recombinant human interleukin 12. *Journal of Immunotherapy*, Vol. 27, No. 6, (Nov-Dec 2004), pp. 452–459

Khan, JA. & Yaquin, S. (2006). Dendritic cell therapy with improved outcome in glioma multiforme-a case report. J Zhejiang Univ Science B, Vol. 7; No. 2, (Feb 2006), pp. 114-117

Lai, A., Tran, A., Nghiemphu, PL., Pope, WB., Solis, OE. et al. (2010). Phase II study of bevacizumab plus temozolomide during and after radiation therapy for patients with newly diagnosed glioblastoma multiforme. *Journal of Clinical Oncology*, Vol. 29, No. 2, (Jan 2010), pp. 142-148

Lehner, B., Schlag, P., Liebrich, W. & Schirrmacher, V. (1990). Postoperative active specific immunization in curatively resected colorectal cancer patients with a virus-modified autologous tumor cell vaccine. *Cancer Immunology Immunotherapy*, Vol. 32, No. 3, pp. 173-178

Liau, LM., Black, KL., Martin NA., Sykes, SN., Bronstein JM. et al. (2000). Treatment of a patient by vaccination with autologous dendritic cells pulsed with allogeneic major histocompatibility complex class I matched tumor peptides. Case report. *Neurosurgical Focus*, Vol. 9, No. 6, (Dec 2000), p. e8

Liau, LM., Prins, RM., Kiertscher, SM., Odesa, SK., Kremen, TJ. et al. (2005). Dendritic cell vaccination in glioblastoma patients induces systemic and intracranial T-cell responses modulated by the local central nervous system tumor microenvironment. *Clinical Cancer Research*, Vol. 11, No. 15, (Aug 2005), pp. 5515–5525

Liu, G., Yuan, X., Zeng, Z., Tunici, P., Ng, H. et al. (2006). Analysis of gene expression and chemoresistance of CD133+ cancer stem cells in glioblastoma. *Mol Cancer*, Vol. 5, (Dec 2006), pp. 67

Lokuta, MA., Maher, J., Noe, KH., Pitha, PM., Shin, ML. & Shin, HS. (1996). Mechanisms of murine RANTES chemokine gene induction by Newcastle disease virus. *J Biol Chem*, Vol. 271, No. 23, (Jan 1996), pp. 13731-13738

Lorence, RM., Roberts, MS., Groene, WS. & Rabin, H. (2001). Replication-competent, oncolytic Newcastle disease virus for cancer therapy. In: *Replication competent viruses for cancer therapy*, Vol. 22, Hernaiz-Driever, Rabkin (eds), pp. 160-182, Karger, Basel

Maes, W., Rosas, G., Verbinnen, B. Boon, L., De Vleeschouwer, S., Ceuppens, JL. & Van Gool, SW. (2009). DC vaccination with anti-CD25 treatment leads to long-term immunity against experimental glioma. *Neurooncology*, Vol. 11, No. 5, (Oct 2009), pp. 529-542

Mandapathil, M., Hilldorfer, B., Szczepanski, MJ., Czystowska, M., Szajnik, M. et al. (2009). Generation and accumulation of immunosuppressive adenosine by human CD4+CD25highFOXP3+ regulatory T cells. *J Biol Chem*, Vol. 285, No. 10, (Mar 2009), pp. 7176-7186

Mailliard, RB., Wankowicz-Kalinska, A., Cai, Q., Wesa, A., Hilkens, CM. et al. (2004). A-Type-1 polarized dendritic cells: A novel immunization tool with optimized CTL-inducing activity. *Cancer Research*, Vol. 64, No. 17, (Sep 2004), pp. 934-5937

Medzhitov, R. (2001). Toll-like receptors and innate immunity. *Nat Rev Immunol*, Vol. 1, No. 2(Nov 2001), pp. 135-45

Mittelbronn, M. Simon, P., Löffler, C., Capper, D., Bunz, B. et al. (2007). Elevated HLAE levels in human glioblastomas but not in grade I to III astrocytomas correlate with infiltrating CD8+ cells. *Journal of Neuroimmunology,* Vol. 189, No. 1-2, (Sep 2007), pp. 50–58

Morse, MA., Mosca, P., Clay, TM. & Lyerly, HK. (2002). Dendritic cell maturation in active immunotherapy strategies. *Expert Opin Biol Ther,* Vol. 2, No. 1, (Jan 2002), pp. 35-43

Morse, MA., Hobeika, AC., Osada, T., Serra, D., Niedzwiecki, D. et al. (2008). Depletion of human regulatory T cells specifically enhances antigen-specific immune responses to cancer vaccines. *Blood,* Vol. 112, No. 3, (Aug 2008), pp. 610-618

Muzio M., Bosisio, D., Polentarutti, N., D´amico, G., Stoppacciaro, A. at al. (2000). Differential expression and regulation of Toll-like receptors (TLR) in human leukocytes: selective expression of TLR3 in dendritic cells. *Journal of Immunology,* Vol. 164, No. 1, (Jun 2000), pp. 5998-6004

Naumov, GN., Bender, E., Zurakowski, D., Kang, SY., Sampson, D. et al. (2006). A model of human tumor dormancy: an angiogenic switch from the angiogenic phenotype. *Journal National Cancer Institute,* Vol. 98, No.5, (Mar 2006), pp. 316-325

Neßelhut, J., Neßelhut, T., Chang, R., Marx, D., Brockmann, W. et al. (2007). Dendritic cell therapy in glioblastoma multiforme. *Journal of Clinical Oncology* 25 (18S) suppl: abstract 3065, Chicago, May-Jun 2007

Neßelhut, J., Lorenzen, D., Marx, D., Chang, RY., Matthes, C. et al. (2009). Cellular immune suppression in cancer patients and its implication for dendritic cell therapy. *Journal of Clinical Oncology* 27 (15s) suppl: abstract 3028, Orlando, May-Jun 2009

Neßelhut, J., Marx, D., Lorenzen, D., Cillien, N., Goebel, W. et al. (2011). Improvement of dendritic cell therapy in glioblastoma multiforme WHO IV by Newcastle disease virus. Abstract 2508, Chicago, June 2011 (in progress)

Nestle, FQ. (2000). Dendritic cell vaccination for cancer therapy. *Oncogene,* Vol. 19, No. 56, (Dec 2000), pp. 6673-6679

Newlands, ES., Stevens, MFG., Wedge, SR., Wheelhouse, RT. & Brock, C. (1997). Temozolomide: a review of its discovery, chemical properties, pre-clinical development and clinical trials. *Cancer Treat Rev,* Vol. 23, No. 1, (Jan 1997), pp. 35-61

Nitta, T., Hishii, M., Sato, K. & Okumura, K. (1994). Selective expression of interleukin-10 gene within glioblastoma multiforme. *Brain Research,* Vol. 649, No. 1-2, (Jun 1994), pp. 122–128

Nizai S., Cupier J., Meyer, B., Bodman-Smith, M., Galustian C. et al. (2009). T-regulatory cell modulation: the future of cancer immunotherapy? *British Journal of Cancer, Vol.* 100, No. 11, (Jun 2009), pp. 1697-1703

Okada, H., Lieberman, FS., Walter, KA., Lunsford, LD., Kondziolka, DS. et al. (2007). Autologous glioma cell vaccine admixed with interleukin-4 gene transfected fibroblasts in the treatment of patients with malignant gliomas. *Journal of Translational Medicine,* Vol. 19, No. 5, (Dec 2007), pp. 67

Okada, H., Kohanbash, G., Zhu, X., Kastenhuber, ER., Hoji, A. et al. (2009). Immunotherapeutic approaches for glioma. *Critical Reviews in Immunology,* Vol. 29, No. 1, pp. 1-42

Okada H., Kalinski P., Ueda R., Hoji, A., Kohanbah G. et al. (2011). Induction of CD8+ T-cell responses against novel glioma-associated antigen peptides and clinical activity by vaccinations with (alpha)-type 1 polarized dendritic cells and polyinosinic-polycytidylic acid stabilized by lysine and carboxymethylcellulose in patients with recurrent malignant glioma. *Journal of Clinical Oncology*, Vol. 29, No. 3, (Jan 2011), pp. 330-336

Pellegatta, S., Poliani, PL., Corno, D., Menghi, F., Ghielmetti, F. et al. (2006). Neurospheres enriched in cancer stem-like cells are highly effective in eliciting a dendritic cell-mediated immune response against malignant gliomas. *Cancer Research*, Vol. 66, No. 21, (Nov 2006), pp. 10247-10252

Peters. JH., Gieseler, R., Thiele, B. & Steinbach, F. (1996). Dendritic cells: from ontogenetic orphans to myelomonocytic descendants. *Immunology Today*, Vol. 17, No. 6, (Jun 1996), pp. 273

Philip, M., Rowley, DA. & Schreiber, H. (2004). Inflammation as a tumor promoter in cancer induction. *Semin Cancer Biol*, Vol. 14, No. 6, (Dec 2004), pp. 433-439

Prins, RM., Soto, H., Konkankit, V., Odesa, SK., Eskin, A. et al. (2011). Gene expression profile correlates with T-cell infiltration and relative survival in glioblastoma patients vaccinated with dendritic cell immunotherapy. *Clinical Cancer Research*, Vol. 17, No. 6, (Mar 2011), pp. 1603-1615

Rainov, NG. & Ren, H. (2003). Oncolytic viruses for treatment of malignant brain tumors. *Acta Neurochir* Suppl. 88, pp. 113-123

Reichard, KW., Lorence, RM., Cascino, CJ., Peeples, ME., Walter, RJ. et al. (1992). Newcastle disease virus selectively kills human tumor cells. *J Surg Res*, Vol. 52, No. 5, (May 1992), pp. 448-453

Ribas, A. Comin-Anduix, B., Chmielowski, B., Jalil, J., de la Rocha, P. et al. (2009). Dendritic cell vaccination combined with CTLA4 blockade in patients with metastatic melanoma. *Clinical Cancer Research*, Vol. 15, No. 19, (Oct 2009), pp. 6267–6276

Romani, N., Reider, D. Heuer, M. et al. (1996). Generation of mature dendritic cells from human blood. An improved method with special regard to clinical applicability. *Journal of Immunology Methods*, Vol. 196, No. 2, (Sep 1996), pp. 1137-1151

Rouard, H., Marquet, J., Léon, A., Maison, P., Haioun, C. et al. (2002). IL-12 secreting dendritic cells are required for optimum activation of human secondary lymphoid tissue T cells. *Journal of Immunotherapy*, Vol. 25, No. 4, (Jul-Aug 2002), pp. 324-333

Rutkowski, S., De Vleeschouwer, S., Kaempgen, E., Wolff, JE., Kühl, J. et al. (2004). Surgery and adjuvant dendritic cell-based tumour vaccination for patients with relapsed malignant glioma, a feasibility study. *British Journal of Cancer*, Vol. 91, No. 9, (Nov 2004), pp. 1656-1662

Sakaguchi, S. (2005). Naturally arising Foxp3-expressing CD25+CD4+ regulatory T cells in immunological tolerance to self and non-self. *Nature Immunology*, Vol. 6, No. 4, (Apr 2005), pp. 345-352

Saikali, S., Avril, T., Collet, B., Hamlat, A., Bansard, JY. et al. (2007). Expression of nine tumour antigens in a series of human glioblastoma multiforme: interest of EGFRvIII, IL-13Rα2, gp100 and TRP-2 for immunotherapy. *Journal of Neurooncology*, Vol. 81, No. 2, (Jan 2007), pp. 139–148

Sallusto, F. & Lanzavecchia, A. (1994). Efficient presentation of soluble antigen by cultured human dendritic cells is maintained by granulocyte/macrophage colony-stimulating factor plus interleukin 4 and downregulated by tumor necrosis factor alpha. *Journal of Experimental Medicine*, Vol. 179, No. 4, (Apr 1994), pp. 1109-1118

Sampson, JH., Archer, GE., Mitchell, DA., Heimberger, AB., Herndon, JE. 2nd et al. (2009). An epidermal growth factor receptor variant III-targeted vaccine is safe and immunogenic in patients with glioblastoma multiforme. *Molecular Cancer Therapeutics*, Vol. 8, No. 10, (Oct 2009), pp. 2773–2779

Schirrmacher, V., Bai, L., Umansky, V., Yu, L., Xing, Y, & Qian, Z. (2000). Newcastle disease virus activates macrophages for anti-tumor activity. *International Journal of Oncology*, Vol. 16, pp. 363-373

Schirrmacher, V. (2005). Clinical trials of antitumor vaccination with an autologous tumor cell vaccine modified by virus infection: improvement of patient survival based on improved antitumor immune memory. *Cancer Immunology Immunotherapy*, Vol. 54, No. 6, Jun 2005), pp. 587-598

Schlag, P., Manasterski, M., Gerneth, T., Hohenberger, P., Dueck, M. et al. (1992). Active specific immunotherapy with Newcastle-disease-virus-modified autologous tumor cells following resection of liver metastases in colorectal cancer. First evaluation of clinical response of a phase II-trial. *Cancer Immunology Immunotherapy*, Vol. 35, No. 5, pp. 325-330

Schnare, M., Barton, GM., Holt, AC., Takeda, K., Akira, S. et al. (2001). Toll-like receptors control activation of adaptive immune responses. *Nature Immunology*, Vol. 2, NO. 10, (Oct 2001), pp. 947-950

Schneider, T., Sailer, M., Ansorge, S., Firsching, R. & Reinhold, D. (2006). Increased concentrations of transforming growth factor beta1 and beta2 in the plasma of patients with glioblastoma. *Journal of Neurooncology*, Vol. 79, No. 1, (Aug 2001), pp. 61-65

Schneider, T., Gerhards, R., Kirches, E. & Firsching, R. (2001). Preliminary results of active specific immunization with modified tumor cell vaccine in glioblastoma multiforme. *Journal of Neuooncology*, Vol. 53, No. 1, (May 2001), pp. 39-46

Schulze, T., Kemmer, W., Weitz, J., Wernecke, KD., Schirrmacher., V. et al. (2009) Efficiency of adjuvant active specific immunization with Newcastle disease virus modified tumor cells in colorectal cancer patients following resection of liver metastases: results of a prospective randomized trial. *Cancer Immunology Immunotherapy*, Vol. 58, No. 1, (Jan 2009), pp.61-69

Seddiki, N., Santner-Nanan, B., Martinson, J., Zaunders, J., Sasson, S. et al. (2006). Expression of interleukin (IL)-2 and IL-7 receptors discriminates between human regulatory and activated T cells. *Journal of Experimental Medicine*, Vol. 203, No. 7, (Jul 2006), pp. 1693-1700

Shah, AC., Benos, D., Gillepsie, GY. & Markert, JM. (2003). Oncolytic viruses: clinical applications as vectors for the treatment of malignant gliomas. *Journal of Neurooncology*, Vol. 65, No. 3, (Dec 2003), pp. 2023-2026

Singh, SK., Clarke, ID., Terasaki, M., Bonn, VE. & Hawkins, C. (2003). Identification of a cancer stem cell in human brain tumors. *Cancer Research*, Vol. 63, No. 18, (Sep 2003), pp. 5821-5828

Steinman, RM. (1991). The dendritic cell system and its role in immunogenicity. *Annual Review of Immunology*, Vol. 9, pp. 271-296

Stewart, LA. (2002). Chemotherapy in adult high-grade glioma: a systematic review and metaanalysis of individual patient data from 12 randomised trials. *Lancet*, Vol. 359, No. 9311, (Mar 2002), pp. 1011-1018

Stupp, R., Gander, M., Leyvraz, S. & Newlands, E. (2001). Current and future developments in the use of temozolomide for the treatment of brain tumours. *Lancet Oncology*, Vol. 2, No. 9, (Sep 2001), pp. 552-560

Stupp, R., Mason, WP., van den Bent, MJ., Weller, M., Fisher, B., et al. (2005). Radiotherapy plus concomitant and adjuvant temozolomide for glioblastoma. *New England Journal of Medicine*, Vol. 352, No. 10, (Mar 2005), pp. 987-996

Stupp, R. & Hegi, ME. (2007). Targeting brain-tumor stem cells. *Nature Biotechnology*, Vol. 25, No. 2, (Feb 2007), pp. 193–194

Tang, J., Flomenberg, P., Harshyne, L., Kenyon, L. & Andrews, DW. (2005). Glioblastoma patients exhibit circulating tumor-specific CD8+ T cells. *Clinical Cancer Research*, Vol. 11, No. 14, (Jul 2005), pp. 5292-5299

Tambuyzer, BR., Ponsaerts, P. & Nouwen, JE. (2009). Microglia: gatekeepers of central nervous system immunology. *Journal of Leukocyte Biology*, Vol. 85, No. 3, (Mar 2009), pp. 352–370,

Termeer, CC., Schirrmacher, V., Brocker, BB. & Becker, JC. (2000). Newcastle disease virus infection induces B7-1/B7-2-independent T-cell costimulatory activity in human melanoma cells. *Cancer Gene Therapy*, Vol. 7, No.2, (Feb 2000), pp. 316-323

Ueda, R., Low, KL., Zhu, X., Fujita, M., Sasaki, K., et al. (2007). Spontaneous immune responses against glioma-associated antigens in a long term survivor with malignant glioma. *Journal of Translational Medicine*, Vol. 19, No. 5, (Dec 2007), pp. 68

Ueda, R., Fujita, M., Zhu, X., Sasaki, K., Kastenhuber, ER. et al. (2009). Systemic inhibition of transforming growth factor-β in glioma-bearing mice improves the therapeutic efficacy of glioma-associated antigen peptide vaccines. *Clinical Cancer Research*, Vol. 15, No. 21, (Nov 2009), pp. 6551–6559

Van Gool, S., Maes, W., Ardon, H., Verschuere, T., Van Cauter, S. & De Vleeschouwer, S. (2009). Dendritic cell therapy of high-grade gliomas. *Brain Pathology*, Vol. 19, No. 4, (Oct 2009), pp. 694–712

Vauleon, E., Avril, T, Collet, B., Mosser, J. & Quillien, V. (2010). Overview of cellular immunotherapy for patients with glioblastoma. *Clinical and Development Immunology*, (Oct 2010), pii: 689171.

Vergati, M., Intrivici, C., Huen, NY., Schlom, J. & Tsang KY. (2010). Strategies for cancer vaccine development. *Journal of Biomedical Biotechnology*, (Jul 2010), pii: 596432

Vieira, PL., de Jong, EC., Wierenga, EA., Kapsenberg, ML. & Kalinski, P. (2000). Development of Th1-inducing capacity in myeloid dendritic cells requires environmental instruction. *Journal of Immunology*, Vol. 164, No. 9, (May 2000), pp. 4507–4512

Visintin, A., Mazzoni, A., Spitzer, JH., Wyllie, DH., Dower, SK. & Segal, DM. (2001). Regulation of Toll-like receptors in human monocytes and dendritic cells. *Journal of Immunology*, Vol. 166, No. 1, (Jan 2001), pp. 249-255

Wagner, S., Csatary, CM., Gosztonyi, G., Koch, HC., Hartmann, C. et al. (2006). Combined treatment of pediatric high-grade glioma with the oncolytic viral strain MTH-68/H and oral valproic acid. *APMIS*, Vol. 114, No. 10, (Oct 2006), pp. 731-743

Walker, G., Laherty, R., Tomlinson, FH., Chuah, T & Schmidt, C. (2008). Results of a phase I dendritic cell vaccine trial for malignant astrocytoma: potential interaction with adjuvant chemotherapy. *Journal of Clinical Neuroscience*, Vol. 15, No.2, (Feb 2008), pp. 114–121

Washburn, B. & Schirrmacher, V. (2002). Human tumor cell infection by Newcastle disease virus leads to upregulation of HLA and cell adhesion molecules and to induction of interferons, chemokines and finally apoptosis. *International Journal of Oncology*, Vol. 21, No. 1, (Jul 2002), pp. 85-93

Washburn, B., Weigand MA., Grosse-Wilde, A., Janke, M., Stahl, H. et al. (2003). TNF-related apoptosis-inducing ligand mediates tumoricidal activity of human monocytes stimulated by Newcastle disease virus. *Journal of Immunology*, Vol. 170, No. 4, (Feb 2003), pp. 1814-1821

Weller, M. & Fontana, A. (1995). The failure of current immunotherapy for malignant glioma. Tumor-derived TGF- β, T-cell apoptosis, and the immune privilege of the brain. *Brain Research Reviews*, Vol. 21, No. 2, (Sep 1995), pp. 128–151

Wheeler, CJ., Das, A., Liu, G., Yu, JS. & Black, KL: (2004). Clinical responsiveness of glioblastoma multiforme to chemotherapy after vaccination. *Clinical Cancer Research*, Vol. 10, No. 16, (Aug 2004), pp. 5316–5326

Wheeler, CJ., Black, KL., Liu, G., Mazer, M., Zhang, X. et al. (2008). Vaccination elicits correlated immune and clinical responses in glioblastoma multiforme patients. *Cancer Research*, Vol. 68, No. 14, (Jul 2008), pp. 5955–5964

Whiteside, TL. & Odoux, C. (2004). Dendritic cellbiology and cancer therapy. *Cancer Immunology Immunotherapy*, Vol. 53, No. 3, (Mar 2004), pp. 240-248

Whiteside, TL. (2008). The tumor microenvironment and its role in promoting tumor growth. *Oncogene*, Vol. 27, No. 45, (Oct 2008), pp. 5904-5912

Wilson, EH., Weninger, W. & Hunter, CA. (2010). Trafficking of immune cells in the central nervous system. *Journal of Clinical Investigation*, Vol. 120, No. 5, (May 2010), pp. 1368–1379

Wischhusen, J., Friese, MA., Mittelbronn, M., Meyermann, R. & Weller, M. (2005). HLA-E protects glioma cells from NKG2D-mediated immune responses in vitro: implications for immune escape in vivo. *J Neuropathol Exp Neurol*, Vol. 64, No. 6, (Jun 2005), pp. 523-528

Wolf, AM., Wolf, D., Steurer, M., Gastl, G., Gunsilius, E. & Grubeck-Loebenstein, B. (2003). Increase of regulatory T cells in the peripheral blood of cancer patients. *Clinical Cancer Research*, Vol. 9, No. 2, (Feb 2003), pp. 606-612

Wollmann, G., Tattersal, P. & van den Pol, AN. (2005). Targeting human glioblastoma cells: comparison of nine viruses with oncolytic potential. *Journal of Virology*, Vol. 79, No. 10, (May 2005), pp. 6005-6022

Woo EY., Chu, CS., Goletz, TJ., Schlienger, K., Yeh, H. et al. (2001). Regulatory CD4 (+) CD25 (+) T cells in tumors from patients with early-stage non-small cell lung cancer and late-stage ovarian cancer. *Cancer Research*, Vol. 61, No. 12, (Jun 2001), pp. 4766-4772

Xu, Q., Liu G., Yuan, X., Xu, M., Wang, H. et al. (2009). Antigen-specific T-cell response from dendritic cell vaccination using cancer stem-like cell-associated antigens. *Stem Cells*, Vol. 27, No. 8, (Aug 2009), pp. 1374-1740

Yamanaka, R., Abe T, Yajima, N., Tsuchiya, N., Homma, J. et al. (2003). Vaccination of recurrent glioma patients with tumour lysate-pulsed dendritic cells elicits immune responses: results of a clinical phase I/II trial. *British Journal of Cancer*, Vol. 89, No. 7, (Oct 2003), pp. 1172-1179

Yamanaka, R., Homma, J., Yajima, N., Tsuchiya, N., Sano, M. et al. (2005). Clinical evaluation of dendritic cell vaccination for patients with recurrent glioma: results of a clinical phase I/II trial. *Clinical Cancer Research*, Vol. 11, No. 11, (Jun 2005), pp. 4160-4167

Yu, JS., Wheeler, CJ., Zeltzer, PM., Ying, H., Finger, DN. et al. (2001). Vaccination of malignant glioma patients with peptide-pulsed dendritic cells elicits systemic cytotoxicity and intracranial T-cell infiltration. *Cancer Research*, Vol. 61, No. 3, (Feb 2001), pp. 842-847

Yu, JS., Liu, G., Ying, H., Yong, WH., Black, KL. & Wheeler. CJ. (2004). Vaccination with tumor lysate-pulsed dendritic cells elicits antigen-specific cytotoxic T-cells in patients with malignant glioma. *Cancer Research*, Vol. 64, No. 14, Jul 2004), pp. 4973-4979

Yung, WK., Albright, RE., Olson, J., Fredericks, R., Fink, K., et al. (2000). A phase II study of temozolomide vs. procarbazine in patients with glioblastoma multiforme at first relapse. *Br J Cancer*, Vol. 83, No. 5, (Sep 2000), pp. 588-593

Zeng, J., Fournier, P. & Schirrmacher, V. (2002). Induction of interferon-alpha and tumor necrosis factor-related apoptosis-inducing ligand in human blood mononuclear cells by hemaglutinin-neuraminidase but not F protein of Newcastle disease virus. *Virology*, Vol. 297, No. 1, (May 2002), pp. 19-30

Zhou, LJ. & Tedder, TF. (1996). CD14+ blood monocytes can differentiate into functionally mature CD83+ dendritic cells. *Proceedings of the National Academy of Sciences of the United States of America*, Vol. 93, No. 6, (Mar 1996), pp. 2588-2592

Zobywalski, A., Javorovic, M., Frankenberger, B., Pohla, H., Kremmer, E. et al. (2007). Generation of clinical grade dendritic cells with capacity to produce biologically active IL-12p70. *Journal of Translational Medicine*, Vol. 12, No. 5, (Apr 2007), pp. 5-18

21

Targeted Therapy for Gliomas: The Oncolytic Virus Applications

Zulkifli Mustafa[1], Hidayah Roslan[2] and Jafri Malin Abdullah[1]
[1]*Universiti Sains Malaysia*
[2]*Universiti Putra Malaysia*
Malaysia

1. Introduction

Cancer now is well described as a genetically defective disease that causes the overgrowth of particular cells. Cancer is phenotypically related to multiple sequential gene mutation and amplification, genetic translocalization, preservation of telomeres and loss of tumor suppressor gene that lead to immortal cell (Sinkovics & Horvath, 2000). In this regard, gliomas are particularly defined as pathological tumors that display histological, immunohistological and ultrastructural evidence of glial differentiation (Maher *et al.*, 2001). Amongst gliomas, glioblastoma multiform (GBM) is one of the most killer cancer and maintains its prevalence despite current millennium intelligent treatment.

Taking advantage of the genetic defects that fuel cancer growth, targeted therapy using viruses to kill mutated or defective-gene cancer cells was investigated. Viruses with oncolytic properties and limited side effects to human were used as miniature biological machine to reach the targeted cancer cells. In this progressing treatment modality, the viruses were specifically studied to reach the targeted cancer without interfering the normal cells, directly inducing cancer cell death or activating the body immune system to infiltrate and mediate the destruction of tumor mass.

Basically, the targeted therapy using virus can be classified into two classes which are *replication-defective* virus that is mainly used as a vehicle for gene therapy by means as a vector for suicide gene delivery and also a *replication-competent* virus (Biederer *et al.*, 2002). Some of the replication-competent viruses that have been studied, focused on its *natural-selective oncotropic* to invade cancerous cells and the others were armed with a genetically engineer technique to activate cell death promoter genes.

As the malignant gliomas are amongst the few rapidly proliferating ones in central nervous system, it is becoming an interesting subject for the study of selective-amplifications virus (Aghi *et al.*, 2006).

In the beginning of this century, it was noted that a patient with cervical carcinoma experienced significant tumor regression after rabies vaccination. In addition, there were reports of remissions of Burkitt's and Hodgkin's lymphomas following natural infection with measles virus. In the 1950s, human trials with several potentially oncolytic viruses were initiated (Evert and Henk G., 2005).

Preclinical studies of oncolytic viruses in gliomas emerged in 1990's where the first attenuated Herpes Simplex Virus and Adenovirus were used followed by oncolytic

Reovirus. To date, four viruses have completed the clinical trials. The viruses are Herpes Simplex Virus (HSV-1, HSV-1716 & HSV-G207), Newcastle Disease Virus (MTH-68/H, NDV-Huj), Adenovirus (Onyx-015) and Reovirus. As the general outcomes of phase 1 trials, the viruses were declared as safe to be injected directly to the brain and no maximum tolerate dose (MTD) were reached. Some anti-glioma activities were also found. Amongst these, NDV showed the most promising benefits with 6 patients showed tumor regression and 3 patients have long term survival (Franz *et al.*, 2010).

In this chapter, taking an example of Newcastle disease virus, we focus on the advantages of virotherapy, targeted pathway in oncolysis mechanism, methodology for virus with oncolytic properties study, and development of tumor model for glioma in a mouse model.

2. Oncolytic virus therapy

Oncolytic virus refer to the virus that kills tumor cells selectively without harming the normal surrounding tissue (Biederer *et al.*, 2002; Franz *et al.*, 2010). As a mode of therapy, oncolytic virus is used to "self-recognize" and infect the mutated cancerous cells which replicates within the infected cells followed by release of new virion that simultaneously amplifies the input dose. New virions later spreads and infect the adjacent cancerous cells. Consequently, infected cells often undergo pathological programmed cell death which also known as apoptosis.

This application modality reflects the application of viruses with *replication-competent* and inheriting the natural selective capability to the cancerous cells. Most studied natural oncotropic viruses are the RNA viruses such as paramyxovirus family including newcastle disease virus (NDV), reovirus, and vesicular stomatitis virus.

Moreover, some viruses were also enhanced with genetic modification by insertion or deletion of therapeutic transgenes respectively (Marianne *et al.*, 2010). Virus can be made tumor selective by modification of the cellular tropism at the level of viral replication in a way that it becomes dependent on specific characteristics of tumor cells for viral replication. This can be achieved by deleting viral genes that are critical for viral replication in healthy cells but are dispensable upon infection of neoplastic cells. Modification of the cellular tropism at the level of cell recognition and binding by altering the viral coat for tumor-selective binding and uptake may also be performed (Evert and Henk G., 2005)

For example, the most common immune-modulatory protein inserted into the oncolytic viruses is the granulocyte-macrophages colony-stimulating factor (GM-CSF) that has been inserted into the adenovirus, herpes simplex virus and vaccinia virus in order to stimulate an inflammatory response within the tumor microenvironment (Marianne *et al.*, 2010) and promoting cell death.

Research of the oncolytic virus also been studied along with current conventional treatments and the virotherapeutics have demonstrated synergy with the approved chemotherapeutics and radiotherapy (Liu *et al*, 2007).

In past decade, the oncolytic viruses have been tested on various human cancer cells in-vitro and animal model with very promising benefits (Schirrmacher and Fournier, 2009). Some of the oncolytic virus been studied and reported in phase 1 against glioma are the herpes simplex virus (HSV), adenovirus, reovirus, and NDV, while the measles virus, vaccinia virus, myxoma virus, polio virus, and vesicular stomatitis virus were at the preclinical level. (Parker *et al.*, 2009)

For NDV, the strain been studied on glioma are the MTH/68H, NDV-HUJ,OV-001, 73-T and V4UPM. The V4UPM is the avirulent strain of ND virus that has been used as a thermostable feed pellet vaccine for poultry. It is been tested to poses excellent oncolytic activity against glioma cell lines. (Zulkifli *et al.*, 2009)

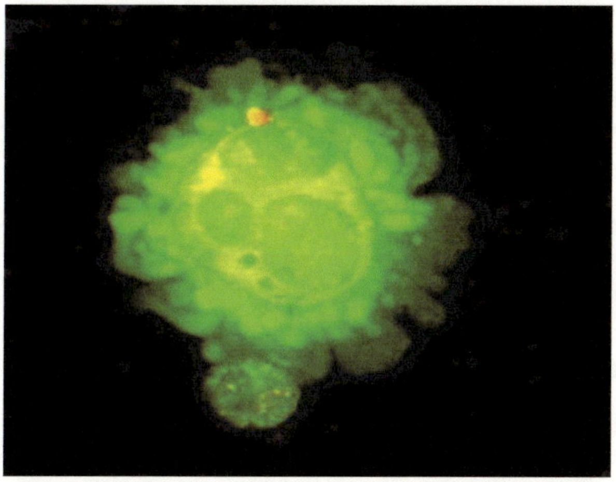

Fig. 1. An example of apoptotic glioma cells infected with newcastle disase virus (40x)

To date, there are 119 patients recruited for clinical trials. HSV (strain G207 & HS-1716), adenovirus (strain ONYX-015), reovirus and NDV (strain NDV-HUJ) have completed the phase 1 clinical trials. NDV strain MTH-68/H reported in several case reports against gliomas. (Franz *et al.*, 2010) .

In the clinical practice, China is reported to be the first country that has approved the oncolytic virus application in 2006. The virus is the genetically modified adenovirus strain H101 that has been reported to enhance anticancer rate response compared to chemotherapy alone.

3. Advantages and disadvantages of viral therapy

In current conventional treatments, gliomas are managed by chemotherapy, resection surgery and also radiation therapy. However, the disease remains incurable. One of the exclusive factors of glioma is the diffuse infiltrative nature of tumor cells into adjacent brain parenchymal. This has led to incomplete resection and regrowth of the cancer. Therefore, oncolytic virus offered promising technique of eradicating the gliomas as it well known to selectively infect only the cancerous cell without harming the normal brain tissue.

As reviewed by Biederer *et al.*, 2002, some of the major advantages of gene therapy and oncolytic virus therapy includes: oncolytic viruses can be engineered by recombinant genetic technology to meet specific targets, pose unique pharmacokinetics properties as its ability to amplify its own input dose and limited side effects to normal tissue. This limited side effect is extended with no adverse effect concerning allergy and asthmatic. (Schirrmacher and Fournier, 2009)

Oncolytic viruses are the foreign body that have innate capacity to stimulate host cytokines for potential anticancer activity. In this regards, some oncolytic viruses infect the target cells of different species and produce non-infectious virion but infected cells will express viral antigens that later attract host antibody against the cancerous cells. (Sinkovics & Horvath, 2000). Tumor cell is immunogenically poor that leads them to escape from being killed by the body immune system. For example, NDV can also infect freshly isolated patient-derived melanoma cells that further lead to increase of viral antigens at the cell surface (Schirrmacher *et al.*, 1999). On the other hand, the different host origin or animal viral are capable of infecting human cells where the pre-existing antibody is low.

Particularly to the reovirus, NDV virus and other simple single stranded RNA virus, their replications are incapable of recombination. In another words, the virus replication does not involve the intermediate DNA steps during their replication and thus no possibility of mutation insertion of viral RNA to host genome. Besides, the virus did not carry the oncogenes.

However, gliomas are always reported with single cell infiltration. Surrounding normal tissue therefore, may inhibit the virus spread that requires cell to cell contact and limits the local treatment implantation.

4. Viral genomic and infection

On the genomic basis, every oncolytic virus is characterized with several proteins that help them to establish the infection to the host cell as well as the cancerous cells.

For the ND virus, it is an avian virus with the genome consisting of 15 kilo base pairs of non-segmented, single-stranded RNA, coded for 6 main structural proteins. These genes namely nucleocapsid (NP), phosphorylation (P), matrix (M), fusion (F), hemaglutinin-neuraminidase (HN), and RNA-dependent RNA polymerase (L) proteins are found to be in 3′ NP-P-M-F-HN-L 5′ arrangement.

The NP protein is the most abundant protein found in the virion. Electron microscopic study reveals that the protein exists as flexible helical structure with a diameter of about 18 nm in length and 1 μm height. Its structure resembles classical morphology with spikes protruding from the central channel (Yusoff and Tan, 2001). Each NP subunits consists of 489 amino acids with molecular mass of about 53 kDa. In viral replication process, NP subunits in association of P and L proteins encapsidate the genomic RNA into RNase-resistant nucleocapsid. This complex, instead of naked viral RNA, becomes the RNA template for transcription and replication processes of the viral RNA genome.

The polycistronic phosphoprotein (P) gene codes for protein of 395 amino acids with a calculated molecular weight of 42 kDa (McGinnes *et al.*, 1988). In the viral transcriptase complex, P protein acts as a cofactor with dual functions; stabilizing the L protein as well as placing the polymerase complex (P:L) on the formed NP:RNA template for mRNA synthesis. Apart from the P protein which is encoded by an unedited transcript of the P gene, NDV was also shown to edit its P gene mRNA to produce V and W proteins. Insertion of one G residue at the conserved editing site (UUUUUCCC, genome sense) will produce the V protein, while insertion of two G residues at the same site will give W protein. The real functions of these two non-structural proteins are yet to be identified but some studies shows that V protein significantly contributes to the virus virulence (Huang Z *et al.*, 2003).

M gene codes for the matrix protein. It can be found between the nucleocapsid and viral envelope proteins. The protein which consists of 371 to 375 amino acids, is considered to be the central organizer of viral morphogenesis such as in making interactions with the cytoplasmic tails of the integral membrane proteins, the lipid bilayer, and the nucleocapsids.

The F gene, an important determinant of NDV pathogenicity, consists of 540 to 580 amino acids which codes for fusion protein or known as fusion glycoprotein Type 1. Virulent and avirulent NDV are characterized by the presence of multibasic and single basic residues in the F_o cleavage site respectively as there is a difference in the amino acid sequences surrounding the precursor F_o for both the virulent and avirulent strain. The amino acid sequences in a virulent strain renders the F protein to be susceptible to cleavage by the host protease and leads to a fatal systemic infection. It was reported that combination of F and HN proteins initiates the NDV infection (McGinnes and Morrison, 2006).

The HN gene codes for hemaglutinin-neuraminidase protein which is the major antigenic determinant of all paramyxoviruses. This multifunctional protein is responsible for attachment to receptors containing sialic acid and neuraminidase (NA) activity. It has been considered that the role of the neuraminidase activity is to prevent self-aggregation of viral particles during budding at the plasma membrane. In addition, HN also has a fusion-promoting activity meaning that coexpression of HN and F is required for cell-cell fusion to be observed.

RNA-dependent RNA polymerase (L) protein is the largest protein in the NDV genome. It consists of 2200 amino acid residues. This protein forms a complex with P protein, and both of these components are required for polymerase activity with NP:RNA templates. The P:L complex can make mRNA *in* vitro that is both capped at its 5′ end and contains a polyA tail at the 3′ end.

Newcastle disease virus initiates infection through attachment of viral membrane to host cell surface receptor, the sialic acid-containing molecule which fused with the viral HN protein. Activated HN protein causes conformational changes to the viral F protein which brings the virion and the host membranes into close proximity (Morrison, 2003). This process allows for the viral nucleocapsid to enter the host cytoplasm. After this step, the nucleocapsid complex (RNA:NP:P:L) directs primary transcription of mRNAs which is complementary to the viral negative strand genome. These mRNA will later serve as templates for further negative strand RNA resulting in genome amplification. Secondary transcription then occurs in the same manner as the primary transcription but using the progeny nucleocapsids instead of the earlier parental's. After transcription is the translation process which produce the viral proteins followed by nucleocapsid assembly, association of P and L proteins, and further encapsidation. All these processes occur in the host cytoplasm. The almost completed virion then moves to the plasma membrane and is released by budding and rendered itself with an envelope coat from the host plasma membrane.

In the oncolytic study, the new NDV's virion was detected as early as 3 hours post infection and apoptotic cell death of glioma was detected via life cell imaging in our study as early as 7 hours post infection. The specific protein of NDV that interacts in the oncotropic mechanism however remains unclear but Elankumaran *et al*, (2007) reported that it was associated with the HN protein.

Schirrmacher and Fournier, 2009 summarised that following the intravenous injection of NDV, the virus was mainly detected in the lung, blood, liver and spleen at 0.5 hour. The amount of virus decreased rapidly over time and reached the detection limit at less than 1 day (blood and thymus), 2 days (kidney), and around 14 days (in lung, liver and spleen).

5. Glioblastoma and oncolytic selective mechanism

The molecular biology of gliomas has provided new insights in the development of brain tumors. These dysregulated cell signalling pathways that have been identified are now becoming the focus of a specific molecular targeted therapy (Chamberline et al., 2006). The

overexpression of these defective genes gives the opportunity to oncolytic virus to infect the gliomas.
In the study of reovirus, the virus infection leads to activation of dsRNA-activated protein kinase (PKR), which phosporylates the a-subunit of eIF-2, resulting in termination in the initiation of translation of viral transcript in normal cells. However, PKR kinase activity is impaired, allowing the virus replication to proceed. Ras-mediated signal transduction is activated in most human cancers due to either mutated Ras or mutated epidermal growth factor receptor (EGFR) (Kirn *et al.*, 2001)). In GBM, 50% was found with EGFR overexpression and high Ras expression especially in the primary GBM. (Aghi M. & Chiocca E.A., 2006)
Oncolytic viruses are believed to replicate and and lyse different malignant cells in vitro and in vivo as a result of an impaired type I interferon response in cancer cells. In Miyakoshi et al study, oncogenes activation in human glioblastoma multiform had increased the activation of protein kinase. This leads to interferon synsthesis and the inhibition of tumoregenesis. (Miyakoshi *et al*, 1990). In gliomas however, the anti-tumor response is impaired by glioma-derivative immunosuppressing factors such TGF-b, IL-10, prostaglandin E2 and gangliosides. TGF-b is the most prominent immunosuppresor that plays a major role in glioma biology whose overexpress and become the hallmark of the gliomas.
On the other hand, normal brain cells response to the viral infections leads to stimulation of the patern-recognition-receptors (PRRs) and later activates the Type 1 interferon.(Franz *et al.*, 2010). The type 1 interferon futher binds and activates the Janus kinases JAK1 and TYK2 which inturns phophorylates the activators for transcription of STAT1 and STAT2. The STAT proteins later heterodimers and forms a complex with IRF9. The complex is known as ISGF3 that futher provides DNA recognition and simultaneously produces the interferon-stimulated genes (IGS) that creates the antiviral state in the target cells and blocks viral replication. In this regards, interferon-beta is the principle antiviral factor secreted by NDV-infected cells. Consequently, the interferon defective tumor cells gives more opportunity for the NDV to effectively replicate compared to normal cell and it is concluded that this replication-competent virus selective mechanism is associated with the defect of the host interferon (Krishnamurthy *et al.*, 2006).This is summarised in the Figure 2 below.
Recently, Puhlmann *et al* has established Rac 1 as a protein which activity is critical for both oncolysis virus sensitivity and autonomous growth behaviour of cancer (Puhlmann *et al.*, 2010). Rac1 plays a role as a pleiotropic regulator of multiple cellular functions including actin skeleton reorganization, gene transcription and cell migration. Rac1 is a key contributor to glioma cell survival, probably via multiple signaling pathways including JNK (Halatsch *et al*, 2009) but is found to be critical for the replication of oncolytic NDV to the highly tumorigenic ras-transformed skin carcinoma cells
However, despite several entry-line association, there are several physicals barriers that is present in the gliomas microenvironment that blocks the virus distribution. The extracellular matrix (ECM), hypoxic region, and high interstitial pressure are amongst the major challenge in achieving lasting oncolytic virus infection (Franz *et al.*, 2010)
Besides that, GBM is currently described with multiple interactive dysregulated cell signalings pathway and this could lead to the inconsistency of outcome (Chamberline et al., 2006) in bigger population target.

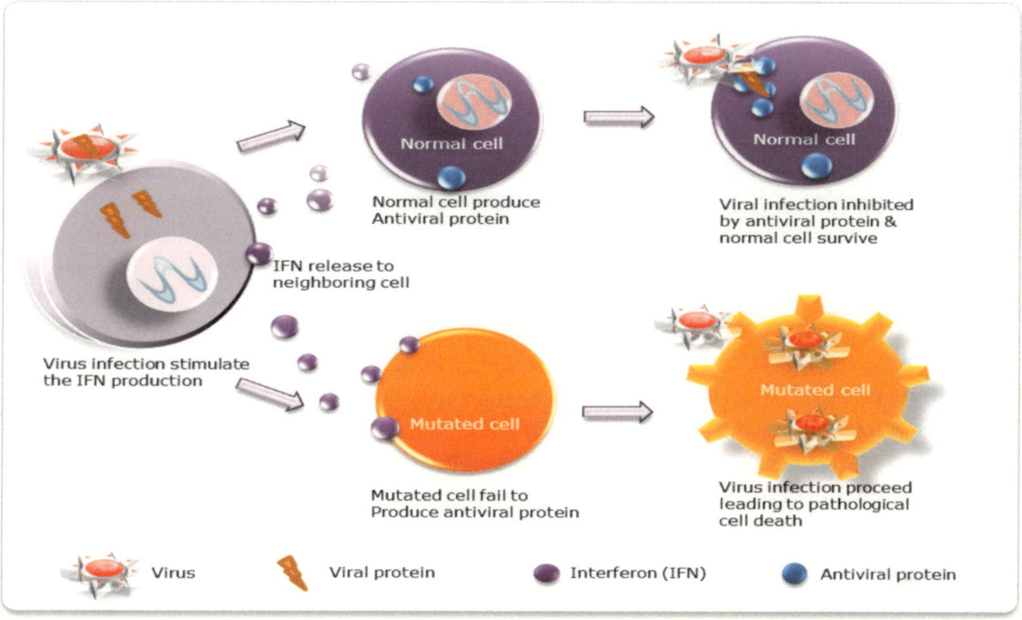

Fig. 2.

6. Cell cycle arrest and pathway

Glioma has been classified according to their hypothesized line of differentiation that is whether they display features of astrocytic, oligodendroglial or ependymal cells. These are graded on the scale of grade one to grade four according to the degree of malignancy judged by histological features. At the molecular level, the mutation that leads to different glioma grades presented with several relevant pathways. In the high grade astrocytoma for example, retinoblastoma mutation is found at approximately 25 percent. In this regard, retinoblastoma is a major regulator of cell cycle progression where mutational inactivation of retinoblastoma leads to unschedule cell cycle entry (Maher *et al.*, 2001).

Cell cycle is a series of cellular events which leads to cell division and replication. Generally, cell cycle mechanism involves 4 different stages; G_1 (gap 1), S (synthesis), G_2 (gap 2) and M (mitosis). G_1 is an interphase between the end of M (mitosis) phase and the beginning of a new cell cycle. At this phase, the cell either prepares to enter the S (synthesis) phase or stops dividing (quiescence). If the cell receives growth signal to replicate, it will move to S phase where it starts synthesizing nucleic acid. Once DNA replication completes, the cell will enter G_2 phase. Here, synthesis of crucial proteins involved in cell division like microtubules occurs and once complete, these cells will move to the M phase and divide itself into 2 daughter cells. All these 4 processes should occur without any disturbance from inside or outside of the cell. Each of the cycle phases is very critical and if anything goes wrong at any stage especially during G_1 and M, they can cause mutations and may lead to cancer. Normal cell usually has several systems to check for errors at each phase and this is known as phase checkpoints.

Transition from G_1 to S phase is controlled mostly by cyclin-dependent kinases (Cdk2, Cdk4, and Cdk6) and their substrates. These Cdks regulate the retinoblastoma family proteins (p107, p130, and pRb) by phosphorylation. Initial partial inactivation of pRb by Cdk4 and Cdk6 induce transcription of E-type cyclins. These cyclins activate Cdk2 which further phosphorylates the pRb and other substrates. The Cdks are regulated by different levels involving interaction with positive and negative partners. Amongst the inhibitors are the Cip/Kip family proteins and one of them is $p27^{Kip1}$. This protein can binds to cyclin D either alone or when complexed to its catalytic subunit CDK4. By doing so, it inhibits catalytic activities (phosphorylation) of CDK4 towards pRB protein. It was reported that phosphorylation at the Thr187 of $p27^{KIP1}$ by Cyclin E/CDK2 complex promotes its degradation by recognition of this phosphorylated $p27^{KIP1}$ by SCF(Skp2) which has the E3 ubiquitin ligase activity (Ungermannova *et al.*, 2005). Degradation of $p27^{KIP1}$ starts the generation of cyclin A-dependent kinase activity which will push the cells from G phase to S phase in the cell cycle. In several studies done in viral infections which induces cell cycle arrest, it was found that the level of this inhibitor protein increases significantly after infection, which leads to arrest of the cell replication process.

A successful introduction of viral genome into a host cell usually causes chaos in the host system and ends-up with the production of viral genome instead of host. Studies done on certain viruses revealed that these viruses are able to stop the host cellular replication mechanism namely cell cycle arrest which may render the virus with advantages in taking over the whole machinery system. This cell arrest is usually associated with elevation or suppression of players in the cell cycle from members of cyclins, CDKs, and inhibitors. For instance, infection of influenza A virus A/WSN/33 (H1N1) causes changes in the host protein expression level of cyclin E and cyclin D1, as well as p21 which are amongst the key molecules of cell cycle (He *et. al.*, 2010). Besides that, p27 is one of the protein involve in the retinoblastoma pathway where glioma cell lines exhibit an inverse corelation between the level of p27 protein and proliferation index (Maher *et al.*, 2001) that could be investigated as a rational component target in cell cycle arrest.

Many other viruses were also reported to cause cell cycle arrest upon infection such as measles virus, human immunodeficiency virus-type 1 (HIV-1), and herpesvirus. Our recent findings on NDV infection also reveal the potential of this virus to block cell cycle in tumor cells.

7. Methods

7.1 Virus propagation

Avirulent NDV propagation is carried out in the Class II laboratory (Laboratory Biosafety Level). Generally, the egg shell is cleaned with 70% ethanol and then candling is done to ensure that the embryo is still alive. Then a mark is made slightly above the air-sac where the mark is pricked with a 21G needle. Through this tiny hole dilution of NDV in PBS is introduced into the allantoic fluid cavity. The hole is then sealed with melting wax and the egg is incubated at 37°C for 48 to 72 hours (subjected to viral virulence) to allow for the viral propagation as well as the embryo growth.

Prior to allantoic fluid collection, the embryo is killed by placing it at 4°C for about 5 hours. Besides killing the embryo, this cold temperature also shrinks the blood capillary inside the egg, thus, extracting the allantoic fluid would be easier. Allantoic fluid is then collected and clarified at 8,000 x *g* for 30 minutes to remove the debris such as red blood cells and yolk if any. Further centrifugation at 20,000 x *g* for 2 and half hours will precipitate the virus at the

bottom of the centrifuge tube. The pellet is then re-suspended in NTE or PBS buffer according to further work specifications.
Virus obtained at this stage can be used in work like HA, HI and other several tests but not for infection and other works that need pure virus application. Virus purification is achieved by separating the virus from other tiny contaminants in the viral suspension through glucose gradient. Special ultracentrifuge with vacuum function is needed for this process since the virus will be spinning at 38,000 x *g* for 4 hours to get better separation. Band containing virus is then identified and extracted for further centrifugation at the same speed in 2 hours. This will pellet the virus at the bottom of the tube. Pure virus pellet is now re-suspended in NTE or PBS buffer and kept at -20°C or -80°C for longer storage.

7.2 In vitro cytotoxic study

Cell lines were cultured in the media and supplemented according to supplier recommendations. For the cytotoxicity study, adapted from the method by Zulkifli *et al.*, 2009, the normal and glioma cell lines were seeded at 1 x 10^5 in 96-well plate and incubated overnight in 37°celcius incubator supplemented with 5% CO_2 gas. Following the attachment of the cells next day, the media was changed. The cells later treated with virus at MOI of log_{10} serial concentrations and incubated for 24, 48 and 72 hours. Relative cell viability later tested with 3-(4,5-dimethylthiazol-2-yl)-5-(3-carboxymethoxyphenyl)-2-(4-sulfophenyl)-2H-tetrazolium (MTS) reagent. The absorbance values were expressed as a percentage and the sigmoidal dose response curve were plotted versus virus dose. The EC50 achieved by the curve represents the dose of virus that reduces the maximal light absorbance capacity of an exposed cell culture by 50% and is proportional to the percentage of cells killed by the virus.

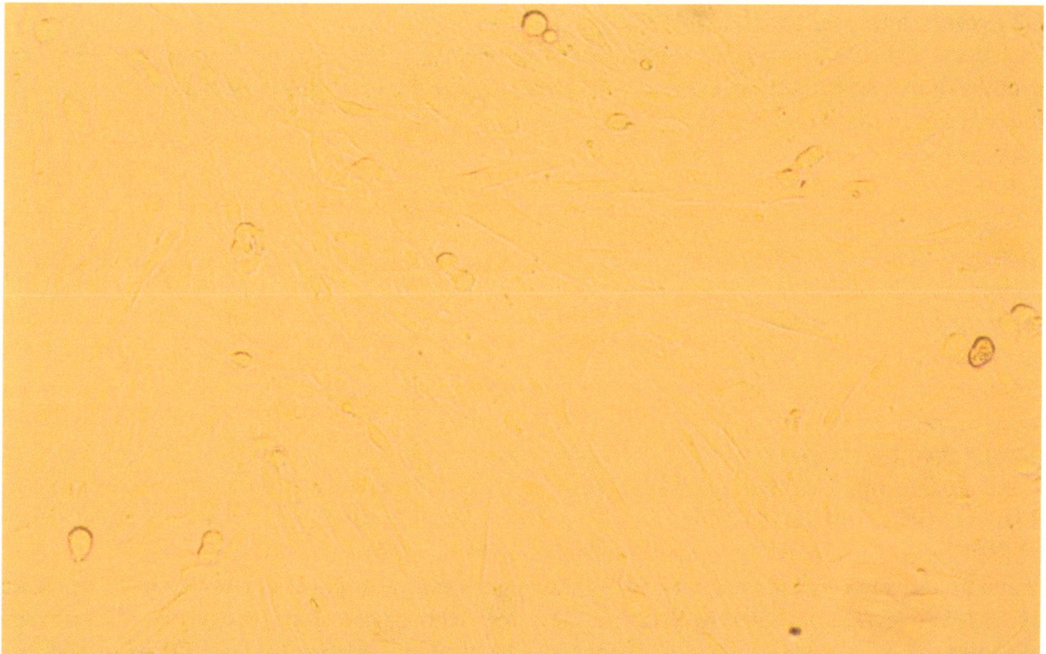

Fig. 3. Confluence glioma cell line in cell culture

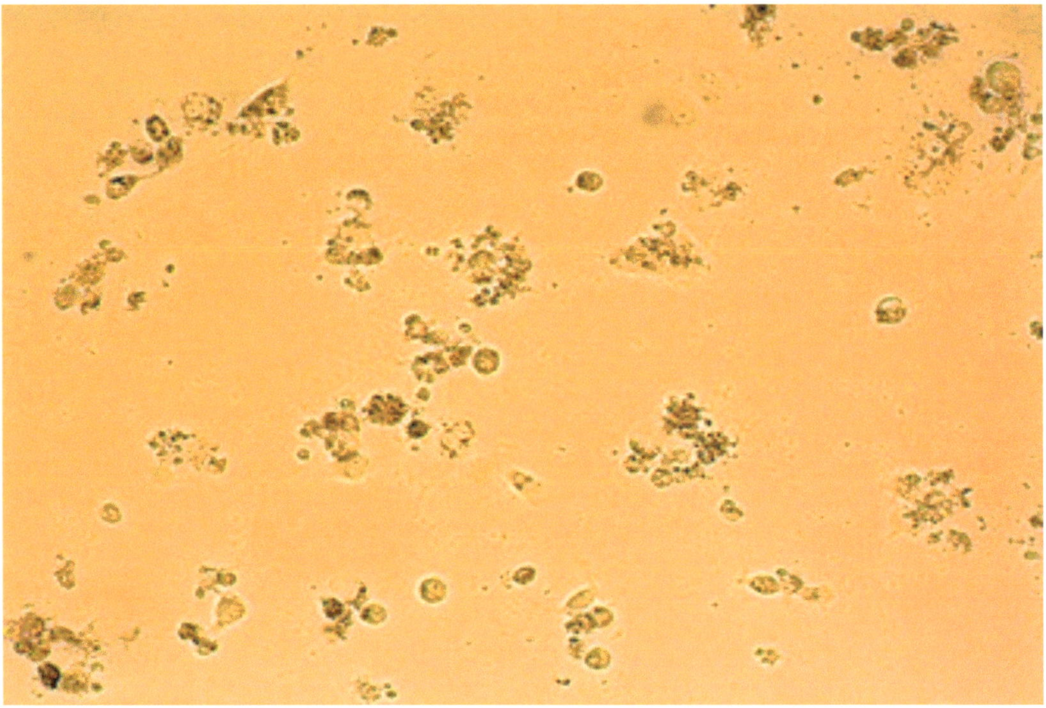

Fig. 4. Apoptotic glioma cells after 48 hours infection with newcastle disease virus

7.3 Protein analysis by SDS-PAGE

Cell cycle process occurs by interactions of many protein players. These proteins are produced at specific rate and amount to meet the purpose; overexpression or reduction in the amount suggests for disturbance or changes in the cycle process, perhaps causing cell cycle arrest. There are several options that can be carried out in a laboratory in order to find out on this changes of protein expression level, but the established method are the SDS-PAGE and Western blot. These two methods allow researchers to find the difference of specific protein level between different samples qualitatively and even quantitatively.

Sodium dodecyl sulfate polyacrylamide gel electrophoresis (SDS-PAGE) is a technique to separate different proteins based on their size by running proteins through a gel forced by electrical voltage. SDS-PAGE gel consists of two parts; the bottom part namely the resolving gel and the upper part which is the stacking gel. Different percentage of resolving and stacking gels can be prepared depending on the size of protein of interest but the standard percentage in most practice is 12% resolving gel and 5% stacking gel. A 12 % resolving gel was prepared first by mixing 30% acrylamide solution, 1.5M Tris (pH 8.8), 10% (w/v) SDS in distilled water, 10% (w/v) ammonium persulfate (APS) in distilled water, deionized water (dH_2O) and N,N,N',N'-Tetramethylethylenediamine (TEMED) in a clean beaker and immediately poured into a set of SDS-PAGE gel casting apparatus (Bio-Rad, USA) to an appropriate level. Immediately after this step, appropriate amount of n-butanol was layered onto the gel and it was left for 45 minutes at room temperature to solidify. After butanol layer was removed and rinsed with dH_2O, stacking gel was prepared by mixing 30% Acrylamide solution, 0.5M Tris (pH 6.8), 10% (w/v) SDS in distilled water, 10% (w/v) APS in distilled water, dH_2O, and TEMED in a clean beaker. This mixture was then mixed properly and immediately layered on top of the resolving gel. A comb was inserted into the stacking gel and everything was allowed to set for about 45 minutes. Then the comb was removed carefully and the glass plates holding the gel was transferred into an inner chamber of Mini Protean-3 Cell electrophoresis tank (BioRad, USA). About 400 ml SDS-PAGE running buffer consisting of 0.025 M Tris, 0.192 M glycine, and 0.1% (w/v) SDS in distilled water (pH 8.3) was prepared and poured into the inner chamber until full while the rest was emptied into the electrophoresis tank.

Samples were then prepared by mixing the cell lysate with 2X sample buffer [125 mMTris-HCl (pH 6.8), 4% SDS, 20% glycerol, 0.0.2% Bromophenol blue, 10% 2-mercaptoethanol (added fresh before use)] at the ratio 1:1 and the mixture was boiled for 5 minutes. After that, the mixture was loaded into SDS-PAGE gel and electrophoresed at 180V for 50 minutes.

7.4 Western blotting and chemiluminescence

Separated proteins in SDS-PAGE gel was then transferred using Western blotting. Briefly, the gel was removed carefully and layered onto a polyvinylidene fluoride (PVDF) placed at the middle of 4 filtered paper. Protein in the gel was transferred by electrical charges attraction at 100V for 1h in a protein wet transfer tank filled with Towbin's transfer buffer [25 mMTris, 190 mM glycine (pH 8.0), 20% (v/v) methanol]. After that, blocking step was carried out by soaking the PVDF in 5% milk diluents for 1h at room temperature or overnight at 4°C. The membrane was washed in TBST buffer [50 mMTris-HCl, 150 mMNaCl, 0.01 Tween 20] 3 times (5 minutes each time) to remove the blocking reagent. Specific protein detection was achieved by incubating the membrane in primary antibody for 1h at room temperature. The membrane was then washed with TBST buffer 3 times (5 minutes each) before it was incubated in secondary antibody conjugated with horseradish peroxidase (HRP) for another 1 h at room temperature. After that, the membrane was washed again with TBST for 3 times (5 minutes each wash).

Protein band of interest was obtained by chemiluminescence method. Reagents from Supersignal West Pico Chemiluminescent Substrate or Supersignal West Dura Chemiluminescent Substrate (Pierce, Thermo Scientific, USA) kit were added onto the membrane for 5 minutes incubation period, allowing for the HRP from the secondary antibody to bind to the substrate and fluoresce. This signal was then captured onto a film in an autoradiography cassette (Fisher Scientific, PA) and developed by a film developer machine (AFP Imaging Corp, USA). These bands can be compared quantitatively using software like Image J. Data used for the purpose of comparison helps in identifying the changes in protein expression level and further other changes or disturbance in the pathway involved.

7.5 Development of glioma model in mouse

Growing the glioma model is one of the critical issue in brain tumor therapy study. One of the common model is the xenograft implant of glioma cell line into the immunosuppresive mouse. Some of the advantages of the implant model are the predictable growth rate of the tumor and it is reproducible in term of location besides the precise histology features. The implant model however fails to give the characteristic of single cell infiltration.

The glioma model in the nude mouse were done according to Zulkifli *et al.* In brief, actively growing glioma cell lines such as DBTRG.05MG and U-87MG were harvested from culture flask, counted at 1 x 10^7 in the PBS and subcutaneously injected to a flank of female 6-weeks old homozygous nu/nu Balb/c mice. Tumors grows until they were clearly growing and palpable measuring (by digital caliper) at $20mm^3$ were obtained. Tumor size is measured using the ellipsoid formula (Length x Width x Height x 0.5) (Tanaka *et al.*) twice weekly .All animal were kill when they lost 25% of their body weight or had difficulty in ambulating, feeding or grooming. The experiments must be conducted according to guidelines and approval by respective animal ethic committee.

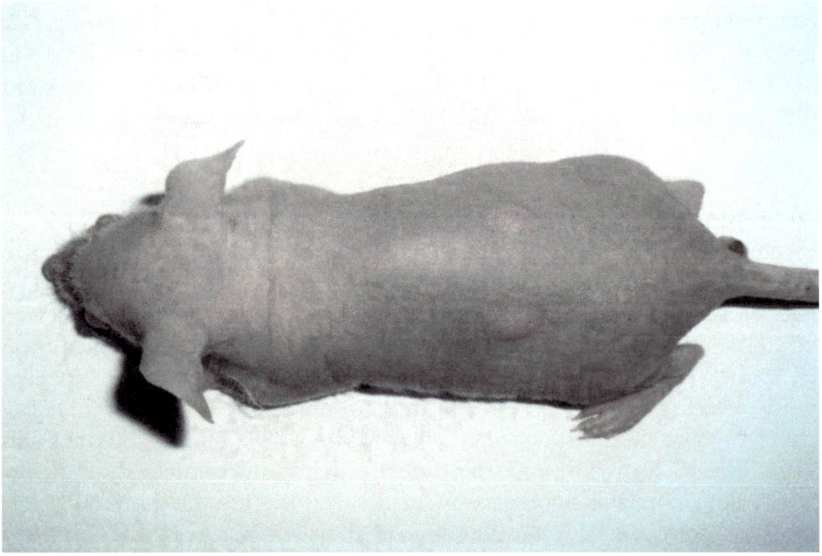

Fig. 5. The glioma growth on the nude mouse flank.

8. Conclusion

The oncolytic virus therapy is now amongst the fastest growing study compare to other salvage therapy as the current progress giving great potential in treating various cancer.

Specific relationship of virus with tumors however shows wide variable thus multiple dosages and optimum temperature have to be specifically studied. Besides that, current outcomes of oncolytic viruses studies show the direction of specific virus to be used for the specific cancers.

9. Acknowledgment

We would like to thank National Cancer Council of Malaysia (MAKNA) for continuous grant support for the oncolytic virus development for brain tumor treatment.

10. References

Aghi M. & Chiocca E.A. Gene therapy for glioblastoma multiform. *Neurosurg Focus*, Vol 20, (4) : E18 April 2006

Bart Evert and Henk G van der Poel (2005). Repliation-Selective oncolytic viruses in the treatment of cancer. *Cancer Gene Therapy*, Vol 12. Pp 141-161

Biederer C., Ries S., Brandts C.H., & McCormick F. (2002) Replication-Selective virus for cancer therapy. *Journal Molecular Medicine*, Vol 80, pp 163-175

Chamberline M.C. (2006). Treatment options for glioma. *Neurosurg. Focus*, Vol 20, (4):E2 April,2006

Elankumaran S., Rockemann D., & Samal Siba.K. (2006) Newcastle disease virus exerts oncolysis by both intrinsic and extrinsic caspase-dependent pathways of cell death. *Journal of virology*. Vol 80, No 15, August 2006. Pp 7522-7534

Franz J. Zemp, Juan Carlos Corredor, Xueqing Lung, Daniel A. Muruve, Peter A, Forsyth (2010): Oncolytic viruses as experimental treatments for malignant gliomas: Using a scourge to treat a devil. *Cytokine & Growth Factors reviews* Vol 21. Pp 103-117

Gerd R. Silberhumer, Peter Brader, Joyce Wong, Inna S. Serganova, Mithat Gonen, Segundo Jaime Gonzales, Ronald Blasberg, Dmitriy Zamarin, and Yuman Fong (2010): Genetically Engineered Oncolytic Newcastle Disease Virus Effectively Induces Sustained Remission of Malignant Pleural Mesothelioma: *Molecular Cancer Therapeutic*;9(10) October 2010 pg 2761-2769

Halatsch M.E., Löw S., Mursch K., Hielsche T., Schmidt U., Unterberg A., Vougioukas V.I., and Feuerhake F.R , (2009) Candidate genes for sensitivity and resistance of human glioblastoma multiforme cell lines to erlotinib *Journal Neurosurg* 111:Pp 211–218,

He, Y., Xu, K., Keiner, B., Zhou, J., Czudai, V., Li, T., Chen, Z., Liu, j., Klenk, H., SHu, Y.L., Sun, B. (2010). Influenza A virus replication induces cell cycle arrest in G_0/G_1 phase. *Journal of Virology* Vol 84. Pp 12832-12840.

Huang, Z., Krishnamurthy, S., Panda, A. and Samal, S.K. (2003). Newcastle disease virus V protein is associated with viral pathogenesis and functions as an alpha interferon antagonist. *Journal of Virology* 77:8676-8685

Junji Miyakoshi, Kelly D. Dobler, Joan Allalunis-Turner, John D.S. McKean, Kenneth Petruk, Peter B. R. Allen, Keith N. Aronyk, Bryce Weir, Debbie Huyser-Wierenga, Dorcas Fulton, Raul C. Urtasun, and Rufus S. Day III (1990): Absence of IFNA and IFNB Genes from malignant glioma cell lines and lack of correlation with cellular sensitivity to interferon: *Cancer research* 50,1990. Pp 278-283.

Kirn D., Martuza R.L., & Zwiebel J. (2001) Replication-selective virotherapy for cancer: Biological principles, risk management and future directions. *Nature Medicine*, Volume 7, No 7, July 2001, pp 781-787

Liu T.C, Galanis E., & Kirn D. (2007) Clinical trial results with oncolytic virotherapy: a century of promise, a decade of progress. *Nature Clinical Practice Oncology*. Volume 4, No 2, February 2007 pp 101-117

Lori W. McGinnes, Homer Pantua, Julie Reitter and Trudy G. Morrison (2006) : Newcastle Disease Virus: Propagation, Quantification, and Storage; *Current Protocols in Microbiology* (2006) 15F.2.1-15F.2.18

Maher E.A., Furnari F.B., Bachoo R.M., Rowitch D.H., Louis D.N., Cavenee W.K., & DePinho R.A. (2001) Malignant Glioma: genetics and biology of a grave matter. *Genes & Dev.* Vol 15 pp 1311-1333

Marianne M. Stanford, John C. Bell, Markus J.V., Vaha-Koskela (2010): Novel Oncolytic viruses: Riding High on the next wave? : *Cytokine & Growth Factors Reviews* Vol 21. Pp 177-183.

McGinnes, L.W, Mcquain, C. and Morrison, T. (1988). The P protein and the nonstructural 38k and 29k proteins of Newcastle disease virus are derived from the same open reading frame. *Virology* 164. Pp 256-264.

McGinnes, L.W. and Morrison, T.G. (2006). Inhibition of receptor binding stabilizes Newcastle disease virus HN and F protein-containing complexes. *Journal of Virology* 80:2894-2903.

Morrison, T.G. (2003). Structure and function of a paramyxovirus fusion protein. *Biochimicaet Biophysica Acta* 1614:73-84.

Omar A.R., Ideris A., Ali A.M., Othman F., Yusoff K., Abdullah J.M., Wali H.S.M., Zawawi M., & Meyyappan N. (2003) An overview of the development of newcastle disease virus as an anti-cancer therapy. *Malaysia Journal of Medical Sciences*. Volume 10 No 1, January 2003 pp 4-12

Parato K., Senger D., Forsyth P.A.J., & Bell J.C. (2005) Recent progress in the battle between oncolytic viruses and tumors. *Nature Review Cancer*, Volume 5, December 2005. Pp 965-976

Parker J.N., Bauer D.F., Cody J.J. and Markert J.M. (2009). Oncolytic Viral Therapy of Malignant Glioma. *The Journal of the American Society for Experimental NeuroTherapeutics*. July, 2009 Vol. 6, 558–569

Puhlmann J., F Puehler, D Mumberg, P Boukamp and R Beier (2010): Rac1 is require for oncolytic NDV replication in human cancer cells and establishes a link between tumorigenesis and sensitivity to oncolytic virus: *Oncogene* Vol 29. Pp 2205-2216.

Sateesh Krishnamurthy, Toru Takimoto, Ruth Ann Scroggs, and Allen Portner (2006): Differentially Regulated Interferon Response Determines the Outcome of Newcastle Disease Virus Infection in Normal and Tumor Cell Lines: *Journal of Virology*, June 2006. Pp.5145-5155.

Schirrmacher V. & Fournier P. (2009). Newcastle Disease Virus: A Promising Vector for Viral Therapy, Immune Therapy, and gene Therapy of Cancer. *Methods in Molecular Biology, Gene therapy of Cancer* Vol 42. Pp 565-605

Schirrmacher V., Haas C., Bonifer R., Ahlert T., Gerhards R. & Ertel C. (1999) Human tumor cell modification by virus infection: an efficient and safe way to produce cancer vaccine with pleiotropic immune stimulatory properties when using Newcastle disease virus. *Gene Therapy*, Vol 6, pp 63-73

Sinkovics J.G. & Horvath J.C. (2000). Newcastle disease virus (NDV): brief history of its oncolytic strains. *Journal of Clinical Virology*, Volume 16, (2000) pp 1-15

Ungermannova, D., Gao, Y. And liu, X. (2005). Ubiquitination of $p27_{KIP1}$ requires physical interaction with cyclin E and probable phosphate recognition by SKP2. *The Journal of Biological Chemistry*, Vol 280(34). Pp 30301-30309.

Yusoff, K. and Tan, W.S. (2001). Newcastle disease virus: macromolecules and opportunities. *Avian Pathology* Vol 30. Pp 439-455.

Zulkifli, M.M., Hilda,S.S., Manaf, A. A., Abdullah, J., Ideris, A., Hasnan, J. (2009) In vitro and In Vivo Studies of Newcastle Disease Virus (NDV) strain V4UPM against Experimental Human Malignant Glioma *Neurological Research*, Volume 31, Number 1, February 2009 , pp. 3-10(8)

22

Development of a DNA-Based Vaccine for Treatment of an Intracerebral Tumor

Terry Lichtor and Roberta P Glick
Rush University Medical Center
USA

1. Introduction

1.1 Treatment limitations of patients with breast cancer metastatic to the brain

Although technical advances have resulted in marked improvement in the ability to diagnose and treat primary breast cancer, brain metastases constitute a common and increasing occurrence associated with considerable morbidity and mortality [Lin et al., 2008; Smedby et al., 2009]. The present standard treatment modalities including surgical resection, cranial irradiation and systemic chemotherapy each have serious adverse side effects and limits in efficacy. The few long-term survivors are inevitably left with cognitive deficits and other disabilities [Heimans & Taphoorn, 2002]. The existence of blood-brain and blood-tumor barriers impedes drug delivery to the tumor. Finally the low therapeutic index between tumor sensitivity and toxicity to normal brain severely limits the ability to systemically deliver therapeutic doses of drugs or administer focal radiation therapy to the tumor. New treatment strategies are urgently needed.

1.2 Transfer of genomic DNA from one cell type to another alters both the genotype and the phenotype of cells that take up the exogenous DNA

Classic studies indicate that transfection of genomic DNA from one cell type to another results in integration of the transferred DNA and stable alteration of the genotype of the recipient cells. The transferred genes are replicated as the cells divide and are expressed. In one study the genome of adenine phosphoribosyltransferase-deficient mouse cells was modified to express the missing enzyme by transfer of DNA from mouse cells whose genome included the gene for the missing enzyme [Wigler et al., 1979]. Analogous findings were observed for membrane-associated determinants. In another study genomic DNA from human cells was transferred into polio virus-receptor-negative mouse cells and the transfected cells expressed the missing receptor [Mendersohn et al., 1986]. Others [Barraclough et al., 1998; Chen et al., 1997] used this approach to identify genes involved in metastasis. Another approach involved the generation of stable transfectants of mouse fibroblasts [Hsu et al., 1984; Kavathas & Herzenberg, 1983]. The transfected cells expressed human membrane T cell antigens, HLA determinants, and B2-microglobulin. The expression of the transferred human genes by the transfected cells was stable and long-term (more than six months). The proportion of the transfected mouse cells that expressed the human gene of interest was surprisingly large--in the range of 1/500. The importance of these findings for development of DNA-based tumor vaccines is that the transfer of genomic DNA into cells resulted in the expression of genes specifying missing enzymes, genes controlling cell proliferation and metastasis, and genes specifying membrane associated determinants. An analogous approach can be used to prepare a vaccine for use in patients with malignant gliomas. Genes specifying tumor associated antigens (TAAs) that fail to provoke anti-tumor immunity can become highly immunogenic antigenic determinants if they are expressed by highly immunogenic cells.

1.3 Multiple mutant/dysregulated genes in cancer cells specify TAAs

A major rationale for the use of DNA-transfer to prepare vaccines for use in cancer therapy is that the vaccine expresses an array of multiple altered genes which define the malignant phenotype. Genetic instability in cancer cells is responsible for the formation of TAAs. TAAs such as β-catenin [Robbins et al., 1996], gp100, Melan A/Mart-1 and tyrosinase in melanoma [de Vries et al., 1997] are differentiation antigens whose expression is dysregulated in cancer cells. Mutant genes also specify TAAs [van der Bruggen et al., 1991]. For example Boon found that a point mutation in a gene in P815 murine mastocytoma cells specified a tumor-rejection antigen [Boon et al., 1994]. Thus, the malignant cell-population is characterized by the presence of numerous TAAs, some of which are unique and others are differentially expressed by cancer cells but all are strong potential targets of immune-mediated attack.

1.4 DNA from the patient's neoplasm is the ideal source of tumor antigens for immunotherapy

Since the total number of different TAAs within the population of malignant cells is large and diverse, successful therapy will depend upon the use of a vaccine that is capable of inducing immunity to the broad array of tumor antigens that characterizes the patient's cancer. Therapy based on the induction of immunity to a single antigen, or peptide, is less likely to be successful. Multi-epitope vaccines are expected to be more efficacious than single-epitope vaccines [Stevenson et al., 2004]. This is especially the case for malignant astrocytomas, where clinically relevant TAAs, i.e., immunity to TAAs that leads to tumor rejection, have not been identified.

1.5 Characteristics of the modified cell line used as the recipient of tumor DNA

Among other advantages of this approach, the cells chosen as DNA-recipients can be selected for their ability to enhance the immune response. The expression of both syngeneic and allogeneic MHC-determinants by the DNA recipient cells is important in order to obtain an optimum anti-tumor response [deZoeten et al., 2002]. The syngeneic determinants provide a restriction element for direct presentation of TAAs to CTLs of the host. Allogeneic antigens served as potent immune adjuvants. Numerous investigators found that the immunogenic properties of cancer cells could be enhanced if the cells were modified to express allogeneic MHC-determinants [Fearon et al., 1988; Gattoni-Celli et al., 1988; Hammerling et al., 1986; Hui et al., 1989; Nabel et al., 1996; Ostrand-Rosenberg et al., 1990]. The modified cells, which ordinarily proliferate in syngeneic immunocompetent recipients, were recognized as "foreign" and were rejected. In the mouse, immunization with tumor cells altered by the introduction and expression of allogeneic class I genes led to immune-mediated rejection of the malignant cells and the induction of protective anti-tumor immunity. However, the introduction of genes specifying allogeneic determinants into cells from a primary neoplasm is technically challenging and not always successful. In contrast, transfer of DNA from the tumor into highly immunogenic syngeneic/allogeneic cells is consistently and reliably achieved.

1.6 Important advantages of preparing a vaccine by transfer of DNA from the patient's neoplasm into nonmalignant fibroblasts

A vaccine prepared by transfer of DNA from the patient's neoplasm into highly immunogenic, nonmalignant human fibroblasts has a number of important advantages. A major advantage is that the cells used as recipients of the DNA can be selected for special properties, which will enhance the anti-tumor immune response. Since the recipient cells are capable of prolonged proliferation *in vitro*, and the transferred DNA is replicated as the cells divide, only a small quantity of DNA from the neoplasm is required to generate the vaccine. In addition, the number of transfected fibroblasts can be expanded as needed to obtain sufficient quantities for repeated immunizations of the cancer patient. The fibroblasts used as DNA-recipients will also express allogeneic class I determinants which is a desirable feature since this leads to an augmented immune response. In addition a cell line derived from the patient's primary neoplasm does not have to be established, which is the case if genes specifying cytokines, allogeneic MHC-determinants, co-stimulatory molecules or other immune-augmenting properties are to be introduced into the autologous tumor cells. The establishment of tumor cell lines, especially cell lines derived from astrocytomas, is technically difficult, often not feasible and may not be representative of the tumor cell population as a whole. Furthermore hybrid cell vaccines prepared by fusion of tumor cells with antigen presenting cells pose similar concerns [Gong et al., 1997; Liang & Cohen, 1976, 1977]. Immunization with tumor cells modified to secrete immune-augmenting cytokines such as IL-2 and GM-CSF has been investigated and shown to result in the development of generalized MHC-restricted anti-tumor immune responses in animal models. However tumor cells are also a source of immunosuppressive factors, which inhibit the anti-tumor activity of the effector cells [Strand & Galle, 1998; Whiteside & Rabinwich, 1998]. The DNA-based vaccines are successful because a full complement of genes is transferred to the recipient cells which results in a robust signal for the development of anti-tumor immune responses.

1.7 Advantages of DNA-based vaccines relative to other types of vaccines

A number of different vaccination strategies are currently being evaluated [Ashley et al., 1997; Condon et al., 1996; Gilboa et al., 1998; Nair et al., 1998; Nestle et al., 1998; Tighe et al., 1998]. The approaches to vaccination with TAAs include those based on: a) defined antigens or antigenic peptides, b) tumor cell lysates or lysate fractions, and c) whole irradiated tumor cells or apoptotic tumor cell bodies. Clinical trials involving vaccines prepared using TAAs or TAA-derived epitopes presented by APCs or fed to dendritic cells (DCs) have shown some promising results. However, defined antigens have to be identified and purified, a tremendous effort requiring an "antigen discovery" approach. The quantity of purified antigen must be increased, to enable multiple immunizations of the cancer patient. While new TAAs are being discovered, the question of which TAA to be used in the vaccine is uncertain and extensively debated. The heterogeneity of antigen expression in the tumor cell population is likely to be a concern. Some tumor cells may not express the antigen chosen for therapy. In one study for example, it was found that expression of known tumor antigens such as gp100 and tyrosinase was variable in different melanoma lesions in the same patient [de Vries et al., 1997]. Not all the malignant cells in the patient's neoplasm expressed these determinants. Since the tumor cell population is heterogeneous, tumor cells that fail to express the defined antigen chosen for therapy are likely to escape destruction by the activated immune system.

The major advantage of vaccines prepared by transfer of tumor DNA into nonmalignant fibroblasts is that TAAs do not have to be purified or produced in large quantities. In comparison with protein vaccines, DNA-based vaccines provide prolonged expression and direct presentation of tumor antigens which results in robust and long-lasting activation of the immune system. From a practical point of view, these vaccines are easy and relatively inexpensive to prepare. Unlike other strategies, vaccines can be prepared from only a limited quantity of tumor-derived DNA, which can be obtained from small surgical specimens (vaccines can routinely be prepared from 50 µg of DNA). Furthermore, the recipient fibroblasts can be selected to meet the requirement for rapid expansion in culture and MHC restriction. The DNA-based vaccines offer a number of important advantages, which greatly encourage their further development for cancer immunotherapy.

1.8 Disadvantages of transfer of tumor-derived DNA transfer into fibroblasts for expression of TAAs

While vaccination based on transfer of tumor-derived DNA into highly immunogenic cells has a number of advantages, there are concerns as well. Since the proportion of total DNA that specifies TAAs is likely to be small, it is possible that a large number of the transfected cells may not express TAAs or may express TAAs at low levels. This concern is minimized, however, by preclinical data which indicate that the proportion of the cells that take-up tumor DNA and express TAAs is sufficient to induce an effective anti-tumor immune response and to significantly increase survival [Lichtor et al., 2008]. Another concern related to therapy with DNA-based vaccines is that genes specifying normal "self" antigens are likely to be expressed by the DNA-transfected cells, creating a danger that autoimmune disease might develop, although this has not been observed thus far. Inbred mice immunized with the DNA-based vaccine or tumor-bearing mice injected with therapeutic DNA-based vaccines failed to exhibit adverse effects [Lichtor et al., 2006]. Of course, protocols that depend upon the use of tumor cell-extracts, peptide eluates of tumor cells, fusion cells, cDNAs or RNAs derived from tumor cells are subject to the same concern. In DNA-based vaccines, genes encoding determinants expressed by non-neoplastic cells are likely to be present in the largest proportion relative to genes specifying TAAs. While the use of purified tumor antigen in the form of cDNA or polynucleotide vaccines specific for known TAAs eliminates this concern, those types of vaccines are dependent on the selection of the most "relevant" vaccinating epitope, as discussed above. It is also conceivable that a cellular vaccine, including one using nonmalignant fibroblasts might grow in the patient, forming a tumor. Conceivably, a transforming oncogene or a defective tumor suppressor gene might be transferred to a normal cell, provoking a neoplasm although this has not been observed. Overall, the disadvantages of DNA-based vaccines are few and are certainly no more difficult to overcome than those associated with other types of experimental tumor-vaccines.

1.9 Defects in TAA presentation by tumor cells

Defects in presentation of TAAs by tumor cells have been described in both murine as well as human tumors [Ohlen et al., 1990; Restifo et al., 1991]. They can result in tumor cell "escape" from host immunity. One mechanism is the loss of MHC determinants, which results in the impaired ability of the tumors to present TAAs. Loss of MHC antigen expression in several murine tumors is correlated with an increase in the malignant properties of the cells [Cohen & Kim, 1994]. Melanomas that recurred in mice treated with a vaccine prepared by transfer of DNA from murine melanoma cells into mouse fibroblasts were deficient in expression of MHC class I determinants [Kim & Cohen, 1994]. Primary and especially metastatic cells may have global or selective down-regulation of class I or class II HLA antigens, due to mutations in β2 microglobulin or TAP genes and thus they may fail to present TAAs in an immunogenic form to immune cells. Even if the host generates tumor-specific CTLs, the effector cells may not be able to eliminate the tumor. In addition to a failure to express HLA antigens, tumors may not express co-stimulatory molecules resulting in an inadequate immune response to TAAs by the host. Immunization with a DNA-based vaccine can overcome certain of these tumor "escape" mechanisms.

Significance

The most compelling reason for the vaccination strategy involving DNA-based cellular vaccines is the current lack of effective therapy for patients with malignant brain tumors such as breast cancer metastatic to the brain. This is verified by the dismal survival statistics, which have remained essentially unchanged for 30 years. Immunization with a vaccine that induces strong anti-tumor responses is an attractive addition or possibly even an alternative to conventional therapies. The DNA-based vaccines described in this review have shown remarkable therapeutic efficiency and survival benefits in some initial murine preclinical studies.

2. Experimental section

2.1 Treatment of intracerebral breast cancer in C3H mice by immunization with syngeneic/allogeneic fibroblast transfected with DNA from breast cancer cells

Whether results obtained by transfer of DNA from a tumor cell line into mouse fibroblasts can be applied to tumors that develop spontaneously is uncertain. Conclusions based on a model system involving tumor cell lines may not apply to neoplasms that arise spontaneously in patients. The appearance of spontaneous breast neoplasms in C3H mice provides an opportunity to investigate this question. DNA isolated from a breast neoplasm that arose spontaneously in the mammary gland of a C3H ($H\text{-}2^K$) mouse in our animal colony (SB5b breast carcinoma cell line) was transferred into mouse fibroblasts ($H\text{-}2^k$). To increase their immunogenic properties and to ensure rejection, the fibroblasts were modified to express $H\text{-}2K^b$ determinants beforehand. $H\text{-}2K^b$ determinants are allogeneic in C3H mice. The results indicated that C3H mice with intracerebral breast cancer treated solely by immunization with fibroblasts transfected with DNA from the same spontaneous breast neoplasm survived significantly longer ($p<0.005$) than mice in various control groups [Lichtor et al., 2005].

2.2 T cell mediated toxicity toward intracerebral breast cancer in mice immunized with syngeneic/allogeneic transfected fibroblasts modified to secrete IL-2, GM-CSF or IL-18

An MTS cytotoxicity assay was used to detect the presence of T cells reactive with breast cancer cells in mice injected i.c. with the mixture of SB5b cells and the modified, DNA-transfected fibroblasts. MTS is a tetrazolium compound which is bioreduced by viable cells into a formazan product that can be detected at 490 mm. The T cells obtained from the spleens of the injected mice were analyzed two weeks after the i.c. injection of the cell mixture. The results indicated that the cytotoxic response of greatest magnitude was in mice injected i.c. with the mixture of SB5b cells and transfected fibroblasts modified to secrete IL-2 or GM-CSF [Lichtor et al., 2005]. Lesser cytotoxic effects were present in mice injected i.c. with SB5b cells and transfected fibroblasts modified to secrete IL-18.

2.3 The proportion of T cells responsive to tumor cells in mice bearing an intracerebral tumor immunized intracerebrally with syngeneic/allogeneic transfected fibroblasts modified to secrete IL-2, IL-18 or IL-2 + IL-18

An ELISPOT-IFN-γ assay was used to determine the proportion of splenic T cells reactive with SB-5b cells in mice immunized with transfected fibroblasts modified to secrete IL-2, IL-18 or both IL-2 and IL-18. The animals were injected i.c. with a mixture of 1.0 X 10^4 SB-5b breast carcinoma cells and 1.0 X 10^6 treatment cells consisting of LMK^bIL-2/SB5b, LMK^bIL-18/SB5b, or a mixture of LMK^bIL-2/SB5b and LMK^bIL-18/SB5b cells. The animals were sacrificed at two weeks and an ELISPOT assay was done using the spleen cells to detect IFN-γ secretion in the presence of SB-5b tumor cells and antibodies against various T-cell subsets. The results indicate that the cellular anti-breast carcinoma immune response was mediated by $CD4^+$, $CD8^+$ and NK/LAK cells [Lichtor et al., 2005]. Although IL-18 secreting cells did not produce a significant anti-tumor immune response as detected with the ELISPOT assay, the combination of IL-2 with IL-18 secreting cells did result in an enhancement of the anti-tumor responses in comparison to animals that were treated with IL-2 secreting cells alone.

2.4 Increased numbers of responding T-cells were detected in the spleens and cervical lymph nodes of naïve mice or mice with i.c. breast cancer injected into the brain with cells from the immuno^{high} pool

An enrichment strategy for the vaccine was developed based on the hypothesis that if aliquots of a transfected cell population were divided into smaller populations, some populations by chance would contain more highly immunogenic cells than others. The populations with higher numbers of immunogenic cells could be identified by their stronger immunogenic response against SB5b cells in C3H/He mice. Two subpools that stimulated immunity to the greatest (immuno^{high} pool) and least (immuno^{low} pool) extents after three rounds of enrichment were selected for further study.

To determine if systemic anti-tumor immunity was generated in tumor-free mice injected i.c. with cells from the immuno^{high} pool, cervical lymph node and spleen cells from the injected mice were analyzed by ELISPOT IFN-γ assays for responding T cells. Naïve C3H/He mice received 2 i.c. injections at weekly intervals of 1.0 X 10^6 cells from the immuno^{high} pool. One week after the second injection, mononuclear cells from the spleens and cervical lymph nodes of the immunized mice were analyzed for the presence of T cells responsive to the breast cancer cells. As controls, an equivalent number of cells from the non-selected master pool or cells from the immuno^{low} pool were substituted for cells from the immuno^{high} pool. As additional controls, the same protocol was followed except that the mice were injected i.c. with equivalent numbers of SB5b cells, with LMK^b cells or with media. Mice injected with SB5b tumor cells received only one injection. The results from the cervical lymph nodes (figure 1) indicated that the highest number of responding cells was in mice injected i.c. with cells from the immuno^{high} pool ($p < 0.005$ vs. cells from mice in any of the other groups). Similar results were found in studies using the spleen cells from these animals [Lichtor et al., 2008].

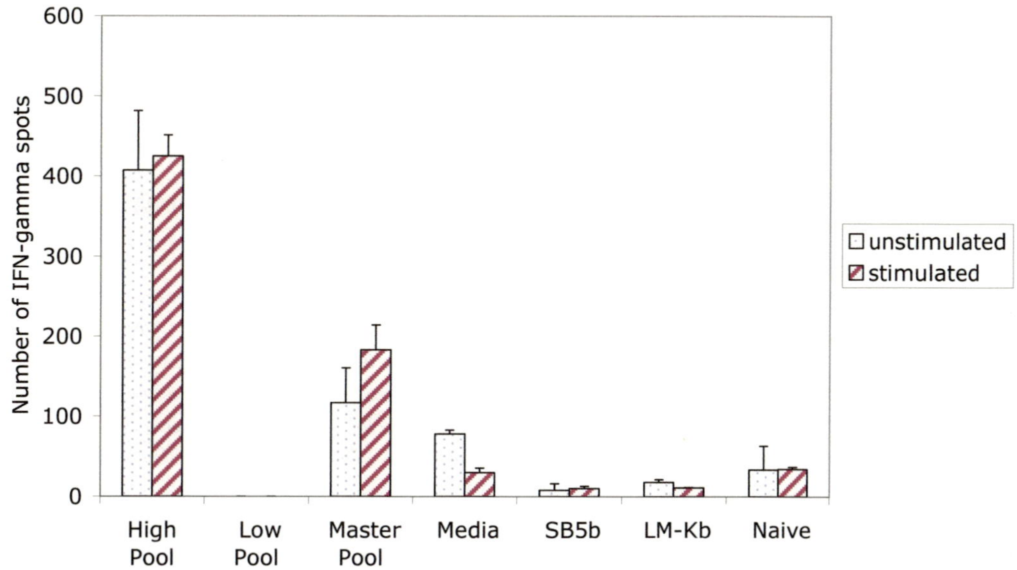

Fig. 1. Development of anti-tumor immunity in cervical lymph nodes from naïve mice injected intracerebrally with an enriched cellular vaccine. ELISPOT IFN-γ assays for responding T cells in the cervical lymph nodes of mice injected i.c. with cells from the immuno^{high} pool. Naïve C3H/He mice received intracerebral injections through a small burr hole two times at weekly intervals with 1.0 X 10^6 cells from the immuno^{high} pool of transfected cells. One week after the second injection, mononuclear cells from the cervical lymph nodes of the injected mice were analyzed by ELISPOT IFN-γ assays for responding T cells. As controls, cells from the non-enriched master pool (LMIL-2K^b/SB5b) or cells from the immuno^{low} pool were substituted for cells from the immuno^{high} pool. As additional controls, the same protocol was followed except that the mice were injected i.c. with media or with equivalent numbers of either SB5b or LMK^b cells, or the mice were not injected. The animals injected i.c. with SB5b cells alone were injected only once. In some instances, SB5b cells (stimulated) were added to the cervical lymph node cell suspensions 16 hrs before the ELISPOT IFN-γ assays were performed (the ratio of spleen cells : SB5b cells = 10:1). In this assay the number of IFN-γ spots/10^6 cervical lymph node cells is measured. Error bars represent one standard deviation. $p < 0.005$ for the difference in the number of spots in the group injected with high pool LMIL-2K^b/SB5b cells co-incubated with SB5b cells versus any of the other groups.

ELISPOT IFN-γ assays were also used to determine the number of responding T cells in the spleens of mice with i.c. breast cancer injected into the tumor bed with cells from the immuno^{high} pool [Lichtor et al., 2008]. A micro cannula was placed into the right frontal lobe of C3H/He mice. SB5b cells (1.0 X 10^4 in 10 μl) were introduced into the brain through the cannula. On days two and nine following, the animals were injected through the cannula into the tumor bed with 1.0 X 10^6 cells from the immuno^{high} pool. As controls, the same procedure was followed except that the cells from the non-enriched master pool or cells from the immuno^{low} pool were substituted for cells from the immuno^{high} pool. As additional controls, the tumor bearing mice were injected into the tumor bed with equivalent numbers of non DNA-transfected LMK^b cells or the mice were injected with SB5b cells alone. The results indicate that the highest number of responding T cells were in the spleens of tumor-bearing mice injected i.c. with cells from the immuno^{high} pool ($p < 0.05$ versus the number of responding spleen cells in mice injected with cells from the master pool and $p < 0.005$ versus the number of spots obtained from any of the other groups).

2.5 T-reg cells are relatively deficient in the spleens of mice with i.c. breast cancer injected into the tumor bed with cells from the immuno^{high} pool

T-reg cells (regulatory T cells) are potent inhibitors of natural antitumor immunity. The success of immunotherapeutic protocols may depend upon the relative numbers of T-reg cells and cytotoxic T lymphocytes in tumor-bearing animals and patients. Quantitative RT-PCR for Foxp3, a transcription factor characteristic of T-reg cells, was used to determine the relative proportions of T-reg cells in the spleens and brains of mice with i.c. breast cancer injected into the tumor bed with cells from the immuno^{high} pool of transfected cells. Naïve C3H/He mice were injected i.c. with 5.0 X 10^4 SB5b cells along with 1.0 X 10^6 cells from the immuno^{high} pool of transfected cells. One week later, the animals received a second i.c. injection of cells from the immuno^{high} pool through the same burr hole alone. As controls, the same procedure was followed except that the mice were injected with equivalent numbers of SB5b cells and cells from the non-enriched master pool or the immuno^{low} pool. The results indicate that $CD4^+/CD25^+/Foxp3^+$ T-reg cells were relatively deficient in the spleens but not in the brains of animals injected with cells from the immuno^{high} pool [Lichtor et al., 2008]. An analysis by FACS of the spleens of the injected animals revealed a relative deficiency of $CD4^+/CD25^+$ T cells and a corresponding increase in the relative numbers of $CD8^+$ cells in the spleens of mice injected i.c. with cells from the immuno^{high} pool.

3. Discussion

Despite standard therapeutic approaches, the survival of patients with primary or metastatic tumors to the brain has not improved significantly in more than thirty years. There is an urgent need for new and more effective forms of treatment. Immunotherapy, designed to stimulate immunity to the autologous tumor, is under active investigation for a number of different histologic types of cancer. The enhanced immunotherapeutic properties of a vaccine prepared by transfer of a cDNA expression library derived from breast cancer cells into a mouse fibroblast cell line appears to have great potential in treatment of intracerebral tumors. As the transferred cDNA integrates spontaneously into the genome of the recipient cells, replicates as the cells divide and is expressed, the vaccine could be prepared from small amounts of tumor tissue, enabling treatment at an early stage of the disease, when tumor tissue is available in only limited amounts and the tumor is most susceptible to immune-based therapy. However, like other cellular tumor vaccines, only a small proportion of the transfected cell population was expected to have incorporated cDNA fragments that specified tumor antigens. A novel enrichment strategy has also been developed to increase the proportion of immunotherapeutic cells in the vaccine.

A number of different strategies have been attempted to develop vaccines that generate enhanced anti-tumor immune responses in mice and patients with intracerebral neoplasms involving the central nervous system. Vaccines have been prepared by "feeding" antigen presenting (dendritic) cells apoptotic bodies from tumor cells or tumor cell lysates. Introduction of tumor cell-derived RNA into dendritic cells is another approach which has been developed. Immunization with dendritic cells "fed" derivatives of tumor cells or transfected with tumor-RNA can result in the induction of immune responses against the broad array of tumor antigens expressed by the population of malignant cells including tumors of neuroectodermal origin [O et al, 2002; Rosenberg et al., 2004]. In patients, immunization with autologous dendritic cells transfected with mRNA from malignant glioma elicited tumor-specific $CD8^+$ cytotoxic T-lymphocyte (CTL) responses against the patient's malignant cells [Kobayashi et al., 2003]. Although results of dendritic cell immunotherapy have demonstrated promise in animal models, clinical trials have been disappointing thus far [Rosenberg et al., 2004].

Other tumor vaccination strategies have been used including modification of neoplastic cells to generate anti-tumor immune responses [Colombo et al., 1991; Gansbacher et al., 1990; Golumbek et al., 1991; Mullen et al., 1992]. Immunization with tumor cells modified to secrete immune-augmenting cytokines such as IL-2 and GM-CSF has resulted in the development of generalized MHC-restricted anti-tumor immune responses in animal models [Cavallo et al., 1993; Connor et al., 1993; Dranoff et al., 1993; Marincola et al., 1994; Ohlen et al., 1990, Tahara et al., 1994]. Selective tumor regression was observed in experimental animals and patients receiving immunotherapy alone, in support of the potential of this type of treatment for patients with malignant disease [Valmori et al., 2000]. The effects of cytokine expression by central nervous system tumors (CNS) were examined initially using glioma cells that were engineered to secrete IL-4 [Yu et al., 1993]. In these studies it was demonstrated that IL-4 transduced glioma cells resulted in the development of anti-tumor immune responses. Delivery of an IFN-β expression plasmid by cationic liposomes to the CNS tumor site was also found to induce significant anti-CNS tumor immunity in pre-clinical models [Liu et al., 2002]. Use of a high-titer adenoviral vector encoding IL-12 is another strategy that was reported to induce anti-tumor responses in a glioma model [Liu et al., 2002]. Epidermal growth factor variant III is a common alteration of the epidermal growth factor receptor found in human tumors, and a peptide vaccine has now proceeded to phase 1 and 2 clinical trials in patients bearing a malignant glioma with the ability of inducing potent T- and B-cell immunity and prolongation of survival [Sampson et al., 2008; Li et al., 2010].

In addition to immunotherapy, other gene therapy strategies have been attempted in the treatment of brain tumors. For example genetically modified, conditionally-replicating Herpes Simplex Virus Type 1 vectors with anti-tumor activity have been used with some encouraging results in Phase I and Phase II clinical trials [Cassady & Parker, 2010]. RNA interference therapy has also been shown to exhibit some therapeutic effects in pre-clinical and clinical studies in patients with gliomas [Guo et al., 2010]. High grade gliomas have been shown to express an IL-13 receptor that differs from the natural IL-13 receptor, and some pre-clinical and clinical trials have been undertaken using an adenoviral vector encoding a mutated human IL-13 fused to pseudomonas exotoxin that specifically binds to the IL-13 receptor [Candolfi et al., 2010]. Antisense oligodeoxynucleotides which target mRNA encoding TGF-beta2, a cytokine secreted by brain tumors with immunosuppressive activity, have been used in a series of Phase I and II clinical trials along with an international Phase III study with some success [Hau et al., 2009]. Finally one of the problems using large viruses in treating brain tumors is that the viruses have a limited capacity to infiltrate into the brain, but recently it has been shown that neural stem cells infected with replicating adenovirus can be used to enhance intratumoral distribution of the oncolytic vectors into a malignant glioma in comparison with virus injection alone [Tyler et al., 2009].

Previous studies indicated that transfection of genomic DNA from the malignant cells into a fibroblast cell line resulted in stable integration and expression of the transferred DNA [Cohen, 2001; Lichtor et al., 2005; Lichtor et al., 2006; Lichtor et al., 2008]. Both the genotype and the phenotype of the cells that took up the exogenous DNA were altered as portions of the transferred DNA were expressed. Immunization of tumor-bearing mice with the DNA-based vaccine resulted in the induction of cell mediated immunity directed toward the type of tumor from which the DNA was obtained, and prolongation of survival, consistent with the expression of an array of TAA by the transfected cells. This was the case for mice with melanoma, squamous cell carcinoma and in mice with breast cancer [Chopra et al., 2006; deZoeten et al., 2002; Lichtor et al., 2008]. Multiple undefined genes specifying TAA that characterize the malignant cell population were expressed by cells that took up DNA from the tumor. The number of vaccine cells could be expanded as required for multiple immunizations. In addition, the recipient cells can also be modified before DNA-transfer to increase their immunogenic properties, as for example, by the introduction of genes specifying immune-augmenting cytokines or allogeneic MHC-determinants, which act as strong immune adjuvants.

4. Conclusions

To be successful, every remaining tumor cell in the patient must be eliminated. It is unlikely that a single form of therapy is capable of achieving this goal. However immunotherapy in combination with surgery, radiation therapy and chemotherapy will likely find a place as a new and important means of treatment for patients with brain tumors. A major advantage of DNA-based vaccines is that they do not require protein purification or its production and yet they are able to elicit robust and long-lasting activation of the immune response, which results in tumor rejection. From a practical point of view, these vaccines are easy to prepare and they are relatively inexpensive. Only a limited quantity of tumor-derived DNA is required, which can be obtained from small surgical specimens. The enrichment strategy enables the generation of highly immunogenic pools of transfected cells with enhanced immunotherapeutic properties.

Thus DNA-based vaccines offer a number of advantages, which greatly encourage their further development for cancer immunotherapy in general and specifically for treatment of breast cancer metastatic to the brain.

5. References

Ashley, D.M.; Faiola, B.; Nair, S.; Hale, L.P.; Bigner, D.D.; Gilboa, E. (1997). Bone marrow-generated dendritic cells pulsed with tumor extracts or tumor RNA induce antitumor immunity against central nervous system tumors. *J Exp Med,* Vol. 186, pp. 1177-1182.

Barraclough, R.; Chen, H.J.; Davies, B.R.; Davies, M.P.; Ke, Y.; Lloyd, B.H.; Oates, A.; Rudland, P.S. (1998). Use of DNA transfer in the induction of metastasis in experimental mammary systems. *Biochem Soc Symp*, Vol. 63, pp. 273-294.

Boon, T.; Cerottini, J.C.; Van den Bynde, B.; van derBruggen, P.; van Pel, A. (1994). Tumor antigens recognized by T lymphocytes. *Ann Rev. Immunol.*, Vol. 12, pp. 337-365.

Candolfi, M., Xiong, W., Yagiz, K., Liu, C., Muhammad, A.K., Puntel, M., Foulad, D., Zadmehr, A., Ahlzadeh, G.E., Kroeger, K.M., Tesarfreund, M., Lee, S., Debinski, W.,

Sareen, D., Svendsen, C.N., Rodriguez, R., Lowenstein, P.R., Castro, M.G. Gene therapy-mediated eelivery of targeted cytotoxins for glioma therapeutics. *Pro. Natl. Acad. Sci. U.S.A.*, Vol. 107; 20021-20026.

Cassady, K.A.; Parker J.N. (2010). Herpesvirus vectors for therapy of brain tumors. *Open Virol J.*, Vol. 4, pp 103-108.

Cavallo, F.; Pierro, F.D.; Giovarelli, M.; Gulino, A.; Vacca, A.; Stoppacciaro, A.; Forni, M.; Modesti, A.; Forni, G. (1993). Protective and curative potential of vaccination with interleukin-2-gene-transfected cells from a spontaneous mouse mammary adenocarcinoma. *Cancer Res.*, Vol. 53, pp. 5067-5070.

Chen, H.; Ke, Y.; Oates, A.J.; Barraclough, R.; Rudland, P.S. (1997). Isolation of and effector for metastasis-inducing DNAs from a human metastatic carcinoma cell line. *Oncogene*, Vol. 14, pp. 1581-1588.

Chopra, A., Kim, T.S., O-Sullivan, I., Martinez, D., Cohen, E.P. (2006). Treatment of squamous carcinoma in mice with a vaccine enriched for cells that induce immunity to squamous carcinoma—a new vaccination strategy. *Int J Cancer*, Vol. 119, pp. 339-348.

Cohen, E.P. (2001). DNA-based vaccines for the treatment of cancer—an experimental model. *Trends Mol Med.*, Vol. 7, pp. 175-179.

Cohen, E.P.; Kim, T.S. (1994). Neoplastic cells that express low levels of MHC class I determinants escape host immunity. *Seminars in Cancer Biology.* Academic Press, London Vol. 5, pp. 419-428.

Colombo, M.P.; Ferrari, G.; Stoppacciaro, A.; Parenza, M.; Rodolfo, M.; Mavilio, F.; Parmiani, G. (1991). Granulocyte colony-stimulating factor gene transfer suppressed tumorigenicity of a murine adenocarcinoma *in vivo*. *J. Exp. Med.*, Vol. 173, pp. 889-897.

Condon, C.; Watkins, S.C.; Celluzi, C.M.; Thompson, K.; Falo, L.D. Jr. (1996). DNA-based immunization by in vivo transfection of dendritic cells. *Nature Med.*, Vol. 2, pp. 1122-1128.

Connor, J.; Bannerji, R.; Saito, S.; Heston, W.; Fair, W.; Gilboa, E. (1993). Regr ession of bladder tumors in mice treated with interleukin 2 gene-modified tumor cells. *J. Exp. Med.*, Vol. 177, pp. 1127-1134.

de Vries, T.J.; Fourkour, A.; Wobbes, T.; Verkroost, G.; Ruiter, D.J.; van Muijen, G.N.P. (1997). Heterologous expression of immunotherapy candidate proteins gp100, MART-1 and tyrosinase in human melanoma cell lines and in human melanocytic lesions. *Cancer Res*, Vol. 57, pp. 3223-3229.

deZoeten, E.F., Markovic, D., Cohen, E.P. (2002). An optimum anti-melanoma response in mice immunized with fibroblasts transfected with DNA from mouse melanoma cells requires the expression of both syngeneic and allogeneic MHC-determinants. *Gene Ther.*, Vol. 9, pp. 1163-1172.

Dranoff, G.; Jaffee, E.; Lazenby, A.; Golumbek, P.; Levitsky, H.; Brose, K.; Jackson, V.; Hamada, H.; Pardoll, D.; Mulligan, R.C. (1993). Vaccination with irradiated tumor cells engineered to secrete murine granulocyte-macrophage colony-stimulating factor stimulates potent, specific and long-lasting anti-tumor immunity. *Proc Nat. Acad Sci USA.*, Vol. 90, pp. 3539-3543.

Fearon, E.R.; Itaya, T.; Hunt, B.; Vogelstein, B.; Frost, P. (1988). Induction in a murine tumor of immunogenic tumor variants by transfection with a foreign gene. *Cancer Res.*, Vol. 48, pp. 2975-2980.

Gansbacher, B.; Bannerji, R.; Daniels, B.; Zier, K.; Cronin, K.; Gilboa, E. (1990). Retroviral vector-mediated gamma-interferon gene transfer into tumor cells generates potent and long lasting antitumor immunity. *Cancer Res.*, Vol. 50, pp. 7820-7825.

Gattoni-Celli, S.; Willett, C.G.; Rhoads, D.B.; Simon, B.; Strauss, R.M.; Kirsch, K.; Isselbacher, K.J. (1988). Partial suppression of anchorage-independent growth and tumorigenicity in immunodeficient mice by transfection of the H-2 class I gene H-$2L^d$ into a human colon cancer cell line (HCT). *Proc. Natl. Acad. Sci. USA*, Vol. 85, pp. 8543-8547.

Gilboa, E.; Nair, K.; Lyerly, H.K. (1998). Immunotherapy of cancer with dendritic cell-based vaccines. *Cancer Immunol. Immunother.*, Vol. 46, pp. 82-87.

Golumbek, P.T.; Lazenby, A.J.; Levitsky, H.I.; Jaffee, L.M.; Karasuyama, H.; Baker, M.; Pardoll, D.M. (1991). Treatment of established renal cancer by tumor cells engineered to secrete interleukin-4. *Science*, Vol. 254, pp. 713-716.

Gong, J.; Chen, D.; Kashiwaba, M.; Kufe, D. (1997). Induction of antitumor activity by immunization with fusions of dendritic and carcinoma cells. *Nat. Med.*, Vol. 3, pp. 558-561.

Guo, D.; Wang, B.; Han, F., Lei T. (2010). RNA interference therapy for glioblastoma. *Expert Opin. Biol. Ther.*, Vol. 10, pp 927-936.

Hammerling, G.J.; Klar, D.; Katzav, S.; Segal, S.; Feldman, M.; Wallich, R.; Hammerling, A. (1986). Manipulation of metastasis and tumour growth by transfection with histocompatibility class I genes. *J. Immunogen.*, Vol. 13, pp. 15-157.

Hau, P., Jachimczak, P., Bogdahn, U. (2009). Treatment of malignant gliomas with TGF-beta2 antisense oligonucleotides. *Expert Rev Anticancer Ther.*, Vol. 9, pp. 1663-1674.

Heimans, J.J.; Taphoorn, M.J. (2002). Impact of brain tumour treatment on quality of life. *J Neurol*, Vol. 249, pp. 955-960.

Hsu, C.; Kavathas, P.; Herzenberg, L.A. (1984). Cell surface antigens expressed on L cells transfected with whole DNA from non-expressing and expressing cells. *Nature*, Vol. 312, pp. 68-69.

Hui, K.M.; Sim, T.F.; Foo, T.T.; Oei, A-A. (1989). Tumor rejection mediated by transfection with allogeneic class I histocompatibility gene. *J. Immunol*, Vol. 143, pp. 3835-3843.

Kavathas, P.; Herzenberg, L.A. (1983). Stable transformation of mouse LM cells (a transformed fibroblast cell line) for human membrane T-cell differentiation antigens, HLA and B2 microglobulin: Selection by fluorescence-activated cell sorting. *Proc. Natl. Acad. Sci. (USA)*, Vol. 80, pp. 524-528.

Kim, T.S; Cohen, E.P. (1994). MHC antigen expression by melanomas recovered from mice treated with allogeneic mouse fibroblasts genetically modified for interleukin-2 secretion and the expression of melanoma-associated antigens. *Cancer Immunol Immunother.*, Vol. 38, pp. 185-193.

Kobayashi, T.; Yamanaka, R.; Homma, J.; Tsuchiya, N.; Yajima, N.; Yoshida, S.; Tanaka, R. (2003). Tumor mRNA-loaded dendritic cells elicit tumor-specific $CD8^+$ cytotoxic T cells in patients with malignant glioma. *Cancer Immunol Immunother.*, Vol. 52, pp. 632-637.

Li, G., Mitra, S., Wong, A.J. (2010). The epidermal growth factor variant III peptide vaccine for treatment of malignant gliomas. *Neurosurg. Clin. N. Am.*, Vol 21: 87-93.

Liang, W.; Cohen, E.P. (1976). Resistance to murine leukemia in mice rejecting syngeneic somatic hybrid cells. *J. Immunol*, Vol. 116, pp. 623-628.

Liang, W.; Cohen, E.P. (1977). Resistance to murine leukemia in mice receiving simultaneous injections of syngeneic hybrid and parental neoplastic cells. *J. Immunol.*, Vol. 118, pp. 903-908.

Lichtor, T., Glick, R.P., Feldman, L.A., Osawa, G., Hardman, J., O-Sullivan, I., Cohen, E.P. (2008). Enhanced Immunity to Intracerebral Breast Cancer in Mice Immunized with a cDNA-Based Vaccine Enriched for Immunotherapeutic Cells. *Journal of Immunotherapy*, Vol. 31, pp. 18-27.

Lichtor, T.; Glick, R.P.; Lin, H.; O-Sullivan, I.; Cohen, E.P. (2005). Intratumoral injection of IL-secreting syngeneic/allogeneic fibroblasts transfected with DNA from breast cancer cells prolongs the survival of mice with intracerebral breast cancer. *Cancer Gene Therapy*, Vol. 12, pp. 708-714.

Lichtor, T., Glick, R.P., O-Sullivan, I., Cohen, E.P. (2006). Antigenic Differences Between Normal and Malignant Cells as a Basis for Treatment of Intracerebral Neoplasms Using a DNA-Based Vaccine. *Current Genomics*, Vol. 7, pp. 253-261.

Lin, N.U., Claus, E., Sohl, J., Razzak, A.R., Arnaout, A., Winer, E.P. (2008). Sites of distant recurrence and clinical outcomes in patients with metastatic triple-negative breast cancer: high incidence of central nervous system metastases. *Cancer*, Vol. 113, pp. 2638-2645.

Liu, Y.; Ehtesham, M.; Samoto, K.; Wheeler, C.J.; Thompson, R.C.; Villarreal, L.P.; Black, K.L.; Yu, J.S. (2002). In site adenoviral interleukin 12 gene transfer confers potent and long-lasting cytotoxic immunity in glioma. *Cancer Gene Ther.*, Vol. 9, pp. 9-15.

Marincola, F.M.; Shamamian, P.; Alexander, R.B.; Gnarra, J.R.; Turetskaya, R.L.; Nedospasov, S.A.; Simonis, T.B.; Taubenberger, J.K.; Yannelli, J.; Mixon, A. (1994). Loss of HLA haplotype and down-regulation in melanoma cell lines. *J Immunol.*, Vol. 153, pp. 1225-1237.

Mendersohn, C.; Johnson, B.; Lionetti, K.A.; Nobis, P.; Wimmer, E.; Racaniello, V.R. (1986). Transformation of a human poliovirus receptor gene into mouse cells. *Proc Natl Acad Sci (USA)*, Vol. 83, pp. 7845-7849.

Mullen, C.A.; Coale, M.M.; Levy, A.T.; Stetler-Stevenson, W.G.; Liotta, L.A.; Brandt, S.; Blaese, R.M. (1992). Fibrosarcoma cells transduced with the IL-6 gene exhibit reduced tumorigenicity, increased immunogenicity, and decreased metastatic potential. *Cancer Res.*, Vol. 52, pp. 6020-6024.

Nabel, G.J.; Gordon, D.; Bishop, D.K.; Nickoloff, B.J.; Yang, Z-Y.; Aruga, A.; Cameron. M.J.; Nabel, EG; Chang, AE. (1996). Immune response in human melanoma after transfer of an allogeneic class I major histocompatibility complex gene with DNA-liposome complexes. *Proc. Natl. Acad. Sci. (USA),* Vol. 93, pp. 15388-15393.

Nair, S.K.; Boczkowski, D.; Morse, M.; Cumming, R.I.; Lyerly, H.K.; Gilboa, E. (1998). Induction of primary carcinoembryonic antigen (CEA)-specific cytotoxic T lymphocytes in vitro using human dendritic cells transfected with RNA. *Nat Biotechnol*, Vol. 16, pp. 364-369.

Natsume, A.; Mizuno, M.; Ryuke, Y.; Yoshida, J. (1999). Antitumor effect and cellular immunity activation by murine interferon-beta gene transfer against intracerebral glioma in mouse. *Gene Ther.*, Vol. 6, pp. 1626-1633.

Nestle, F.O.; Alijagic. S.; Gilliet, M.; Sun, Y.; Grabbe, S.; Dummer, R.; Burg, G.; Schadendorf, D. (1998). Vaccination of melanoma patients with peptide-or-tumor lysate-pulsed dendritic cells. *Nature Med*, Vol. 4, pp. 328-332.

O, I.; Ku, G.; Ertl, H.C.J.; Blaszczyk-Thurin, M. (2002). A dendritic cell vaccine induces protective immunity to intracranial growth of glioma. *Anticancer Res.*, Vol. 22, pp. 613-622.

Ohlen, C.; Bastin, J.; Ljunggren, H.G.; Foster, L.; Wolpert, E.; Klein, G.; Townsend, A.R.M., Karre, K. (1990). Resistance to H-2-restricted but not to allo-H-2-specific graft and cytotoxic T lymphocyte responses in lymphoma mutant. *J. Immunol.*, Vol. 145, pp. 52-58.

Ostrand-Rosenberg, S.; Thakur, A.; Clements, V. (1990). Rejection of mouse sarcoma cells after transfection of MHC class II genes. *J. Immunol*, Vol. 144, pp. 4068-4071.

Restifo, N.P.; Esquivel, F.; Asher, A.L.; Stottre, H.; Barth, J.R.; Bennink, J.R.; Mule, J.J.; Yewdell, J.W.; Rosenberg, S.A. (1991). Defective presentation of endogenous antigens by a murine sarcoma: Implications for the failure of an anti tumor immune response. *J. Immunol.*, Vol. 147, pp. 1453-1458.

Robbins, P.F.; El-Gamil, M.; Li, Y.F.; Kawakami, Y.; Loftus, D.; Appella, E.; Rosenberg S.A. (1996). A mutated β-catenin gene encodes a melanoma-specific antigen recognized by tumor-infiltrating lymphoyctes. *J. Exp. Med.*, Vol. 183, pp. 1185-1192.

Rosenberg, S.A.; Yang, J.C.; Restifo, N.P. (2004). Cancer immunotherapy: moving beyond current vaccines. *Nat Med.*, Vol. 10, pp. 909-915.

Sampson, J.H., Archer, G.E., Mitchell, D.A., Heimberger, A.B., Bigner, D.D. (2008). Tumor-specific immunotherapy targeting the EGFRvIII mutation in patients with malignant glioma. *Semin. Immunol.*, Vol. 20, pp. 267-275.

Smedby, K.E., Brandt, L., Bäckland M.L., Blomqvist, P. (2009). Brain metastases admissions in Sweden between 1987 and 2006. *Br J Cancer*, Vol. 101, pp. 1919-1924.

Stevenson, F.K., Ottensmeier, C.H., Johnson, P., Zhu, D., Buchan, S.L., McCann, K.J., Roddick J.S., King, A.T., McNicholl, F., Savelyeva, N, Rice, J. (2004). DNA vaccines to attack cancer. *Proc Natl Acad Sci USA*, Vol. 101, pp. 14646-14652.

Strand, S.; Galle, P.R. (1998). Immune evasion by tumors: involvement of the CD95 (APO-1/Fas) system and its clinical implications. *Mol. Med. Today*, Vol. 4, pp. 63-68.

Tahara, H.; Zeh, H.J.; Storkus, W.J.; Pappo, I.; Watkins, S.C.; Gubler, U.; Wolf, S.F.; Robbins, P.D.; Lotze, M.T. (1994). Fibroblasts genetically engineered to secrete interleukin 12 can suppress tumor growth and induce antitumor immunity to a murine melanoma *in vivo*. *Cancer Res.*, Vol. 54, pp. 182-189.

Tighe, H.; Corr, M.; Roman, M.; Raz, E. (1998). Gene vaccination: plasmid DNA is more than just a blue print. *Immunol. Today*, Vol. 19, pp. 89-97.

Tyler, M.A., Ulasov, IV, Sonabend, A.M., Nandi, S., Han, Y. Marler, S., Roth, J., Lesniak, M.S. (2009). Neural stem cells target intracranial glioma to deliver an oncolytic adenovirus in vivo. *Gene Ther.*, Vol. 16; pp. 262-278.

Valmori, D.; Levy, F.; Miconnet, I.; Zajac, P.; Spagnoli, G.C.; Rimoldi, D.; Lienard, D.; Cerundolo, V.; Cerottini, J.C.; Romero, P. (2000). Induction of potent antitumor CTL responses by recombinant vaccinia encoding a melon-A peptide analogue. *J Immunol.*, Vol. 164, pp. 1125-1131.

van der Bruggen, P.; Traversari, C.; Chomez, P.; Lurquin. C.; Deplaen. B.; Van den Bynde, B.; Knuth, A.; Boon, T. (1991). A gene encoding an antigen recognized by cytolytic T lymphocytes on a human melanoma. *Science*, Vol. 254, pp. 1643-1647.

Whiteside, T.L.; Rabinowich, H. (1998). The role of Fas/FasL in immunosuppression induced by human tumors. *Cancer Immunol. Immunother*, Vol. 46, pp. 175-184.

Wigler, M.; Pellicer, A.; Silverstein, S.; Axel, R.; Urlaub, 0.; Chasm, L. (1979). DNA-mediated transfer of the adenine phosphoribosyltransferase locus into mammalian cells. *Proc. Natl. Acad. Sci. (USA)*, Vol. 76, pp. 1373-1376.

Yu, J.S.; Wei, M.X.; Chiocca, E.A.; Martuza, R.L.; Tepper, R.I. (1993). Treatment of glioma by engineered interleukin 4-secreting cells. *Cancer Research*, Vol. 53, pp. 3125-3128.

Gene Therapy of Glioblastoma Multiforme - Clinical Experience on the Use of Adenoviral Vectors

Thomas Wirth and Seppo Ylä-Herttuala
University of Eastern Finland
Finland

1. Gene therapy

1.1 Definition of gene therapy

According to the European Medicines Agency (EMA), a gene therapy medicinal product means "a biological medicinal product that contains an active substance, which contains or consists of a recombinant nucleic acid used in or administered to human beings with a view of regulating, replacing, adding or deleting a genetic sequence, as well as if its therapeutic, prophylactic or diagnostic effect relates to the recombinant nucleic acid sequence it contains, or to the products of genetic expression of this sequence". Simplified, in the current meaning gene therapy is the transfer of nucleic acids to somatic cells of a patient to result in a therapeutic effect. Generally, gene therapy can be classified into two categories - somatic gene therapy and germ line gene therapy. The difference between these two approaches is that in somatic gene therapy the genetic material is inserted to selected target cells, but the genetic information is not passed along to the next generation, whereas in germ line gene therapy the genetic information is passed on to the next generation. The classification of gene therapy into these two categories is of importance, since as up to day legislation allows gene therapy only to somatic cells.

1.2 History of gene therapy

In 1952, Zinder and Lederberg introduced a new term "transduction" as to describe the transfer of genetic material to cells. They demonstrated that a phage (i.e. a virus that was referred to as a filterable agent) of *Salmonella typhimurium* can carry DNA from one bacterium to another (Zinder & Lederberg, 1952). Furthermore, they pointed out that the active "filtrate" (i.e. phage) could transfer (i.e. transduce) many hereditary traits from one bacteria strain to another strain. This was a very interesting and important finding, as it explained how bacteria of different species could gain resistance to the same antibiotic very quickly. This basic understanding that phages could transfer genetic materials was soon extended also to eukaryotic viruses and a decade later after Zinder and Lederbergs discovery, Howard Temin found that specific genetic mutations as a result of virus infection could be inherited (Temin, 1961). He observed in his experiments that chicken cells infected with the Rous sarcoma virus (RSV) stably inherited viral specific gene mutations that contained the information for the generation of RSV progenies. As in the case of Zinder's and Lederberg's study, this observation was of great importance, as it unveiled the conundrum that genetic information would flow only from DNA to RNA. As the Rous sarcoma virus is a RNA virus, Temin's study showed that information could also flow from RNA to DNA, which subsequently led to the discovery of RNA-dependent DNA polymerases. Furthermore, it was realized that the acquisition of the new characteristic was stably inherited and that this was through the chromosomal insertion of the foreign genetic material (Sambrook et al, 1968).

It was obvious that viruses had properties that could be very useful in delivering genes into cells of interest. Accumulating evidences of successful cell transformation studies gave rise to the thought that genetic engineering may become a novel means for treating genetic diseases. In 1966, Edward Tatum published a paper arguing that viruses could effectively be used for modulating somatic cells and hence be a intriguing tool for gene therapy (Tatum, 1966). Of course, it was also clear that it would be necessary to strip those viruses from their pathology causing genes and replace them with a therapeutic gene or genes. Unfortunately, at that time appropriate tools for recombinant DNA technologies were not established yet. However, this did not prevent some scientists to continue working with viruses. A couple of years later after Edward Tatum's paper, Rogers et al. demonstrated an initial proof-of-concept of virus mediated gene transfer. In this study, they provided proof that a transfer of a foreign genetic material is possible by using viruses. Rogers et al. used the tobacco mosaic virus as a vector vehicle to introduce a polyadenylate stretch to the viral RNA (Rogers & Pfuderer, 1968). Motivated by the results and the hypothesis that viruses might be useful tools to introduce genetic material to cells, they went even further. Several years later, the same group performed the first direct human gene therapy trial. In that study, they used the wild-type Shope papilloma virus with the intention to introduce the gene for arginase into two girls suffering from a urea cycle disorder (Terheggen et al, 1975, Rogers et al, 1973). Based on their previous studies, they believed that the Shope papilloma virus encoded the gene for arginase activity and that this gene could be transferred by introducing the virus to the patients. Unfortunately, the outcome of the trial was negative. There was no change, neither in the arginine levels, nor in the clinical course of the hyperargininemias. Later on, after sequencing of the virus genome, it turned out that the Shope papilloma virus genome does not encode an arginase.

The study by Rogers et al. already initiated discussions about the ethical aspects and rationality of gene therapy. But it was at the latest, when Martin Cline performed a study to treat thalassaemia patients, when a big ethical debate was initiated. In that study, bone marrow cells from thalassaemia patients were taken and transfected ex vivo with plasmids containing the human globulin gene, after which these cells were re-introduced to the patients (Beutler, 2001, MacMillan, 1982). The problem, however, was that Cline had not received permission to perform those studies from the UCLA Institutional Review Board, as well as there were clear concerns about the efficacy of this therapy, since earlier animal studies demonstrated negative results (Beutler, 2001, Mercola et al, 1980). As a result, it became clear that human gene therapy would be technically, as well as ethically more complex than it was expected. Serious technical hurdles to effective gene therapy were apparent. Firstly, since of the lack of appropriate tools for recombinant DNA technology, there was no means to obtain specific functional genes. Secondly, there was no efficient or targeted means by which to deliver or replace a non-functional gene with a functional one to a defective cell. It became clear that in order to have effective therapy, the functional gene needed to be delivered to the right place and in a sufficient amount. Nevertheless, as compared to traditional medicine, gene therapy offered unique possibilities.

The discovery of the existence of integrated proviruses of viral RNA genome and the reverse transcriptase lead to the development of new and more efficient retroviral vectors. This was expected to overcome some of the barriers of chemical transfection. Several experiments proved that retroviral vectors could be used to complement genetic defects and correct disease phenotype in human cell culture models. They suggested that many human cell types are amenable to retrovirus mediated gene transduction (Goncalves, 2005). The development of adenoviral vectors further improved transduction efficiency. In comparison to retroviral vectors, adenoviruses are able to transduce both dividing and non-dividing cells, however, resulting in a more transient expression profile.

The initial targets for gene therapy were mainly monogenic disorders such as enzyme defects associated with metabolic diseases; namely Lesch-Nyhan syndrome, adenosine deaminase (ADA) deficiency, familial hyper-cholesterolaemia of low density lipoprotein (LDL) receptor deficiency, α1-antitrypsin deficiency, clotting factor deficiencies and Gaucher disease. Indeed, excellent results were obtained from ADA deficiency and adrenoleukodystrophy treatments with retroviral vectors (Aiuti et al, 2009, Cartier et al, 2009), but also failures were reported. One of the best known cases is the one of Jesse Gelsinger in 1999. Gelsinger suffered from a partial deficiency of ornithine transcarbamylase (OTC), a liver enzyme that is required for the removal of excessive nitrogen from amino acids and proteins. He was treated with adenoviral vectors encoding for the ornithine transcarbamylase gene. Four days after the treatment Jesse Gelsinger died from multiorgan failure. He was the first patient in whom death could be directly attributed to the viral vector used for treatment.

From the inception of gene therapy, cancer has been a major target. It is by far the most common disease area where gene therapy is applied to, composing over 60% of all ongoing clinical gene therapy trials worldwide, followed by cardiovascular diseases and making up close to 10% of all trials (Figure 1). The first clinical trial on cancer started in 1990, where patients with advanced melanoma were treated with tumour infiltrating lymphocytes genetically modified *ex-vivo* to express tumour necrosis factor (Rosenberg et al, 1990). Since then, many cancer types have been targeted with gene therapy including brain, lung, breast, pancreatic, liver, colorectal, prostate, bladder, head and neck, ovarian and renal cancer (Figure 1) (Wirth et al, 2009).

Up to year 2010, more than 1700 approved gene therapy clinical trials worldwide have been conducted or are still ongoing, but so far neither the Food and Drug Administration (FDA), nor the EMA have approved any human gene therapy product for commercial use. One of the major hurdles has been how to get the relevant genetic material into a sufficient number of target cells, and how to avoid the transduction of non-target cells (i.e. how to target the gene transfer vector to cells of interest)?

2. Gene transfer methods

Different methods for gene delivery have been studied and used. They can be grouped into three different categories: 1) physical, 2) viral and 3) non-viral methods. Examples of physical methods are electroporation, ultrasound and gene gun delivery. In the viral or non-viral gene transfer methods, a biological (a virus) or a synthetic (liposomes or nanoparticles) vector is used as a vehicle to deliver the genetic material into the cells. In the clinical trials the most commonly used gene transfer vectors have been adenovirus, retrovirus and naked/plasmid DNA (Figure 2). Even though lentiviral vectors represent currently only a small percentage of the viral vectors being used, they have been intensively studied and may be a promising candidate in future gene therapy strategies.

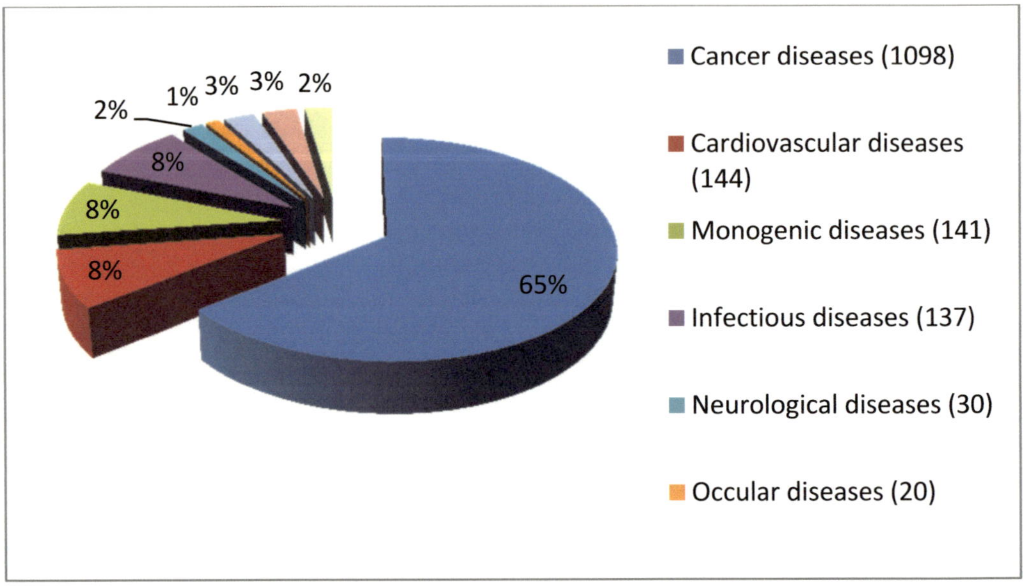

Fig. 1. The graph shows the different indications that have been addressed by gene therapy in clinical trials. Even though initial studies have been conducted on monogenetic diseases, cancer became soon after a major interest, with up to date consisting 65% of all clinical trials. The reasons for this are the highly unmet medical need in cancer therapy, as well as its big market size. Also, the ethical acceptance of gene therapy as a therapeutic modality is a factor that surely has supported the shift from monogenetic diseases to cancer.

There are three main methods that have been utilized to deliver a genetic material into the brain: 1) Stereotactic intracerebral inoculation by craniotomy, 2) intrathecal or intraventricular administration and 3) intravascular administration of the gene transfer vector. Of those three methods, the stereotactic inoculation by craniotomy is the most commonly used strategy (Wirth & Yla-Herttuala, 2006). Genetic material can be delivered also by *ex-vivo* gene transfer approach, in which gene transduction is performed outside the patient (i.e. *ex vivo*), into previously isolated autologous cells, which are re-introduced back to the patient. Even though the intracerebral injection of gene transfer vectors is the simplest approach for local gene therapy, this method still faces obstacles that remain to overcome. The direct intraparenchymal injection is limited by the small volumes that can be administered into focal areas. Also, the diffusion of the gene transfer vectors is minimal, i.e. they do not significantly penetrate into brain parenchyma, which may restrict the transduction to only a few micrometers from the injection site (Rainov & Kramm, 2001). Convection enhanced delivery is a method to improve the spread of the gene transfer vector within the tissue by maintaining a pressure gradient during interstitial infusion (Bidros et al, 2010). In this method multiple catheters are placed within the tumour and the vector solution is infused at a continuous and slow rate (Bidros et al, 2010). However, there is still discussion about, whether convection enhanced delivery really improves transduction efficiency (Bidros et al, 2010, ter Horst et al, 2006). One of the limitations of direct intratumoural administration is that it is possible to do only with solid tumours. In case of systemic administration of the gene transfer vector, targeting of the vector specifically to the tumour cells or restricting the expression of the transgene to tumour cells is essential (Bourbeau et al, 2007).

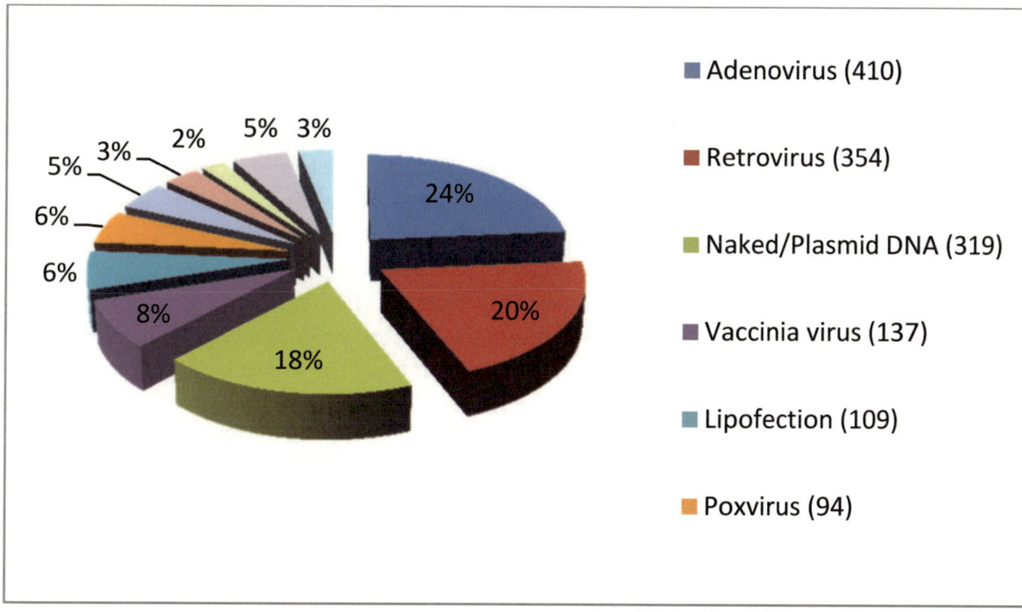

Fig. 2. The graph shows the different gene transfer vectors used in clinical settings. By far, adenoviral, retroviral and naked plasmid/DNA have been the most commonly used gene transfer vectors.

Viral vectors are considered as the most effective of all gene delivery methods for *in-vivo* gene transfer. Commonly used viral vectors for brain cancer gene therapy includes retrovirus, herpes simplex virus, adenovirus and adeno-associated virus (Figure 2). Apart from these, baculovirus, New Castles' Disease virus, polio virus, semliki forest virus, measles virus, lentivirus, reovirus and vaccinia virus have also been used as vectors. In most of these vectors, the viral genome has been genetically modified to make them replication defective and non-pathogenic and to make space for the transgene. However, in the oncolytic viruses the viral genome has been modified to give them the ability to specifically replicate only within tumour cells that would lead to the lyses of the tumour cells. Some of the new viral vectors have the ability to replicate only once within the target cells without the ability to disseminate, thereby aiming at increasing the transgene copy number and expression within the transduced cells.

2.1 Adenoviruses as a gene transfer vector

Adenoviral vectors have been widely utilized for gene therapy studies both in preclinical and clinical settings. To date, more than 100 adenovirus serotypes have been classified, of which 51 serotypes are human adenoviruses, divided into seven species (human adenovirus A to F). These classifications are based on their hemagglutination properties, oncogenic potential in newborn hamsters, genomic organization and DNA homology (Sharma et al, 2009). Adenoviruses are non-enveloped, icosahedral viruses of 80 to 1200 nm in diameter.

They contain a linear, double stranded DNA genome of 30 to 40 kb. As gene transfer vectors, they can carry relatively large fragments of foreign DNA. The main components of adenoviruses are the capsid and the core. The homotrimeric hexon capsomers, which are the main constituent of the capsid, form the 20 triangular faces of the icosahedron. Each of the 12 vertices on the adenovirus surface is made up of a penton capsomere. The penton capsomere is composed of a penton base and a fiber protein. The latter forms a spike-shaped protrusion with a terminal globular domain or "knob" that is responsible for the attachment of the virus to its primary receptor. In addition to hexon and penton capsomers, there are several hexon-associated proteins with capsid-stabilizing functions. The double stranded DNA genome is located in the virion core with DNA associated proteins and terminal proteins that serve as a primer for DNA replication.

Human adenoviruses are known to cause a variety of clinical symptoms, depending on their serotypes (Sharma et al, 2009). These include infections of the upper and lower respiratory tract, renal and urinary tract, gastroenteritis and ocular infections. The coxsackie-adenovirus receptor is a 46 kDa type I transmembrane glycoprotein on the surface of many cell types and serves as a primary receptor for human adenoviruses. The knob domain of the homotrimeric fiber binds to the coxsackie-adenovirus receptor, mediating virus attachment to the cell. Subsequently, an Arg-Gly-Asp-motif located on the penton base interacts with a cell surface integrin molecules that play a role as a secondary or internalization receptor and triggers the virus entry via clathrin-dependent receptor mediated endocytosis. In addition to the coxsackie-adenovirus receptor, other receptors, such as class I major histocompatibility complex, heparan sulphate glycosaminoglycans and vascular cell adhesion molecule-1 have been shown to play a role in the viral cell entry. Adenoviruses transduce both dividing and quiescent cells and they provide an efficient, but transient transgene expression. They exist extrachromosomally within the host cell, although the viral DNA migrates into the cell nucleus. Because of their broad host and cell range, adenoviral vectors have been extensively used in experimental models, as well as in clinical protocols.

Adenoviral vectors have been used in suicide gene therapy, anti-angiogenic gene therapy, oncoviral therapy, gene therapy based on immune modulation, gene therapy targeting oncogenes or tumour suppressor genes and gene therapy targeting tumour invasion and apoptosis. In addition, approaches such as gene delivery of antisense or small interference RNAs (siRNA) targeted to growth factors in order to increase the sensitivity of glioma cells to chemotherapeutics or to inhibit migration and invasion of glioma cells have been developed. The most extensively studied and used adenoviral serotype in gene therapy is the serotype 5, causing only mild or asymptomatic infections (Sharma et al, 2009, Raty et al, 2008). In the first generation of adenoviral vectors, the E1 region encoding for early viral proteins is replaced by the transgene, making the vectors replication defective. By deleting the E1 region, a transgene capacity of 4.7-4.9 kb is achieved, which is then further increased to 8.3 kb by deleting the non-essential region E3. To circumvent the problem of the host cellular immune response against the viral proteins produced by other early viral genes, a second generation adenoviral vectors was described, where the E4 region is deleted. This second generation of adenoviral vectors was shown to be safer in terms of causing less apoptosis and inducing to a lesser extent an immune response in vivo. The third generation adenoviral vectors were constructed by deleting additional adenovirus genes, resulting in a so called high-capacity, gutless or helper-dependent adenoviral vectors.

3. Glioblastoma multiforme

Brain tumours can be divided into primary and secondary brain tumours. Primary brain tumours derive from within the brain, whereas secondary brain tumours originate from organs such as lung, breast, colon, skin, kidney and thyroid, which have metastasized to the brain. Primary brain tumours are classified based on histological appearance, resemblance of the tumour cells to embryonic, foetal or differentiated mature cells, growth pattern, radiological features and surgical appearance. The most common and also the most lethal primary brain tumours in adults are gliomas, which account for 60 to 70% of primary tumours. Their overall global incidence lies between 4-6 new cases per 100,000 population per year, which has not changed significantly within the past 30 years (Ohgaki & Kleihues, 2005, Ohgaki, 2009)(Wirth et al, 2009). Current standard therapy of malignant glioma includes surgical resection followed by adjuvant radiotherapy and/or chemotherapy (i.e. temozolomide), which results in an overall mean survival of 14.6 months after diagnosis and a 5-year survival of 9.8% (Stupp et al, 2009). More recently, in May 2009 the FDA approved bevacizumab (an antibody against the growth factor VEGF) for the treatment of glioblastoma multiforme under an accelerated approval process (Cloughesy, 2010). The approval was based on the results of 2 phase II clinical trials that showed bevacizumab reduced the tumour size in some patients. Another recently published phase II trial of single-agent bevacizumab followed by bevacizumab plus irinotecan showed a significant therapeutic activity in patients with recurrent glioblastoma (Friedman et al, 2009). However, the results are somewhat under strong dispute, as the European Medicine Agency (EMA) has recently denied the approval of bevacizumab for the treatment of recurrent high-grade glioma (Balana et al, 2011). Nevertheless, even though the addition of temozolomide to standard therapy, as well as the addition of bevacizumab plus irinotecan as an optional protocol, has significantly improved the survival of glioma patients, there is still a highly unmet medical need for this indication. Even recent trials combining cetuximab (an antibody against the epidermal growth factor receptor) with bevacizumab and irinotecan or the combination of bevacizumab with temozolomide did not improve the overall survival of patients with glioblastoma multiforme (Hasselbalch et al, 2010, Lai et al, 2011). It is the diffusely infiltrating property of these tumours and the resistance to chemotherapy and radiotherapy that makes the therapy mostly ineffective, which ultimately leads to tumour recurrence at some point of time.

3.1 Gene therapy of glioblastoma multiforme

Brain tumours bear several features that make them particularly amenable to gene therapy. Firstly, brain tumours are in most cases single, localized lesions of rapidly dividing cells in a background of non-dividing cells. Secondly, they rarely metastasize outside the central nervous system and if recurrence occurs, it typically happens in the close vicinity of the original lesion. Different gene therapy approaches using different gene transfer vectors for the treatment of malignant gliomas have been studied. These include pro-drug activation/suicide gene therapy, anti-angiogenic gene therapy, oncolytic virotherapy, immune modulation, correction of gene defects, inhibition of tumour invasion, apoptosis induction, gene therapy to enhance chemo- and radiotherapy, myeloprotective gene therapy, antisense and RNA interference (RNAi) based strategies. Although most of these methods have demonstrated promising success in vitro and in pre-clinical studies, only few of them have progressed up to phase III clinical trials.

3.2 Clinical efficacy of adenovirus mediated gene therapy in glioblastoma multiforme

Up to date, 20 registered clinical trials for the treatment of malignant glioma using adenoviral vectors have been conducted or are still ongoing. Different approaches such as suicide gene therapy strategy, interleukin-2, interferon-β, melanoma differentiation associated gene-7/interleukin 24 (mad-7/IL-24), p53, a dominant negative EGF receptor mutant (D-EGFR-CD533), the human soluble FMS-like tyrosine kinase 3 ligand concomitant with Herpes simplex virus-thymidine kinase, a Fas-TNF receptor chimera, p53 and a conditionally replication-competent adenovirus (Delta-24-RGD) have been utilized. The very first clinical gene therapy trial against brain cancer was registered in 1992. In that trial autologous tumour cells were modified ex vivo with retrovirus to express interleukin-2 gene in neuroblastoma. In the following year, brain cancer patients were treated with herpes simplex virus thymidine kinase suicide gene therapy using retrovirus vectors producing cells and concomitant administration of ganciclovir. However, transduction efficiency was a major problem in these trials, resulting in poor therapeutic efficacy. Another problem was that retrovirus producing cells were murine of origin. In comparison to retroviral vectors, adenoviral vectors have shown to have higher transduction efficacy as well as transgene expression (Sandmair et al, 2000a). Adenoviruses transduce both, dividing and quiescent cells, which may provide an important advantage, as not all cancer cells proliferate within the tumour at a given time point. In 1996, Eck et al. published the first phase I clinical trial, where adenovirus Herpes simplex virus-thymidine kinase was used with the intention to patients with recurrent gliomas. However, the first completed trial using adenovirus Herpes simplex virus-thymidine kinase in patients with malignant glioma was published by Sandmair et al. in 2000. In that study, 21 patients were enrolled to compare the efficacy of both, the retrovirus-packaging cells Herpes simplex virus-thymidine kinase and the adenovirus mediated Herpes simplex virus-thymidine kinase gene therapy for the treatment of primary or recurrent gliomas. The mean survival time in the adenovirus Herpes simplex virus-thymidine kinase group was 15 months and significantly longer, when compared to a 7.4 months survival time in the retrovirus-packaging-cells group. The control group, which received adenovirus *LacZ* had a mean survival time of 8.3 months. Although the retrovirus-packaging-cells approaches were found safe, no efficacy was observed in malignant glioma patients. The low gene transfer efficacy with retrovirus and the lack of the treatment response indicated that retroviral Herpes simplex virus-thymidine kinase gene therapy may not be efficient enough in human clinical settings. This was further confirmed by the results from the first randomized, open-labeled, parallel group phase III clinical trial of 248 patients, where Herpes simplex virus-thymidine kinase produced by retroviral producing cells did not result in an improvement of survival (Rainov, 2000). Trask et al. conducted a non-controlled phase I study in which patients with recurrent malignant brain tumours were injected with adenovirus Herpes simplex virus-thymidine kinase with doses ranging from $2x10^9$ to $2x10^{12}$ virus particles via a single stereotactic intratumoural injection (Trask et al, 2000). Despite the occurrence of pronounced central nervous system toxicity in patients receiving the highest dose, adequate safety and feasibility was reported for adenovirus Herpes simplex virus-thymidine kinase gene therapy.

In 2003, a phase I clinical trial published by Lang et al., described the use of adenoviral vactors encoding for the tumour suppressor gene *TP53* to treat patients with recurrent malignant gliomas (Lang et al, 2003). In that study, 15 patients ought to undergo

intratumoural stereotactic injection of the adenoviral vector via an implanted catheter, followed by en bloc resection of the tumour and treatment of the post-resection cavity. Due to the design of the study, the tumour response could not be assessed, but the study demonstrated minimal toxicity. No systemic viral dissemination was observed and a maximum tolerated dose was not reached in this study. Analysis of tumour specimens demonstrated restricted transgene expression close to the injection site. Chiocca et al. published a phase I dose-escalation trial of the oncolytic adenovirus ONYX-015, which preferentially replicates in p53-deficient cells and thereby lyses them (a common feature in tumour cells). In that trial, 24 patients with recurrent malignant glioma were injected with the oncolytic virus with doses ranging from 10^7 to 10^{10} pfu (plaque forming units) in a total of 10 injections into 10 different sites of the cavity of resected tumours. None of the patients experienced serious adverse events related to the virus. However, in this trial the maximum tolerated dose was not reached. All patients showed tumour progression with a median time of 46 days and a median survival time of 6.2 months (Chiocca et al, 2004). One patient with anaplastic astrocytoma had stable disease and two patients who underwent a second resection had lymphocytic and plasmacytoid cell infiltration at the site of injection. Nevertheless, despite a good safety profile, the overall therapeutic efficacy was poor. In another study performed by Chiocca et al., 11 patients were injected with different doses of interferon-β-expressing adenoviruses ranging from $2x10^{10}$ to $2x10^{11}$ viral particles stereotactically into the tumour. This was followed by surgical removal of the tumour 4-8 days later with additional injections of the adenovirus into the tumour bed (Chiocca et al, 2008). Generally, the treatment was well tolerated with only one patient experiencing dose-limiting side effect after post-operative injection with the highest dose. However, all patients had disease progression and/or recurrence within 4 months after the treatment. The median time to tumour progression was 9.3 weeks and the median overall survival was 17.9 weeks.
So far, the only adenoviral vector that has completed a phase III clinical trial (Cerepro®, by Ark Therapeutics Group plc) is based on the suicide gene therapy Herpes simplex virus-thymidine kinase. In that trial, adenoviral vector encoding for Herpes simplex virus-thymidine kinase was injected into the walls of the tumour cavity of glioma patients after the resection of the tumour (Figure 3).
The clinical efficacy of Cerepro® was evaluated first in two separate phase II clinical trials; a phase IIa trial and a phase IIb trial (Sandmair et al, 2000a, Immonen et al, 2004). In the randomized and controlled phase IIb trial published by Immonen, carried out in 36 patients, seventeen patients with operable or recurrent malignant gliomas receiving Herpes simplex virus-thymidine kinase adenoviral vector (Cerepro®) implicated a survival advantage over control patients, who did not receive Cerepro®. The mean survival of the patients in the Cerepro® group (70.6 weeks) was significantly longer ($p<0.0095$) when compared to the standard care group (39.0 weeks) or a historical control group ($P<0.0017$). This study was also historically the first randomized, controlled trial with an adenoviral vector using Herpes simplex virus-thymidine kinase, where an increased survival of the patients was shown when compared to standard therapy. The results from the study were very encouraging and it was concluded that Cerepro® could provide an effective adjuvant treatment for patients with operable primary or recurrent malignant glioma. Therefore, a multicenter, standard care controlled, randomized clinical phase III trial was commenced. However, the results coming out of that trial were not as significant as those from the

previous IIb trial. As a result, suggestions by the European Medicines Agency were given for further clinical evaluation, as they concluded that the data did not provide sufficient evidence of significant clinical benefit compared to current standard treatment.

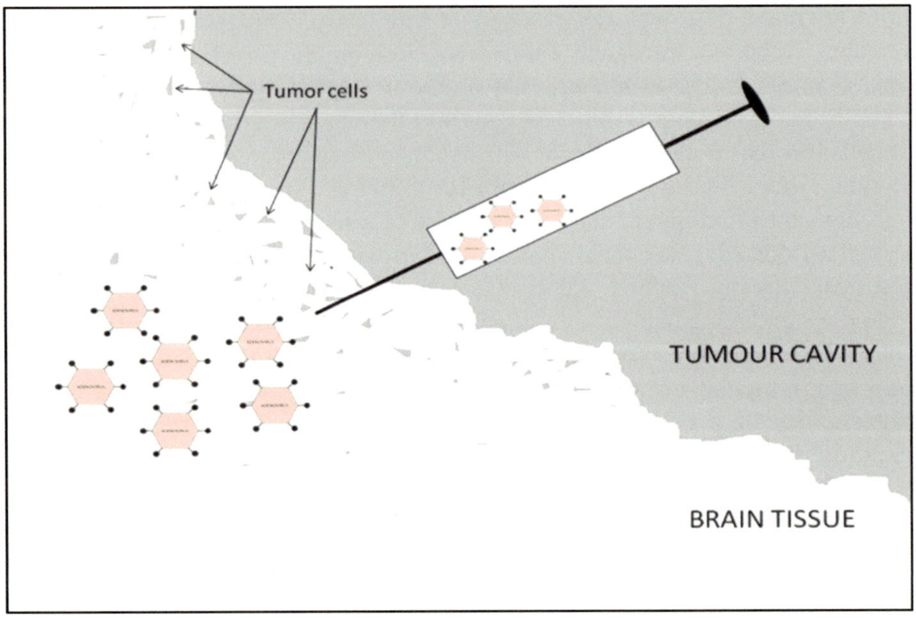

Fig. 3. In case of Cerepro® adenoviral vectors encoding for the Herpes simplex virus-thymidine kinase are injected into the tumour cavity of resected tumours, which is followed by ganciclovir administration. The injection of Cerepro® into the tumour cavity results in the transduction of mainly healthy brain cells, which express the Herpes simplex virus thymidine kinase and converts ganciclovir into ganciclovir-monophosphate. Ganciclovir-monophosphate is than further converted ultimately into ganciclovir-triphosphate, by the cells own kinases, which is toxic to proliferating cells. As the brain does not harbour any proliferating cells other than the tumour cells, Cerepro® does not affect healthy brain cells.

4. Suicide gene therapy

The most common approach in these studies has been the use of the Herpes simplex virus-thymidine kinase gene followed by either ganciclovir or valacyclovir treatment.

Suicide gene therapies can generally be divided into two steps. In the first step, a gene of a foreign enzyme is delivered (via viral vectors) to the tumour where it is to be expressed. In the second step, a non-active pro-drug is administered, which will be selectively metabolized to the active form by the foreign enzyme expressed in the tumour. Ideally, the gene for the enzyme should be expressed exclusively in the tumour cells and should reach a concentration sufficient to activate the pro-drug for a clinical benefit. Several suicide genes have been studied with varying results. Herpes simplex virus-thymidine kinase, Cytosine deaminase (CD)/5-fluorocytosine (5-FC), cytochrome P450/cyclophosphamide (CPA), E.coli purine nucleoside phosphorylase (PNP)/6-methyl-purine-2'-deoxynucleoside, and carboxypeptidase G2 (CPG2)/methotrexate-α-phenylalanine are some of the pro-drug activation systems that have been attempted on brain cancer treatment. Because the foreign enzyme will not be expressed in all cells of the targeted tumour in vivo, a "bystander effect" is required, whereby the pro-drug is cleaved to an active drug that kills not only the tumour cells in which it is formed, but also neighbouring tumour cells that do not express the transgene (Figure 4).

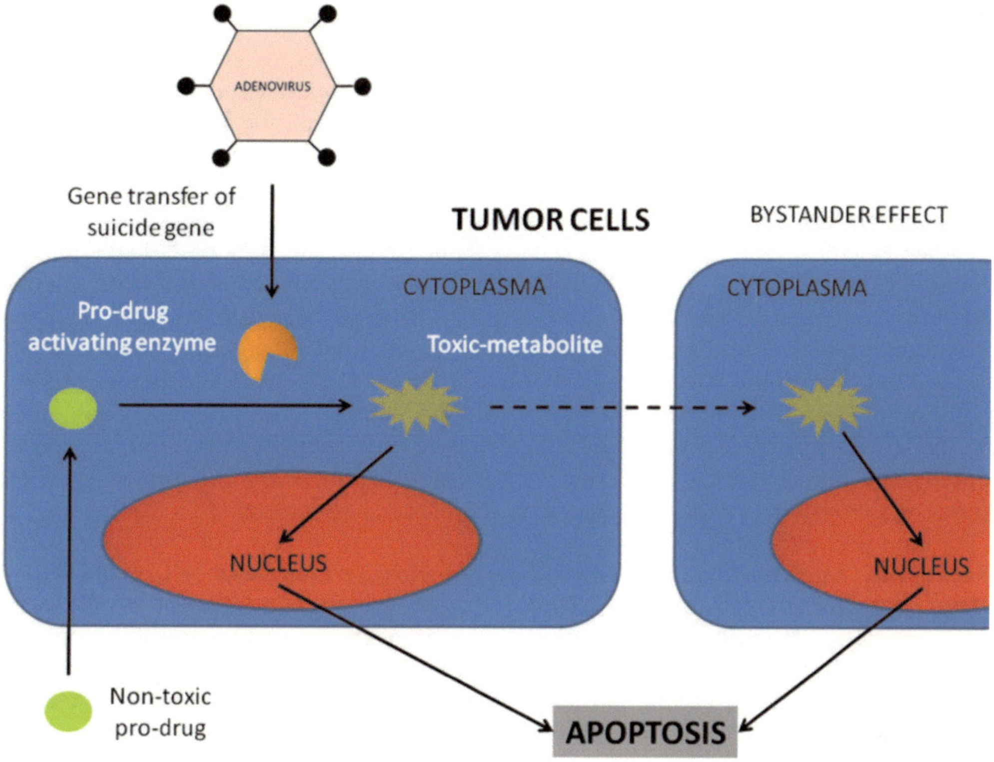

Fig. 4. A schematic presentation of how suicide gene therapy works. First, a suicide gene needs to be introduced into the target cells, after which it will be expressed by the cell. The second step is the administration of a pro-drug, which will be converted into a toxic metabolite by the introduced pro-drug activating enzyme (i.e. the suicide gene), which ultimately leads to cell death. The toxic metabolite can further diffuse passively or actively into neighbouring tumour cells and induce cell death.

4.1 Herpes simplex virus-thymidine kinase / ganciclovir therapy against glioblastoma multiforme

The Herpes simplex virus-thymidine kinase/ganciclovir therapy is based on the pro-drug activating enzyme Herpes simplex virus-thymidine kinase that converts the nucleotide analogue ganciclovir to its toxic metabolite. Apart from malignant glioma, Herpes simplex virus-thymidine kinase/ganciclovir has been studied also in many other cancer types, both in pre-clinical models and in clinical trials. Data from six phase I/II clinical trials using adenoviral vectors encoding for the Herpes simplex virus-thymidine kinase have been published and two of the trials have demonstrated a significant benefit for the treatment of patients with malignant glioma. Despite not observing total cures or complete responses, the prolongation of survival without a deteriorating quality of life in patients with a fatal disease such as glioblastoma multiforme is a strong indication of the therapeutic potential of gene therapy.

Originally, the Herpes simplex virus-thymidine kinase gene was cloned by McKnight in 1980 (McKnight, 1980). This property to kill tumour cells when given ganciclovir was soon realized and led to the idea of using this as a therapeutic strategy to treat solid tumours. The first proof-of-concept of the therapeutic efficacy of the Herpes simplex virus-thymidine kinase/ganciclovir therapy was established ten years later by Moolten and Wells. They used retroviral vectors expressing the Herpes simplex virus-thymidine kinase gene in order to transduce murine sarcoma and lymphoma cells in vivo (Moolten & Wells, 1990). In the initial studies murine fibroblasts transduced with Herpes simplex virus-thymidine kinase retroviral vectors were inoculated intratumourally, followed by ganciclovir treatment (Moolten & Wells, 1990). Ganciclovir is a synthetic acyclic analogue of 2'-deoxy-guanosine, chemically designated as 9-[[2-hydroxy-1-hydroxymethyl)ethoxy]methyl]-guanine. Ganciclovir is known as being the first antiviral drug to be effective in the treatment of cytomegalovirus (CMV) diseases in humans. It is converted to ganciclovir-monophosphate by the Herpes simplex virus-thymidine kinase, which has a 1000 fold higher affinity for ganciclovir than the mammalian form of the enzyme. Cell kinases continue the phosphorylation further and convert the ganciclovir-monophosphate into a ganciclovir-diphosphate and finally to a toxic ganciclovir-triphosphate. Cytotoxic ganciclovir-triphosphate results in the inhibition of the DNA polymerase thus preventing DNA replication (Figure 5).

The Herpes simplex virus-thymidine kinase/ganciclovir therapy is cell cycle dependent, where only dividing cells are affected. This property is considered to be of advantage in cancer therapy, where dividing tumour cells are often surrounded by non-dividing, healthy cells. Moreover, it has been shown that the expression of the non-human enzyme Herpes simplex virus-thymidine kinase and the presence of tumour antigens that become available after the death of the transduced cells are able to induce an antitumoural immune response against the tumour cells. It is believed that both local and systemic immune responses contribute to the overall therapeutic effect of Herpes simplex virus-thymidine kinase/ganciclovir by stimulating the tumour infiltration of CD4+ and CD8+ T cells, natural killer cells and macrophages into the tumour. Furthermore, work by different groups suggests that ganciclovir induced cell killing occurs due to apoptosis through the activation of mitochondrial damage pathways, chromosomal aberrations, and sister chromatin exchange that leads to target cell death due to cell cycle arrest.

As current gene therapy vectors cannot achieve 100% gene transfer efficacy, the bystander effect is essential for an effective anti-tumour therapy. A very important advantage of Herpes simplex virus-thymidine kinase/ganciclovir gene therapy is its bystander effect, where neighbouring non-transduced cells are also exposed to the toxic ganciclovir-triphosphate metabolite (Freeman et al, 1993). Interestingly, it was noticed that also Herpes simplex virus-thymidine kinase-negative cells were killed after exposure to ganciclovir. Moreover, it was found that even with low concentration of Herpes simplex virus-thymidine kinase -positive tumour cells, tumour growth could be prevented (Freeman et al., 1993, Wu et al., 1994, Sandmair et al., 2000b). An experiment conducted by Sandmair et al suggests that 10% of the tumour cells have to be transduced with Herpes simplex virus-thymidine kinase gene in order to achieve a significant tumour regression (Sandmair et al, 2000b). However, this "bystander effect" seems to be dependent on the cell type. The exact mechanism of the "bystander effect" is not completely understood, but several mechanisms have been postulated (van Dillen et al, 2002). For example, it has been observed that the number of gap junctions plays a vital role in this effect. Additionally, it was demonstrated that the number of gap junctions seems to correlate with the efficiency of killing neighbouring cells. There is on the other hand experimental evidence where the release of toxic ganciclovir-triphosphate into the culture medium by dying cells results in apoptosis of non-transduced cells. This was shown to be dependent on ganciclovir-triphosphate accumulation in the surrounding cells and the concentration of ganciclovir in the medium, suggesting that cell-to cell contacts are not essential. Another possible mechanism includes the stimulation of the immune system, endothelial cell transduction leading to disruption of tumour vasculature and phagocytosis of apoptotic vesicles by neighbouring non-transduced cells (van Dillen et al, 2002, Burrows et al, 2002, Kruse et al, 2000).

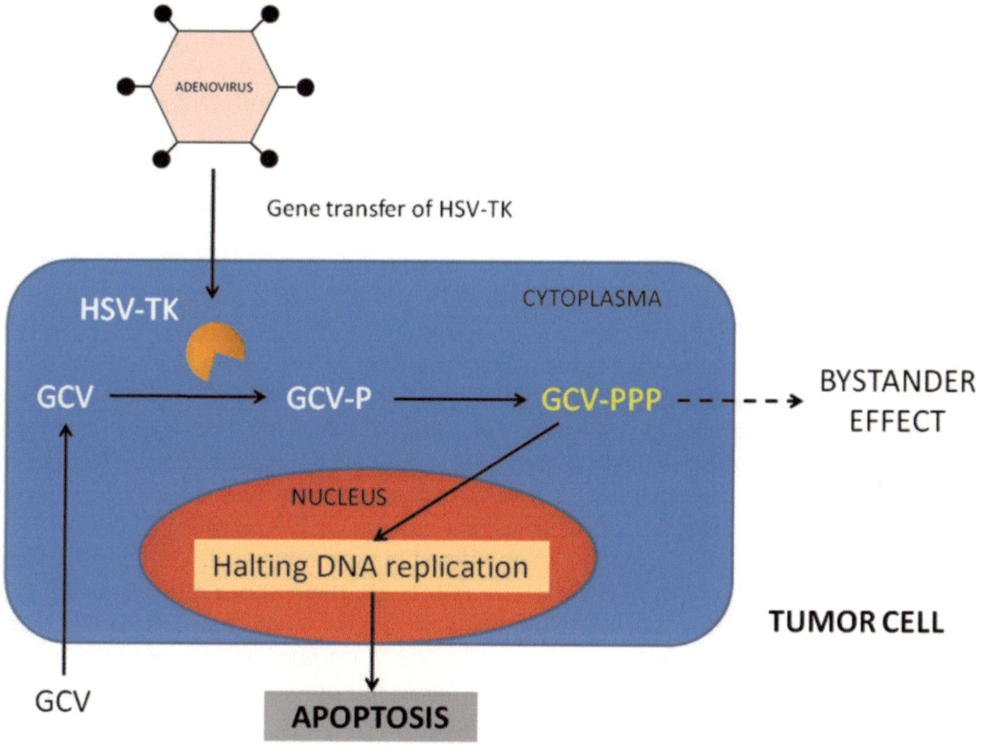

Fig. 5. In Herpes simplex virus-thymidine kinase/ganciclovir gene therapy the gene for the Herpes simplex virus thymidin kinase is introduced into the target cells. After gene transfer the pro-drug ganciclovir is administered to the patient, which is converted by the introduced Herpes simplex virus thymidin kinase into ganciclovir monophosphate. The cells own enzymes than further convert ganciclovir-monophosphat into ganciclovir-biposphate and ganciclovir-triphosphate, being the active molecule.. Ganciclovir tri-phosphate is a nucleotide analogue, which is incorporate into the DNA genome, thereby halting DNA replication.

5. The safety of adenoviral vectors

Adenoviruses are human pathogens and a significant proportion of the human population posses pre-existing antibodies against them. Some serological surveys have shown this to be as high as 40-60% for serotypes 1, 2 and 5 in children, which could rapidly inactivate the systemically administered adenoviral vectors (Verma & Weitzman, 2005). Generally, an adenoviral vector injection will result in an initial non-specific host response with the release of the cytokines tumour necrosis factor-α (TNF-α), interleukins (IL) 1 and 6, followed by a specific cell-mediated immune response directed against the infected cells, mediated by cytotoxic T lymphocytes, monocytes and natural killer cells and a humoral response through activated B cells and CD4+ T lymphocytes. This may give rise to a major obstacle for the efficiency and safety of the use of adenovirus vectors (Barcia et al, 2006, Driesse et al, 1998).

The immune response within the brain towards a viral vector, however, might differ from the response one can see in other organs. Immunologically, the brain can be divided into two compartments and the type of the initiated immune response as a result of viral vector delivery (into the brain) will greatly depend on the compartment into which the viral vector has been delivered. The first immunological compartment consists of the ventricles, meninges and choroid plexi, which all contain cellular, vascular and lymphatic components of the immune system as one can see in most other organs (Galea et al, 2007). The second immunological compartment is the brain parenchyma itself. A hallmark of this compartment is the lack of dendritic cells and lymphatic vessels in it and it is separated from the general circulation by the blood brain barrier, formed by tight intercellular endothelial junctions (Galea et al, 2007, Bechmann et al, 2007). Functionally, this means that the injection of viral vectors into the ventricular systems, for example, will result in the activation of an innate and adaptive immune response, whereas the injection of a viral vector only into the brain parenchyma would result in an innate inflammatory response, but would not trigger a systemic adaptive immune response (Lowenstein et al, 2007). Furthermore, Thomas et al demonstrated in his studies that the innate immune response was dose-dependent and ultimately influenced the duration of the transgene expression (Thomas et al, 2001).

Despite this, the safety data of adenoviral mediated gene therapy collected from different human trials have been uniformly satisfactory. Although, there is not much data about the long-term aspects regarding the safety of adenoviral vectors in humans, several meta-analysis exist demonstrating that adenoviruses have an adequate safety profile in humans. The tolerability towards adenoviral vectors has been acceptable and the side effects have mostly been mild without any serious adverse events related to gene therapy (Wirth et al, 2009, Immonen et al, 2004).

Generally, the main concerns in cancer gene therapy of patients with malignant gliomas are the safety issues when using viruses to deliver the therapeutic genes into the brain. Especially in the case of adenoviruses the inflammatory reactions that might arise in the brain are of concern. In some clinical studies using adenoviruses for gene transfer, evidences of side effects such as increased brain oedema, epileptic seizures and haemorrhages have been demonstrated (Wirth et al, 2009, Immonen et al, 2004). However, these complications have not been related directly to viral mediated gene therapy, but most likely to the advanced disease and the surgical procedures.

The first study evaluating the safety and efficacy of Cerepro® was also the first completed recombinant adenovirus mediated Herpes simplex virus-thymidine kinase gene therapy

trial against malignant glioma in humans (Sandmair et al, 2000a). In order to evaluate the safety of Herpes simplex virus-thymidine kinase therapy serological assessment, i.e. routine blood and urine analysis, as well as tests for the detection of anti-adenoviral antibodies were performed. The study showed that the therapy was well tolerated and no major alterations in routine laboratory tests were observed. No systemic escape of the virus was detected from urine or plasma samples with PCR. Anti-adenovirus antibodies were measured before and two weeks after the gene transfer. A four fold increase in antibodies against the adenoviral vector was detected in four patients. Two of the patients had also short-term transient fever reactions. No severe adverse events related to viral mediated gene therapy were detected in neither of the treatment groups. The most serious adverse events were some elevation in the frequency of epileptic seizures (2 patients), hemiparesis and aphasia (1 patient). Nevertheless, it could not be excluded that these adverse events were related to the mechanical irritation of the operation procedure and the tumour resection itself.
The phase IIb study of Cerepro® showed also a good safety profile with no signs of significant safety concerns. Three patients had transient reversible elevation of liver enzymes; two out of 17 patients in the Cerepro® group developed localized post-operative intracerebral oedema. Adenovirus was detected by PCR in the plasma of two patients three days after gene therapy, but not thereafter. A similar safety profile was seen also in the phase III trial.

6. Ethical considerations of gene therapy based medicines

As a result of the study of Cline and colleagues in 1980, an intense debate about the ethical issues of gene therapy was initiated. It is of no surprise that genetic modification of human beings, even though for therapeutic purposes, would raise many ethical questions. Arguable, gene therapy raises many ethical questions, which is a response to uncertainty and fear towards gene therapy or its possible consequences. It raises concerns about the safety in humans and their offspring, environment safety, its impact on the society in general and whether gene therapy is ethically distinctive from other medical therapies. An example of the social impact of gene therapy based medicine would be, whether it is going to be a treatment modality only accessible to a certain group of people, i.e. people with a higher social status or income. Is it going to be accessible for everyone, in other words will it be covered by the social health care system? How much it will cost? It is of no surprise that opinions and points of views about gene therapy vary from one extreme to another. Cultural as well as religious opinions have a strong impact on these standpoints. Questions, such as which would be the diseases where gene therapy is ethically acceptable or what would be the cost of the therapy, need to be asked in order to justify gene therapy in humans.
Whereas gene therapy is more tolerated for life-threatening diseases, such as cancer or AIDS, it is not tolerated in the correction of learning disorders. The question is what is acceptable and what is not? How about dealing with genetic or chromosomal disorders? Would it be ethically acceptable to practise gene therapy on people with Dawn syndrome? What would be the justification of using gene therapy in the enhancement of some individual physical or mental properties? Somatic gene therapy appears to be more tolerated than germline gene therapy. Currently, legislation allows only gene therapy into somatic cells, even though the distinction between germ-line gene therapy and somatic gene therapy can be questioned. One of the main arguments and at the same time also one of our biggest fears, is the risk of uncontrolled genetic changes produced in an individual by gene

therapy, which in the worst case would be passed also onto the offspring's of the treated person. The fact, that other therapies also can cause genetic alterations is often disregarded. For example, many different mutagenic drugs (e.g. those often used in cancer treatment), as well as radiation therapy may cause genetic alterations and if this mutation happens in germline, it will be passed onto future generations.

There are also technical issues concerning the justification of gene therapy. For example, what are the technical details of the DNA and vector to be used? The technical aspects involved, risks endeavoured by the patient and the fear of human genetic engineering are some of the major reasons why human gene therapy trials have long been difficult to conduct. The use of viral gene transfer vectors, such as lentiviruses has raised scepticism about the safety of these vectors. Non-viral vectors are not yet efficient enough, but have gained better acceptance in the society. In this regard, it seems that gene therapy in cancer is ethically acceptable, whereas the use of genetically modified stem cells is a much more difficult topic. Needless to say, the normal principles of good clinical research apply in the conduct of the ethical evaluation of gene therapy protocols. The integrity and free will of a patient should be respected, all available information for the informed consent should be given and the safety of an individual must be the first concern of the treatment protocols.

7. Conclusion

Currently, most of the gene therapy strategies used are limited to the local administration of the gene transfer vector, or to *ex vivo* gene transfer approaches. For that, malignant glioma represents an attractive target for gene therapy, because of its restricted anatomical location and absence of metastases outside the central nervous system. However, the greatest shortcoming with gene therapy is the low transduction efficiency of the gene transfer vector and its minimal distribution within the tissue. Certainly, the low transduction efficiency can be regarded as a methodological problem to some extent, but still, if one wants to improve the potential scope of gene therapy, the focus needs to be directed towards vector development and improved efficiencies. Furthermore, the concept of using a single agent therapy has been noted as being not as successful as being hoped in achieving a complete cure, and thus, combination therapy with existing conventional modalities or other new therapies may offer additional benefit in cancer gene therapy. There are already encouraging results of combination gene therapy in experimental glioma, where adenoviral mediated Herpes simplex virus-thymidine kinase/ganciclovir therapy has been combined to adenovirally transduced FMS like tyrosine kinase 3 ligand (FLT3L) immunotherapy (King et al, 2008).

Currently, the first gene based products have entered the market. In October 2003, China became the first country to approve the commercial production of a gene therapy drug. Shenzhen SiBiono GenTech (Shenzhen, China), obtained a drug license from the State Food and Drug Administration of China (SFDA; Beijing, China) for its recombinant Ad-p53 gene therapy (Gendicine) for head and neck squamous cell carcinoma (HNSCC). In 2006, the conditionally replicating adenovirus H-101 gained marketing approval for head and neck squamos cell carcinoma - also in China. More recently, Rexin-G, a pathotropic targeted retroviral vector designed to interfere with *cyclin GI* gene by integrating into the host DNA, has recently been approved in the Philippines for the treatment of all solid tumors that are refractory to standard chemotherapy.

8. References

Aiuti, A, Cattaneo, F, Galimberti, S, Benninghoff, U, Cassani, B, Callegaro, L, Scaramuzza, S, Andolfi, G, Mirolo, M, Brigida, I, Tabucchi, A, Carlucci, F, Eibl, M, Aker, M, Slavin, S, Al-Mousa, H, Al Ghonaium, A, Ferster, A, Duppenthaler, A, Notarangelo, L, Wintergerst, U, Buckley, RH, Bregni, M, Marktel, S, Valsecchi, MG, Rossi, P, Ciceri, F, Miniero, R, Bordignon, C and Roncarolo, MG. (2009). Gene therapy for immunodeficiency due to adenosine deaminase deficiency. *N.Engl.J.Med.*, 360. 5, (Jan 29), pp.447-458, 1533-4406; 0028-4793

Balana, C, Etxaniz, O, Buges, C and Martinez, A. (2011). Approval denied by the European Medicines Agency (EMA) for bevacizumab in the treatment of high-grade glioma recurrence: a good idea or a grave error? *Clin.Transl.Oncol.*, 13. 3, (Mar), pp.209-210, 1699-3055; 1699-048X

Barcia, C, Gerdes, C, Xiong, WD, Thomas, CE, Liu, C, Kroeger, KM, Castro, MG and Lowenstein, PR. (2006). Immunological thresholds in neurological gene therapy: highly efficient elimination of transduced cells might be related to the specific formation of immunological synapses between T cells and virus-infected brain cells. *Neuron.Glia Biol.*, 2. 4, (Nov), pp.309-322, 1741-0533; 1740-925X

Bechmann, I, Galea, I and Perry, VH. (2007). What is the blood-brain barrier (not)? *Trends Immunol.*, 28. 1, (Jan), pp.5-11, 1471-4906; 1471-4906

Beutler, E. (2001). The Cline affair. *Mol.Ther.*, 4. 5, (Nov), pp.396-397, 1525-0016; 1525-0016

Bidros, DS, Liu, JK and Vogelbaum, MA. (2010). Future of convection-enhanced delivery in the treatment of brain tumors. *Future Oncol.*, 6. 1, (Jan), pp.117-125, 1744-8301; 1479-6694

Bourbeau, D, Lau, CJ, Jaime, J, Koty, Z, Zehntner, SP, Lavoie, G, Mes-Masson, AM, Nalbantoglu, J and Massie, B. (2007). Improvement of antitumor activity by gene amplification with a replicating but nondisseminating adenovirus. *Cancer Res.*, 67. 7, (Apr 1), pp.3387-3395, 0008-5472; 0008-5472

Burrows, FJ, Gore, M, Smiley, WR, Kanemitsu, MY, Jolly, DJ, Read, SB, Nicholas, T and Kruse, CA. (2002). Purified herpes simplex virus thymidine kinase retroviral particles: III. Characterization of bystander killing mechanisms in transfected tumor cells. *Cancer Gene Ther.*, 9. 1, (Jan), pp.87-95, 0929-1903

Cartier, N, Hacein-Bey-Abina, S, Bartholomae, CC, Veres, G, Schmidt, M, Kutschera, I, Vidaud, M, Abel, U, Dal-Cortivo, L, Caccavelli, L, Mahlaoui, N, Kiermer, V, Mittelstaedt, D, Bellesme, C, Lahlou, N, Lefrere, F, Blanche, S, Audit, M, Payen, E, Leboulch, P, l'Homme, B, Bougneres, P, Von Kalle, C, Fischer, A, Cavazzana-Calvo, M and Aubourg, P. (2009). Hematopoietic stem cell gene therapy with a lentiviral vector in X-linked adrenoleukodystrophy. *Science*, 326. 5954, (Nov 6), pp.818-823, 1095-9203; 0036-8075

Chiocca, EA, Abbed, KM, Tatter, S, Louis, DN, Hochberg, FH, Barker, F, Kracher, J, Grossman, SA, Fisher, JD, Carson, K, Rosenblum, M, Mikkelsen, T, Olson, J, Markert, J, Rosenfeld, S, Nabors, LB, Brem, S, Phuphanich, S, Freeman, S, Kaplan, R and Zwiebel, J. (2004). A phase I open-label, dose-escalation, multi-institutional trial of injection with an E1B-Attenuated adenovirus, ONYX-015, into the peritumoral region of recurrent malignant gliomas, in the adjuvant setting. *Mol.Ther.*, 10. 5, (Nov), pp.958-966, 1525-0016; 1525-0016

Chiocca, EA, Smith, KM, McKinney, B, Palmer, CA, Rosenfeld, S, Lillehei, K, Hamilton, A, DeMasters, BK, Judy, K and Kirn, D. (2008). A phase I trial of Ad.hIFN-beta gene therapy for glioma. *Mol.Ther.*, 16. 3, (Mar), pp.618-626, 1525-0024; 1525-0016

Cloughesy, T. (2010). FDA accelerated approval benefits glioblastoma. *Lancet Oncol.*, 11. 12, (Dec), pp.1120, 1474-5488; 1470-2045

Driesse, MJ, Vincent, AJ, Sillevis Smitt, PA, Kros, JM, Hoogerbrugge, PM, Avezaat, CJ, Valerio, D and Bout, A. (1998). Intracerebral injection of adenovirus harboring the HSVtk gene combined with ganciclovir administration: toxicity study in nonhuman primates. *Gene Ther.*, 5. 8, (Aug), pp.1122-1129, 0969-7128; 0969-7128

Freeman, SM, Abboud, CN, Whartenby, KA, Packman, CH, Koeplin, DS, Moolten, FL and Abraham, GN. (1993). The "bystander effect": tumor regression when a fraction of the tumor mass is genetically modified. *Cancer Res.*, 53. 21, (Nov 1), pp.5274-5283, 0008-5472

Friedman, HS, Prados, MD, Wen, PY, Mikkelsen, T, Schiff, D, Abrey, LE, Yung, WK, Paleologos, N, Nicholas, MK, Jensen, R, Vredenburgh, J, Huang, J, Zheng, M and Cloughesy, T. (2009). Bevacizumab alone and in combination with irinotecan in recurrent glioblastoma. *J.Clin.Oncol.*, 27. 28, (Oct 1), pp.4733-4740, 1527-7755; 0732-183X

Galea, I, Bechmann, I and Perry, VH. (2007). What is immune privilege (not)? *Trends Immunol.*, 28. 1, (Jan), pp.12-18, 1471-4906; 1471-4906

Goncalves, MA. (2005). A concise peer into the background, initial thoughts and practices of human gene therapy. *Bioessays,* 27. 5, (May), pp.506-517, 0265-9247; 0265-9247

Hasselbalch, B, Lassen, U, Hansen, S, Holmberg, M, Sorensen, M, Kosteljanetz, M, Broholm, H, Stockhausen, MT and Poulsen, HS. (2010). Cetuximab, bevacizumab, and irinotecan for patients with primary glioblastoma and progression after radiation therapy and temozolomide: a phase II trial. *Neuro Oncol.*, 12. 5, (May), pp.508-516, 1523-5866; 1522-8517

Immonen, A, Vapalahti, M, Tyynela, K, Hurskainen, H, Sandmair, A, Vanninen, R, Langford, G, Murray, N and Yla-Herttuala, S. (2004). AdvHSV-tk gene therapy with intravenous ganciclovir improves survival in human malignant glioma: a randomised, controlled study. *Mol.Ther.*, 10. 5, (Nov), pp.967-972, 1525-0016

King, GD, Muhammad, AK, Curtin, JF, Barcia, C, Puntel, M, Liu, C, Honig, SB, Candolfi, M, Mondkar, S, Lowenstein, PR and Castro, MG. (2008). Flt3L and TK gene therapy eradicate multifocal glioma in a syngeneic glioblastoma model. *Neuro Oncol.*, 10. 1, (Feb), pp.19-31, 1522-8517; 1522-8517

Kruse, CA, Lamb, C, Hogan, S, Smiley, WR, Kleinschmidt-Demasters, BK and Burrows, FJ. (2000). Purified herpes simplex thymidine kinase retroviral particles. II. Influence of clinical parameters and bystander killing mechanisms. *Cancer Gene Ther.*, 7. 1, (Jan), pp.118-127, 0929-1903

Lai, A, Tran, A, Nghiemphu, PL, Pope, WB, Solis, OE, Selch, M, Filka, E, Yong, WH, Mischel, PS, Liau, LM, Phuphanich, S, Black, K, Peak, S, Green, RM, Spier, CE, Kolevska, T, Polikoff, J, Fehrenbacher, L, Elashoff, R and Cloughesy, T. (2011). Phase II study of bevacizumab plus temozolomide during and after radiation therapy for patients with newly diagnosed glioblastoma multiforme. *J.Clin.Oncol.*, 29. 2, (Jan 10), pp.142-148, 1527-7755; 0732-183X

Lang, FF, Bruner, JM, Fuller, GN, Aldape, K, Prados, MD, Chang, S, Berger, MS, McDermott, MW, Kunwar, SM, Junck, LR, Chandler, W, Zwiebel, JA, Kaplan, RS and Yung, WK. (2003). Phase I trial of adenovirus-mediated p53 gene therapy for recurrent glioma: biological and clinical results. *J.Clin.Oncol.*, 21. 13, (Jul 1), pp.2508-2518, 0732-183X; 0732-183X

Lowenstein, PR, Mandel, RJ, Xiong, WD, Kroeger, K and Castro, MG. (2007). Immune responses to adenovirus and adeno-associated vectors used for gene therapy of brain diseases: the role of immunological synapses in understanding the cell biology of neuroimmune interactions. *Curr.Gene Ther.*, 7. 5, (Oct), pp.347-360, 1566-5232; 1566-5232

MacMillan, P. (1982). The Cline affair. *Nurs.Times*, 78. 9, (Mar 3-9), pp.383, 0954-7762; 0954-7762

McKnight, SL. (1980). The nucleotide sequence and transcript map of the herpes simplex virus thymidine kinase gene. *Nucleic Acids Res.*, 8. 24, (Dec 20), pp.5949-5964, 0305-1048

Mercola, KE, Stang, HD, Browne, J, Salser, W and Cline, MJ. (1980). Insertion of a new gene of viral origin into bone marrow cells of mice. *Science*, 208. 4447, (May 30), pp.1033-1035, 0036-8075; 0036-8075

Moolten, FL and Wells, JM. (1990). Curability of tumors bearing herpes thymidine kinase genes transferred by retroviral vectors. *J.Natl.Cancer Inst.*, 82. 4, (Feb 21), pp.297-300, 0027-8874

Ohgaki, H. (2009). Epidemiology of brain tumors. *Methods Mol.Biol.*, 472. pp.323-342, 1064-3745

Ohgaki, H and Kleihues, P. (2005). Population-based studies on incidence, survival rates, and genetic alterations in astrocytic and oligodendroglial gliomas. *J.Neuropathol.Exp.Neurol.*, 64. 6, (Jun), pp.479-489, 0022-3069; 0022-3069

Rainov, NG. (2000). A phase III clinical evaluation of herpes simplex virus type 1 thymidine kinase and ganciclovir gene therapy as an adjuvant to surgical resection and radiation in adults with previously untreated glioblastoma multiforme. *Hum.Gene Ther.*, 11. 17, (Nov 20), pp.2389-2401, 1043-0342

Rainov, NG and Kramm, CM. (2001). Vector delivery methods and targeting strategies for gene therapy of brain tumors. *Curr.Gene Ther.*, 1. 4, (Nov), pp.367-383, 1566-5232

Raty, JK, Lesch, HP, Wirth, T and Yla-Herttuala, S. (2008). Improving safety of gene therapy. *Curr.Drug Saf.*, 3. 1, (Jan), pp.46-53, 1574-8863

Rogers, S, Lowenthal, A, Terheggen, HG and Columbo, JP. (1973). Induction of arginase activity with the Shope papilloma virus in tissue culture cells from an argininemic patient. *J.Exp.Med.*, 137. 4, (Apr 1), pp.1091-1096, 0022-1007; 0022-1007

Rogers, S and Pfuderer, P. (1968). Use of viruses as carriers of added genetic information. *Nature*, 219. 5155, (Aug 17), pp.749-751, 0028-0836; 0028-0836

Rosenberg, SA, Aebersold, P, Cornetta, K, Kasid, A, Morgan, RA, Moen, R, Karson, EM, Lotze, MT, Yang, JC and Topalian, SL. (1990). Gene transfer into humans--immunotherapy of patients with advanced melanoma, using tumor-infiltrating lymphocytes modified by retroviral gene transduction. *N.Engl.J.Med.*, 323. 9, (Aug 30), pp.570-578, 0028-4793; 0028-4793

Sambrook, J, Westphal, H, Srinivasan, PR and Dulbecco, R. (1968). The integrated state of viral DNA in SV40-transformed cells. *Proc.Natl.Acad.Sci.U.S.A.*, 60. 4, (Aug), pp.1288-1295, 0027-8424; 0027-8424

Sandmair, AM, Loimas, S, Puranen, P, Immonen, A, Kossila, M, Puranen, M, Hurskainen, H, Tyynela, K, Turunen, M, Vanninen, R, Lehtolainen, P, Paljarvi, L, Johansson, R, Vapalahti, M and Yla-Herttuala, S. (2000a). Thymidine kinase gene therapy for human malignant glioma, using replication-deficient retroviruses or adenoviruses. *Hum.Gene Ther.*, 11. 16, (Nov 1), pp.2197-2205, 1043-0342

Sandmair, AM, Turunen, M, Tyynela, K, Loimas, S, Vainio, P, Vanninen, R, Vapalahti, M, Bjerkvig, R, Janne, J and Yla-Herttuala, S. (2000b). Herpes simplex virus thymidine kinase gene therapy in experimental rat BT4C glioma model: effect of the percentage of thymidine kinase-positive glioma cells on treatment effect, survival time, and tissue reactions. *Cancer Gene Ther.*, 7. 3, (Mar), pp.413-421, 0929-1903

Sharma, A, Li, X, Bangari, DS and Mittal, SK. (2009). Adenovirus receptors and their implications in gene delivery. *Virus Res.*, 143. 2, (Aug), pp.184-194, 1872-7492; 0168-1702

Stupp, R, Hegi, ME, Mason, WP, van den Bent, MJ, Taphoorn, MJ, Janzer, RC, Ludwin, SK, Allgeier, A, Fisher, B, Belanger, K, Hau, P, Brandes, AA, Gijtenbeek, J, Marosi, C, Vecht, CJ, Mokhtari, K, Wesseling, P, Villa, S, Eisenhauer, E, Gorlia, T, Weller, M, Lacombe, D, Cairncross, JG, Mirimanoff, RO, European Organisation for Research and Treatment of Cancer Brain Tumour and Radiation Oncology Groups and National Cancer Institute of Canada Clinical Trials Group. (2009). Effects of radiotherapy with concomitant and adjuvant temozolomide versus radiotherapy alone on survival in glioblastoma in a randomised phase III study: 5-year analysis of the EORTC-NCIC trial. *Lancet Oncol.*, 10. 5, (May), pp.459-466, 1474-5488

Tatum, EL. (1966). Molecular biology, nucleic acids, and the future of medicine. *Perspect.Biol.Med.*, 10. 1, (Autumn), pp.19-32, 0031-5982; 0031-5982

Temin, HM. (1961). Mixed infection with two types of Rous sarcoma virus. *Virology*, 13. (Feb), pp.158-163, 0042-6822; 0042-6822

ter Horst, M, Verwijnen, SM, Brouwer, E, Hoeben, RC, de Jong, M, de Leeuw, BH and Sillevis Smitt, PA. (2006). Locoregional delivery of adenoviral vectors. *J.Nucl.Med.*, 47. 9, (Sep), pp.1483-1489, 0161-5505; 0161-5505

Terheggen, HG, Lowenthal, A, Lavinha, F, Colombo, JP and Rogers, S. (1975). Unsuccessful trial of gene replacement in arginase deficiency. *Z.Kinderheilkd.*, 119. 1, pp.1-3, 0044-2917; 0044-2917

Thomas, CE, Birkett, D, Anozie, I, Castro, MG and Lowenstein, PR. (2001). Acute direct adenoviral vector cytotoxicity and chronic, but not acute, inflammatory responses correlate with decreased vector-mediated transgene expression in the brain. *Mol.Ther.*, 3. 1, (Jan), pp.36-46, 1525-0016; 1525-0016

Trask, TW, Trask, RP, Aguilar-Cordova, E, Shine, HD, Wyde, PR, Goodman, JC, Hamilton, WJ, Rojas-Martinez, A, Chen, SH, Woo, SL and Grossman, RG. (2000). Phase I study of adenoviral delivery of the HSV-tk gene and ganciclovir administration in patients with current malignant brain tumors. *Mol.Ther.*, 1. 2, (Feb), pp.195-203, 1525-0016

van Dillen, IJ, Mulder, NH, Vaalburg, W, de Vries, EF and Hospers, GA. (2002). Influence of the bystander effect on HSV-tk/GCV gene therapy. A review. *Curr.Gene Ther.*, 2. 3, (Sep), pp.307-322, 1566-5232

Verma, IM and Weitzman, MD. (2005). Gene therapy: twenty-first century medicine. *Annu.Rev.Biochem.*, 74. pp.711-738, 0066-4154

Wirth, T, Samaranayake, H, Pikkarainen, J, Maatta, AM and Yla-Herttuala, S. (2009). Clinical trials for glioblastoma multiforme using adenoviral vectors. *Curr.Opin.Mol.Ther.*, 11. 5, (Oct), pp.485-492, 2040-3445; 1464-8431

Wirth, T and Yla-Herttuala, S. (2006). Gene technology based therapies in the brain. *Adv.Tech.Stand.Neurosurg.*, 31. pp.3-32, 0095-4829

Wu, JK, Cano, WG, Meylaerts, SA, Qi, P, Vrionis, F and Cherington, V. (1994). Bystander tumoricidal effect in the treatment of experimental brain tumors. *Neurosurgery*, 35. 6, (Dec), pp.1094-102; discussion 1102-3, 0148-396X

Zinder, ND and Lederberg, J. (1952). Genetic exchange in Salmonella. *J.Bacteriol.*, 64. 5, (Nov), pp.679-699, 0021-9193; 0021-9193